Oxford Textbook of

Medical Mycology

Oxford Textbook of
Medical Mycology

Edited by

Christopher C. Kibbler
Centre for Medical Microbiology, University College London, UK

Richard Barton
Mycology Reference Centre, Leeds General Infirmary, UK

Neil A.R. Gow
Aberdeen Fungal Group, MRC Centre for Medical Mycology at the University of Aberdeen, UK

Susan Howell
Mycology Laboratory, St John's Institute of Dermatology, Viapath, London, UK

Donna M. MacCallum
Aberdeen Fungal Group, MRC Centre for Medical Mycology at the University of Aberdeen, UK

Rohini J. Manuel
Public Health Laboratory, National Infection Service,
Public Health England, London, UK

OXFORD
UNIVERSITY PRESS

OXFORD
UNIVERSITY PRESS

Great Clarendon Street, Oxford, OX2 6DP,
United Kingdom

Oxford University Press is a department of the University of Oxford.
It furthers the University's objective of excellence in research, scholarship,
and education by publishing worldwide. Oxford is a registered trade mark of
Oxford University Press in the UK and in certain other countries

First Edition published in 2018

Published in the United States of America by Oxford University Press
198 Madison Avenue, New York, NY 10016, United States of America

British Library Cataloguing in Publication Data
Data available

Library of Congress Control Number: 2017943525

ISBN 978-0-19-875538-8

Oxford University Press makes no representation, express or implied, that the drug dosages in this book are correct. Readers must therefore always check the product information and clinical procedures with the most up-to-date published product information and data sheets provided by the manufacturers and the most recent codes of conduct and safety regulations. The authors and the publishers do not accept responsibility or legal liability for any errors in the text or for the misuse or misapplication of material in this work. Except where otherwise stated, drug dosages and recommendations are for the non-pregnant adult who is not breast-feeding

Links to third party websites are provided by Oxford in good faith and for information only. Oxford disclaims any responsibility for the materials contained in any third party website referenced in this work.

Foreword

I have a fondness for mycology because I have worked all my life on the fungus fission yeast, trying to uncover the mechanisms underlying the control of the eukaryotic cell cycle. Medical mycology is a specialty which has made great strides in recent years and is having increasing influence on the clinical outcomes of individuals with immunocompromising diseases such as leukaemia and AIDS. The mortality of some of their infections is still well over 70%. For example, there are around a million cases of cryptococcosis a year, of which more than 600,000 will result in death. Overall, infections due to fungi occur on a scale similar to malaria, and to many bacterial and viral diseases.

This is a timely comprehensive text on the subject, which has its roots in the British Society for Medical Mycology (BSMM) global Master's programme, and is aimed at both scientists and clinicians. Advances in targeted chemotherapy can be marred by invasive fungal infections, and there is a real need to encourage young scientists and clinicians to fully engage with this specialty. In the last 50 years, we have gone from a time when there was just one broad-spectrum antifungal agent for the treatment of serious invasive disease, to one when there are around 20. Diagnostic methods have been refined and studied in clinical trials, antifungal susceptibility assays are internationally defined and tested, and our understanding of fungal taxonomy and epidemiology has been transformed by molecular biology. There is much to be optimistic about and there is a significant body of knowledge to be assimilated by those working in this area. I think that this Oxford Textbook will go a long way towards achieving this last aspiration.

The editors have recruited international experts to produce up-to-date and detailed chapters aimed at a postgraduate readership. The scope of the book is broad and is divided into six sections, dealing in turn with the basics of mycology, the causative organisms, a systems approach to the mycoses, infections in special populations, diagnostics, and therapy. This book should be a companion for mycology courses and for many scientists and healthcare workers looking to further their knowledge of these topics.

Professor Sir Paul Nurse
Director, The Francis Crick Institute, London

Preface

This book had its genesis in the British Society for Medical Mycology (BSMM) Master's programme. The editors are tutors on this programme and came together with the express idea of producing a suitable textbook to accompany the courses. Hence, the structure of the book is loosely based on the course structure, expanding content in areas of focused study and bringing together recently acquired knowledge in one place.

However, it was apparent that such a book could be a companion for other courses and, indeed, for scientists and clinicians looking to further their knowledge of medical mycology in topics as diverse as cell function, epidemiology, and advanced diagnostics, through to therapeutic drug monitoring in the management of mycoses. As a consequence, the scope of the book is broader and deeper than originally planned and its readership is expected to be much wider. We have, therefore, divided the book into more sections than originally considered, dealing in turn with the basics of mycology (cell function, taxonomy, pathogenesis, immunology, and so on), the causative organisms, a systems approach to the mycoses, infections in special populations, diagnostics, and therapy. To take advantage of this broad remit, the reader should make use of all the different sections. For example, whilst the general principles of therapy are dealt with in the clinical sections, the reader will find more details of the individual drugs and strategies in the therapy section, and more about the causative fungi in the mycology section.

We have recruited a faculty of international experts, many of whom are lecturers on the BSMM programme, to produce up-to-date and detailed chapters aimed at a postgraduate readership, and we are very grateful to them for the time and care they have put into their efforts on your behalf. In addition, I would like to thank my fellow editors and everyone who has been involved with the BSMM course. This *Oxford Textbook of Medical Mycology* is dedicated to them and to the current and former students scattered around the world.

Professor Chris Kibbler
London, January 2018

Contents

List of Abbreviations

AAPCC	American Association of Poison Control Centres
ABLC	amphotericin B lipid complex
ABPA	allergic bronchopulmonary aspergillosis
ABPM	allergic bronchopulmonary mycosis
AFLP	amplified fragment length polymorphism
AFRS	allergic fungal rhinosinusitis
ADI	AIDS-defining illness
AGREE II	Appraisal of guidelines research & evaluation II (system)
AIDS	acquired immune deficiency syndrome
AmB-D	amphotericin B-deoxycholate
APACHE	Acute Physiology and Chronic Health Evaluation (system)
APECED	autoimmune polyendocrinopathy with candidiasis and ectodermal dystrophy
APPH	acute primary pulmonary histoplasmosis
ART	antiretroviral therapy
ATCC	American Type Culture Collection
ATP	adenosine triphosphate
AUC	area under the concentration curve
BAL	bronchoalveolar lavage
BCR	B-cell receptor
BCSH	British Committee for Standards in Haematology
BDG (1→3)	β-D-glucan
bp	base pair
BSMM	British Society for Medical Mycology
cART	combination antiretroviral therapy
CATs	conidial anastomosis tubes
CCPA	chronic cavitary pulmonary aspergillosis
CDC	Centers for Disease Control and Prevention
CFP	cyan fluorescent protein
CFT	complement fixation test
CFTR	cystic fibrosis transmembrane regulator
ChIP-Seq	chromatin immunoprecipitation sequencing
CGB	canavanine-glycine-bromothymol blue (agar)
CGD	chronic granulomatous disease
CLRs	C-type lectin receptors
CMI	cell-mediated immunity
CMV	cytomegalovirus
CNPA	chronic necrotizing pulmonary aspergillosis
CNS	central nervous system
CONSORT	Consolidated Standards of Reporting Trials
COPD	chronic obstructive pulmonary disease
CPA	chronic pulmonary aspergillosis
CRAG	cryptococcal antigen
CRBSI	catheter-related bloodstream infection
CSF	cerebrospinal fluid
CT	computed tomography
CT-PET	CT–positron emission tomography
CVC	central venous catheter
DALI	Defining Antibiotic Levels in Intensive care unit patients (study)
DAPI	4′, 6-diamidino-2-phenylindole (stain)
DCs	dendritic cells
DD	double diffusion (test)
ds	double-stranded
EAPCRI	European *Aspergillus* PCR Initiative
ECIL	European Conference on Infections in Leukaemia
ECOFF	epidemiological cut-off
EDTA	ethylenediaminetetraacetic acid
ECMM	European Confederation of Medical Mycology
EFRS	eosinophilic fungal rhinosinusitis
EIA	enzyme immunoassay
ELBW	extremely low birth weight
ELISA	enzyme-linked immunosorbent assay
EMA	European Medicines Agency
EMRS	eosinophilic mucin rhinosinusitis
ENT	ear, nose & throat services
EORTC	European Organisation for Research and Treatment of Cancer
EQAS	external quality assurance schemes
ESCMID	European Society of Clinical Microbiology and Infectious Diseases
FDA	Food and Drug Administration
FDG PET-CT	18F-fluorodeoxyglucose positron-emission tomography/computed tomography
FEV1	forced expiratory volume in one second
FFPE	formalin-fixed paraffin-embedded
FISH	fluorescence *in situ* hybridization (test)
FLAIR	fluid-attenuated inversion recovery
FRS	fungal rhinosinusitis
GABA	gamma-aminobutyric acid
G-CSF	granulocyte colony-stimulating factor
GFP	green fluorescent protein

GM	galactomannan
GM-CSF	granulocyte-macrophage colony-stimulating factor
GOLD	Global Initiative for Obstructive Lung Disease
GRADE	Grades of Recommendations, Assessment, Development and Evaluation
GUT	gastrointestinally induced transition (yeast cell)
GvHD	graft-versus-host disease
HAART	highly active antiretroviral therapy
HDPs	host defence peptides
H&E	haematoxylin & eosin (stain)
HEPA	high-efficiency particulate air
HIV	human immunodeficiency virus
HLA	human leucocyte antigen
HPLC	high-performance liquid chromatography
HRCT	high-resolution CT
HRT	hormone replacement therapy
HSCT	haematopoietic stem cell transplantation
5-HT	5-hydroxytryptamine
IA	invasive aspergillosis
IARC	International Agency for Research on Cancer
IC	invasive candidiasis
ICD	International Classification of Diseases
ICED	implantable cardiac electronic device
ICN	International Code of Nomenclature
ICP	intracranial pressure
ICPA	International Commission of Penicillium and Aspergillus
ICTF	International Commission on the Taxonomy of Fungi
ICU	intensive care unit
IDSA	Infectious Diseases Society of America
IE	infective endocarditis
IFD	invasive fungal disease
IFI	invasive fungal infection
IFN	interferon
Ig	immunoglobulin
IL	interleukin
IPA	invasive pulmonary aspergillosis
IRIS	immune reconstitution inflammatory syndrome
ITS	internal transcribed spacer (region)
ITU	intensive therapy unit
IVDU	intravenous drug use
KOH	potassium hydroxide
KOH/DMSO	potassium hydroxide/dimethyl sulphoxide
LA	latex agglutination (test)
LAI	laboratory-acquired infection
L-AmB	liposomal amphotericin B
LFA	lateral flow assay
MALDI-TOF	matrix-assisted laser desorption/ionization–time-of-flight (mass spectrometry)
MAPK	mitogen-activated protein kinase
MBL	mannose-binding lectin
MDCT	multi-detector CT
MHC	major histocompatibility complex
MIC	minimum inhibitory concentration
MIP	methylation induced premeiotically
MLST	multi-locus sequence typing
MRI	magnetic resonance imaging
MSG	major surface glycoprotein
mTOR	mammalian target of rapamycin
NA	nucleic acid
NADPH	nicotinamide adenine dinucleotide phosphate
NCF	Nomenclature Committee for Fungi
NETs	neutrophil extracellular traps
NF	nuclear factor
NFAT	nuclear factor of activated T cell
NHEJ	non-homologous end-joining
NICU	neonatal intensive care unit
NK	natural killer (cells)
NLRs	NOD-like receptors
NOX	NADPH oxide
OCP	oral contraceptive pill
ODI	optical density index
PAMP	pathogen-associated molecular pattern
PAS	periodic acid-Schiff
PASH	periodic acid Schiff-haematoxylin (stain)
PCM	paracoccidioidomycosis
PCN	percutaneous nephrostomy
PCP	*Pneumocystis* pneumonia
PCR	polymerase chain reaction
PD	peritoneal dialysis
PHE	Public Health England
PJI	prosthetic joint infection
PMN	polymorphonuclear
PNA	peptide nucleic acid
POC	point-of-care (tests, etc.)
Pra1	pH-regulated antigen
PRRs	pattern recognition receptors
QoE	quality of evidence
RAPD	random amplified polymorphic DNA
RCT	randomized controlled trial
RFP	red fluorescent protein
RIP	repeat-induced point mutation
ROS	reactive oxygen species
rRNA	ribosomal ribonucleic acid
RT	reverse transcriptase
RVVC	recurrent vulvovaginal candidiasis
SAB	Sabouraud's glucose–peptone agar
SAFS	severe asthma with fungal sensitization
Saps	secreted aspartyl proteinases
SCARE	Surveillance Collaboration on *Aspergillus* Resistance in Europe
SIGN	Scottish Intercollegiate Guideline Network
SNPs	single-nucleotide polymorphisms
SoR	strength of recommendation
SOT	solid organ transplant
SOWgp	spherule outer wall glycoprotein
STAT	signal transducer and activator of transcription
STIR	short tau inversion recovery
TB	tuberculosis
TCR	T-cell receptor
TDM	therapeutic drug monitoring
T-DNA	transfer DNA
Th cell	T helper cell
TLRs	toll-like receptors
$\%T_{MIC}$	percentage of time plasma drug concentrations exceed the MIC over a 24-hour dosing interval

TMP-SMX	trimethoprim-sulphamethoxazole
TNF	tumour necrosis factor
TOR	target of rapamycin
TP	tube precipitin (test)
TRANSNET	Transplant-Associated Infection Surveillance Network
Tregs	regulatory T cells
UTI	urinary tract infection
UV	ultraviolet
VNTR	variable number tandem repeats
VVC	vulvovaginal candidiasis
WBC	white blood cell
WGS	whole-genome sequence
YFP	yellow fluorescent protein

List of Contributors

H. Ruth Ashbee, School of Molecular and Cellular Biology, University of Leeds, UK

Matthijs Backx, Public Health Wales Microbiology Division, University Hospital of Wales, Cardiff, UK

Rosemary A. Barnes, Infection and Immunity, School of Medicine, Cardiff University, University Hospital of Wales, Cardiff, UK

Richard Barton, Mycology Reference Centre, Leeds General Infirmary, Leeds, UK

Tihana Bicanic, Institute for Infection and Immunity, St George's, University of London, UK

Andrew M. Borman, Public Health England National UK Mycology Reference Laboratory, Bristol, UK

Rosie E. Bradshaw, Institute of Fundamental Sciences, Massey University, Palmerston North, New Zealand

Mary E. Brandt, Mycotic Diseases Branch, Centers for Disease Control and Prevention, Atlanta, GA, USA

Alistair J.P. Brown, Aberdeen Fungal Group, MRC Centre for Medical Mycology at the University of Aberdeen, UK

Gordon D. Brown, Aberdeen Fungal Group, MRC Centre for Medical Mycology at the University of Aberdeen, UK

Arunaloke Chakrabarti, Postgraduate Institute of Medical Education and Research, Chandigarh, India

Heather L. Clark, University of California, Irvine, CA, USA

Angela Ahlquist Cleveland, Mycotic Diseases Branch, Centers for Disease Control and Prevention, Atlanta, GA, USA

Joanne Cleverley, Department of Radiology, Royal Free Hospital, London, UK

Christopher P. Conlon, Nuffield Department of Medicine, University of Oxford, UK

Oliver A. Cornely, Department I of Internal Medicine, University Hospital of Cologne, Germany, Cologne Excellence Cluster on Cellular Stress Responses in Aging-Associated Diseases (CECAD), and Clinical Trials Centre Cologne, ZKS Köln, University of Cologne, Germany, German Centre for Infection Research, Partner Site Bonn-Cologne, Germany

Laura Cottom, NHS Greater Glasgow and Clyde Health Board, Glasgow, UK

Manuel Cuenca-Estrella, Instituto de Salud Carlos III, Madrid, Spain

Ivy M. Dambuza, Aberdeen Fungal Group, MRC Centre for Medical Mycology at the University of Aberdeen, UK

Blandine Denis, Service des maladies infectieuses et tropicales, Hôpital Saint Louis, AP-HP Paris, France UMR S 1136, INSERM et Sorbonne Universités, UPMC Univ Paris 06, Paris, France

David W. Denning, University Hospital of South Manchester NHS Foundation Trust, Manchester, UK

Sarah Drake, University of Leeds and Leeds Teaching Hospitals NHS Trust, Leeds, UK

Paul S. Dyer, School of Life Sciences, University of Nottingham, Nottingham, UK

Stuart Flanagan, Department of Infection and Immunology, Royal London Hospital, London, UK

Beatriz L. Gómez, School of Medicine and Health Sciences, Universidad del Rosario, Bogotá, Colombia

Angel González, Basic and Applied Microbiology Research Group (MICROBA), School of Microbiology, Universidad de Antioquia, Medellín, Colombia

Neil A.R. Gow, Aberdeen Fungal Group, MRC Centre for Medical Mycology at the University of Aberdeen, UK

Catriona L. Halliday, Clinical Mycology Reference Laboratory, Centre for Infectious Diseases and Microbiology Laboratory Services, NSW Pathology, ICPMR, Westmead Hospital, Westmead, NSW, Australia

Thomas S. Harrison, Institute for Infection and Immunity, St George's, University of London, UK

Roderick J. Hay, Skin Infection Clinic, King's College Hospital NHS Trust, Denmark Hill, London, UK

Susan Howell, Mycology Laboratory, St John's Institute of Dermatology, Viapath, London, UK

Bernhard Hube, Department of Microbial Pathogenicity Mechanisms, Leibniz Institute for Natural Product Research and Infection Biology – Hans Knöll Institute (HKI), Jena, Germany

Samantha E. Jacobs, Transplantation-Oncology Infectious Diseases Program, Division of Infectious Diseases, Weill Cornell Medical Center, New York, NY, USA

Darius Armstrong James, National Heart and Lung Institute, Imperial College London, UK

Elizabeth M. Johnson, Public Health England National UK Mycology Reference Laboratory, Bristol, UK

Brian L. Jones, NHS Greater Glasgow and Clyde Health Board, Glasgow, UK

Christopher C. Kibbler, Centre for Medical Microbiology, University College London, UK

Sarah E. Kidd, National Mycology Reference Centre, SA Pathology, Adelaide, SA, Australia

Philipp Koehler, Department I of Internal Medicine, University Hospital of Cologne, Germany Cologne Excellence Cluster on Cellular Stress Responses in Aging-Associated Diseases (CECAD), and Clinical Trials Centre Cologne, ZKS Köln, University of Cologne, Germany

Chris Kosmidis, University Hospital of South Manchester NHS Foundation Trust, Manchester, UK

Oliver Kurzai, National Reference Center for Invasive Fungal Infections, Leibniz Institute for Natural Product Research and Infection Biology – Hans Knöll Institute (HKI), Jena, Germany

Fanny Lanternier, Université Paris-Descartes, Centre d'Infectiologie Necker-Pasteur, Hôpital Necker-Enfants Malades, Paris, France Centre National de Référence Mycoses Invasives et Antifongiques, Unité de Mycologie Moléculaire, Institut Pasteur, Paris, France

Rebecca Lester, University of Liverpool, Liverpool, UK

Russell E. Lewis, Infectious Diseases Unit, S. Orsola-Malpighi Hospital, Department of Medical and Surgical Sciences, University of Bologna, Bologna, IT

Chris Linton, Public Health England National UK Mycology Reference Laboratory, Bristol, UK

Shawn R. Lockhart, Mycotic Diseases Branch, Centers for Disease Control and Prevention, Atlanta, GA, USA

Olivier Lortholary, Université Paris-Descartes, Centre d'Infectiologie Necker-Pasteur, Hôpital Necker-Enfants Malades, Paris, France Centre National de Référence Mycoses Invasives et Antifongiques, Unité de Mycologie Moléculaire, Institut Pasteur, Paris, France

Sebastian B. Lucas, Department of Histopathology, St Thomas' Hospital, London, UK

Donna M. MacCallum, Aberdeen Fungal Group, MRC Centre for Medical Mycology at the University of Aberdeen, UK

Damien Mack, Division of Infection and Immunity, University College London, UK

Rohini J. Manuel, Public Health Laboratory, National Infection Service, Public Health England, UK

Eileen K. Maziarz, Department of Medicine, Duke University School of Medicine, Durham, NC, USA

Rajal K. Mody, Mycotic Diseases Branch, Centers for Disease Control and Prevention, Atlanta, GA, USA

Eavan G. Muldoon, Mater Misericordiae University Hospital, Dublin, Ireland

Carol A. Munro, Aberdeen Fungal Group, MRC Centre for Medical Mycology at the University of Aberdeen, UK

Frank C. Odds, Aberdeen Fungal Group, MRC Centre for Medical Mycology at the University of Aberdeen, UK

Shara Palanivel, Royal Free London NHS Foundation Trust, and Royal National Orthopaedic Hospital, Stanmore, London, UK

Michael D. Palmer, Public Health England (PHE) National Mycology Reference Laboratory, Bristol, UK

Eric Pearlman, Case Western Reserve University, Cleveland, OH, USA

John R. Perfect, Department of Medicine, Duke University School of Medicine, Durham, NC, USA

Nick D. Read, Manchester Fungal Infection Group, Division of Infection, Immunity and Respiratory Medicine, University of Manchester, UK

Anna Reed, Royal Brompton and Harefield NHS Trust, London, UK

Angela Restrepo, Corporación para Investigaciones Biológicas (CIB), Medellín, Colombia

John H. Rex, F2G, Ltd., Eccles, UK; CARB-X, Boston, MA; Rex Life Sciences LLC, Wellesley, MA

Thomas R. Rogers, Department of Clinical Microbiology, Trinity College Dublin, St James's Hospital Campus, Dublin 8, Ireland

Jonathan Sandoe, University of Leeds and Leeds Teaching Hospitals NHS Trust, Leeds, UK

Silke Schelenz, Department of Microbiology, Royal Brompton Hospital, London, UK

Shila Seaton, National External Quality Assessment Service (NEQAS), National Infection Service, Public Health England, Colindale, London, UK

Anand Shah, Fungal Disease Immunobiology, Imperial College London, UK

Gillian S. Shankland, School of Medicine, Dentistry and Nursing, University of Glasgow, UK

Catherine B. Small, Transplantation-Oncology Infectious Diseases Program, Division of Infectious Diseases, Weill Cornell Medical Center, New York, NY, USA

Stephanie J. Smith, Barts Health National Health Service Trust, London, UK

Jack D. Sobel, Wayne State University, School of Medicine, Detroit, MI, USA

Jeanette Wagener, Aberdeen Fungal Group, MRC Centre for Medical Mycology at the University of Aberdeen, UK

Thomas J. Walsh, Transplantation-Oncology Infectious Diseases Program, Division of Infectious Diseases, Weill Cornell Medical Center, New York, NY, USA

David W. Warnock, Faculty of Biology, Medicine and Health, University of Manchester, UK

Simon Warren, Royal Free London NHS Foundation Trust, London, UK

Adilia Warris, Aberdeen Fungal Group, MRC Centre for Medical Mycology at the University of Aberdeen, UK

P. Lewis White, Public Health Wales, Microbiology, Cardiff, University Hospital of Wales, Cardiff, UK

Duncan Wilson, Aberdeen Fungal Group, MRC Centre for Medical Mycology at the University of Aberdeen, UK

SECTION 1

The principles of medical mycology

CHAPTER 1

Introduction to medical mycology

David W. Warnock

Changing patterns of fungal diseases

Over the last four decades, the spectrum of fungal disease has evolved, to the extent that a medical mycologist who retired in the 1970s would find the discipline today almost unrecognizable. Until that time, few groups of fungi were regarded as pathogenic for humans or animals. These few included the aetiologic agents of the common superficial diseases, dermatophytosis and mucosal candidiasis, but these were not seen as serious. There were also several well-recognized subcutaneous mycoses, including chromoblastomycosis, mycetoma, and sporotrichosis, but these were largely a problem in the tropics and subtropics. The principal systemic mycoses—aspergillosis, candidiasis, and cryptococcosis—were largely untreatable and usually fatal. However, these diseases were regarded as uncommon. Furthermore, *Pneumocystis jirovecii* infection was not even recognized to be a fungal disease.

Many factors have contributed to the emergence of fungal diseases as an increasingly important problem. As with other microbial infections, these have included: medical progress and changes in healthcare practices; changes in the environment; increased international travel and commerce; and the development of antimicrobial drug resistance (Institute of Medicine 1992). This chapter will highlight the importance of fungi as human pathogens and discuss the challenges they pose for global public health and for healthcare.

The biggest single change in the pattern of fungal disease since the 1970s has been the emergence of opportunistic mycoses, such as aspergillosis and candidiasis, as major causes of life-threatening infection in immunocompromised individuals. These diseases now constitute the predominant group of fungal infections seen in healthcare settings, and a number of them have emerged as problems of global significance. However, the impact of these infections on human health is not widely recognized, and deaths resulting from these diseases are often overlooked (Brown et al. 2012).

For all of its benefits, medical progress has led to an expanding population of susceptible hosts with impaired immune defences against infection. These individuals are at heightened risk for many serious fungal diseases, including aspergillosis, candidiasis, cryptococcosis, mucormycosis, and pneumocystosis. The most significant emergence of opportunistic fungal infections worldwide has occurred in people living with human immunodeficiency virus (HIV) infection. Before the widespread usage of anti-retroviral therapy, up to 80% of HIV-infected individuals developed mucosal candidiasis, while many were diagnosed with cryptococcosis, histoplasmosis, pneumocystosis, or other lethal fungal diseases including *Talaromyces (Penicillium) marneffei* infection. While the numbers have diminished significantly in the developed world since the late 1990s, many countries in sub-Saharan Africa and Asia remain highly affected by the AIDS (acquired immune deficiency syndrome) pandemic, and there are few signs of a decline in the importance of the mycoses.

Other emerging populations at risk for serious fungal diseases have included those who have received immunosuppressive medications or invasive medical interventions. These groups include patients receiving critical care and those who are undergoing organ or stem cell transplantation. With new developments in the management of the underlying disorders, the populations at risk for fungal disease are constantly evolving. For example, in the endemic regions of the United States, histoplasmosis has become one of the most frequent life-threatening infections in patients being treated with tumour necrosis factor (TNF)-alpha blockers for diseases such as rheumatoid arthritis, inflammatory bowel disease, and various dermatological conditions (Hage et al. 2010).

In addition to infections acquired in hospitals and other healthcare settings, there has also been a marked increase in the incidence of several of the community-acquired systemic mycoses that are endemic in the Americas, particularly coccidioidomycosis. Thousands of cases of this disease, caused by two closely related soil-dwelling fungi—*Coccidioides immitis* and *Coccidioides posadasii*—are now reported each year in the endemic regions of the south-western United States, mostly from Arizona and California. Massive population growth, urban development, and consequent changes in land-use patterns have contributed to this trend, as has the seasonal migration of increasing numbers of previously unexposed persons from non-endemic areas of the United States (Park et al. 2005). Many of these individuals are older, with underlying chronic illnesses and debilitation, and consequently are at greater risk of developing the more serious forms of coccidioidomycosis.

Our current understanding of the geographic distribution of coccidioidomycosis in the United States is largely based on the results of skin testing conducted in the 1950s. However, since 2010, unrelated cases of the disease have been recognized in growing numbers of eastern Washington State residents, far to the north of the known geographic range (Marsden-Haug et al. 2013). Epidemiological and microbiological findings, including whole-genome sequencing analysis, indicate that these infections were acquired in Washington State, exposure likely having occurred during soil disruption

(Litvintseva et al. 2015). The reasons for this recent emergence of coccidioidomycosis are not clear, but possible explanations for the presence of *Coccidioides* include recent extreme weather events and/or climate change. The extensive drought that has affected California may have resulted in the production of contaminated dust that spread fungal spores to the North. It is also possible that *Coccidioides* has been established in Washington for some time, but infrequent human exposure and/or lack of awareness among physicians delayed its recognition. The retrospective detection of cases of the disease among animals lends support to this hypothesis (Marsden-Haug et al. 2013). Nonetheless, whatever the precise cause, it is clear that factors such as anthropogenic dispersal, animal host movement, and climatic changes conducive to colonization may influence the endemic ranges of fungal pathogens.

While coccidioidomycosis remains a regional problem, cryptococcosis is an emerging fungal disease of global importance. Virtually all cases of cryptococcosis are caused by *Cryptococcus neoformans* and the closely related species *Cryptococcus gattii*. The former has a worldwide distribution, particularly in soil and avian habitats. In contrast, *C. gattii* is found in association with trees, and until recently, its geographic range was thought to be limited to the tropics and subtropics. However, since 1999, human and animal cases of *C. gattii* infection have been reported with increasing frequency on Vancouver Island in western Canada, and the outbreak has since spread to mainland British Columbia and to the adjacent states of Washington, Oregon, Idaho, and California in the United States. The outbreak has been associated with significant ill-health and high rates of death among those infected (Harris et al. 2011).

The recent emergence of *C. gattii* in a temperate region suggests that the pathogen may have adapted to a new climatic niche, or that climatic warming may be creating a more hospitable environment for its development. However, the possibility that environmental conditions supportive of *C. gattii* are broader than previously suspected cannot be discounted. Nonetheless, the rapid geographic expansion of this fungal pathogen has raised concerns that *C. gattii* infections could emerge as an even greater threat to public health. This is underscored by evidence that human activity has contributed to the dispersal of the outbreak (Kidd et al. 2007).

International travel and tourism is another factor that has affected the pattern of fungal diseases. The number of reported outbreaks and sporadic cases of histoplasmosis and coccidioidomycosis has increased among individuals who normally reside in places far distant from the areas where these diseases are endemic. The largest number of travel-related mycoses has been reported from US residents, many of whom have acquired an infection while visiting an endemic area within North or Central America or, less commonly, in South America, Africa, or Asia (Panackal et al. 2002). Travel-related infections have also been reported among European visitors to the United States and Latin America (Buitrago et al. 2011). With increasing numbers of visitors and immigrants to the United States from Asia, reports of travel- and migration-related mycoses are beginning to emerge from India and China. Healthcare providers increasingly need to consider these diseases in their differential diagnosis when treating returning travellers with a febrile respiratory illness.

Estimating the burden of fungal diseases

Despite general agreement that the mycoses are becoming more important, our understanding of the true magnitude of the burden posed by these diseases and their socioeconomic impact remains largely incomplete. Understanding the burden of different fungal diseases is important because it will allow meaningful comparisons to be made between these infections and other important diseases. Only then will it be possible to persuade policy makers of the benefits to be derived from allocating resources to diagnosing, treating, and preventing the mycoses.

The first step in developing estimates of the burden of any disease is to obtain epidemiological surveillance data regarding its incidence and prevalence. In the case of fungal diseases, our efforts have been undermined by the limited amounts of data available, and in many instances, by the ways in which these data were acquired. Most public health agencies, with the exception of the US Centers for Disease Control and Prevention (CDC), do not conduct any active epidemiological surveillance for fungal diseases. Usually, this is because these diseases are seen as low priorities, and because active surveillance is labour-intensive and expensive to perform. The CDC has conducted active population-based surveillance for *Candida* bloodstream infections (Cleveland et al. 2015) and cryptococcosis (Mirza et al. 2003), and performed prospective surveillance for invasive fungal infections among haematopoietic stem cell and solid-organ transplant recipients (Kontoyiannis et al. 2010; Pappas et al. 2010). Similar active surveillance programmes have been reported from other countries, mostly in Europe, but few have been sustainable in the long term.

Passive surveillance, which relies on healthcare providers and laboratories to submit information to public health agencies, is less expensive to conduct than active surveillance, but is not ideal in relation to fungal diseases. Because these infections are not usually transmissible from person to person, there is minimal incentive for healthcare providers to report cases since no immediate public health action needs to be taken. In the United States, only coccidioidomycosis is a notifiable disease, and reporting is only required in states where it is endemic (Arizona, California, Nevada, New Mexico, Texas, and Utah) and about 15 others. In other developed countries, such as the United Kingdom and France, there are ongoing, informal reporting schemes for some fungal infections, but these are limited in scope. There are no data from many parts of the developing world.

Even when all diagnosed cases of a disease are reported, most surveillance systems do not capture the total burden of that disease in a population. This is because some of those affected do not seek medical care, or because specimens are not obtained from all cases, or because the appropriate tests are not performed. Given the limitations of current tests, it seems probable that invasive fungal infections are under-diagnosed. If these infections are also under-reported, it must be assumed that the existing surveillance data underestimate the incidence and prevalence of these diseases.

Numerous studies have been conducted to measure the global burden of infectious diseases, but few have focused on the mycoses. Among the first to do so was one from the CDC that estimated the yearly global burden of cryptococcal meningitis in persons with HIV infection to be nearly one million cases (Park et al. 2009). The region with the greatest number of cases was sub-Saharan Africa, with 720,000 cases, followed by South and Southeast Asia with 120,000 cases. In addition, almost 625,000 deaths were estimated to occur globally, mostly occurring in sub-Saharan Africa, with over 500,000 deaths annually. These estimates of the global burden of cryptococcosis involved major extrapolations from the available epidemiological data. Nonetheless, they are important because they showed that the disease was one of the leading causes of death among people with HIV infection. In sub-Saharan Africa, cryptococcosis was estimated to cause more deaths than tuberculosis.

Much effort is currently being devoted to developing similar global burden of disease estimates for other mycoses. This work has served to highlight the many gaps in current surveillance data and the methodological limitations involved. Until additional data and more refined methods become available, it will be essential to exercise caution when reviewing published estimates of the burden of ill health and death caused by fungal diseases.

Improving the diagnosis of fungal diseases

Determining the infectious agent responsible for a patient's illness remains fundamental to evidence-based treatment and care decisions. Among the challenges in dealing with opportunistic invasive fungal diseases—with many caused by unusual environmental fungi—none is more critical than early diagnosis of these infections. Improved laboratory diagnostic tools that allow earlier implementation of appropriate therapy have the potential to affect healthcare decisions to a degree well out of proportion to their cost (Institute of Medicine 2000).

In the developed world, new diagnostic approaches, such as fungal antigen tests and fungal nucleic acid detection, offer great promise for diseases such as aspergillosis, candidiasis, and pneumocystosis. However, even as more of these tools become commercially available, interpreting the test findings still calls for a high level of mycological competence. The new diagnostic procedures that have been developed have not yet had a significant impact in many clinical laboratories, largely because they have not been standardized and validated, and because there remains a lack of consensus on their performance characteristics. These complexities, combined with subtle clinical presentations, continue to result in delayed diagnosis and may compromise clinical care (Brown et al. 2012).

In the under-developed and developing countries, where the burden of fungal disease is highest, many clinical laboratories are small and poorly equipped, and may be staffed by individuals with minimal training. Furthermore, they are often inaccessible to many patients. In these settings, inexpensive but dependable point-of-care (POC) diagnostic tests can make a tremendous difference to the cost and quality of healthcare. A new POC dipstick test for detection of cryptococcal antigen in urine or blood has improved the capacity for diagnosis of cryptococcal meningitis in sub-Saharan Africa (Kabanda et al. 2014), and a similar approach could transform the diagnosis and management of AIDS-associated histoplasmosis throughout South America (Nacher et al. 2013). Setting priorities and ensuring that these tests are developed and implemented in the most efficient way will be challenging. With widened access to improved diagnostics, it may be possible to reduce the burden of these and other fungal diseases to the lower levels seen in the developed world.

Improving the therapy of fungal diseases

Just as improved diagnostics may help to reduce the morbidity and mortality associated with fungal diseases, so may better therapeutics. The rising incidence of serious opportunistic fungal infections has brought about an increased use of existing antifungal agents and has stimulated the search for new ones. The last two decades have seen the introduction of an important new class of antifungal agents (the echinocandins), the expansion of an established class of agents (the azoles), and the development of novel methods for delivering established agents (lipid-based formulations of amphotericin B).

In the developed world, the new drugs that have been introduced have changed the standards of care for the treatment of many invasive fungal diseases, particularly aspergillosis and candidiasis, yet patient outcomes remain disappointing (Ostrosky-Zeichner et al. 2010). This is due, in large part, to the lack of early antifungal therapy resulting from delays in disease diagnosis and fungal identification. The available drugs also suffer from restrictions in spectrum of activity, in bioavailability in target tissues, and in routes of administration. Further complications include toxicity, undesirable drug interactions, and the emergence of drug resistance. Unfortunately, few antifungal drugs are currently in active development. This is because fewer companies are now developing antimicrobials of any type, and because the global market for antifungal drugs is not predicted to give a sufficiently large financial return to attract the needed investment.

In the developing world, many antifungal drugs are either unavailable or simply unaffordable. While fluconazole is available in almost all countries, amphotericin B is not. This is despite the older drug often being life-saving in the management of cryptococcal meningitis and disseminated histoplasmosis. Moreover, while there is mounting evidence for the benefit of flucytosine (5-fluorocytosine)-containing combination therapy for cryptococcosis, access to the drug in sub-Saharan Africa and Asia, where disease burden is greatest, is inadequate at present (Loyse et al. 2013). Coordinated efforts from governmental and international stakeholders are needed to develop, disseminate, and implement antifungal treatment guidelines, to encourage generic drug production and facilitate registration, and to widen access to these agents.

Evolving problems of drug resistance

In general, acquired resistance to antifungal drugs has been a much less common problem than antibacterial drug resistance. In the 1990s, long-term use of fluconazole to treat oral candidiasis in people with HIV infection led to the widespread emergence of resistant strains of *Candida albicans*, which were associated with treatment failure and relapse. However, with the advent of more effective antiretroviral therapy, a dramatic decline occurred in the rates of oral colonization and symptomatic infection, and this was accompanied by falling rates of azole drug resistance (Martins et al. 1998).

First described in 2009, *Candida auris* has since been reported from at least 12 countries across four continents (Vallabhaneni et al. 2016). This emerging pathogen has caused large outbreaks of invasive infection following transmission in healthcare settings (Schelenz et al. 2016) and it appears to be increasing in prevalence, at least in some countries such as India, where it now accounts for almost 5% of *Candida* bloodstream infections among patients receiving intensive care (Chakrabarti et al. 2015).

Candida auris is of concern because it is often resistant to multiple antifungal drugs. In one recent report, 50 of 54 isolates (93%) from South Asia, South Africa, and South America were found to be resistant to fluconazole, while 54% were resistant to voriconazole,

35% to amphotericin B, 7% to echinocandins, and 6% to flucytosine (Lockhart et al. 2017). Moreover, 41% of isolates were resistant to two or more classes of antifungal agents, a feature not seen in other clinically important *Candida* species. Whole genome sequencing analysis has demonstrated that isolates became grouped into unique clades by geographic region, suggesting nearly simultaneous and recent, independent emergence of *C. auris* on three continents, rather than spread from a single geographic source (Lockhart et al. 2017). Although data on antifungal prescribing practices are difficult to obtain, anecdotal evidence suggests that empirical and prophylactic use of antifungal agents has been increasing, and this supports the hypothesis that antifungal selection pressure may, in part at least, be responsible for the emergence of *C. auris*.

More recently, azole resistance in *Aspergillus fumigatus* has emerged as a potential global public health concern. Many of these resistant isolates appear to have been acquired as such from the environment as an unintended consequence of agricultural fungicide use (Vermeulen et al. 2013). Others have been recovered from patients with chronic lung disease during long-term azole treatment (Howard et al. 2009; Mortensen et al. 2011). Although evidence for a causal role of agricultural triazole use in resistance development is accumulating, definitive proof is lacking. Putative azole-resistant environmental strains of *A. fumigatus* have been recovered from patients across Europe and are now also being reported from Asia, the Middle East, Africa, and Australia. Similar strains have recently been identified among *A. fumigatus* isolates collected in US institutions (Wiederhold et al. 2016).

Taken as a whole, these developments have potentially serious consequences for patient management. In the case of *Candida auris*, treatment options may be limited. Implementation of strict infection control measures and rapid detection of cases may be the best options to contain hospital-acquired transmission (Schelenz et al. 2016). However, when traditional biochemical methods are used, *C. auris* is often misidentified, most commonly as *C. haemulonii*. Specialized methods, such as MALDI-TOF MS (matrix-assisted laser desorption/ionization–time-of-flight mass spectrometry) or molecular identification, are required and these may not be immediately available in countries where resources are limited, and where access to antifungals other than fluconazole may also be restricted.

For azole-resistant *Aspergillus fumigatus*, dose-escalation of mould-active azoles, such as voriconazole and posaconazole, will be inadequate, and the outcome of azole–echinocandin combination treatment at best uncertain. New molecular diagnostic tools are urgently needed to allow rapid detection of resistance mechanisms in both culture-positive and -negative patients. Ongoing investment in surveillance programmes, such as the Surveillance Collaboration on *Aspergillus* Resistance in Europe (SCARE) network (van der Linden et al. 2015), will be critical for monitoring trends in the incidence and prevalence of azole resistance and for detecting the emergence of new resistance mechanisms.

Improving the prevention of fungal diseases

Antifungal chemoprophylaxis is currently one of the most promising prevention strategies for the prevention of fungal infections. It can provide protection to susceptible individuals, such as transplant recipients and patients receiving intensive care, although this is not always economically or medically justified, especially if the cost is high and the perceived benefit does not outweigh the risk of adverse drug interactions or selection for resistance. Expert guidelines, based on evidence from well-designed clinical trials, support the use of targeted prophylaxis in various high-risk patient groups (Maertens et al. 2011). There is, however, an almost complete lack of genetic and other prognostic biomarkers that would allow identification of those individuals at greatest risk.

Cryptococcosis is among the most common causes of meningitis in sub-Saharan Africa, and is a leading cause of death among people with HIV infection. Although prophylaxis is not a cost-effective means of preventing infection, targeted pre-emptive treatment with fluconazole has emerged as a highly promising approach to managing the disease (Meya et al. 2015). This has become feasible with the advent of a simple POC dipstick test that can detect cryptococcal antigen several weeks before overt signs of meningitis develop. The substantial public-health benefits of screening people with HIV for cryptococcal infection when they access healthcare have recently been confirmed in a large clinical trial in Tanzania and Zambia (Mfinanga et al. 2015). Broader implementation of this 'screen and treat' approach in countries with a high burden of cryptococcosis could save thousands of lives each year.

Vaccination is the ultimate tool for the prevention and control of infectious disease. Unfortunately, there are no vaccines in clinical use for any fungal disease. This is despite the development of vaccines against a number of fungal pathogens, including several that have proven effective in animal models. Few have been translated to human clinical trials because the target market is perceived to be too small to justify the costs of manufacturing and testing a vaccine in today's rigorously controlled clinical research environment.

Conclusion

Fungal diseases exact a tremendous toll in terms of human life and healthcare costs in both the developed and the developing world. This chapter has outlined several areas that require attention if we are to improve this dismal situation. Firstly, ongoing surveillance programmes need to be established for a range of fungal diseases, both on a national basis and within individual sentinel medical centres, if we are to determine the true magnitude of the burden posed by these mycoses. Until more precise estimates become available, it will be difficult to convince policy makers that fungal diseases are common and that the burden they impose on public health and medical care is large and rising. Only then will it become possible to obtain the investment needed to stimulate scientific interest in combating and preventing these diseases.

Secondly, better and more rapid diagnostics need to be developed to allow earlier implementation of appropriate antifungal therapy. Development of such tools would also facilitate the gathering of accurate epidemiological surveillance data. Although better diagnostics may not prevent fungal diseases, simpler and easier diagnosis may lead to increased numbers of patients being successfully treated for mycoses, and this may in turn reduce the burdens of ill health and death. If access to affordable diagnostics can be increased in the developing world, it may be possible to reduce the fungal disease burden to levels seen in the developed world.

Thirdly, there is an ongoing need for safer and more effective antifungal drugs, and to translate the growing understanding of fungal immunopathogenesis into novel immunotherapeutic strategies, especially for the treatment of opportunistic fungal infections in susceptible individuals. In under-developed and developing countries, improved access to low-cost antifungal drugs is a critically important issue. Wider availability may ultimately be of benefit not only for invasive infections, such as cryptococcosis and histoplasmosis, but also for diseases such as mycetoma and fungal keratitis, which can have devastating economic consequences for those affected. Finally, new strategies are needed to slow the emergence of antifungal drug resistance.

References

Brown GD, Denning DW, Gow NAR, Levitz SM, Netea MG and White TC (2012) Hidden killers: human fungal infections. *Sci Transl Med* 4: 165rv13.

Buitrago MJ, Bernal-Martinez L, Castelli MV, Rodriguez-Tudela JL and Cuenca-Estrella M (2011) Histoplasmosis and paracoccidioidomycosis in a non-endemic area: a review of cases and diagnosis. *J Travel Med* 18: 26–33.

Chakrabarti A, Sood P, Rudramurthy SM, et al. (2015) Incidence, characteristics and outcome of ICU-acquired candidemia in India. *Intensive Care Med* 41: 285–95.

Cleveland AA, Harrison LH, Farley MM, et al. (2015) Declining incidence of candidemia and the shifting epidemiology of *Candida* resistance in two US metropolitan areas, 2008-2013: results from population-based surveillance. *PLoS ONE* 10: e120452. doi:10.1371/journal.pone.0120452

Hage CA, Bowyer S, Tarvin SE, Helper D, Kleiman MB and Wheat LJ (2010) Recognition, diagnosis, and treatment of histoplasmosis complicating tumor necrosis factor blocker therapy. *Clin Infect Dis* 50: 85–92.

Harris JR, Lockhart SR, Debess E, et al. (2011) *Cryptococcus gattii* in the United States: clinical aspects of infection with an emerging pathogen. *Clin Infect Dis* 53: 1188–95.

Howard SJ, Cerar D, Anderson MJ, et al. (2009) Frequency and evolution of azole resistance in *Aspergillus fumigatus* associated with treatment failure. *Emerg Infect Dis* 15: 1068–76.

Institute of Medicine (1992) *Emerging Infections: Microbial Threats to Health in the United States* (Washington, DC: National Academy Press).

Institute of Medicine (2000) *Medicare Laboratory Payment Policy: Now and in the future* (Washington, DC: National Academy Press).

Kabanda T, Siedner MJ, Klausner JD, Muzoora C and Boulware RR (2014) Point-of-care diagnosis and prognostication of cryptococcal meningitis with the cryptococcal antigen lateral flow assay on cerebrospinal fluid. *Clin Infect Dis* 58: 113–16.

Kidd SE, Bach PJ, Hingston AO, et al. (2007) *Cryptococcus gattii* dispersal mechanisms, British Columbia, Canada. *Emerg Infect Dis* 13: 51–7.

Kontoyiannis DP, Marr KA, Park BJ, et al. (2010) Prospective surveillance for invasive fungal infections in hematopoietic stem cell transplant recipients, 2001-2006: overview of the Transplant-Associated Infection Surveillance Network (TRANSNET) database. *Clin Infect Dis* 50: 1091–100.

Litvintseva AP, Marsden-Haug N, Hurst S, et al. (2015) Valley fever: finding new places for an old disease: *Coccidioides immitis* found in Washington State soil associated with recent human infection. *Clin Infect Dis* 60: e1–3.

Lockhart SR, Etienne K, Vallabhaneni S, et al. (2017) Simultaneous emergence of multidrug resistant *Candida auris* on 3 continents confirmed by whole genome sequencing and epidemiological analyses. *Clin Infect Dis* 64: 134–40.

Loyse A, Dromer F, Day J, Lortholary O and Harrison TS (2013) Flucytosine and cryptococcosis: time to urgently address the worldwide accessibility of a 50-year-old antifungal. *J Antimicrob Chemother* 68: 2435–44.

Maertens J, Marchetti O, Herbrecht R, et al. (2011) European guidelines for antifungal management in leukemia and hematopoietic stem cell transplant recipients: summary of the ECIL 3–2009 update. *Bone Marrow Transplant* 46: 709–18.

Marsden-Haug, N, Goldoft M, Ralston, C, et al. (2013) Coccidioidomycosis acquired in Washington State. *Clin Infect Dis* 56: 847–50.

Martins MD, Lozano-Chiu M and Rex JH (1998) Declining rates of oropharyngeal candidiasis and carriage of *Candida albicans* associated with trends towards reduced rates of carriage of fluconazole-resistant *C. albicans* in human immunodeficiency virus-infected patients. *Clin Infect Dis* 27: 1291–4.

Meya DB, Rajasingham R, Nalintya E, Tenforde M and Jarvis JN (2015) Preventing cryptococcosis: shifting the paradigm in the era of highly active antiretroviral therapy. *Curr Trop Med Rep* 2: 81–9.

Mfinanga S, Chanda D, Kivuyo SL, et al. (2015) Cryptococcal meningitis screening and community-based early adherence support in people with advanced HIV infection starting antiretroviral therapy in Tanzania and Zambia: an open-label, randomized controlled trial. *Lancet* 385: 2173–82. doi: 10.1016/S0140-6736(15)60164-7

Mirza SA, Phelan M, Rimland D, et al. (2003) The changing epidemiology of cryptococcosis: an update from population-based active surveillance in 2 large metropolitan areas, 1992-2000. *Clin Infect Dis* 36: 789–94.

Mortensen KL, Jensen RH, Johansen HK, et al. (2011) *Aspergillus* species and other molds in respiratory samples from patients with cystic fibrosis: a laboratory-based study with focus on *Aspergillus fumigatus* azole resistance. *J Clin Microbiol* 49: 2243–51.

Nacher N, Adenis A, McDonald S, et al. (2013) Disseminated histoplasmosis in HIV-infected patients in South America: a neglected killer continues on its rampage. *PLoS Negl Trop Dis* 7: e2319.

Ostrosky-Zeichner L, Casadevall A, Galgiani JN, Odds FC and Rex JH (2010) An insight into the antifungal pipeline: selected new molecules and beyond. *Nat Rev Drug Discov* 9: 719–27.

Panackal AA, Hajjeh RA, Cetron MS and Warnock DW (2002) Fungal infections among returning travelers. *Clin Infect Dis* 35: 1088–95.

Pappas PG, Alexander BA, Andes DR, et al. (2010) Invasive fungal infections among organ transplant recipients: results of the Transplant-Associated Infection Surveillance Network (TRANSNET). *Clin Infect Dis* 50: 1101–11.

Park BJ, Sigel K, Vaz V, et al. (2005) An epidemic of coccidioidomycosis in Arizona associated with climatic changes, 1998-2001. *J Infect Dis* 191: 1981–7.

Park BJ, Wannemuehler KA, Marston BJ, et al. (2009) Estimation of the current global burden of cryptococcal meningitis among persons living with HIV/AIDS. *AIDS* 23: 525–30.

Schelenz S, Hagen F, Rhodes JL, et al. (2016) First hospital outbreak of the globally emerging *Candida auris* in a European hospital. *Antimicrob Resist Infect Control* 5: 35. doi: 10.1186/s13756-016-0132-5

Vallabhaneni S, Kallen A, Tsay S, et al. (2016) Investigation of the first seven reported cases of *Candida auris*, a globally emerging invasive, multidrug-resistant fungus—United States, May 2013-August 2016. MMWR Morb Mortal Wkly Rep 65: 1234–7.

van der Linden JW, Arendrup MC, Warris A, et al. (2015) Prospective multicenter international surveillance of azole resistance in *Aspergillus fumigatus*. *Emerg Infect Dis* 21: 1041–4.

Vermeulen E, Lagrou K and Verweij PE (2013) Azole resistance in *Aspergillus fumigatus*: a growing public health concern. *Curr Opin Infect Dis* 26: 493–500.

Wiederhold NP, Gil VG, Gutierrez F, et al. (2016) First detection of TR34 L98H and TR46 Y121F T289A Cyp51 mutations in *Aspergillus fumigatus* isolates in the United States. *J Clin Microbiol* 54: 168–71.

CHAPTER 2

Fungal taxonomy and nomenclature

Andrew M. Borman

Introduction to fungal taxonomy and nomenclature

Fungi can be uni- or multicellular. Unicellular organisms which divide by budding have traditionally been referred to as yeasts, whereas multicellular fungi (moulds) exist as filament-like hyphae which grow via apical extension to form a mycelial mat. However, moulds and yeasts are not taxonomically valid divisions, and many medically important endemic fungi exhibit thermal or nutritional dimorphism allowing them to interconvert between morphologically distinct yeast (or spherule) and mould forms. The fungal kingdom is vast and ancient. Of the estimated 1–10 million species (Cannon 1997; Blackwell 2011; Hawksworth 2001), only approximately 1% has been formally described and named. Of the small proportion of fungi that have been named, less than a thousand are commonly reported as the agents of animal and human infections, with only a small proportion of these being capable of eliciting disease in immunocompetent hosts (Guarro et al. 1999).

Classical, phenotype-based taxonomy

Fungal reproduction can be asexual (mitosis), resulting in the production of usually large numbers of asexual spores (conidia) that are essentially identical to the parent and permit spread to, and colonization of, new geographic niches, or sexual (resulting from hyphal and nuclear fusion followed by meiosis) (Alexopoulos et al. 1996). Historically, the identification and hierarchical classification of filamentous fungi have been based on examination of their microscopic morphology, and in particular their reproductive structures (Ainsworth et al. 1973; Sutton 1973; Kendrick 1979; Weresub and Hennebert 1979; Sutton 1980; Subramanian 1983; Sugiyama 1987; Hennebert 1991; Reynolds and Taylor 1993; Hawksworth 1994; Guarro et al. 1999). On the basis of the types of sexual structures that fungi can be induced to form, the kingdom was divided into a limited number of distinct phyla—the Ascomycota, Zygomycota, and Basidiomycota—for fungi with recognized sexual (teleomorph) forms (Figures 2.1 and 2.2). The sexual spores of Ascomycota (ascospores) are typically produced in sacs (asci) contained in large, thick-walled structures called ascocarps (although some species produce single, solitary ascospores). Basidiomycota species produce sexual basidiospores borne on basidia which are often contained within macroscopic fruiting bodies (basidiomata) typical of mushrooms, toadstools, smuts, and bracket fungi. Conversely, fungi classified in the phylum Zygomycota produce single, thick-walled, sexual zygospores which are often highly ornamented. However, with a few notable exceptions, most fungi are heterothallic and will only undergo sexual reproduction when two independent, compatible isolates are present (Figure 2.2), and often in unique environmental conditions. Thus a fourth form-division, the Deuteromycota (or Fungi Imperfecti), was created to encompass all those fungi for which a sexual form (teleomorph) had not been described or could not be induced (Figure 2.2) (reviewed in Talbot 1971; Kendrick 1981; Seifert 1993). A similar classification into Ascomycota, Zygomycota, and Basidiomycota could be achieved on the basis of examination of the anamorph (asexual) forms of the fungi, including the presence of specific hyphal structures (septa, clamp connections) and the types of asexual spores formed and their method of production (conidiogenesis) in laboratory cultures (Figure 2.1) (Hughes 1953;. The hyphae of Zygomycota species are hyaline (colourless), broad, and ribbon-like and possess few to no septa (pauci-septate), and asexual conidia (termed sporangiospores) are typically produced inside large sac-like structures (sporangia). Conversely, the hyphae of filamentous Ascomycota species (many medically important Ascomycota species are yeasts) are narrow and highly septate, and may be either hyaline or dematiaceous (brown). Ascomycota species typically produce large numbers of conidia in culture on appropriate media, although the precise mechanism of conidiogenesis varies dramatically. Finally, species of the filamentous Basidiomycota, whilst producing hyphae similar to those of the Ascomycota, rarely produce conidia in culture, and most often present as rapidly growing floccose (fluffy) white colonies. However, upon careful examination, the hyphae can be distinguished from those of the Ascomycota by the presence of clamp connections (Alexopoulos et al. 1996; Figure 2.1) and, occasionally, delicate lateral projections termed spicules. It should, however, be noted that most medically important Basidiomycota species have anamorph states that are spherule (yeasts) rather than hyphal in form.

Although there is a staggering diversity in conidial forms and mechanisms of production, especially amongst the Ascomycota, different fungi have undergone either convergent or divergent evolution, with the result that many genetically unrelated species have very similar conidial characteristics, while other genetically similar species have vastly different morphological appearances. To further complicate matters, since fungi are of interest to a wide range of scientists (medical mycologists, geneticists, phytopathologists,

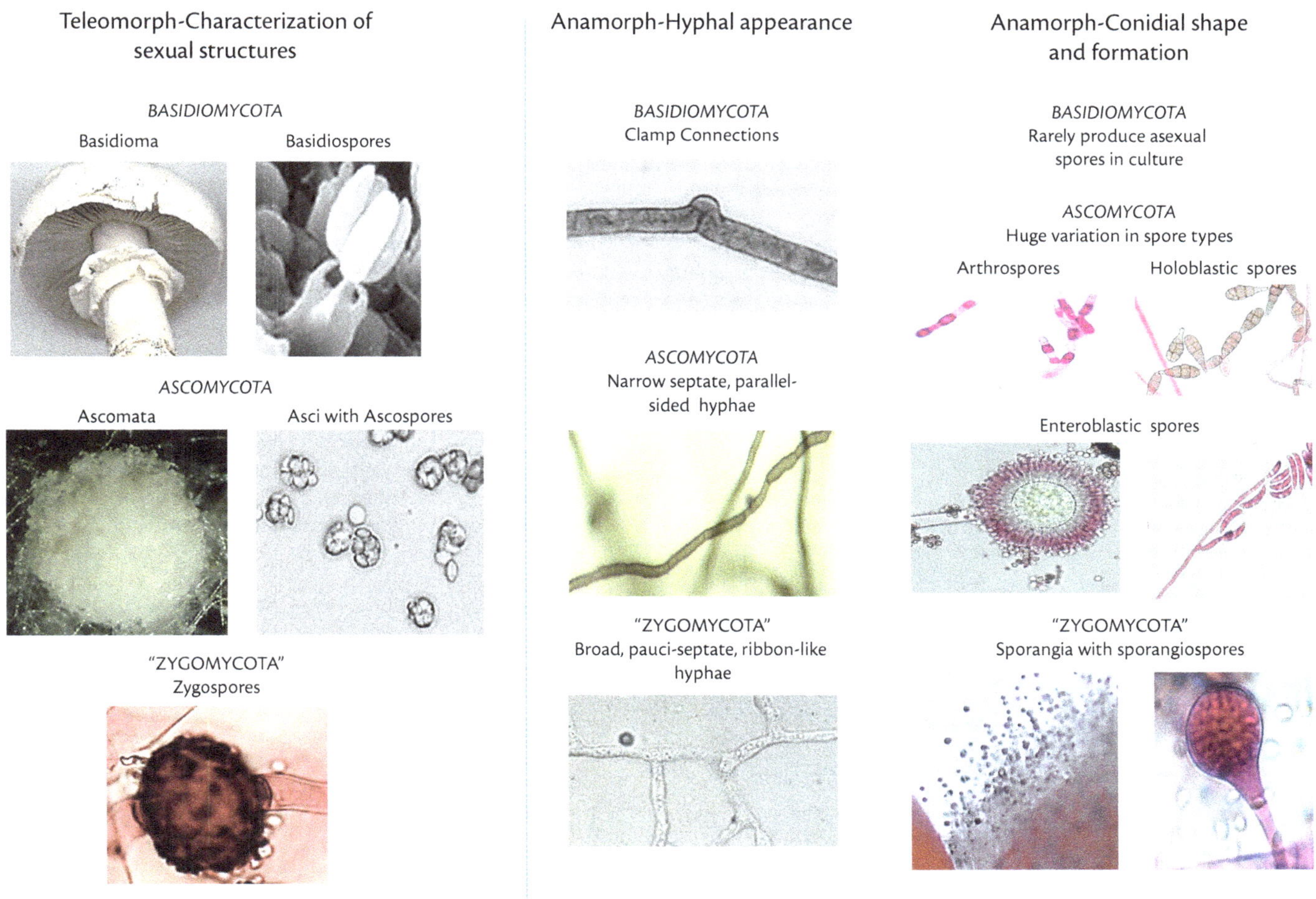

Figure 2.1 Approaches to fungal identification and taxonomy. Common features of the sexual cycles (left-hand side) and asexual cycles (right-hand side) of Basidiomycota, Ascomycota, and 'Zygomycota'.
Reproduced courtesy of Andrew M. Borman.

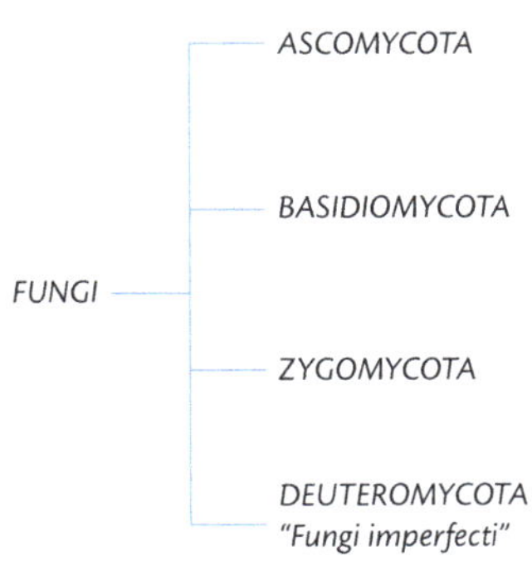

Figure 2.2 Traditional separation of the fungal kingdom into three phyla (Ascomycota, Basidiomycota, Zygomycota) and the form-division Deuteromycota for those fungi without a known sexual stage.

the biotechnology industry, and so on) and the sexual and asexual forms of fungi often develop independently of each other with little obvious morphological relatedness, a single genetic entity may have been described and named independently several times (Weresub and Pirozynski 1979).

Molecular approaches to identification and taxonomy

Since it is well established that different fungal species have dramatically varied antifungal susceptibility profiles (see, for example, Pfaller et al. 1998), the accurate identification of the agents of human infections is essential for appropriate patient management. However, many fungal isolates from deep and chronic infections do not produce conidia in the laboratory, rendering their conventional identification impossible. The advent of rapid and cost-effective approaches for extracting and analyzing fungal DNA has vastly facilitated the accurate identification of clinically important isolates, and has also permitted a greater taxonomic understanding of the fungal kingdom. Molecular analyses involving PCR (polymerase chain reaction) amplification and sequencing of conserved regions of the fungal genome encoding the rRNA (ribosomal ribonucleic acid) genes have permitted pan-fungal approaches to fungal identification (reviewed in Borman et al. 2008), and indeed the internal transcribed spacer region 1 (ITS1) has been proposed and accepted as an excellent candidate for fungal DNA barcoding (Balajee et al. 2009; Schoch et al. 2012). More sophisticated approaches examining additional protein-coding gene loci have permitted the development of multi-locus sequence typing and fungal strain typing (reviewed in Peterson 2012). However, a more immediate impact of such approaches has been the radical and continual revision of the fungal tree of life based on a phylogenetic approach to species recognition (see Hawksworth 2006 for review) where DNA sequence similarity is used to define species boundaries.

On the basis of such approaches, the fungal kingdom is now known to comprise at least seven phyla (Glomeromycota, Blastocladiomycota, Chytridiomycota, Neocallimastigomycota, and Microsporidia—with the retention of Ascomycota and Basidiomycota, which now constitute the sub-kingdom Dikarya (Figure 2.3; Hibbett et al. 2007). Organisms previously ascribed to the Deuteromycota can now be sequenced and their correct positions in the fungal kingdom ascertained. More dramatically, the phylum Zygomycota has been disbanded, after molecular approaches demonstrated unequivocally that it was polyphyletic. The fungi previously classified in the phylum Zygomycota are now spread between the phylum Glomeromycota, and four subphyla *incertae sedis* (of uncertain position): the Mucoromycotina, Entomophthoromycotina, Kickxellomycotina, and Zoopagomycotina, with most of the medically important members contained in the order Mucorales within Mucoromycotina (Hoffmann et al. 2013; Figure 2.3).

The phylum Ascomycota has now been divided into three subphyla, which comprise at least 14 classes and 60 orders (Figure 2.4). The subphylum Taphrinomycotina to date contains only one medically important fungal genus, *Pneumocystis*, which is formally located within the fungal kingdom. The subphylum Saccharomycotina contains a single medically important order, Saccharomycetales, which encompasses most pathogenic ascomycetous yeasts. The remainder of the medically important ascomycete genera are classed within the subphylum Pezizomycotina, and are divided between at least 14 orders, including: the Capnodiales (*Cladosporium* and related genera); the Pleosporales (*Alternaria, Bipolaris, Curvularia, Exserohilum, Ulocladium*, and many of the agents of dark-grain eumycetoma); the Chaetothyriales (*Cladophialophora, Exophiala, Fonsecaea, Phialophora, Ramichloridium*, and *Rhinocladiella*); the Eurotiales (*Aspergillus, Penicillium, Paecilomyces, Rasamsonia,*

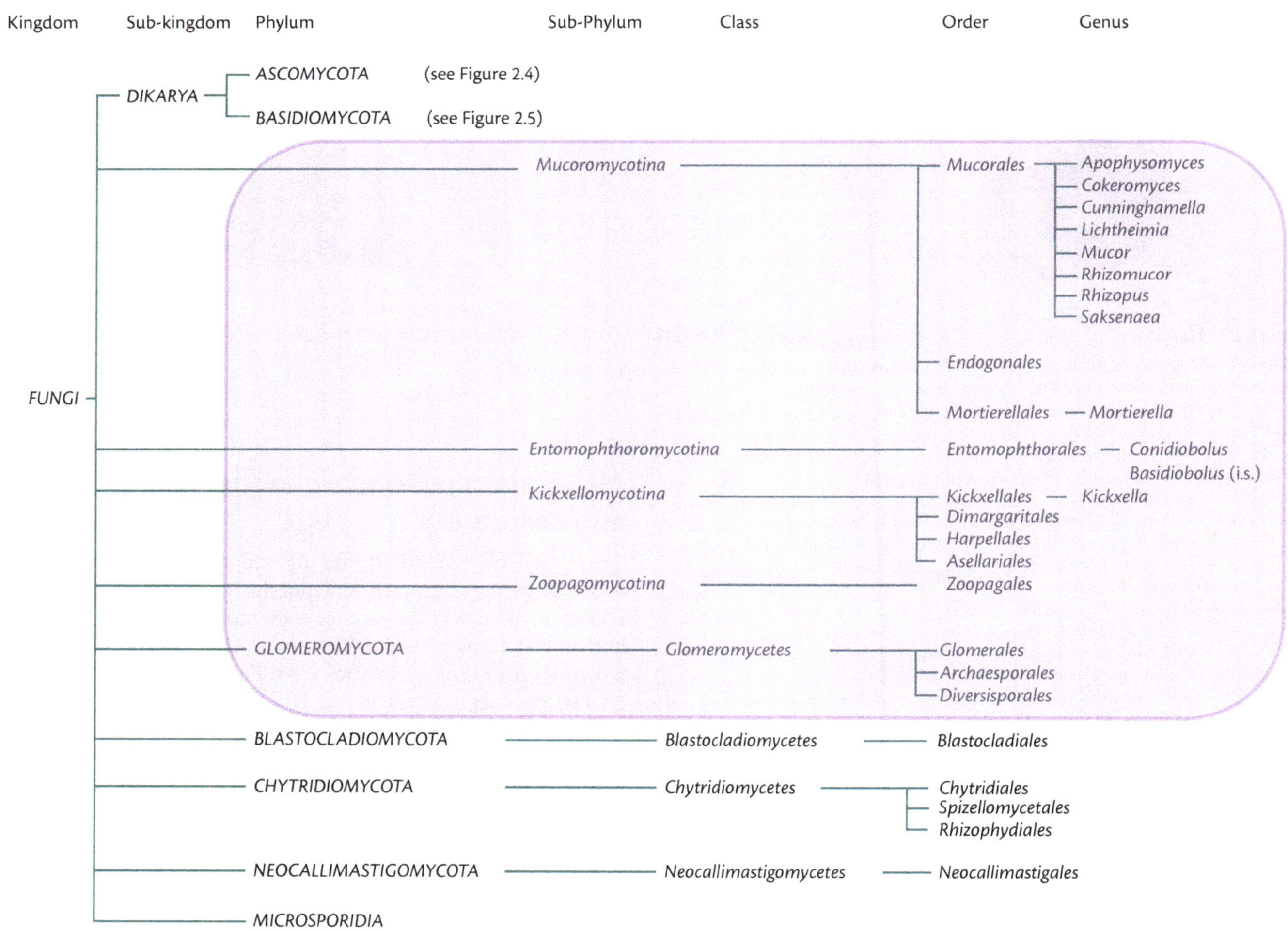

Figure 2.3 Recent taxonomy of the fungal kingdom. Organisms previously accommodated in the phylum 'Zygomycota' are highlighted in the blue-shaded lozenge. The positions of the more common, medically important mould genera are shown.

Source: data from Hibbett D. M. et al., 'A Higher-Level Phylogenetic Classification of the Fungi', *Mycological Research*, Volume 111, pp. 509–47. Published by Elsevier Ltd, http://www.sciencedirect.com/science/article/pii/S0953756207000615

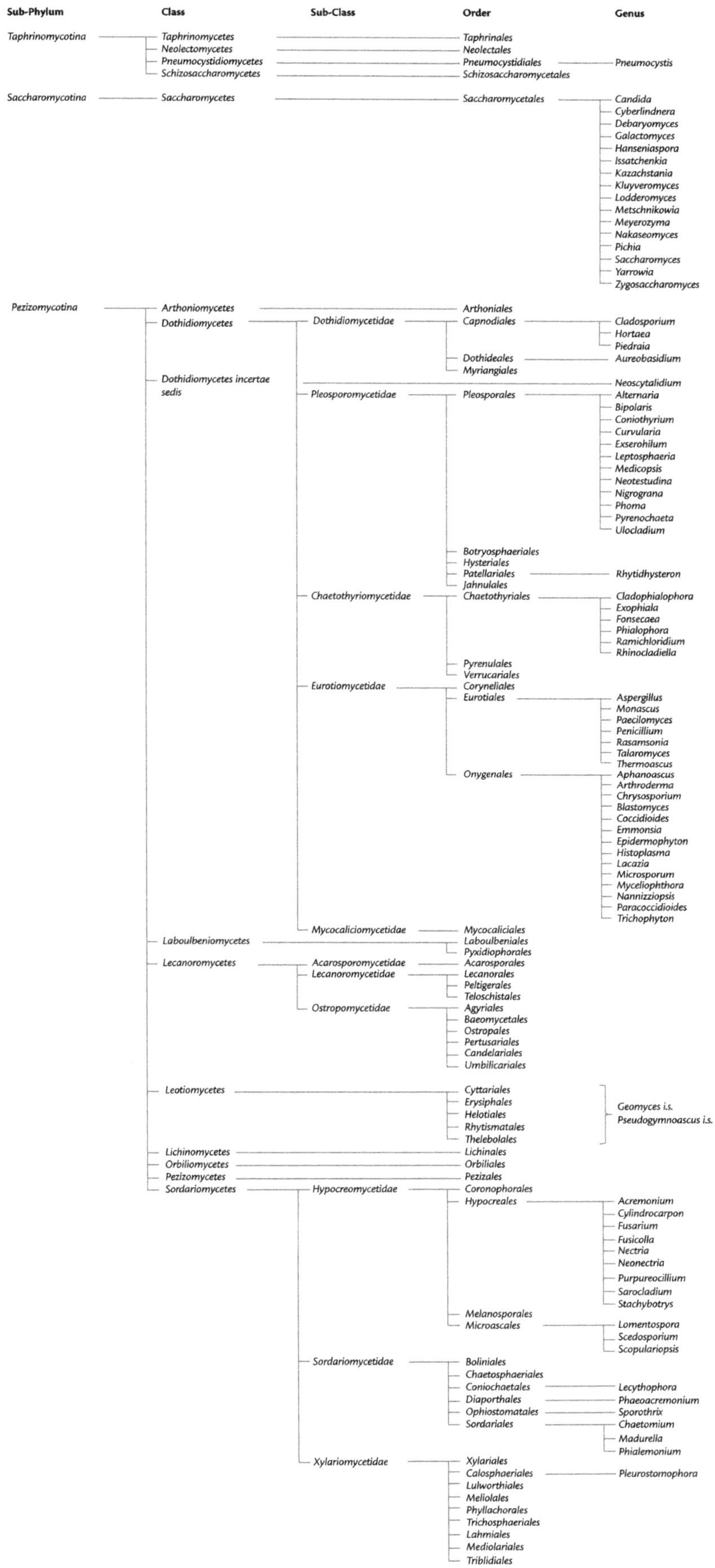

Figure 2.4 Revised taxonomy of the Ascomycota. The position of medically relevant genera is shown.

Talaromyces, and Thermoascus); the Onygenales (the dermatophytes [*Trichophyton, Microsporum, Epidermophyton*, and fungi with *Arthroderma* teleomorphs], the thermally dimorphic fungi with Ajellomyces teleomorphs [*Blastomyces, Coccidioides, Emmonsia, Histoplasma, and Paracoccidioides*], *Chrysosporium, Lacazia, Myceliophthora*, and *Nannizziopsis*); the Hypocreales (*Acremonium* and allied genera, *Fusarium* and allied genera, *Purpureocillium*, and *Stachybotrys*); the Microascales (*Lomentospora, Scedosporium*, and *Scopulariopsis*); the Sordariales (*Chaetomium, Madurella, and Phialemonium*); the Dothideales (*Aureobasidium*); the Patellariales (*Rhytidhysteron*); the Coniochaetales (*Lecythophora*); the Diaporthales (*Phaeoacremonium*); the Ophiostomatales (*Sporothrix*); and the Calosphaeriales (*Pleurostomophora*). Even with this greatly revised taxonomy, some medically important ascomycete genera (*Neoscytalidium, Geomyces, Pseudogymnoascus*) remain *incertae sedis*, pending molecular analyses of more of the fungal kingdom (Figure 2.4).

Finally, the phylum Basidiomycota contains three subphyla (Pucciniomycotina, Ustilaginomycotina, and Agaricomycotina) and at least 46 orders (Figure 2.5). To date, only around a dozen basidiomycete genera have been formally associated with human infections (Figure 2.5), and these are restricted to five orders. Order Sporidiales (Pucciniomycotina) contains the basidiomycete yeast genera *Rhodotorula* and *Sporobolomyces; Trichosporon* and *Cryptococcus* are classified in the order Tremellales (Agaricomycotina); *Bjerkandera, Coprinus, Irpex, Hormographiella,*

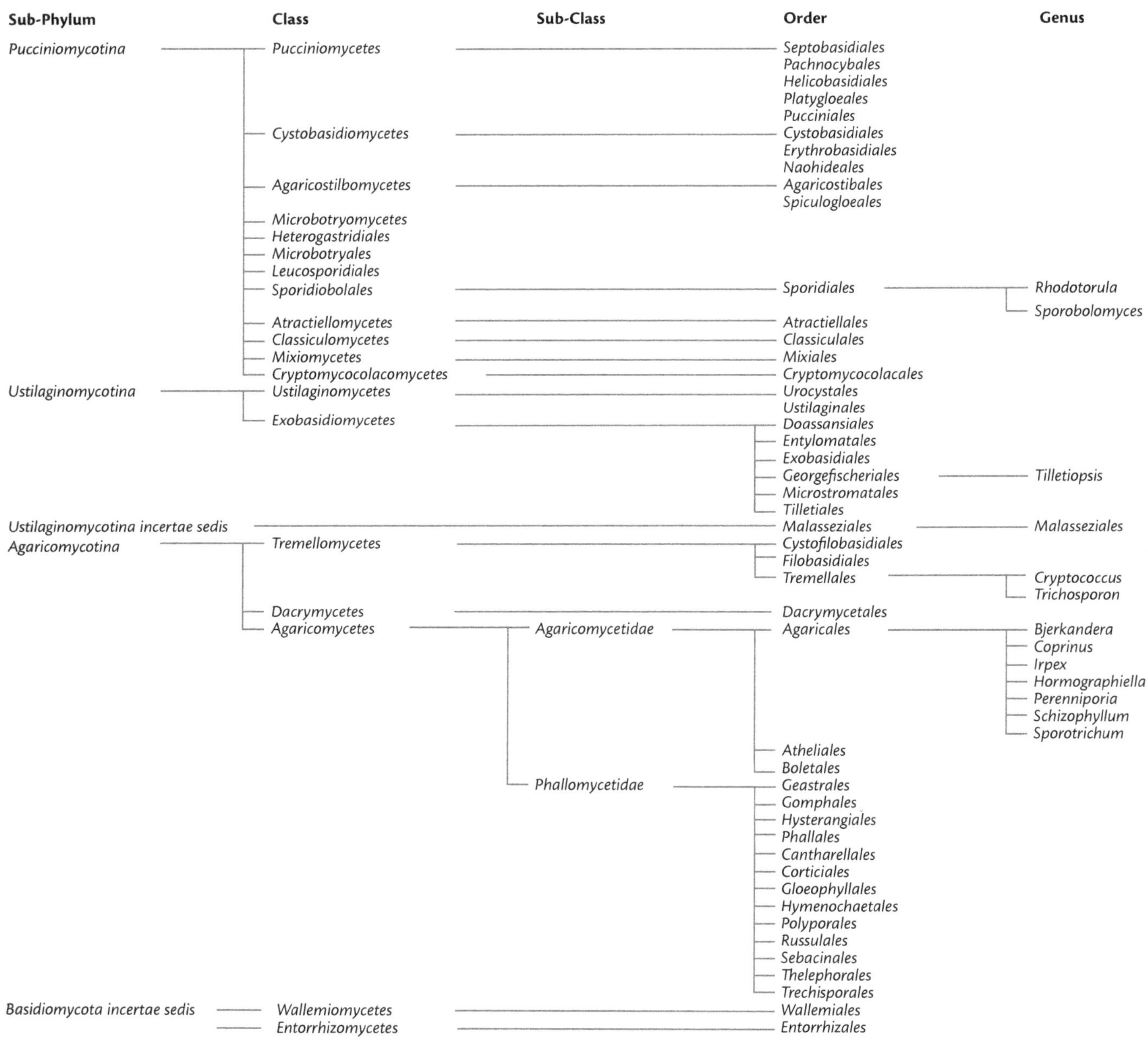

Figure 2.5 Revised taxonomy of the Basidiomycota. The position of medically relevant genera is shown.

Perenniporia, *Schizophyllum*, and *Sporotrichum* reside within the order Agaricales (Agaricomycotina); and *Tilletiopsis* is classified within the order Georgefischeriales (Ustilaginomycotina). The fifth order, the Malasseziales (*Malassezia* spp.), is also a member of the subphylum Ustilaginomycotina, but its exact position remains to be determined (Figure 2.5).

A further repercussion of the widespread adoption of molecular approaches to fungal identification and classification is the discovery of cryptic species (species which can only be distinguished by DNA sequencing) within many medically important morphospecies (reviewed in Hawksworth 2006). It is now accepted that *Aspergillus fumigatus* is a species complex that encompasses in excess of 40 cryptic species (reviewed in Johnson and Borman 2009), and a similar number of cryptic species have been discovered in the *Fusarium solani* species complex (see, for example, Short et al. 2013). In some cases, certain cryptic species have been reported to have altered antifungal susceptibility profiles (Balajee et al. 2005; Borman et al. 2008), whereas in others discrimination to species level within a species complex appears to be less medically important (Borman et al. 2013). Nevertheless, regardless of the medical relevance, the demonstration of cryptic species in most medically important genera has further added to the complexity of fungal taxonomy and nomenclature (see below).

Impact of molecular approaches on fungal nomenclature

Fungal nomenclature is governed by strict rules established by the International Code of Nomenclature (ICN) for algae, plants, and fungi. Under the ICN dictates, a name for a fungal species is only valid if it is in Latin binomial form, has been submitted to the MycoBank database, and has a living culture (usually of the type strain) permanently preserved in an accepted culture collection. Fungal name changes have always been permitted, and historically concerned the most commonly encountered fungal species which had been described and named independently many times by different authorities, only for those isolates later to be demonstrated to be identical and thus the names synonymous (Figure 2.6). Under such circumstances, the earliest valid name was usually retained. Molecular approaches to fungal identification have, to some extent, facilitated this process, as fungi which are genetically indistinguishable should, in theory, be synonymous. However, there are

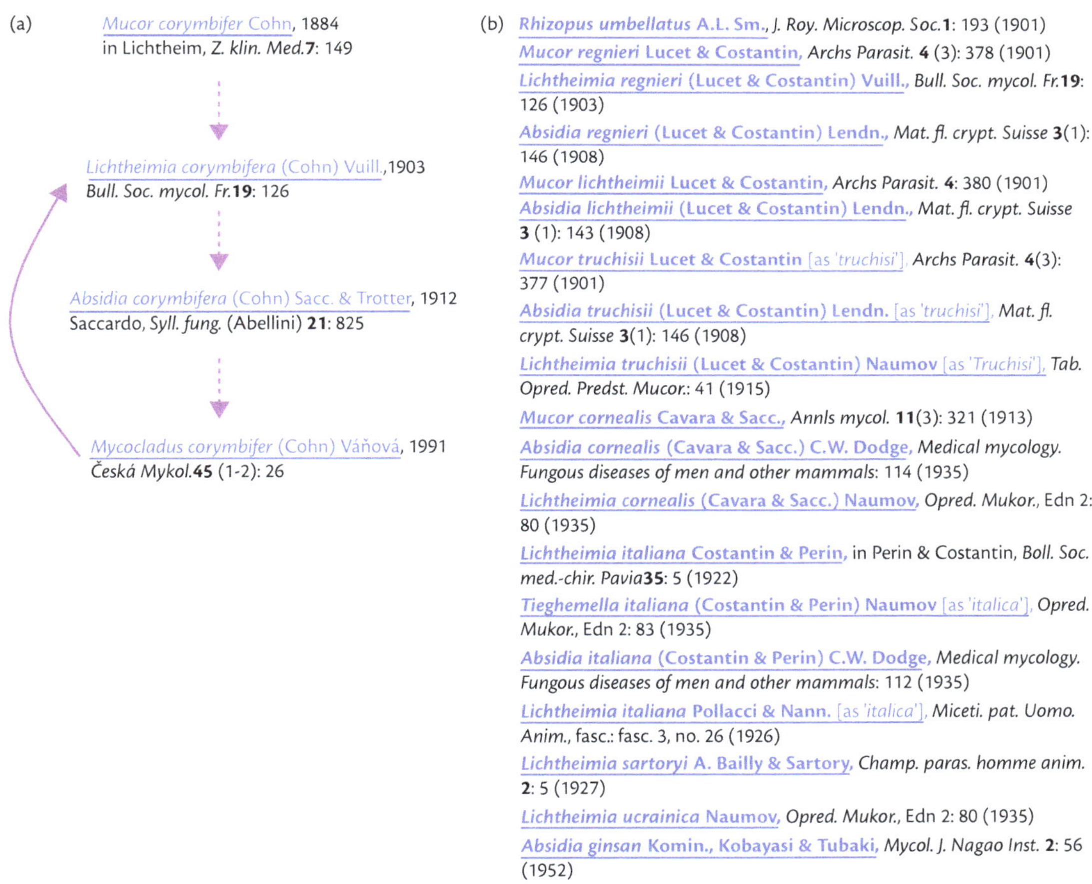
(a)
Mucor corymbifer Cohn, 1884
in Lichtheim, Z. klin. Med.7: 149
Lichtheimia corymbifera (Cohn) Vuill.,1903
Bull. Soc. mycol. Fr.19: 126
Absidia corymbifera (Cohn) Sacc. & Trotter, 1912
Saccardo, Syll. fung. (Abellini) 21: 825
Mycocladus corymbifer (Cohn) Váňová, 1991
Česká Mykol.45 (1-2): 26
(b)
Rhizopus umbellatus A.L. Sm., J. Roy. Microscop. Soc.1: 193 (1901)
Mucor regnieri Lucet & Costantin, Archs Parasit. 4 (3): 378 (1901)
Lichtheimia regnieri (Lucet & Costantin) Vuill., Bull. Soc. mycol. Fr.19: 126 (1903)
Absidia regnieri (Lucet & Costantin) Lendn., Mat. fl. crypt. Suisse 3(1): 146 (1908)
Mucor lichtheimii Lucet & Costantin, Archs Parasit. 4: 380 (1901)
Absidia lichtheimii (Lucet & Costantin) Lendn., Mat. fl. crypt. Suisse 3 (1): 143 (1908)
Mucor truchisii Lucet & Costantin [as 'truchisi'], Archs Parasit. 4(3): 377 (1901)
Absidia truchisii (Lucet & Costantin) Lendn. [as 'truchisi'], Mat. fl. crypt. Suisse 3(1): 146 (1908)
Lichtheimia truchisii (Lucet & Costantin) Naumov [as 'Truchisi'], Tab. Opred. Predst. Mucor.: 41 (1915)
Mucor cornealis Cavara & Sacc., Annls mycol. 11(3): 321 (1913)
Absidia cornealis (Cavara & Sacc.) C.W. Dodge, Medical mycology. Fungous diseases of men and other mammals: 114 (1935)
Lichtheimia cornealis (Cavara & Sacc.) Naumov, Opred. Mukor., Edn 2: 80 (1935)
Lichtheimia italiana Costantin & Perin, in Perin & Costantin, Boll. Soc. med.-chir. Pavia35: 5 (1922)
Tieghemella italiana (Costantin & Perin) Naumov [as 'italica'], Opred. Mukor., Edn 2: 83 (1935)
Absidia italiana (Costantin & Perin) C.W. Dodge, Medical mycology. Fungous diseases of men and other mammals: 112 (1935)
Lichtheimia italiana Pollacci & Nann. [as 'italica'], Miceti. pat. Uomo. Anim., fasc.: fasc. 3, no. 26 (1926)
Lichtheimia sartoryi A. Bailly & Sartory, Champ. paras. homme anim. 2: 5 (1927)
Lichtheimia ucrainica Naumov, Opred. Mukor., Edn 2: 80 (1935)
Absidia ginsan Komin., Kobayasi & Tubaki, Mycol. J. Nagao Inst. 2: 56 (1952)

Figure 2.6 The taxonomic (**a**) and nomenclatural (**b**) 'merry-go-round'.

a The principal taxonomic revisions of *Lichtheimia corymbifera*; dashed arrows indicate temporary changes, and the solid arrow indicates the final (hopefully) taxonomic position.

b Some of the various nomenclatural synonyms of *L. corymbifera* over the past century.

Source: data from Index Fungorum, accessible at http://www.indexfungorum.org/.

Table 2.1 Accepted and likely future nomenclatural changes to human pathogenic fungi. The original name(s) by which the species was described, intermediary (transitional) name(s), and the currently accepted name(s) are shown. Note that in many cases, the name commonly employed by clinicians and mycologists is a transitional name and not the original name. In most cases the species epithet has been retained to limit nomenclatural confusion

Original name(s)	Intermediary name(s)	Currently accepted name(s)
Acremonium strictum/kiliense		*Sarocladium strictum/kiliense*
Cadophora richardsiae	*Phialophora richardsiae*	*Pleurostomophora richardsiae*
Diplorhinotrichum gallopavum	*Ochroconis gallopava*	*Verruconis gallopava*
Drechslera australiensis/hawaiiensis	*Bipolaris australiensis/hawaiiensis*	*Curvularia australiensis/hawaiiensis*
Fusarium lichenicola	*Cylindrocarpon lichenicola*	*Fusarium lichenicola*
Geomyces destructans		*Pseudogymnoascus destructans*
Lomentospora prolificans	*Scedosporium inflatum/Scedosporium prolificans*	*Lomentospora prolificans*
Mucor corymbifer	*Lichtheimia corymbifera/* *Absidia corymbifera/* *Mycocladus corymbifer*	*Lichtheimia corymbifera*
Penicillium argillaceum	*Geosmithia argillacea*	*Rasamsonia argillacea*
Penicillium lilacinum	*Paecilomyces lilacinus*	*Purpureocillium lilacinum*
Penicillium marneffei		*Talaromyces marneffei*
Pyrenochaeta mackinnonii		*Nigrograna mackinnonii*
Pyrenochaeta romeroi		*Medicopsis romeroi*
Ramichloridium mackenziei		*Rhinocladiella mackenziei*
Ramularia destructans	*Cylindrocarpon destructans*	*Ilyonectria destructans*
Sporotrichum pannorum	*Geomyces pannorum*	*Pseudogymnoascus pannorum*
Trichosporon capitatum	*Geotrichum capitatum/Blastoschizomyces capitatus*	*Saprochaete capitata*
Torula dimidiata	*Hendersonula toruloidea/Scytalidium dimidiatum/* *Fusicoccum dimidiatum*	*Neoscytalidium dimidiatum*

caveats to this approach, especially when genomic regions that are fairly conserved are employed to establish phylogenetic relationships with fungi that have diverged more recently. For example, initial approaches for examining dermatophyte phylogeny using conserved loci could not distinguish *Trichophyton tonsurans*, an anthropophilic agent of tinea capitis in humans, from *T. equinum*, a zoophilic cause of horse ringworm (reviewed in Borman and Summerbell 2015). Further studies using additional loci did, however, demonstrate that the two are distinct genetically as well as morphologically and clinically. Similar discussions continue regarding *T. rubrum*, the principal cause of tinea pedis and tinea unguium in developed countries, and *T. soudanense*, an agent almost exclusively of tinea capitis that originated on the African sub-continent (Borman and Summerbell 2015). Thus, fungal taxonomy and nomenclature remain something of a battleground between the 'lumpers' (who propose to synonymize fungal species with quite distinct geographic niches, different morphological appearances, and even spectra of clinical presentations) and the 'splitters' (who use very precise genetic loci to demonstrate innumerable cryptic species within morpho-species that are morphologically and clinically indistinguishable).

A second acceptable reason for fungal name changes is when studies demonstrate that a species should not remain in its current genus. Effectively, when a new fungal genus is erected, it is done so around a type species, with additional different species being accommodated in the genus over time. Molecular approaches have demonstrated that in many cases, these additional species are quite unrelated to the type species, and have clearly undergone considerable convergent phenotypic evolution. For example, *Absidia corymbifera*, which had been retained as a valid name for nearly a century, was shown to be genetically distinct from *Absidia repens*, the type of the genus, and was briefly renamed *Mycocladus corymbifer*, before attaining its final genetically compatible nomenclatural resting place as *Lichtheimia corymbifera*, a name by which it had been briefly known from 1903 (Figure 2.6). In such cases, wherever possible, the species epithet is retained (after adjusting according to the rules of Latin grammar), in an attempt to minimize nomenclatural confusion. Other examples include *Scytalidium dimidiatum* (now *Neoscytalidium dimidiatum*), which is genetically distant from the type species *S. lignicola*, and *Paecilomyces lilacinus* (now *Purpureocillium lilacinum*), which is not even in the same fungal class as *P. variotii*, the type species of the genus (Figure 2.4).

For other common fungi, a more cautious approach has been proposed. Since the type species of *Aspergillus* is *A. glaucus*, on the basis of phylogenetic approaches most other *Aspergillus* species should therefore be removed from the genus, and renamed with their teleomorph names, which, according to convention, should take precedence over anamorph names. This would result in at least nine new teleomorph genera to encompass the other former members of *Aspergillus* (reviewed in Samson et al. 2014). Similarly, the type species of *Fusarium* is *F. sambucinum*, which has a *Gibberella* teleomorph. Thus, all those current *Fusarium* species which have teleomorphs other than *Gibberella* should be removed, including *Fusarium solani* (teleomorph *Haematonectria haematococca*) and *Fusarium dimerum*. However, several large working groups, containing many of the scientists who originally demonstrated the polyphyletic natures of these two genera, have proposed that the status quo be maintained in the face of phylogenetic evidence, to 'preserve established research connections' in the diverse communities interested in *Fusarium* (Geiser et al. 2013) and 'maintain the prevailing, broad concept of *Aspergillus*' (Samson et al. 2014). Although at odds with much molecular phylogenetic evidence, this nomenclatural obfuscation, which is supported by the International Commission of Penicillium and Aspergillus (ICPA), will certainly reduce confusion in medical mycology, where accepted nomenclatural changes have to be filtered down to clinicians. A non-exhaustive list of accepted and likely future nomenclatural changes to common medically important fungi can be found in Table 2.1, although this is likely to be subject to considerable change.

One fungus = one name

The existence of both anamorph and teleomorph states that share little morphological relatedness for many medically important fungi, and which have often been described separately many years apart, has resulted in many fungal species having several names. In 2011, the 'Amsterdam Declaration' (Hawksworth et al. 2011) proposed a substantial modification of Article 59 of the code of nomenclature that would enforce the abandonment of dual nomenclature in fungi. From January 2013, it was declared that each fungus must retain a single name, with the decisions on which names should be retained being taken, or at least ratified by, the Nomenclature Committee for Fungi (Hawksworth 2011). The pre-existing convention, by which the teleomorph name should always take precedence, could certainly lead to considerable confusion in the medical mycology community, which has widely ignored the convention previously as it was usually the anamorph state that was isolated in the laboratory. To somewhat soften the blow to medical mycologists, additional changes to the code included the instruction to 'follow the principle of priority of publication when selecting the generic name to adopt', which seemingly ends the previous precedence of teleomorph over anamorph, with the caveat 'except where the younger generic name is far better known'. To further lessen unnecessary and transient nomenclatural instability, working groups and committees established under the auspices of the International Commission on the Taxonomy of Fungi (ICTF) and the Nomenclature Committee for Fungi (NCF) will propose lists of retained (protected) and rejected names for key genera, with only definitive changes being ratified. Whilst this might seem like a satisfactory fix, it still has its adversaries (Gams and Jaklitsch 2011), who argue that if this applies at both the genus and species level, then numerous new combinations or specific conservation proposals would be required, and that many important teleomorph genera would also be abolished. There is also the question of who should decide, and how, whether an anamorph or teleomorph name is more popular. Suggestions that have been explored to date include the use of internet search engines to examine the number of 'hits' against a given fungal name (ICPA). Whatever the final decisions, it is inevitable that fungal nomenclature is heading for stormy waters, which hopefully in the end will lead to a more stable and scientifically robust taxonomic understanding of the fungal kingdom.

Disclaimers

To the author's knowledge, the taxonomic affiliations described in this chapter were correct at the time of press. Considerable further taxonomic changes affecting several orders have been proposed since the time of writing. The most clinically important taxonomic and nomenclatural revisions affect the Onygenales, with substantial changes to proposed nomenclature for the agents of dermatophytosis and the hazard group 3 pathogens in Ajellomycetaceae. Comprehensive overviews of these changes can be found in de Hoog et al. (2017) and Dukik et al. (2017).

References

Ainsworth GC, Sparrow FK and Sussman AS (ed.) (1973) *The Fungi: An Advanced Treatise*, IVA: A Taxonomic Review with Keys: Ascomycetes and Fungi Imperfecti (London: Academic Press), 1–7.

Alexopoulos CJ, Mims CW and Blackwell M (1996) *Introductory Mycology* (4th edn, New York: John Wiley & Sons), 868 pp.

Balajee SA, Borman AM, Brandt ME, et al. (2009) Sequence-based identification of Aspergillus, Fusarium and the Mucorales in the clinical mycology laboratory: where are we and where should we go from here? *J Clin Microbiol* 47: 877–84.

Balajee SA, Gribskov JL, Hanley E, Nickle D and Marr KA (2005) *Aspergillus lentulus* sp. nov., a new sibling species of *A. fumigatus*. *Eukaryot Cell* 4: 625–32.

Blackwell M (2011) The Fungi: 1,2,3 ... 5.1 million species? *Am J Bot* 98: 426–38.

Borman AM, Linton CJ, Miles S-J and Johnson EM (2008) Molecular identification of pathogenic fungi. *J Antimicrob Chemother* 61: i7–i12.

Borman AM, Petch R, Linton CJ, Palmer MD, Bridge PD and Johnson EM (2008) *Candida nivariensis*, an emerging pathogenic fungus with multidrug resistance to antifungal agents. *J Clin Microbiol* 46: 933–8.

Borman AM and Summerbell RC (2015) *Trichophyton, Microsporum, Epidermophyton*, and agents of superficial mycoses, *in*: J Jorgensen, M Pfaller, K Carroll, et al., eds, *Manual of Clinical Microbiology* (11th edn, Washington, DC: ASM Press), 2128–52.

Borman AM, Szekely A, Linton CJ, Palmer MD, Brown P and Johnson EM (2013) Epidemiology, antifungal susceptibility, and pathogenicity of *Candida africana* isolates from the United Kingdom. *J Clin Microbiol* 51: 967–72.

Cannon PF (1997) Strategies for rapid assessment of fungal diversity. *Biodivers Conserv* 6: 669–80.

Dukik K, Muñoz JF, Jiang Y, et al. (2017) Novel taxa of thermally dimorphic systemic pathogens in the Ajellomycetaceae (Onygenales). *Mycoses* 60: 296–309.

Gams W and Jaklitsch W [& 77 signatories] (2011) A critical response to the 'Amsterdam Declaration'. *Mycotaxon* 116: 1–12.

Geiser DM, Aoki T, Bacon CW, et al. (2013) One fungus, one name: defining the genus *Fusarium* in a scientifically robust way that preserves longstanding use. *Phytopathology* 103: 400–8.

Guarro J, Gene J and Stchigel AM (1999) Developments in fungal taxonomy. *Clin Microbiol Rev* 12: 454–500.

Hawksworth DL (ed.) (1994) *Ascomycete Systematics: Problems and perspectives in the nineties* (Plenum Press: New York).

Hawksworth DL (2001) The magnitude of fungal diversity: the 1.5 million species estimate revisited. *Mycol Res* 105: 1422–32.

Hawksworth DL (2006) Pandora's mycological box: molecular sequences vs. morphology in understanding fungal relationships and biodiversity. *Rev Iberoam Micol* 23: 127–33.

Hawksworth DL (2011) A new dawn for the naming of fungi: impacts of decisions made in Melbourne in July 2011 on the future publication and regulation of fungal names. *MycoKeys* 1, 7–20; *IMA Fungus* 2: 155–62.
Hawksworth DL, Crous PW, Redhead SA, et al. [& 69 signatories] (2011) The Amsterdam declaration on fungal nomenclature. *IMA Fungus* 2: 105–12; *Mycotaxon* 116: 491–500.
Hennebert GL (1991) Art-59 and the problem with pleoanamorphic fungi. *Mycotaxon* 40: 479–96.
Hibbett DM, Binder M, Bischoff JF, et al. (2007) A higher-level phylogenetic classification of the Fungi. *Mycol Res* 111: 509–47.
Hoffmann K, Jpawłowska J, Walther G, et al. (2013) The family structure of the Mucorales: a synoptic revision based on comprehensive multigene-genealogies. *Persoonia* 30: 57–76.
de Hoog GS, Dukik K, Monod M, et al. (2017) Toward a novel multilocus phylogenetic taxonomy for the dermatophytes. *Mycopathologia* 182: 5–31.
Hughes SJ (1953) Conidiophores, conidia and classification. *Canadian Journal of Botany* 315: 577–659.
Johnson EM and Borman AM (2009) Identification of *Aspergillus* at the species level: the importance of conventional methods; microscopy and culture, *in*: A Pasqualotto, ed., *Aspergillus and Aspergillosis* (New York: Springer Press), 55–74.
Kendrick B (ed.) (1979) *The Whole Fungus: The sexual-asexual synthesis*, Vols 1–2 (Ottowa: National Museums of Canada).
Kendrick B (1981) The history of conidial fungi, *in*: GT Cole and B Kendrick, eds, *Biology of Conidial Fungi* (New York: Academic Press), 3–18.
Peterson SW (2012) Aspergillus and Penicillium identification using DNA sequences: barcode or MLST? *Appl Microbiol Biotechnol* 95: 339–44.
Pfaller MA, Jones RN, Messer SA, Edmond MB and Wenzel RP (1998) National surveillance of nosocomial blood stream infection due to species of *Candida* other than *Candida albicans*: frequency of occurrence and antifungal susceptibility in the SCOPE Program. *Diagn Microbiol Infect Dis* 31: 327–32.
Reynolds DR and Taylor JW (eds) (1993) *The Fungal Holomorph: Mitotic, meiotic and pleomorphic speciation in fungal systematics* (Oxfordshire: CABI International).
Samson RA, Visagie CM, Houbraken J, et al. (2014) Phylogeny, identification and nomenclature of the genus *Aspergillus*. *Stud Mycol* 78: 141–73.
Schoch CL, Seifert KA, Huhndorf S, et al.; Fungal Barcoding Consortium; Fungal Barcoding Consortium Author List (2012) Nuclear ribosomal internal transcribed spacer (ITS) region as a universal DNA barcode marker for Fungi. *Proc Natl Acad Sci USA* 109: 6241–46.
Seifert KA (1993) Integrating anamorphic fungi into the fungal system, *in*: DR Reynolds and JW Taylor, eds, *The Fungal Holomorph: Mitotic, Meiotic and Pleomorphic Speciation in Fungal Systematics* (Oxfordshire: CABI International), 79–85.
Short DP, O'Donnell K, Thrane U, et al. (2013) Phylogenetic relationships among members of the *Fusarium solani* species complex in human infections and the descriptions of *F. keratoplasticum* sp. nov. and *F. petroliphilum* stat. nov. *Fungal Genet Biol* 53: 59–70.
Subramanian CV (1983) *Hyphomycetes: Taxonomy and biology* (London: Academic Press).
Sugiyama J (ed.) (1987) *Pleomorphic Fungi: The diversity and its taxonomic implications* Tokyo: Kodansha Ltd), 325 pp.
Sutton BC (1973) Coelomycetes, *in*: GC Ainsworth, FK Sparrow and AS Sussman, eds, *The Fungi: An advanced treatise*, vol. IVA—*A Taxonomic Review with Keys: Ascomycetes And Fungi Imperfecti* (New York: Academic Press), 513–82.
Sutton BC (1980) *Coelomycetes—Fungi Imperfecti with pycnidia, acervuli and stromata* (Kew, Surrey: Commonwealth Mycological Institute).
Talbot PHB (1971) *Principles of Fungal Taxonomy* (London: Macmillan), 274 pp.
Weresub LK and Hennebert GL (1979) Anamorph and teleomorph: terms for organs of reproduction rather than karyological phases. *Mycotaxon* 8: 181–6.
Weresub LK and Pirozynski KA (1979) Pleomorphism of fungi as treated in the history of mycology and nomenclature, *in*: B Kendrick, ed., *The Whole Fungus: The sexual-asexual synthesis*, vol. 1 (Ottowa: National Museums of Canada), 17–30.

CHAPTER 3

Physiology and metabolism of fungal pathogens

Neil A.R. Gow and Alistair J.P. Brown

Fungal metabolism

Fungi are defined as 'aerobic, characteristically mycelial heterotrophs'. In fact, for medically relevant species, many develop as yeasts in the human body. They also share the ability to be able to grow at body temperature, often at rather low oxygen tensions. Nevertheless, they must obtain all their nutrients from their human host. Indeed, the ability to assimilate and metabolize available nutrients, and to survive local environmental stresses in diverse niches in the human body, largely differentiates human-pathogenic from non-pathogenic fungal species.

Collectively, fungal pathogens can colonize, grow, and infect almost all parts of the human body, including hair; skin; oral cavity, gut, and vaginal mucosa; epithelial and endothelial cell layers; blood; and tissues. These microenvironments differ significantly in terms of their local oxygen and CO_2 partial pressures, nutrients, and the presence or absence of other competing microbes and immune cells. Consequently, adaptive physiological responses are required to cope with these niche-specific challenges. Many nutrients must be wrestled from the host or obtained by the destruction of barriers and organized tissues that are protected by innate and adaptive immunological forces.

Obtaining nutrients from the human host

Central metabolic pathways have largely been conserved in pathogenic fungi (Han et al. 2011), with the exception of *Pneumocystis* species. These obligate pathogens appear to have shed amino acid biosynthetic pathways, and instead they scavenge these essential precursors of protein synthesis from the host (Hauser et al. 2010). Other fungal pathogens, such as *Candida albicans,* are commensals that co-exist with their hosts for most of the time without inflicting damage. Pathogenic *Candida* species interact with bacteria on the skin, in the gut, in the oral cavity, and on the vaginal lumen. The endogenous microbiota itself represents part of the protective immunity of the host, since these other microbes compete for nutrients and host binding sites and produce molecules that inhibit fungal growth. Nutrients in the gut are quickly absorbed by bacterial microbial flora and human epithelial cells, and the nutrient profile and oxygen tension differ substantially in the small and large intestine. Recently it was shown that *C. albicans* generates a specific cell type (called a GUT (gastrointestinally induced transition) cell) that augments its ability to exist as a commensal in the bowel (Pande et al. 2013). The GUT-specific transcriptome has been shown to upregulate genes involved in the metabolism of short-chain fatty acids and other micronutrients that are enriched in the large intestine. In addition, this host niche is anaerobic, resulting in increased iron bioavailability. Consequently, *C. albicans* GUT cells downregulate iron-acquisition genes, to prevent the toxicity caused by iron excess (Pande et al. 2013). Genes encoding several virulence factors are also downregulated in GUT cells, implying that this cell type is adapted for commensalism rather than pathogenicity. Dermatophytes may also downregulate processes that promote invasion beyond the dermal layers with a view to sustaining long-term colonization of keratin-rich outer surfaces. Metabolism has therefore not always been evolutionarily tuned to promoting maximum host destruction.

Glucose is the preferred carbon source for most fungi, but its concentration varies substantially within the body. Blood glucose concentrations are maintained at around 0.06–0.1% (3–5 mM), but they are around 0.5% in the vaginal lumen, and lower than 1 mM in the phagosome of macrophages (Owen and Katz 1999). Consequently, following phagocytosis, the metabolism of *C. albicans* switches from glycolysis towards fatty acid β-oxidation, the glyoxylate cycle, and gluconeogenesis. Indeed, the glyoxylate pathway enzymes isocitrate lyase and citrate synthase are upregulated following phagocytosis (Lorenz and Fink 2001), and *C. albicans* null mutants that lack glyoxylate pathway genes display attenuated virulence (Lorenz and Fink 2001; Mιramón et al. 2012). In contrast, when *C. albicans* grows in host organs such as the kidney, both glycolytic and glyoxylate cycle genes are activated, suggesting that fungal cells are subjected to heterogeneous microenvironments with differing carbon sources in these complex niches (Barelle et al. 2006; Wilson et al. 2009). The non-fermentable carboxylic acid, lactic acid, exists in significant concentrations in both the gastrointestinal and vaginal tracts, and enzymes required for its metabolism are important for *Candida* species to be able to colonize the gut. Key metabolic regulators such as the glycolytic activator Tye7 are also required for gut colonization (Lavoie et al. 2010).

Non-glucose-based (alternative) carbon sources can be gained by active hydrolysis of host proteins or phospholipids, and many fungal pathogens produce secreted proteases, lipases, and phospholipases that degrade high molecular weight host molecules into assimilatable amino acids, fatty acids, and other carbon sources. Exposure to glucose enhances the oxidative stress resistance of *C. albicans* (Rodaki et al. 2009). Also, cells pre-grown on oleic acid are more virulent than those grown on glucose or amino acids in

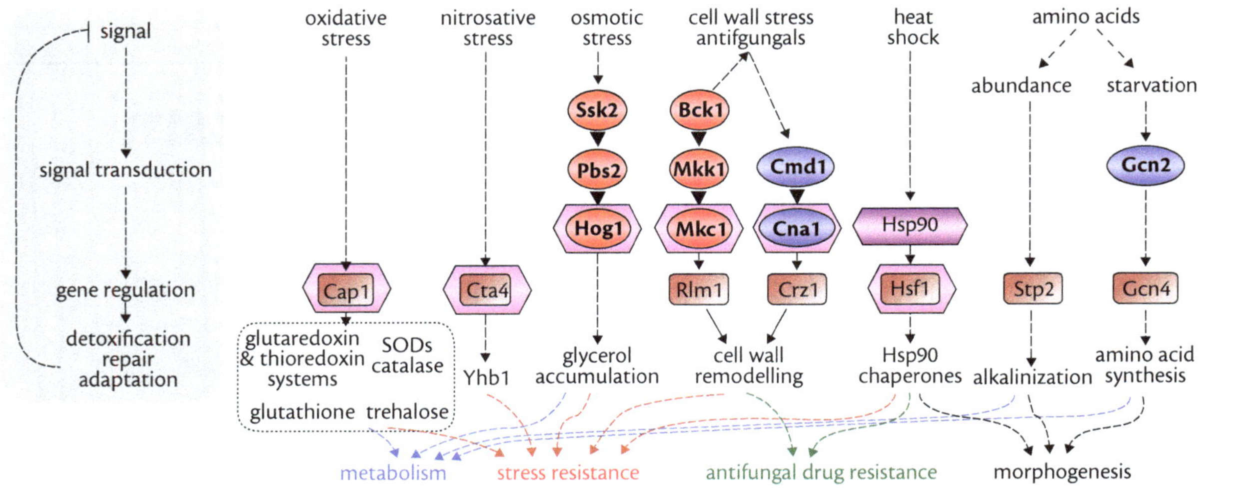

Figure 3.1 Multiple signalling pathways mediate link metabolism to stress adaptation, morphogenesis, and antifungal drug resistance. Transcription factors are highlighted in grey boxes, components of MAP kinase modules in red ovals, and other types of regulator (protein kinase or phosphatase) in blue ovals. Hsp90 is represented in a purple hexagon, and Hsp90 client proteins, the activity of which might be modulated by temperature (see text), are shown with a background purple hexagon.

Reproduced courtesy of Alistair J. P. Brown.

a vaginal infection model (Ene et al. 2012). Moreover, growth on different carbon sources has been shown to alter virulence in a systemic mouse model.

Unlike, *S. cerevisiae, C. albicans* is able to assimilate both lactate and oleic acid in the presence of glucose (Brown et al. 2014b), essentially making it more metabolically versatile. In the absence of glucose, *C. albicans* can grow efficiently on amino acids. This leads to local increases in ambient pH through the excretion of excess ammonia, and this local alkalinization triggers hyphal development (Vylkova and Lorenz 2014), a key virulence trait (Figure 3.1). Adaptive metabolic responses are intertwined with *C. albicans* virulence traits: the amino acid starvation response is mechanistically linked to yeast-hypha morphogenesis through the global regulator Gcn4 (Tripathi et al. 2002) (Figure 3.1).

Micronutrient acquisition and restriction

Certain micronutrients, such as iron and zinc, are generally present at very low concentrations in host niches, and hence are rate limiting for growth *in vivo*. This is partly because the host has evolved strategies to restrict microbial access to these micronutrients and thereby prevent pathogen proliferation (Potrykus et al. 2013). This process has been called nutritional immunity. To counteract this micronutrient limitation, pathogenic fungi have evolved efficient micronutrient scavenging mechanisms.

Iron is essential for the host and for fungal pathogens alike. Consequently, *Candida, Aspergillus, Cryptococcus*, and other fungal pathogens have multiple mechanisms for promoting iron acquisition from the human host (Almeida et al. 2008; Potrykus et al. 2014). *A. fumigatus* produces iron chelators, called siderophores, that have a high affinity for iron and help transport it into the cell. Although *Candida albicans* and *Cryptococcus neoformans* do not produce siderophores, they have the potential to exploit siderophores produced by bacteria. In *A. fumigatus*, the SidA siderophore is important for growth under iron-replete conditions *in vivo*, although this fungus also has a reductive iron assimilatory mechanism that also facilitates *in vivo* survival (Johnson 2008; Schrettl et al. 2010; Chen et al. 2011). However, siderophore production dominates iron acquisition during pathogenesis (Schrettl et al. 2010).

The acquisition of iron from transferrin or ferritin requires the presence of ferric reductases, copper oxidase(s), and iron permeases (Potrykus et al. 2014). Iron can also be acquired from haemoglobin—for example, after *C. albicans* hyphae bind to erythrocytes, releasing haem and subsequently iron. *Candida* can also bind and extract iron from transferrin and from the host iron storage protein ferritin via the hyphal cell wall protein Als3 (Almeida et al. 2008). This haem–iron acquisition pathway is upregulated during the progression of systemic *Candida* infections (Potrykus et al. 2013). The availability of iron is strongly influenced by pH, with alkaline pH resulting in higher levels of non-soluble ferric ion. Accordingly, the pH-sensing *RIM101* pathway is involved in the transcriptional regulation of genes on the reductive iron assimilation pathway (Cornet and Gaillardin 2014).

Other trace metals—including zinc, manganese, and copper—are essential for the growth and survival of fungal pathogens (Potrykus et al. 2013). A novel zinc acquisition 'zincophore' pathway, not dissimilar to the iron siderophores mechanism, has been identified in *C. albicans*. This involves secretion of a specific zinc-binding pH-regulated antigen 1 (Pra1) (Citiulo et al. 2012). In *C. albicans* the zinc transporters are differentially regulated in response to pH, Zrt1, and Pra1, being operational under neutral-alkaline conditions, and with Zrt2 being upregulated under acidic conditions (Wilson 2015). Interestingly, pathogenic fungi that exist in geographical regions with acidic soils lack Pra1 homologues (e.g. *Histoplasma*), whereas those that inhabit regions with non-acidic soils contain Pra1 homologues (e.g. *Coccidioides*) (Wilson 2015).

Counteracting imposed stresses

Fungal pathogens, including *Candida* species, attempt to neutralize the reactive oxygen and nitrogen species generated in the phagosome of macrophages and neutrophils by producing detoxifying enzymes (e.g. superoxide dismutases and catalases), buffering agents (such as glutathione and thioredoxin), and proteins that repair oxidative and nitrosative damage and promote protein refolding. *C. albicans* upregulates these protective functions by activating key stress pathways such as the Hog1 MAP kinase and Cap1 pathways, as well as the heat shock transcription factor Hsf1 pathway (Enjalbert et al. 2006; Brown et al. 2012) (Figure 3.1), thereby mitigating against phagocyte killing (Eissenberg et al. 1993) mediated by host NADPH (nicotinamide adenine dinucleotide phosphate) oxidase and other oxidative damaging agents. Phagosomal toxins can also be neutralized by glutathione, which is converted by reactive oxidative and nitrosative species to glutathione disulphide and S-nitrosoglutathione, respectively. These adducts are then recycled back to glutathione (Tillmann et al. 2015). Furthermore, *C. albicans* can also neutralize the acidic pH of the phagosome via ammonia extrusion. Mutants that lack Stp2, a transcriptional activator of the amino acid permease genes that are required for this alkalinization process *in vitro*, display an impaired ability to escape macrophage killing (Vylkova et al. 2014) (Figure 3.1).

The ability of fungal pathogens to colonize and infect the host is dependent on metabolic processes to generate osmolytes such as glycerol, which protect against osmotic stress, antioxidants such as glutathione, which defend against oxidative and nitrosative stresses, and the general stress protectant trehalose (Brown et al. 2014b). Glucose metabolism can enhance oxidative stress survival, which may prime cells for attack by macrophages and neutrophils prior to their phagocytosis (Brown et al. 2014b). Carbon metabolism can also affect other aspects of virulence including tolerance to osmotic stress and antifungal drug exposure (Rodaki et al. 2009; Perez et al. 2013). For example, lactate-grown cells of *C. albicans* were more resistant to osmotic stress, amphotericin B and caspofungin, and less resistant to azoles, compared with glucose-grown cultures (Ene et al. 2012). In part, these changes reflect modifications to the fungal cell wall. Therefore, changes in metabolism that accompany the natural history of an infection have many consequences for disease and antifungal chemotherapy (Brown et al. 2014a; Whittington et al. 2014).

Sensing and responding to host signals

To detect and respond to dynamic changes in host nutrients, stresses, and other host signals, fungal cells deploy a series of highly conserved signal transduction pathways that counter environmental challenges with appropriate cellular responses (Figure 3.1). The core environmental stress response has, however, been rewired in some fungal pathogens in a manner that reflects their pathogenesis. Of these, mitogen-activated protein kinase (MAPK) cascades, AP-1-like transcriptional responses, and calcium–calcineurin signalling are all critical in coordinating the environment with growth and stress responses (Rispail et al. 2009; Nikolaou et al. 2009; Brown et al. 2012; Bahn and Jung 2013). Many conserved proteins on these pathways are required for fungal virulence. These pathways are activated by a range of stimuli and result in alterations to the cell cycle, morphogenesis, and cell wall and stress pathways (Figure 3.1) through the activation of specific transcription factors and other regulators. The Hog1 MAPK pathway confers resistance to a wide range of stresses, including osmotic and oxidative stresses, by regulating protective functions at transcriptional and post-transcriptional levels (Enjalbert et al. 2006). The Mkc1 MAPK pathway protects against cell wall stresses and some antifungal drugs by controlling the expression of cell wall remodelling functions (Walker et al. 2008). The AP-1-like transcription factor, Cap1, upregulates genes that protect against oxidative stress and antifungal drugs (Znaidi et al. 2009). Meanwhile, the calcium–calcineurin signalling pathway mediates cell wall remodelling in response to the damage induced by antifungal drugs (Sanglard et al. 2003; Walker et al. 2008). The activities of these pathways appear to be modulated in response to ambient temperature by the molecular chaperone Hsp90 (Leach et al. 2012a, b) (Figure 3.1), which might be significant in the febrile patient.

Metabolic adaptation influences fungal virulence

In addition to promoting efficient growth through effective nutrient assimilation (see 'Obtaining nutrients from the human host') and enhancing immune evasion (see 'Metabolism modulates immune surveillance'), metabolic adaptation affects fungal pathogenicity by modulating the expression of key virulence factors (Figure 3.2) (Gow and Hube 2012; Ene et al. 2013; Brown et al. 2014b). Metabolic changes are seen in host niches during the course of fungal infections, for example in *C. albicans* and *Aspergillus fumigatus* (Barelle et al. 2006; McDonagh et al. 2008). Also, pathogens such as *Cryptococcus* and *Paracoccidioides* display major transcriptional and metabolic reprogramming following phagocytic exposure (Fan et al. 2005; Tavares et al. 2007; Kronstad et al. 2013). *Histoplasma* also displays distinct transcriptional programmes for its infectious and pathogenic states (Inglis et al. 2013). Key metabolic regulators are closely coupled to the regulation of virulence. These include Gcn4 (see 'Obtaining nutrients from the human host' (Tripathi et al. 2002)), and also TOR (target of rapamycin)—a major regulator of growth that is important for virulence, morphogenesis, and fluconazole tolerance resistance (Cutler et al. 2001; Lee et al. 2012; Su et al. 2013). Consequently, many mutations that affect central

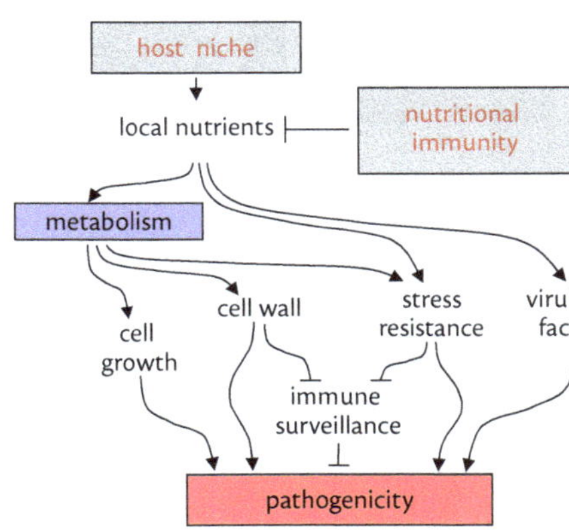

Figure 3.2 Metabolism influences the pathogenicity of *C. albicans* at multiple levels. Host niches differ significantly with respect to the local nutrients they offer and invading fungus (see text). Nutritional immunity is a mechanism by which the host attempts to deprive invading microbes of essential micronutrients such as iron.

metabolism also have direct or indirect effects on the expression of virulence factors and pathogenicity, as well as cell wall and stress resistance (Lorenz and Fink 2001; Brega et al. 2004; Martinez and Ljungdahl 2005; Barelle et al. 2006; Noble et al. 2010; Whittington et al. 2014).

Cell walls and cellular morphogenesis

Physiological changes induced by the host can result in alterations to the overall cell shape of the fungus and in the architecture and composition of the cell wall (Figure 3.3). Switches in cell morphology between budding, pseudohyphal, hyphal, and other growth forms contribute to the virulence of fungal pathogens (Sudbery et al. 2004; Gow and Hube 2012). Much attention has been paid to hyphal development in *C. albicans,* but both budding and filamentous forms are required for its virulence (Sudbery et al. 2004; Gow et al. 2012). In contrast, pathogens such as *Histoplasma* and *Cryptococcus* grow in budding forms during host colonization and infection. Additional morphological forms contribute to fungal pathogenicity. For example, giant *Cryptococcus* 'titan' cells and large *C. immitis* spherules, such as *C. albicans* hyphae, exceed the size that phagocytes can easily ingest (Zaragosa and Nielsen 2013), and therefore are more likely to escape immune surveillance.

Fungal cell walls are highly responsive to changing environmental conditions, and alterations in the cell wall result in changes in antifungal drug sensitivity and in their immunological profile (Netea et al. 2008; Walker et al. 2008; Marakalala et al. 2013; Brown et al. 2014a). Fungal pathogens also have mechanisms for evading detection and killing by phagocytes—for example, by producing inhibitors of chemotaxis or phagocytosis; secreting decoy molecules; inducing stress-protection pathways (see 'Counteracting imposed stresses'); interfering with the phagosome maturation process; or escaping from phagocytes by inducing their own expulsion or by lysing the captor.

Most fungi have a characteristic core cell wall architecture comprising an inner structural layer of β-glucans and chitin and an outer wall of glycosylated proteins or, in the case of *Cryptococcus*, a thick gelatinous capsule composed of two polysaccharides, glucuronoxylomannan and galactoxylomannan. For *Cryptococcus*, the capsule thickness is enhanced by *in vivo* growth conditions (Zaragosa and Nielsen 2013). The architecture and physical properties of the *C. albicans* cell wall, which represents a protective barrier against many toxic enzymes, are also strongly influenced by the growth conditions. For example, lactate-grown cells of *C. albicans* have a much thinner inner cell wall (Figure 3.3) and marked differences in the cell wall proteome (Ene et al. 2012, 2014). Many cell wall remodelling enzymes are also affected by the carbon source for growth, and their activity influences important phenotypes such as cell wall porosity, hydrophobicity, and elasticity (Ene et al. 2015). Therefore, as *C. albicans* cells adapt to local carbon sources, this adaptation leads to major changes in the cell wall that are likely to directly affect the physiology of the cells in different host niches

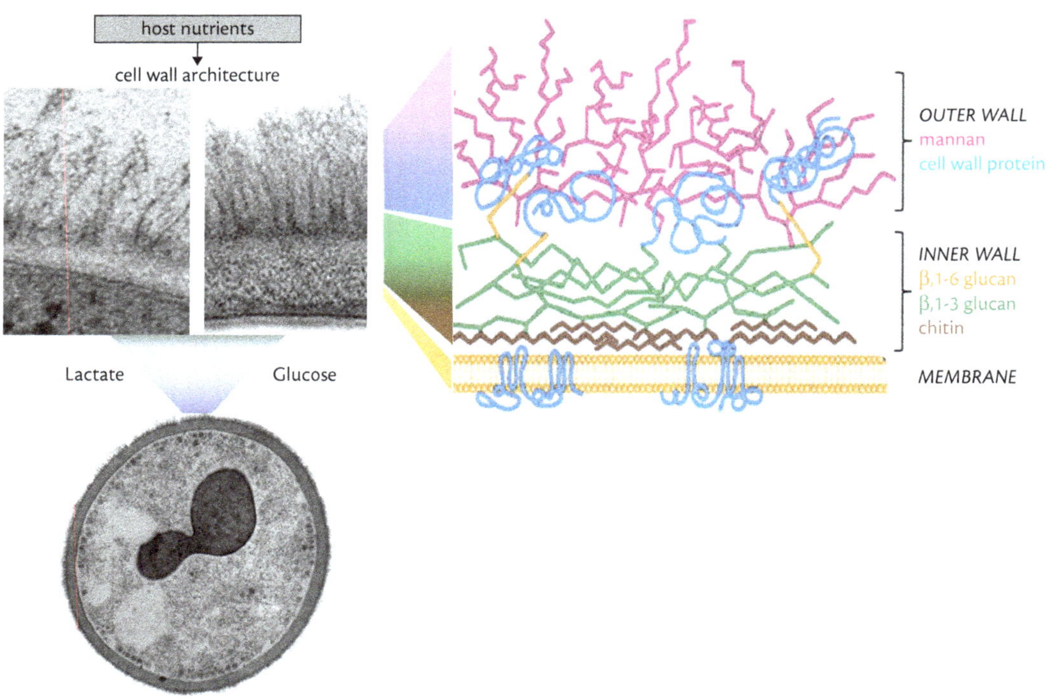

Figure 3.3 Host nutrients influence cell wall architecture in *C. albicans*. The cartoon on the right illustrates the molecular structure of the *C. albicans* cell wall. The transmission electron micrographs on the left highlight the major architectural differences in the cell wall between glucose- and lactate-grown *C. albicans* cells.

Adapted with permission from Gow, N. A. R. et al., 'Candida albicans morphogenesis and the host defence: discriminating invasion from colonization,' *Nature Reviews Microbiology*, Volume 10, Issue 2, pp. 112–22, Copyright © 2011, Rights Managed by Nature Publishing Group; and *Trends in Microbiology*, Volume 22, Issue 11, Brown, A. J. P. et al., 'Metabolism impacts Candida immunogenicity and pathogenicity at multiple levels,' pp. 614–22, Copyright © 2014 The Authors. Published by Elsevier Inc. Reproduced under Creative Commons Attribution 3.0 Unported (CC BY 3.0).

such as the bloodstream or vagina (Brown et al. 2014a; Whittington et al. 2014).

Metabolism modulates immune surveillance

Many of the major pathogen-associated molecular patterns, which are recognized by pattern recognition receptors on host immune cells, are located at the cell surface. It has now been demonstrated that the physiological status of a fungal cell can significantly modulate the recognition, phagocytosis, and cytokine profile of interacting immune cells (Figure 3.2) (Netea et al. 2008; Gow et al. 2012; Marakalala et al. 2013). For example, lactate-grown *C. albicans* cells do not induce such strong inflammatory immune responses as glucose-grown cells (Ene et al. 2013), with monocytes inducing more interleukin(IL)-10 and less IL-17. Lactate-grown *C. albicans* cells are also ingested less efficiently by macrophages, and those that are phagocytosed are more adept at escaping or killing the phagocyte.

Carbon metabolism also influences the function of immune cells. A switch from oxidative phosphorylation to aerobic glycolysis (also termed the 'Warburg effect') is crucial for proliferating lymphocytes (Delgoffe et al. 2011), and subsequently for anti-*Candida* responses such as the differentiation of T cells to protective Th17 subtypes. Also, innate inflammatory responses require succinate and a robust glycolytic profile (Tannahill et al. 2013). In addition, tryptophan catabolism of gut mucosal cells, promoting IL-22 production by myeloid cell types, leads to more effective intestinal immunity and protection against *C. albicans* (Zelante et al. 2013). Therefore, central metabolism affects the physiological status of the interacting phagocytes as well as their fungal targets, thereby influencing the outcome of interactions between fungal pathogens and the innate immune system.

Conclusion

Fungal virulence and pathogenicity have often been investigated in terms of specific virulence factors and fitness attributes that individual fungal pathogens possess and that are not shared with commensal fungi. However, highly conserved aspects of central metabolism are also important for fungal pathogens. Indeed, unbiased experimental approaches, such as comprehensive genetic screens and genome-wide transcriptional profiling, have highlighted the central importance of effective metabolic and physiological adaptation to host niches for fungal colonization and infection (Figure 3.2). Fungal pathogens must be quick to adapt to a multitude of local changes in host microenvironments. Metabolic flexibility is critical for their survival in the human host.

References

Almeida RS, Brunke S, Albrecht A, et al. (2008) The hyphal-associated adhesin and invasin Als3 of *Candida albicans* mediates iron acquisition from host ferritin. *PLoS Pathog* 4: e1000217.

Bahn Y-S and Jung K-W (2013) Stress signaling pathways for the pathogenicity of *Cryptococcus*. *Eukaryot Cell* 12: 1564–77.

Barelle CJ, Priest CL, MacCallum DM, Gow NAR, Odds FC and Brown AJP (2006) Niche-specific regulation of central metabolic pathways in a fungal pathogen. *Cell Microbiol* 8: 961–71.

Brega E, Zufferey R and Mamoun CB (2004) *Candida albicans* Csy1p is a nutrient sensor important for activation of amino acid uptake and hyphal morphogenesis. *Eukaryot Cell* 3: 135–43.

Brown AJP, Brown GD, Netea MG and Gow NAR (2014a). Metabolism impacts *Candida* immunogenicity and pathogenicity at multiple levels. *Trends Microbiol* 22: 614–22.

Brown AJP, Budge S, Kaloriti D, et al. (2014b) Stress adaptation in a pathogenic fungus. *J Exp Biol* 217: 144–55.

Brown AJP, Haynes K, Gow NAR and Quinn J (2012) Stress responses in *Candida*, *in*: CJ Clancy and RA Calderone, eds, *Candida and Candidiasis* (2nd edn, Washington DC: ASM Press), 225–42.

Chen C, Pande K, French SD, Tuch BB and Noble SM (2011) An iron homeostasis regulatory circuit with reciprocal roles in *Candida albicans* commensalism and pathogenesis. *Cell Host Microbe* 10: 118–35.

Citiulo F, Jacobsen ID, Miramon P, et al. (2012). *Candida albicans* scavenges host zinc via Pra1 during endothelial invasion. *PLoS Pathog* 8: e1002777.

Cornet M and Gaillardin C (2014) pH signaling in human fungal pathogens: a new target for antifungal strategies. *Eukaryot Cell* 13: 342–52.

Cutler S, Pan X, Heitman J and Cardenas ME (2001) The TOR signal transduction cascade controls cellular differentiation in response to nutrients. *Mol Biol Cell* 12: 4103–13.

Delgoffe GM, Pollizzi KN, Waickman AT, et al. (2011). The kinase mTOR regulates the differentiation of helper T cells through the selective activation of signaling by mTORC1 and mTORC2. *Nat Immunol* 12: 295–303.

Eissenberg LG, Goldman WE and Schlesinger PH (1993). *Histoplasma capsulatum* modulates the acidification of phagolysosomes. *J Exp Med* 177: 1605–11.

Ene IV, Brunke S, Brown AJP and Hube B (2014). Metabolism in fungal pathogenesis, *in*: A Casadevall, A Mitchell, J Berman, et al., eds, *Human Fungal Pathogens* (New York: CSHL Press). doi: 10.1101/cshperspect.a019695

Ene IV, Cheng SC, Netea MG and Brown AJP (2013). Growth of *Candida albicans* cells on the physiologically relevant carbon source, lactate, affects their recognition and phagocytosis by immune cells. *Infect Immun* 81: 238–48.

Ene IV, Heilmann CJ, Sorgo AG, et al. (2012). Carbon source-induced reprogramming of the cell wall proteome and secretome modulates the adherence and drug resistance of the fungal pathogen *Candida albicans*. *Proteomics* 12: 3164–79.

Ene IV, Walker LA, Schiavone M, et al. (2015) Cell wall remodelling enzymes modulate fungal cell wall elasticity and osmotic stress resistance. *MBio* 6: e00986–15

Enjalbert B, Smith DA, Cornell MJ, et al. (2006) Role of the Hog1 stress-activated protein kinase in the global transcriptional response to stress in the fungal pathogen *Candida albicans*. *Mol Biol Cell* 17: 1018–32.

Fan W, Kraus PR, Boily MJ and Heitman J (2005) *Cryptococcus neoformans* gene expression during murine macrophage infection. *Eukaryot Cell* 4, 1420–33.

Gow NAR and Hube B (2012) *Candida albicans* cell wall structure: relationship with commensalism and invasion. *Curr Opin Microbiol* 15: 406–12.

Gow NAR, van de Veerdonk FL, Brown AJP and Netea MG (2012) *Candida albicans* morphogenesis and host defence: discriminating invasion from colonization. *Nat Rev Microbiol* 10: 112–22.

Han TL, Cannon RD and Villas-Boas SG (2011). The metabolic basis of Candida albicans morphogenesis and quorum sensing. *Fungal Genet Biol* 48: 747–63.

Hauser PM, Burdet FX, Cisse OH, et al. (2010). Comparative genomics suggests that the fungal pathogen *Pneumocystis* is an obligate parasite scavenging amino acids from its host's lungs. *PLoS One* 5: e15152.

Inglis DO, Voorhies M, Hocking Murray DR and Sil A (2013) Comparative transcriptomics of infectious spores from the fungal pathogen *Histoplasma capsulatum* reveals a core set of transcripts that specify infectious and pathogenic states. *Eukaryot Cell* 12: 828–52.

Johnson L (2008) Iron and siderophores in fungal–host interactions. *Mycol Res* 112: 170–83.

Kronstad JW, Hu G and Jung WH (2013) An encapsulation of iron homeostasis and virulence in *Cryptococcus neoformans*. *Trends Microbiol* 21: 457–65.

Lavoie H, Hogues H, Mallick J, et al. (2010) Evolutionary tinkering with conserved components of a transcriptional regulatory network. *PLoS Biol* 8: e1000329.

Leach MD, Budge S, Walker L, Munro C, Cowen LE and Brown AJP (2012a) Hsp90 orchestrates transcriptional regulation by Hsf1 and cell wall remodelling by MAPK signalling during thermal adaptation in a pathogenic yeast. *PLoS Pathog* 8: e1003069.

Leach MD, Klipp E, Cowen LE and Brown AJP (2012b) Hsp90—a biological transistor that tunes cellular outputs to thermal inputs. *Nat Rev Microbiol* 10: 693–704.

Lee H, Lamichhane A-K, Garraffo M, Kwon-Chung JK and Chang Y-C (2012) Involvement of PDK1, PKC and TOR signaling pathways in basal fluconazole tolerance in *Cryptococcus neoformans*. *Mol Microbiol* 84: 130–46.

Lorenz MC and Fink GR (2001) The glyoxylate cycle is required for fungal virulence. *Nature* 412: 83–6.

McDonagh A, Fedorova ND, Crabtree J, et al. 2008. Sub-telomere directed gene expression during initiation of invasive aspergillosis. *PLoS Pathog* 4: e1000154.

Marakalala MJ, Vautier S, Potrykus J, et al. (2013). Differential adaptation of *Candida albicans in vivo* modulates immune recognition by Dectin-1. *PLoS Pathog* 9: e1003315.

Martinez P and Ljungdahl PO (2005) Divergence of Stp1 and Stp2 transcription factors in Candida albicans places virulence factors required for proper nutrient acquisition under amino acid control. *Mol Cell Biol* 25: 9435–46.

Miramón P, Dunker C, Windecker H, et al. (2012). Cellular responses *of Candida albicans* to phagocytosis and the extracellular activities of neutrophils are critical to counteract carbohydrate starvation, oxidative and nitrosative stress. *PLoS One* 7: e52850.

Netea MG, Brown GD, Kullberg B-J and Gow NAR (2008) An integrated model of pattern recognition of *Candida albicans* in innate immunity. *Nat Rev Microbiol* 6: 67–78.

Nikolaou E, Agrafioti I, Stumpf M, Quinn J, Stansfield I and Brown AJP (2009) Phylogenetic diversity of stress signalling pathways in fungi. *BMC Evol Biol* 9: 44.

Noble SM, French S, Kohn LA, Chen V and Johnson AD (2010) Systematic screens of a Candida albicans homozygous deletion library decouple morphogenetic switching and pathogenicity. *Nat Genet* 42: 590–8.

Owen DH and Katz DF (1999) A vaginal fluid simulant. *Contraception* 59: 91–5.

Pande K, Chen C and Noble SM (2013) Passage through the mammalian gut triggers a phenotypic switch that promotes *Candida albicans* commensalism. *Nat Genet* 45: 1088–91.

Perez JC, Kumamoto CA and Johnson AD (2013) *Candida albicans* commensalism and pathogenicity are intertwined traits directed by a tightly knit transcriptional regulatory circuit. *PLoS Biol* 11: e1001510.

Potrykus J, Ballou ER, Childers DS and Brown AJP (2014) Conflicting interests in the pathogen-host tug of war: fungal micronutrient scavenging versus mammalian nutritional immunity. *PLoS Pathog* 10: e1003910.

Potrykus J, Stead D, MacCallum DM, et al. (2013). Fungal iron availability during deep seated candidiasis defined by a complex interplay of systemic and local events. *PLoS Pathog* 9: e1003676.

Rispail R, Soanes DM, Ant C, et al. (2009) Comparative genomics of MAP kinase and calcium–calcineurin signalling components in plant and human pathogenic fungi. *Fungal Genet Biol* 46: 287–98.

Rodaki A, Bohovych IM, Enjalbert B, et al. (2009) Glucose promotes stress resistance in the fungal pathogen, *Candida albicans*. *Mol Biol Cell* 20: 4845–55.

Sanglard D, Ischer F, Marchetti O, Entenza J and Bille J (2003) Calcineurin A of *Candida albicans*: involvement in antifungal tolerance, cell morphogenesis and virulence. *Mol Microbiol* 48: 959–76.

Schrettl M, Beckmann N, Varga J, et al. (2010) HapX-mediated adaptation to iron starvation is crucial for virulence of *Aspergillus fumigatus*. *PLoS Pathog* 6: e1001124.

Su C, Lu Y and Liu H (2013) Reduced TOR signaling sustains hyphal development in *Candida albicans* by lowering Hog1 basal activity. *Mol Biol Cell* 24: 385–97.

Sudbery P, Gow NAR and Berman J (2004) The distinct morphogenic states of *Candida albicans*. *Trends Microbiol* 12: 317–25.

Tannahill GM, Curtis AM, Adamik J, et al. (2013) Succinate is an inflammatory signal that induces IL-1β through HIF-1α. *Nature* 496: 238–42.

Tavares AHFP, Silva SS, Dantas A, et al. (2007) Early transcriptional response of *Paracoccidioides brasiliensis* upon internalization by murine macrophages. *Microbes Infect* 9: 583–90.

Tillmann AT, Strijbis K, Cameron G, et al. (2015). Contribution of Fdh3 and Glr1 to glutathione redox state, stress adaptation and virulence in *Candida albicans*. *PLoS One* 10: e0126940.

Tripathi G, Wiltshire C, Macaskill S, Tournu H, Budge S and Brown AJP (2002) CaGcn4 co-ordinates morphogenetic and metabolic responses to amino acid starvation in *Candida albicans*. *EMBO J* 21: 5448–56.

Vylkova S and Lorenz MC (2014) Modulation of phagosomal pH by *Candida albicans* promotes hyphal morphogenesis and requires Stp2p, a regulator of amino acid transport. *PLoS Pathog* 10: e1003995.

Walker LA, Munro CA, de Brujin I, et al. (2008) Stimulation of chitin synthesis rescues *Candida albicans* from echinocandins. *PLoS Pathog* 4: e1000040.

Whittington A, Gow NAR and Hube B (2014) From commensal to pathogen: *Candida albicans*, *in*: O Kurzai, ed., *The Mycota*, XII: Human Fungal Pathogens (Heidelberg: Springer-Verlag), 3–18.

Wilson D (2015) An evolutionary perspective on zinc uptake by human fungal pathogens. *Metallomics* 7: 979–85.

Wilson D, Thewes S, Zakikhany K, et al. (2009) Identifying infection-associated genes of *Candida albicans* in the postgenomic era. *FEMS Yeast Res* 9: 688–700.

Zaragosa O and Nielsen K (2013) Titan cells in Cryptococcus neoformans: cells with a giant impact. *Curr Opin Microbiol* 16: 409–13.

Zelante T, Iannitti RG, Cunha C, et al. (2013). Tryptophan catabolites from microbiota engage aryl hydrocarbon receptor and balance mucosal reactivity via interleukin-22. *Immunity* 39: 372–85.

Znaidi S, Barker KS, Weber S, et al. (2009) Identification of the *Candida albicans* Cap1p regulon. *Eukaryot Cell* 8: 806–20.

CHAPTER 4

Fungal cell structure and organization

Nick D. Read

Introduction to fungal cells

The main types of 'cells' produced by human pathogenic fungi are hyphae, yeast cells, and spores. The majority of fungi produce filamentous hyphae, some produce yeast cells, and almost all produce spores. Fungi produce a wide range of different types of hyphae, yeast cells, and spores. This chapter focuses on describing the structure and organization of these different cell types with an emphasis on those produced by human fungal pathogens. A discussion of the highly specialized cells produced by the obligate, fungal pathogens *Pneumocystis* and Microsporidia are beyond the scope of this review.

Hyphae

The majority of fungi are moulds, which are characterized by producing filamentous hyphae. Different types of hyphae possess unique combinations of structural, behavioural, and functional attributes. The vegetative hypha at the periphery of a colony is a tip-growing cellular element that undergoes regular branching, is commonly multinucleate, and usually produces septa (cross walls). The mass of vegetative hyphae in the colony of a filamentous fungus is referred to as a *mycelium.* Many (but not all) filamentous fungi undergo prolific cell fusion within the colony to form a complex interconnected hyphal network (Figure 4.1).

Mycologists commonly describe hyphae as 'cells' in a very loose sense that, strictly speaking, is incorrect. Problems can be encountered when using the term 'cell' in the context of a hypha. This is because the hypha in a vegetative colony, except during its earliest stages of development, is not like a 'classical cell' as is typical of animals and plants. Thus a hypha is not usually a discrete, uninucleate unit of protoplasm bounded by a plasma membrane and cell wall/extracellular matrix. This is further complicated by most true filamentous fungi forming hyphae with septa that commonly, but not invariably, possess central pores. These septal pores can be open, allowing cytoplasmic and organelle transport between adjacent hyphal compartments, or blocked, preventing such movement. If these septal pores are occluded, we can consider the hyphal compartment to be a true cell. However, because the colonies of true filamentous fungi frequently have extensive regions in which there is cytoplasmic continuity between multiple hyphal compartments, the fungal colonies (or parts thereof) are often referred to as having a *supracellular* state (Read 2007). However, in contrast to this, the hyphae of *Candida albicans* are composed of true, uninucleate compartmentalized cells that are not connected via their cytoplasm.

Hyphae exhibit extraordinary developmental versatility, phenotypic plasticity, and diverse functionality. They serve key roles in colony establishment, exploration, and invasion of their environment (including that of the host); nutrient mobilization by secreting extracellular digestive enzymes; uptake of nutrients from the environment; translocation of nutrients and water within the colony; defence of their occupied substratum by producing antibiotics; long-distance signalling; and reproduction, dispersal, and survival by the formation of spores. To fulfil these diverse functions, hyphae, or different regions of individual hyphae, can become specialized, which in turn is manifested by differences in their structure and organization (Read 1994).

Hyphae can be involved in producing complex multicellular tissues and organs, but these are formed in a fundamentally different way to those found in animals and plants. Multicellular development at this level involves hyphal aggregation and adhesion, followed by specialization and septation of hyphal compartments within the aggregate. A wide range of multicellular structures resulting from hyphal aggregation are formed by fungi, including sclerotia and both asexual and sexual fruit bodies (Read 1994; Lord and Read 2011). Similar processes of complex multihyphal, multicellular development are also involved during infection, with the formation of biofilms and fungal balls by *Aspergillus fumigatus* in the lungs (Beauvais and Latgé 2015).

Most research on fungal hyphae has focused on understanding the growth and cell biology of vegetative hyphae at the colony periphery in a monoculture in, or on, a homogeneous, artificial nutrient growth medium (Figure 4.1). These hyphae are generally regarded as the sole contributors to the radial extension of a mature colony of a filamentous fungus (Moore et al. 2011). Most mycologists' perception of what a hypha is, how it is organized, how it grows, and how it functions is largely based on studies of these hyphae at the margin of an expanding colony. However, it is clear that there are other types of less understood specialized hyphae, including germ tubes which emerge from spores and are involved in colony establishment, and hyphae that produce spores. Hyphae can also be specialized for invading host tissue (e.g. the flattened frond-like hyphae of dermatophytes that grow between skin cells and the perforating organs that dermatophytes produce to penetrate

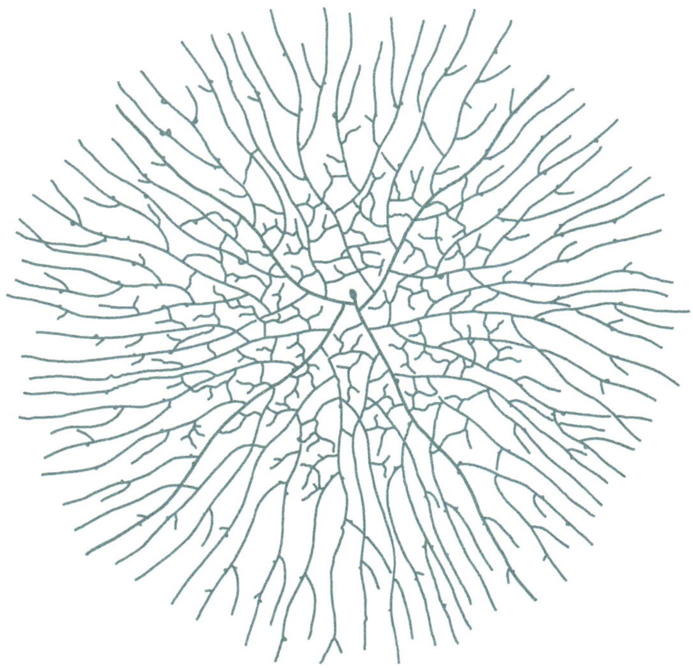

Figure 4.1 Morphology of a radially expanding colony of the basidiomycete *Coprinus sterquilinus* derived from a single spore. It shows an outer peripheral zone in which the hyphae avoid each other (negative tropisms) and a subperipheral region in which certain hyphal branches home towards each other and anastomose to form an interconnected network of hyphae. Expansion of the colony outwards is limited to tip growth of leading hyphae at the periphery of the colony.

hair; Kanbe and Tanaka 1982). These specialized hyphae typically have a different organization and/or mode of growth to the much studied, leading hyphae at the colony periphery.

Hyphae contain the full gamut of organelles that are common to eukaryotic animal and/or plant cells (e.g. cell walls, nuclei, mitochondria, endoplasmic reticulum, Golgi apparatus, endosomal vacuoles, various types of vesicles, and peroxisomes). They may also contain organelles (e.g. the Woronin body) or organelle complexes (e.g. the apical multivesicular body called the Spitzenkörper) that are specific to certain fungi (Figure 4.2). Within the apical compartment of an actively growing hypha, and sometimes to a lesser extent in subapical compartments, many of these organelles are markedly polarized in their distribution with the Spitzenkörper located at the hyphal apex (Figures 4.2–4.5).

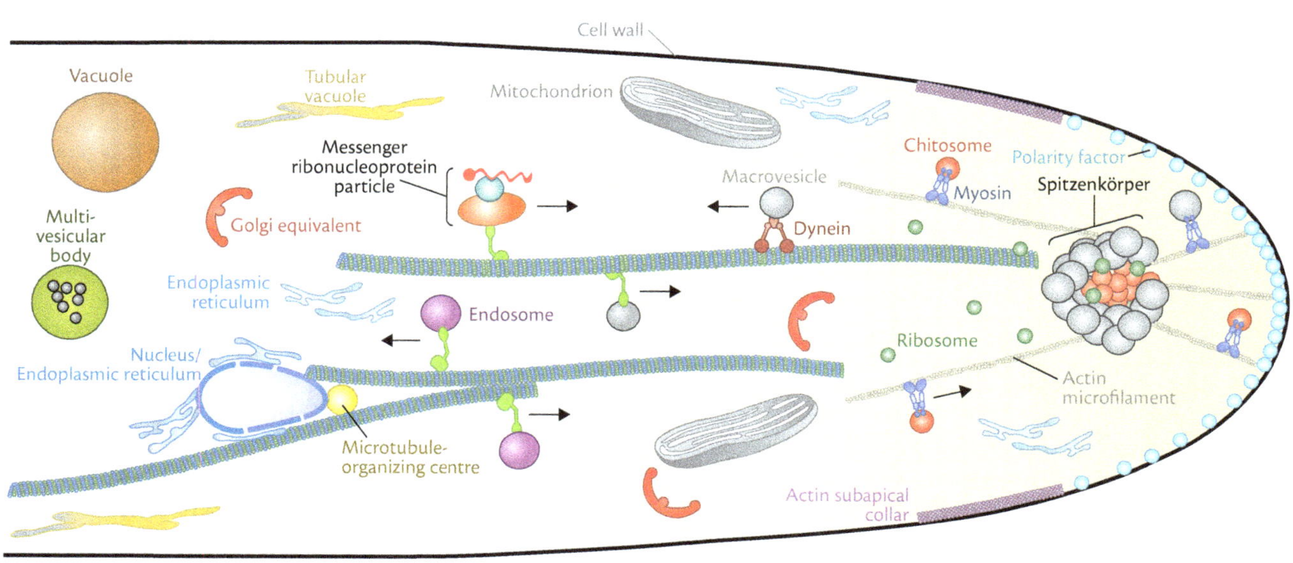

Figure 4.2 Diagrammatic representation of a hyphal apex showing the major components participating in tip growth (see text for details).

However, the distribution of the individual organelles is typically very dynamic and varies between different fungal taxa (Roberson et al. 2010).

The Spitzenkörper

The mature vegetative hyphae at the periphery of an established colony elongate by means of tip growth. This process involves highly polarized secretion and cell wall synthesis that is restricted to a region occupying only a few micrometres at the apices of the extending hyphae (Riquelme 2013; Schultzhaus and Shaw 2015). Tip growth in the vegetative hyphae of most filamentous fungi (with the notable exception of the zygomycetes) is intimately associated with the behaviour of a multicomponent structure dominated by vesicles collectively known as the *Spitzenkörper* (from the German for 'apical body') (Riquelme 2013; Riquelme and Sanchez-Leon 2014). This structure is usually only found within the tip of a growing hypha, and its precise position within the hyphal tip is coincident with the subsequent direction of hyphal growth. These critical observations of Spitzenkörper behaviour were noted in pioneering live-cell imaging studies of hyphal growth by Girbardt in the 1950s, in which he was able to monitor Spitzenkörper dynamics in unstained hyphae using phase-contrast microscopy (Bartnicki-Garcia 2015). After visualization by transmission electron microscopy, the Spitzenkörper was found to correlate with a large accumulation of vesicles of different sizes, with large vesicles (*macrovesicles*, 70–90 nm in diameter) usually surrounding small vesicles (*microvesicles*, 30–40 nm in diameter) (Figure 4.2). A region within the centre of the Spitzenkörper (the 'core') is largely devoid of vesicles and rich in the cytoskeletal protein actin. The vesicles are believed to be mostly secretory in function, and different vesicles in some fungi have been shown to contain different cell wall synthesizing enzymes. In particular, in the ascomycete *Neurospora crassa*, chitin synthase is associated with a class of microvesicles called chitosomes, whilst two β-1,3 glucan synthases have been found to be localized to macrovesicles (Riquelme and Sanchez-Leon 2014, 2015; Bartnicki-Garcia 2015). However, in another fungus, the basidiomycete plant pathogen *Ustilago maydis*, two different chitin synthases, and a β-1,3 glucan synthase, have all been shown to be present in a single microvesicle (Schuster et al. 2016).

Since the 1990s, the ability to label the Spitzenkörper and its individual components with fluorescent dyes and fluorescent proteins has greatly facilitated analysis of the structure and function of the Spitzenkörper (Figures 4.3 and 4.4). Overall, the Spitzenkörper is generally regarded as a 'vesicle supply centre', the dynamic behaviour of which regulates the initiation, maintenance, and direction of hyphal growth. More specifically, the vesicle supply centre is viewed as a moveable distribution centre for vesicles involved in cell surface expansion, the mathematical basis of which has been elegantly modelled (Bartnicki-Garcia et al. 1989; Bartnicki-Garcia 2002). Because the vegetative hypha grows at its tip, the history of the behaviour and activity of the Spitzenkörper as a vesicle supply centre is manifested in the morphology of hyphae and the mycelium that they generate.

The Spitzenkörper is also the primary response element to environmental signals that influence hyphal morphogenesis (Read 2007). Hyphal growth responds extremely sensitively and quickly (sometimes within seconds) to a myriad of signals within the changing, heterogeneous microenvironments through which hyphae explore and invade. The hyphae of pathogens respond to chemical and physical signals from the host that can be used as cues to assist the successful penetration and invasion of host tissue. These environmental stimuli rapidly modify the behaviour and activity of the Spitzenkörper. The speed of these responses clearly shows that transcriptional regulation is not initially involved, but that in many cases receptors in the apical plasma membrane must connect through signal transduction machinery to the responding Spitzenkörper, which seems to be dynamically tethered to the plasma membrane.

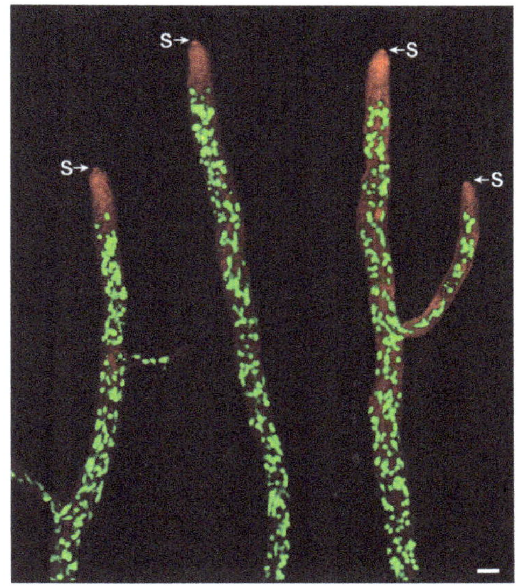

Figure 4.3 Multinucleate hyphae in branching vegetative hyphae at the periphery of a colony of *Neurospora crassa*. Nuclei (green) were labelled with green fluorescent protein, and membranes stained with FM4-64 (red). Note the Spitzenkörper (arrows) at the tips of the growing hyphae and branches that have formed subapically. The extension of these hyphae is restricted to a few micrometres at these hyphal tips. Also note that there is a 20–25 μm region devoid of nuclei just behind the hyphal tips. Bar = 10 μm.

Reprinted from *Fungal Genetics and Biology*, Volume 41, Issue 10, Freitag M. et al., 'GFP as a tool to analyze the organization, dynamics and function of nuclei and microtubules in Neurospora crassa,' pp. 907–20, Copyright © 2004, with permission from Elsevier, http://www.sciencedirect.com/science/journal/10871845

Hyphal growth of the human pathogen *Candida albicans* responds to the physical properties and microtopography of the surface on which it grows—a process termed *thigmotropism*. These thigmotropic responses can facilitate tissue invasion—as has been compellingly demonstrated in a number of fungal plant pathogens (Brand and Gow 2012). Thigmotropism is demonstrated most elegantly on artificial, microfabricated surfaces that are devoid of host chemical signals. *Candida* hyphae in contact with a surface have an asymmetrical 'nose-down' tip morphology, and the Spitzenkörper of these hyphae is located close to the underlying surface that is being sensed (Figure 4.4). This contrasts with the typical symmetrical *hyphoid* shape, with a centrally located Spitzenkörper, which is characteristic of growing hyphal tips that are not contact-sensing (Figures 4.3 and 4.5a). Furthermore, the *Candida* Spitzenkörper responds very rapidly and dynamically to physical obstacles encountered by the hypha, and this is manifested in the pattern of its subsequent growth and morphogenesis (Thomson et al. 2015; Figure 4.4).

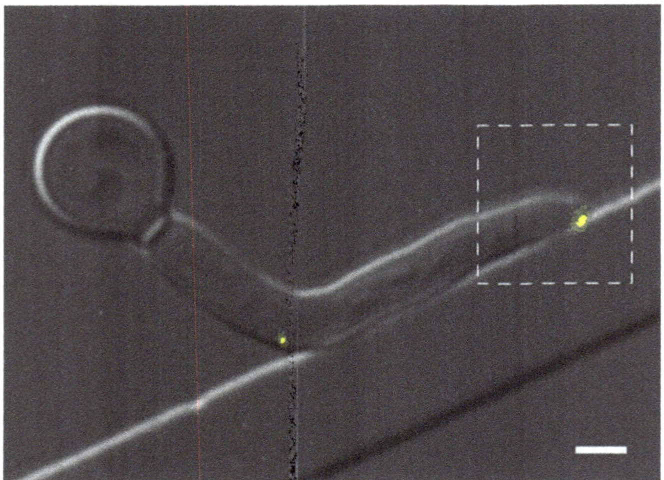

Figure 4.4 Hyphal tips of *Candida albicans* responding thigmotropically to an artificial microfabricated ridge. Note the 'nose'-down morphology of the hypha growing against the ridge and the asymmetrically located Spitzenkörper (yellow) labelled with yellow fluorescent protein (fused to the light chain myosin protein Mlc1). Bar = 2 μm.

Secretory pathways involved in hyphal growth

The classical view of the polarized secretory process that underlies hyphal tip growth is that proteins are synthesized on the endoplasmic reticulum and then transported to closely associated Golgi apparatus within which they are glycosylated. The proteins are then packaged up in secretory vesicles budded off from the Golgi apparatus and transported along cytoskeletal elements to the Spitzenkörper, from which they are targeted to the apical plasma membrane (Schultzhaus and Shaw 2015). As indicated earlier, different cell wall synthesizing enzymes can be delivered to the hyphal tip in different secretory vesicles, or they can be delivered to the tip in the same vesicle. The advantage of the latter is that the enzymes are exocytosed at the same site on the apical plasma membrane, thus establishing a local focus of coordinated cell wall synthesis (Schuster et al. 2016). There are also other secretory pathways in hyphae about which we understand little, including the secretion involved in subapical branch formation, septum formation, and even intercalary growth (Read 2011).

In contrast to animal and plant Golgi apparatus, fungal Golgi bodies are uniquely not organized as stacks of flattened cisternae (or dictyosomes). Instead, the Golgi bodies of fungi appear as single tubular, and often fenestrated, cisternae that vary in shape from cup-like to planar bodies (Roberson et al. 2010; Pantazopoulou et al. 2014). However, they are functionally equivalent to the stacked Golgi bodies of other organisms and are thus often referred to as *Golgi equivalents* (Figure 4.2). It should be noted that the Golgi bodies in fungal cells are commonly incorrectly portrayed in textbooks as stacked cisternae.

Cell polarity regulation

Significant insights into the molecular basis of hyphal tip growth have been acquired in recent years (Riquelme 2013; Riquelme and Sanchez-Leon 2014). In hyphal tips, cell-end marker (landmark) proteins mark sites on the plasma membrane for polarized growth. Sterol-rich domains in the plasma membrane are believed to regulate the positioning of these cell-end markers (Takeshita et al. 2014). Rho GTPases are recruited to the landmarked plasma membrane regions (Fischer et al. 2008) and are essential regulators of cell polarity in fungi and other eukaryotes (Arkowitz and Bassilana 2015). Two other important macromolecular complexes within the hyphal tip that partially co-localize with the Spitzenkörper are the *polarisome* and the *exocyst*. The polarisome is a key multiprotein complex involved in regulating the actin cytoskeleton and secretory machinery required for polarized hyphal growth, whilst the exocyst is composed of proteins that regulate secretory vesicle docking and fusion with the plasma membrane (Riquelme et al. 2014; Schultzhaus and Shaw 2015).

Cell wall

The fungal cell wall is a highly regulated, dynamic organelle surrounding the fungal cell. It serves numerous important essential roles including: (1) determining and maintaining the morphology and integrity of developing fungal cells; (2) allowing the fungal cell to generate a high turgor to aid fungal cell growth, penetration, and invasion of the environment; (3) protecting fungal cells against changes in external osmotic pressure and other environmental stresses; and (4) providing a dynamic interface between the fungal cell and its surrounding environment (Bowman and Free 2006; Latgé 2007; Osherov and Yarden 2010). All of these roles are important in fungal pathogenesis. It is thus not surprising that one class of antifungal drugs (the echinocandins) target a cell wall synthesizing enzyme (β-1,3 glucan synthase) (see Chapter 46).

Fungal cell walls comprise a cross-linked network of chitin, glucans, other polysaccharides, and glycoproteins (Latgé 2007;

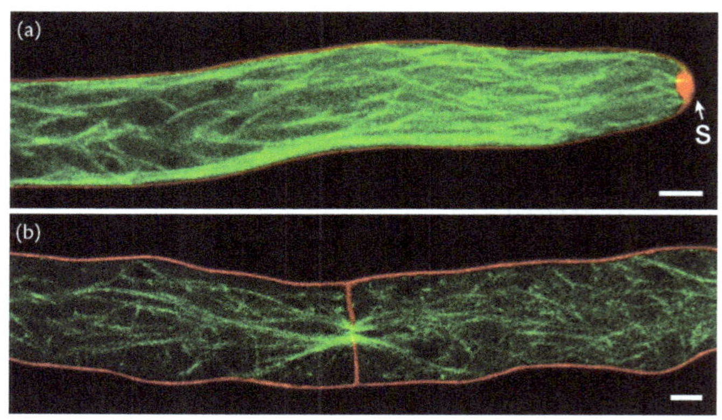

Figure 4.5 Spitzenkörper, microtubules, and septum within vegetative hyphae at the colony periphery of *Neurospora crassa*. Microtubules were labelled with the green fluorescent protein, and the Spitzenkörper and plasma membrane were stained with the membrane-selective dye FM4-64.

a Growing hyphal tip. Note the high concentration of longitudinally orientated microtubules extending into the stained Spitzenkörper (S).

b Subapical hyphal region a few compartments back from the apical compartment. Microtubules have been forced into closer proximity to each other by the inward growing septum. Bars = 5 μm.

Osherov and Yarden 2010; see Figure 3.3). The precise composition, however, varies considerably between different fungal species and is highly regulated and sensitive to environmental changes. Indeed, the surface chemistry of the cell walls of fungal pathogens have been described as a 'moving target' helping these fungi to avoid recognition by the host immune system (Erwig and Gow 2016). The structure, composition, and mechanical properties of the cell wall also vary considerably along the length of a polarized hypha. At the growing hyphal tip the cell wall is thin (~50 nm) and plastic, though it becomes thicker (< ~250 nm) and more rigid with further cell wall synthesis and crosslinking of its components. Septa are also composed of typically thick cell walls bordered by plasma membrane (Roberson et al. 2010).

Cytoskeleton

There are three main cytoskeletal elements in fungi: microtubules, actin microfilaments, and septins. Microtubules and actin microfilaments form a dynamic interconnected, interacting system throughout the cytoplasm and play a variety of roles, including the formation of spindles—allowing chromosome segregation during nuclear division—and nuclear positioning—providing tracks for the transport of secretory vesicles to hyphal tips and for the intracellular movement of organelles and protein complexes (Xiang and Oakley 2010). The transport of secretory vesicles from their sites of formation to the Spitzenkörper, and then probably to their sites of fusion with the plasma membrane, occurs along microtubules and/or actin microfilaments. In true filamentous fungi (e.g. *Aspergillus*), microtubules are believed to be primarily responsible for the long-distance transport of secretory vesicles to the Spitzenkörper (Figure 4.5a; Xiang and Oakley 2010; Schultzhaus et al. 2016). Actin microfilaments are also concentrated in the Spitzenkörper core of both types of vegetative hyphae, where they are associated with the actin nucleating protein, formin (Berepiki et al. 2011).

The transport of secretory vesicles and other intracellular cargo along cytoskeletal elements is driven by motor proteins (Figure 4.2). Kinesin and dynein motor proteins transport cargo along microtubules (Xiang and Oakley 2010; Egan et al. 2012) whilst myosin motor proteins transport cargo along actin microfilaments (Xiang and Oakley 2010). Hydrolysis of ATP (adenosine triphosphate) leads to conformational changes in the motor proteins resulting in coordinated 'walking' of the motor protein along the cytoskeletal element.

Septins form protein complexes with each other and further assemble into supramolecular structures such as filaments and rings. These structures can allow septins to function in localizing other proteins within different regions of cells either by providing a scaffold to which other proteins can attach themselves or by providing a diffusion barrier for molecules. As a result, septins are particularly important in compartmentalizing membrane domains and generating cell asymmetry such as during polarized hyphal growth (Khan et al. 2015).

Endocytosis

Besides secretion (i.e. exocytosis of secretory vesicles) playing a critical role in hyphal growth, another essential process involving vesicle trafficking in fungal cells is endocytosis (Steinberg 2014; Schultzhaus and Shaw 2015). Endocytosis is a mechanism by which endocytic vesicles are budded off the cytoplasmic side of the plasma membrane, allowing plasma membrane molecules, extracellular molecules, and fluids to be taken up by fungal cells. It plays important roles in the internalization of membrane proteins and lipids for degradation, the recycling of these membrane molecules back to the plasma membrane, and the uptake of certain signal molecules. F-actin is involved in endocytic vesicle assembly and is commonly visualized as actin patches. These actin patches are particularly concentrated in a collar associated with the plasma membrane behind the Spitzenkörper (Figure 4.2), where localized endocytosis is believed to play an important role in membrane recycling back to the hyphal tip during tip growth (Berepiki et al. 2011; Schultzhaus and Shaw 2015).

Endocytic vesicles fuse with an organelle called the early endosome, which acts as a molecular sorting compartment by directing molecules for degradation in the vacuole or recycling them back to the plasma membrane. Endosomes are extraordinarily dynamic in fungal hyphae and exhibit rapid bidirectional movement that involves a complex interplay between the motor proteins kinesin and dynein along microtubules. There is growing evidence that endosomes perform other important functions in hyphae. For example, they have been shown to shuttle proteins between the hyphal tip and the subapical vacuoles in which they are degraded. They have also been found to deliver other molecules and protein complexes to the hyphal tip. These molecular cargoes include the protein synthesis machinery, mRNA, and peroxisomes, which can 'hitchhike' on endosomes (Higuchi and Steinberg 2015; Salogiannis et al. 2016).

Hyphal branching

Hyphae undergo branch formation. This is an essential feature serving different roles during colony development. Branching allows hyphae to increase their surface area to maximize nutrient acquisition from their surrounding environment. Hyphal branches can also differentiate to serve different specialized functions to those of their parent hyphae (e.g. cell fusion or spore formation). The predominant form of hyphal branching is subapical (Figures 4.1 and 4.3), but apical branching can also occur in some fungi. Interestingly, apical branching has not been observed in the hyphae of the filamentous yeast *C. albicans*. Branching is influenced by external and internal factors, but the mechanism by which branch initiation is regulated is little understood. It clearly involves the establishment of polarized growth from a new site along a hypha, and its formation involves much of the machinery involved in the maintenance of tip growth (Harris 2008). The leading hyphae and their lateral branches at the colony periphery tend to strongly avoid each other (a negative tropism) by some unknown mechanism of intercellular signalling. This process serves to space these hyphae and branches apart, which minimizes their competition for nutrients from the environment (Figures 4.1 and 4.3).

Septa

As indicated earlier, fungal hyphae typically possess septa. They are formed periodically along the hypha and are mostly initiated in the extending apical hyphal compartment. Septa in some species are produced in the vicinity of hyphal branches, whilst in other species they are not (Harris 2008). An actomyosin ring (containing F-actin and myosin) forms adjacent to the plasma membrane at a site at which a septum will subsequently form. It then contracts and guides plasma membrane invagination and localized cell wall synthesis resulting from localized secretion in this region (Figure 4.5b;

Berepiki et al. 2011; Mourino-Perez 2013). Hyphal septa in true filamentous fungi are not normally complete and retain a septal pore. Although these pores are initially open, allowing cytoplasmic and organelle movement between adjacent compartments, they can become blocked by specialized plugs. Septal pore occlusion will physically isolate adjacent hyphal compartments and promote cell specialization. Hyphal damage can potentially cause catastrophic cell death within the interconnected mycelial network. However, filamentous ascomycetes possess peroxisome-derived, septal pore-associated crystalline organelles known as Woronin bodies, which ameliorate this risk. When a hypha is ruptured, a Woronin body rapidly blocks the pore to stem the loss of protoplasm (Jedd and Chua 2000; Dhavale and Jedd 2007). In some species, Woronin bodies also commonly block septal pores in the absence of damage. In *Aspergillus niger*, this process promotes cell heterogeneity, and thus multicellular differentiation, whilst limiting the long-distance movement of cytoplasm and organelles within the mycelium (Bleichrodt et al. 2012, 2015). In other species (e.g. *N. crassa*), the majority of septal pores in the mycelium are open, which can result in the very rapid bulk flow of cytoplasm and organelles in older parts of the colony (Lew 2011; Pieuchot et al. 2015). Other types of septal pore plugs are observed in ascomycete and basidiomycete fungi, and these can also play important roles in the selective communication between hyphal compartments and/or multicellular differentiation (Lai et al. 2012). The septa of hyphae of the filamentous yeast *C. albicans* each possess a single, extremely small (25 nm) micropore which can, at best, only provide very selective communication between the hyphal compartments (Gow et al. 1980). In fungi belonging to the Mucorales, however, septa are rarely formed (Roberson et al. 2010).

Hyphal fusion

Prolific vegetative cell fusion is common in many true filamentous fungi (e.g. *Neurospora crassa*; Read et al. 2010), though rare in others (e.g. *A. nidulans*; Schultzhaus et al. 2016), and has not been reported in filamentous yeasts (e.g. *C. albicans*). The mechanistic basis of this type of cell fusion has been extensively analyzed in the fungal model *N. crassa* (Read et al. 2010, 2012; Herzog et al. 2015), but it also occurs in human pathogens such as *Fusarium oxysporum* (Ruiz-Roldán et al. 2010). During colony initiation, cell fusion involves the formation of specialized cell protrusions, or short hyphae, called *conidial anastomosis tubes* (CATs), whilst in older regions of the colony specialized *fusion hyphae* develop as branches from the main hyphae. The CATs/fusion hyphae undergo chemotropism towards each other and anastomose to form complex interconnected networks of germlings/hyphae within the developing colony (Figure 4.1). Hyphal fusion can serve various roles including the sharing of nutrient and water resources between different regions of a colony. Recent evidence in studies on plant pathogens has indicated that cell fusion may also be important in facilitating horizontal gene/chromosome transfer, which may increase genetic diversity and allow pathogens to acquire new virulent traits (Ma et al. 2010; Roper et al. 2011, 2013; Ishikawa et al. 2012).

Nuclei

Hyphal compartments of vegetative hyphae in most species (e.g. *A. nidulans*) are multinucleate (e.g. Hickey and Read 2009; Figure 4.3), though in some (e.g. *C. albicans*) they are uninucleate (Thomson et al. 2016). However, in others (e.g. *F. oxysporum*), hyphal compartments can be uninucleate during colony initiation and then later become multinucleate (Shahi et al. 2015). The number of nuclei within a multinucleate hyphal compartment varies considerably and can be up ~100 (Roper et al. 2011). In *A. nidulans*, there has been shown to be a relationship between the ratio of hyphal cytoplasmic volume and the number of nuclei with a mechanism operating that triggers mitosis when the ratio between the two exceeds a critical value. Nevertheless, there is usually no strict relationship between multinucleate nuclear division and septation in hyphae, and the hyphal compartments do not undergo 'cell' separation as observed in the cell cycle of uninucleate yeast cells. For this reason, the term *duplication cycle* was introduced to describe the hyphal equivalent to the cell cycle of uninucleate yeast, animal, and plant cells (Harris 1997).

Nuclei most commonly undergo mitoses in hyphal compartments in the colony periphery, although mitotic nuclear divisions are also observed in older regions of the fungal mycelium (Ishikawa et al. 2013; Shahi et al. 2015). In some species (e.g. *C. albicans*), only the apical hyphal compartment remains mitotically active (Thomson et al. 2016). Three basic types of mitotic nuclear division have been described in multinucleate hyphae (Gladfelter 2006): (1) synchronous mitoses, where all nuclei within a hyphal compartment divide simultaneously; (2) parasynchronous mitoses, where nuclear division is initiated in one hyphal region and then a wave of mitoses travels down the hypha, resulting in sequential nuclear division; and (3) asynchronous mitoses, in which individual nuclei seem to divide independently of neighbouring nuclei. Some species have only been observed to undergo one of these division patterns, whilst others exhibit two, or even all three, patterns (Gladfelter 2006; Ishikawa et al. 2013; Shahi et al. 2015).

Fungal mitoses can be 'closed' or 'semi-open'. In closed mitosis, the nuclear envelope remains intact throughout nuclear division and is exhibited by the budding yeast and filamentous fungi that undergo asynchronous nuclear division (e.g. *N. crassa*; Roca et al. 2010). In semi-open mitosis, components of the nuclear envelope transiently break down during mitosis (De Souza and Osmani 2009).

Vacuoles

Fungal vacuoles are acidic organelle compartments with features in common with plant vacuoles and mammalian lysosomes. They have multiple functions including being involved in many aspects of cellular homeostasis, membrane trafficking, signalling, nutrition, storage of polyphosphates and amino acids, removal of toxic compounds from the cytoplasm, and autophagy (Veses et al. 2008).

The morphology of vacuoles varies significantly between being highly dynamic, pleiomorphic tubular structures through to small vesicular, to larger spherical/ovoid, structures which—in distal hyphal regions—can fill whole hyphal compartments. Vacuolar morphologies vary considerably depending on the species, age of the hyphal compartment within which they reside, and the nutrient status of the medium (Veses et al. 2008; Bowman and Bowman 2010). In *A. nidulans* and many true filamentous fungi, tubular vacuolar compartments are concentrated behind hyphal tips, whilst the spherical/ovoid vacuoles are often more prevalent in older hyphal compartments (Hickey and Read 2009). In some species a dynamic, interconnected vacuolar network can be continuous over a very long distance along the length of a hypha and can play roles in mediating long-distance nutrient transport and signalling within the fungal mycelium (Veses et al. 2008; Bowman and Bowman 2010).

An important function of vacuoles is in *autophagy*, which involves the degradation and turnover of proteins and organelles. In one type of autophagy (*macroautophagy*), cytoplasm and organelles are sequestered in double-membrane bounded vesicles called *autophagosomes*, which dock and fuse with vacuoles, allowing their contents to be broken down by vacuolar hydrolases (Bowman and Bowman 2010). Autophagy and vacuolation can be extensive in old regions of fungal colonies, and autophagy-mediated degradation may provide an efficient means to recycle and translocate the contents of aging hyphae for the benefit of the rest of the mycelium (Shoji and Craven 2011).

Yeast cells

Yeast cells are typically uninucleate single cells that reproduce vegetatively by processes involving septation and separation of daughter cells that can occur either by budding or by binary fission. The budding yeast *Saccharomyces cerevisiae* and the fission yeast, *Schizosaccharomyces pombe,* have been studied extensively as eukaryotic models, particularly in relation to the cell cycle and cell polarization (Alberts et al. 2014; Martin and Arkowitz 2014). Many important fungal pathogens produce yeast cells, and most of these (e.g. *Candida, Cryptococcus, Histoplasma, Blastomyces*, and *Paracoccidioides*) propagate themselves during infection by budding (Figure 4.6), with the notable exception of the yeast cells of *Penicillium* (*Talaromyces*) *marneffei*, which reproduce by binary fission (Boyce and Andrianopoulos 2013). Besides producing yeast cells, most of these pathogens are described as *dimorphic* or filamentous yeasts because, under certain conditions, they can produce hyphae (Gauthier 2015). Indeed, some species (notably *C. albicans*) are often called *polymorphic* because they also form *pseudohyphae*, which more closely resemble yeast cells than hyphae.

Yeast cells lack the extreme developmental versatility, phenotypic plasticity, and diverse functionality of hyphae, and thus are not well adapted to exploring and invading the vast array of heterogeneous microenvironments (including hosts) inhabited by filamentous fungi. Nevertheless, yeast cells have a higher surface area to volume ratio than hyphae and are capable of higher metabolic rates and more rapid production of biomass in nutrient-rich environments. Furthermore, the separation of yeast cells can allow their rapid dissemination within aqueous environments (e.g. the human bloodstream) (Read 1994).

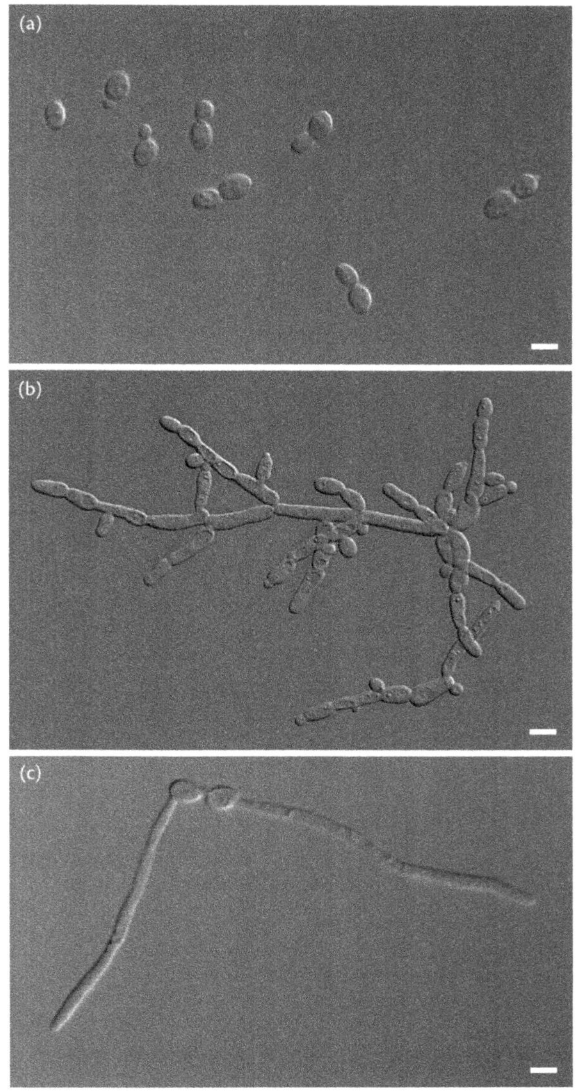

Figure 4.6 Polymorphic *Candida albicans*.

a Budding yeast cells.

b Pseudohyphae composed of elongated budding yeast cells that have not separated.

c Hyphae. Bar = 5 µm.

Reproduced courtesy of Darren Thomson.

Yeast cell budding and growth

The yeast cells and pseudohyphae of *C. albicans* are similar to those of *S. cerevisiae* in shape, size, and cell cycle events (Lew and Reed 1995; Berman 2006). In common with the initiation of polarized growth in hyphae, the initiation of polarized growth in yeast cells involves the recruitment of Rho GTPases to a landmarked plasma membrane region at the site of subsequent bud emergence. This is coupled to the orientation of actin cables and polarized distribution of cortical actin patches to this site. Following the initial polarized outgrowth of the bud there is a switch to isotropic growth to produce the ellipsoidal daughter cell, and this is associated with an unpolarized, even distribution of actin patches over the whole yeast cell cortex. When the daughter cell is fully expanded and the two cells are about to undergo cytokinesis, a septin ring and the actin patches congregate at the site of cytokinesis, where the polarized deposition of cell wall material is required for septation to occur before the cells finally separate. The cortical actin patches are the sites of endocytosis that are in close proximity to distinctly separate sites of exocytosis. In budding yeast cells, secretory vesicles and other organelles are only transported along actin cables, whilst—in contrast to the situation in hyphae—microtubules are restricted to just playing a role in nuclear positioning, spindle formation, and the segregation of chromosomes during nuclear division. Nuclei divide across the motherbud neck (i.e. the site of septation), in contrast to nuclear division in multinucleate hyphae, which is not directly linked to septation. Yeast cell septa are complete (i.e. lack septal pores). *Bud scars* remain on the surfaces of yeast cells following daughter cell separation, and subsequent buds form at other sites on the yeast cell surface (Martin and Arkowitz 2014).

Pseudohyphae

These are formed by budding yeast cells remaining attached after cytokinesis and becoming elongated. Subsequent budding of these attached cells results in highly branched structures with constrictions between each cell (Figure 4.6b). Mechanical agitation easily disrupts the attachment between pseudohyphal cells (Berman 2006; Veses and Gow 2009; Sudbery 2011).

Dimorphism

The ability to exhibit dimorphic switching between a yeast and a hyphal growth form (Figure 4.6c) is a key feature of many human fungal pathogens. In *C. albicans*, both morphological forms, as well as pseudohyphae, are important for virulence and have distinct functions during the different stages of disease development, including adhesion, invasion, damage, dissemination, immune evasion, and the host response (Jacobsen et al. 2012). Furthermore, during infection, *C. albicans* produces highly structured biofilms composed of yeast cells, pseudohyphae, and hyphae encased in an extracellular matrix (Nobile and Johnson 2015; Soll and Daniels 2016) The majority of other important dimorphic pathogens (e.g. *Histoplasma, Blastomyces* and *Paracoccidioides*) produce only yeast cells at 37°C and thus are the sole vegetative cells involved in human infection (Boyce and Andrianopoulos 2015; Gauthier 2015).

The Cryptococcus capsule and extracellular vesicles

Cryptococcus is another very important human fungal pathogen that grows inside the host as budding yeast cells. The main characteristic feature of yeast cells of *Cryptococcus* is the formation of a polysaccharide capsule around a melanized cell wall (Figure 4.7). The capsule grows in size within the host and is considered to be the main virulence factor of *C. neoformans* because it has multiple effects on the host, including inhibiting phagocytosis by macrophages and modulating the host's innate and adaptive immune responses (Zaragoza et al. 2009; O'Meara and Alspaugh 2012). The complex capsule polysaccharide is synthesized within the cell and is then transported by means of extracellular vesicles through the cell wall to the capsule surface. Fungal extracellular vesicles were first discovered in *C. neoformans* (Rodrigues et al. 2007; Rodrigues et al. 2015). It is becoming increasingly clear that extracellular vesicles are part of a general mechanism of macromolecule export by yeast cells and hyphae. They can have a varied cargo, including nucleic acids, toxins, lipoproteins, and enzymes, some of which can be involved in virulence (Nimrichter et al. 2016).

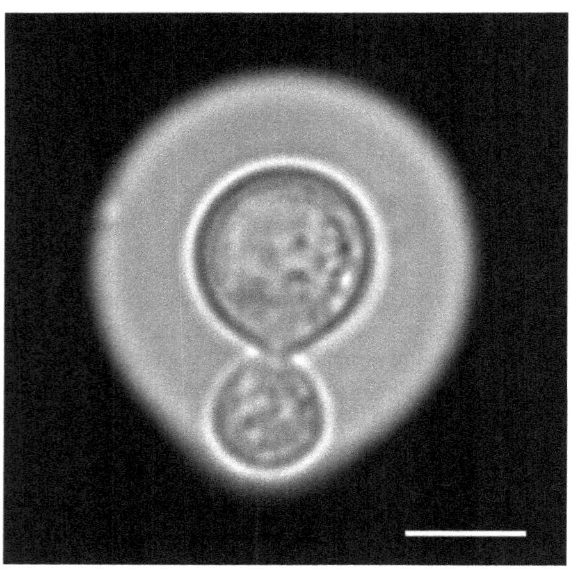

Figure 4.7 Budding *Cryptococcus gattii* yeast cell surrounded by extensive capsule after staining with India ink. Bar = 5 μm.
Reproduced courtesy of Ewa Bielska.

Titan cells

A striking morphological phenomenon of *C. neoformans* yeast cells, which are typically 5–7 μm in diameter, is that they can undergo a transition to form so-called 'titan cells', which can be up to 100 μm in diameter (Zaragoza and Nielsen 2013). These giant yeast cells have greatly thickened cell walls and capsules with a different structure, and are especially effective at dampening the host response (O'Meara and Alspaugh 2012).

Yeast cell mating

This process has been studied in considerable depth in the yeast models *S. cerevisiae and S. pombe* (Merlini et al. 2016) and is similar up until the cell fusion stage in *C. albicans* (Lockhart et al. 2003). The difference relates to the mating cells of *S. cerevisiae* and *S. pombe* being haploid whilst those of *C. albicans* are diploid. In all three yeasts, cells of opposite mating type secrete peptide pheromones (α and **a** factors) to signal mating, and respond by each growing a mating projection (a process known as *shmooing*) towards a potential mate. Following contact, the two partner cells fuse. In *S. cerevisiae* and *S. pombe*, cell fusion is followed by nuclear fusion to form a diploid cell, which can reproduce vegetatively by budding in rich medium. However, when these diploid cells are starved of nutrients, they undergo meiosis to produce four-walled, haploid ascospores. Whether *C. albicans* can undergo meiosis, however, remains an open question. Nevertheless, in this yeast there is clear evidence for a parasexual cycle whereby diploid cells mate to form tetraploid cells, which subsequently lose chromosomes in a random but concerted manner to return to the diploid state (Nobile and Johnson 2007).

Spores

Fungal spores are discrete cellular structures produced by virtually all fungi. Their form varies considerably and they can be unicellular or, as a result of septation, multicellular. They can be derived either asexually, when they are collectively termed *mitospores* (e.g. sporangiospores, conidia, and chlamydospores), or sexually, when they are called *meiospores* (e.g. ascospores, zygospores, basidiospores) (Moore-Landecker 2011; Money 2015). The types of spores and spore-producing structures, including multihyphal fruit bodies, are important features used in fungal classification, and the spore types produced by many fungal pathogens can assist in their identification (see Chapter 2).

Fungal spores serve reproductive, dispersal, and/or survival functions, and this is commonly reflected in their varied structure and

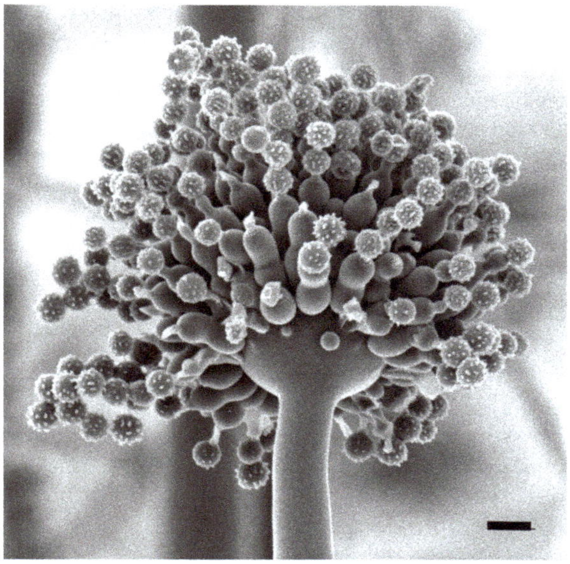

Figure 4.8 Asexual apparatus of *Aspergillus niger*. Note the chains of conidia produced from bottle-shaped phialides (conidiogenous cells) borne on top of a conidiophore, which is swollen at its apex to form a vesicle. Image obtained by low-temperature scanning electron microscopy. Bar = 5 μm.

Reproduced with permission from Read N. D., 'Low-temperature scanning electron microscopy of fungi and fungus-plant interactions,' pp. 17–29. In: Mendgen K. and Lesemann D. (eds.) *Electron Microscopy of Plant Pathogens*, Springer-Verlag, Berlin, Germany, Copyright © 1991.

organization. All spores produced by human fungal pathogens are non-motile (i.e. lack flagella), and some (e.g. conidia and sporangiospores) are produced in very large numbers and released into the air in their natural environment outside the host. An important pathogenicity determinant of airborne spores that initiates infection via lung inhalation is their small size (typically <3 μm in width), which allows them to penetrate deep into lungs to the level of alveoli.

The different types of fungal spores, along with their mechanisms of formation, modes of dispersal, and functions, have been recently reviewed (Money 2015). The following sections focus on the main spore types (see 'Conidia', 'Chlamydospores', 'Sporangiospores', 'Endospores', and 'Basidiospores') encountered in human fungal diseases and the roles that their structure and organization play in the disease process.

Conidia

These are the main mitospores produced by ascomycete pathogens (e.g. *A. fumigatus, P. marneffei, Fusarium spp.,* and dermatophyte pathogens). Some pathogens (e.g. *Fusarium spp., Histoplasma capsulatum*, and many dermatophytes) develop morphologically distinct *microconidia* and *macroconidia* (Webster and Weber 2007). Conidia are derived from specialized *conidiogenous cells* differentiated from hyphae. There are two basic types of conidium development: *blastic* and *thallic* conidiogenesis (Webster and Weber 2007; Moore et al. 2011; Money 2015; see also Chapter 2).

In *blastic conidiogenesis*, conidia are formed in a yeast bud-like manner from the tips or the sides of conidiogenous cells or from the spores at the ends of chains of conidia. In some fungi the conidiogenous cell is termed a *phialide* and is borne on a conidiophore stalk which is swollen at its apex to form a so-called *vesicle* (Figure 4.8). Spores formed by this blastic mechanism are often referred to as *blastospores*. However, the term 'blastospore' is commonly loosely used by medical mycologists for other cell types produced in a budding manner. For instance, the budding yeast cells of *C. albicans* are sometimes described as blastospores that, during dimorphic switching, 'germinate' to produce germ tubes/hyphae, whilst in the basidiomycete *C. neoformans*, budding yeast cells formed directly from hyphae are called blastospores (Lin and Heitman 2006). The genetic control of blastic conidiogenesis, and its regulation by environmental factors (particularly light), has been intensively studied in *A. nidulans and N. crassa* (Ebbole 2010; Park and Yu 2012).

In *thallic conidiogenesis*, individual hyphal compartments of a pre-existing hypha differentiate into conidia, and this culminates in their physical separation by binary fission or hyphal fragmentation. Spores of this type are often referred to as *arthrospores* and are important infectious agents in pathogens such as *Coccidioides* and many dermatophytes.

Chlamydospores

These are typically large, spherical, thick-walled, pigmented mitospores that are produced singly or in chains either at hyphal tips or in subapical hyphal regions. They are produced by a wide range of human fungal pathogens, including *C. albicans, C. neoformans, Fusarium spp.*, and many dermatophytes (e.g. Staib and Mourschäuser 2006; Leslie and Xu 2010), and can survive harsh environmental conditions.

Sporangiospores

These are mitospores produced by cytoplasmic cleavage coupled with cell wall synthesis within a multinucleate *sporangium* that is borne on a specialized hyphal stalk called a *sporangiophore*. They are the infectious agents of members of the Mucorales (Webster and Weber 2007; Reiss et al. 2012).

Endospores

These are a unique type of fungal mitospore produced by the ascomycete pathogens *Coccidioides immitis* and *C. posadasii* in the lungs from a large (<80 μm in width), specialized, multinucleate walled structure called a *spherule*. The spherule develops from an inhaled arthroconidium that undergoes isotropic growth, and repeated nuclear divisions, followed by the progressive segmentation of the spherule protoplasm to form 100–300 walled, uninucleate endospores. When spherules rupture, the endospores are released and are each capable of developing into a new spherule within the host (Huppert et al. 1982; Reiss et al. 2012).

Basidiospores

These are haploid meiospores produced externally from specialized cells derived from hyphae called *basidia*. In *C. neoformans* the basidiospores are produced in chains and are believed to be important infectious agents, along with desiccated yeast cells, that are inhaled into the lungs (Lin and Heitman 2006).

Spore cell walls

Besides providing the spore with protection and morphology, spore cell walls also play other roles during infection. For example, in *A. fumigatus*, the surface of the dormant spore cell wall is covered in a hydrophobic layer of hydrophobin rodlet proteins that masks their recognition by the host immune system (Aimanianda et al. 2009).

Melanin on the spore surface also contributes to them being immunologically inert and can additionally inhibit the phagocytic killing process by macrophages (Bayry et al. 2014).

Spore germination

Spores released into the air rapidly dehydrate and thus have a low water content and no metabolic activity, and are therefore dormant. This dormancy may be broken simply by the spore becoming rehydrated and exposed to favourable conditions for germination. In other cases, spores may impose a longer period of dormancy on themselves once they have arrived at a suitable site for germination. One common cause of this is when spores release a germination self-inhibitor that prevents germination at high spore concentrations as a way of reducing competition for nutrient resources (Ugalde and Rodriguez-Urra 2014).

Spores can germinate to produce specialized hyphae called germ tubes, involved in colony establishment (Figure 4.9), and often other specialized cell protrusions/short hyphae termed conidial anastomosis tubes, which function in fusing together conidial germlings (see 'Hyphal fusion'). Some (e.g. basidiospores of *C. neoformans*) germinate by budding to produce yeast cells (Lin and Heitman 2006). Prior to germination, spores commonly undergo a period of isotropic growth which, in some fungi (e.g. *Aspergillus*), is very accentuated (d'Enfert 1997). Numerous changes in gene expression and biochemical changes occur during the germination process (Kasuga et al. 2005), and many of the same proteins involved in regulating hyphal tip growth also regulate the polarized emergence of a germ tube. Spores can be uninucleate (e.g. conidia of *Aspergillus*; Harris 1999) or multinucleate (e.g. macroconidia of *N. crassa*; Roca et al. 2010); however, mitotic nuclear division is not usually essential for germination, although the two processes are often coupled (Harris 1999; Ishikawa et al. 2013). A recognizable Spitzenkörper is not always evident at the site of germ tube emergence, but develops as the germ tube matures before differentiating into a vegetative hypha (Araujo-Palomares et al. 2007). Marked avoidance responses (negative tropisms) are typically observed between germinating spores that are close to each other. Initially, germ tubes emerge at sites on the spore surface that are as far as possible from the sites of germination on adjacent spores. The growing germ tubes also avoid adjacent germ tubes (Figure 4.9), which is akin to the hyphal avoidance response at the colony periphery (Figures 4.1 and 4.3), and which should similarly reduce competition between adjacent germ tubes for nutrient resources. The chemical identity of the avoidance factor(s) released by spores, germ tubes, and vegetative hyphae has not yet been determined.

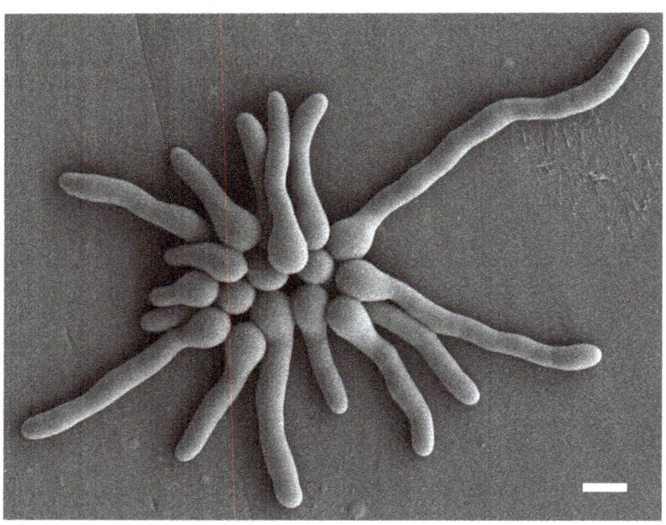

Figure 4.9 Germinating conidia of *Aspergillus fumigatus* growing on cellophane overlying agar growth medium. Note that germ tubes growing out from the aggregated conidia are exhibiting avoidance responses (negative tropisms). Image obtained by low-temperature scanning electron microscopy. Bar = 10 μm. Reproduced courtesy of Kathryn M. Lord and Nick D. Read.

Acknowledgements

Thanks are due to Drs Geoff Robson and Darren Thomson for helping me identify recent literature on the topic of this chapter, to Darren and Dr Kathryn Lord for providing unpublished images, and to Darren for assisting in the preparation of the figures.

References

Aimanianda V, Bayry J, Bozza S, et al. (2009) Surface hydrophobin prevents immune recognition of airborne fungal spores. *Nature* 460: 1117–21.

Alberts B, Johnson A, Lewis J, et al. (2014) *Molecular Biology of the Cell* (6th edn, New York: Garland Science).

Araujo-Palomares CL, Castro-Longoria E and Riquelme M (2007) Ontogeny of the Spitzenkörper in germlings of *Neurospora crassa*. *Fungal Genet Biol* 44: 492–503.

Arkowitz RA and Bassilana M (2015) Regulation of hyphal morphogenesis by Ras and Rho small GTPases. *Fungal Biol Rev* 29: 7–19.

Bartnicki-Garcia S (2002) Hyphal tip growth: outstanding questions, *in*: HD Osiewacz, ed., *Molecular Biology of Fungal Development* (New York: Marcel Dekker, Inc.), 29–58.

Bartnicki-Garcia S (2015) Manfred Girbardt and Charles Bracker: outstanding pioneers in fungal microscopy. *Nat Microbiol* 13: 52–57.

Bartnicki-Garcia S, Hergert F and Gierz G (1989) Computer simulation of fungal morphogenesis and the mathematical basis for hyphal tip growth. *Protoplasma* 153: 46–57.

Bayry J, Beaussart A, Dufrêne YF, et al. (2014) Surface structure characterization of *Aspergillus fumigatus* conidia mutated in the melanin synthesis pathway and their human cellular response. *Infect Immun* 82: 3141–53.

Beauvais A and Latgé J-P (2015) *Aspergillus* biofilm *in vitro* and *in vivo*. *Microbiol Spectra* 3: doi 10.1128/microbiolspec.MB-0017-2015

Berepiki A, Lichius A and Read ND (2011) Actin organization and dynamics in filamentous fungi. *Nat Rev Microbiol* 9: 876–87.

Berman J (2006) Morphogenesis and cell cycle progression in Candida albicans. *Curr Opin Microbiol* 9: 595–601.

Bleichrodt R-J, Hulsman M, Wösten HAB and Reinder MJT (2015) Switching from a unicellular to multicellular organization in an *Aspergillus niger* hypha. *MBio* 6: e00111-15.

Bleichrodt R-J, van Veluw GJ, Recter B, Maruyama J-I, Kitamoto K and Wösten HAB (2012) Hyphal heterogeneity in *Aspergillus oryzae* is the result of dynamic closure of septa by Woronin bodies. *Mol Microbiol* 86: 1334–44.

Bowman EJ and Bowman BJ (2010) Vacuoles in filamentous fungi, *in*: KA Borkovich and D Ebbole, eds, *Cellular and Molecular Biology of Filamentous Fungi* (Washington DC: American Society of Microbiology), 179–90.

Bowman SM and Free SJ (2006) The structure and synthesis of the fungal cell wall. *Bioessays* 28: 799–808.

Boyce K and Andrianopoulos A (2013) Morphogenetic circuitry regulating growth and development in the dimorphic pathogen *Penicillium marneffei*. *Eukaryot Cell* 12: 154–60.

Boyce K and Andrianopoulos A (2015) Fungal dimorphism: the switch from hyphae to yeast is a specialized morphogenetic adaptation allowing colonization of a host. *FEMS Microbiol Rev* 39: 797–811.

Brand AC and Gow NAR (2012) Tropic orientation responses in pathogenic fungi, *in*: J Pérez-Martin and A Di Pietro, eds, *Morphogenesis and Pathogenicity in Fungi*, 22: *Topics in Current Genetics* (Berlin: Springer-Verlag), 21–41.

Buller AHR (1931) *Researches on Fungi*, Vol. 4 (London: Longman).

d'Enfert C (1997) Fungal spore germination: insights from the molecular genetics of *Aspergillus nidulans* and *Neurospora crassa*. *Fungal Genet Biol* 21: 163–72.

De Souza CP and Osmani SA (2009) Double duty for nuclear proteins—the price of more open forms of mitosis. *Trends Genet* 25: 545–54.

Dhavale TJ and Jedd G (2007) The fungal Woronin body, *in*: RG Howard and NAR Gow, eds, *The Mycota*, 8: *Biology of the Fungal Cell* (Berlin: Springer-Verlag), 87–96.

Ebbole D (2010) The conidium, *in*: KA Borkovich and D Ebbole, eds, *Cellular and Molecular Biology of Filamentous Fungi* (Washington DC: American Society of Microbiology), 577–90.

Egan MJ, McClintock MA and Reck-Peterson SL (2012) Microtubule-based transport in filamentous fungi. *Current Opin Microbiol* 15: 637–45.

Erwig LP and Gow NAR (2016) Interactions of fungal pathogens with phagocytes *Nat Rev Microbiol* 14: 163–79.

Fischer R, Zekert N and Takeshita N (2008) Polarized growth in fungi—the interplay between the cytoskeleton, positional markers and membrane domains. *Mol Microbiol* 68: 813–26.

Freitag M, Hickey PC, Raju NB, Selker EU and Read ND (2004) GFP as a tool to analyze the organization, dynamics and function of nuclei and microtubules in *Neurospora crassa*. *Fungal Genet Biol* 41: 907–20.

Gauthier GM (2015) Dimorphism in fungal pathogens of mammals, plants and insects. *PLoS Pathog* 11: e1004608.

Gladfelter A (2006) Nuclear anarchy: asynchronous mitosis in multinucleated fungal hyphae. *Current Opin Microbiol* 9: 547–52.

Gow NAR, Gooday GW, Newsam RJ and Gull K (1980) The ultrastructure of septum in *Candida albicans*. *Curr Microbiol* 4: 357–59.

Harris SD (1997) The duplication cycle of Aspergillus nidulans. *Fungal Genet Biol* 22: 1–12.

Harris SD (1999) Morphogenesis is coordinated with nuclear division in germinating *Aspergillus nidulans* conidiospores. *Microbiology* 145: 2747–56.

Harris SD (2008) Branching of fungal hyphae: regulation, mechanisms and comparison with other branching systems. *Mycologia* 100: 823–32.

Herzog S, Schumann MR and Fleiβner A (2015) Cell fusion in *Neurospora crassa*. *Curr Opin Microbiol* 28: 53–9.

Hickey PC and Read ND (2009) Imaging living cells of *Aspergillus in vitro*. *Med Mycol* 47: S110–19.

Higuchi Y and Steinberg G (2015) Early endosomes motility in filamentous fungi: how and why they move. *Fungal Biol Rev* 29: 1–6.

Huppert M, Sun SH and Harrison JL (1982) Morphogenesis throughout saprobic and parasitic cycles of *Coccidioides immitis*. *Mycopathologia* 22: 107–22.

Ishikawa FH, Souza E, Read ND and Roca MG (2013) *Colletotrichum lindemuthianum* exhibits different patterns of nuclear division at different stages in its vegetative life cycle. *Mycologia* 105: 795–801.

Ishikawa FH, Souza E, Shoji J, et al. (2012) Heterokaryon incompatibility is suppressed following conidial anastomosis tube fusion in a fungal plant pathogen. *PLoS One* 7: e31175.

Kanbe T and Tanaka K (1982) Ultrastructure of the invasion of human hair *in vitro* by the keratinophilic fungus *Microsporum gypseum*. *Infect Immun* 38: 706–15.

Kasuga T, Townsend JP, Tian C, et al. (2005) Long-oligomer microarray profiling in *Neurospora crassa* reveals the transcriptional program underlying biochemical and physiological events of conidial germination. *Nucleic Acids Res* 33: 6469–85.

Khan A, McQuilken M and Gladfelter AS (2015) Septins and generation of asymmetries in fungal cells. *Annu Rev Microbiol* 69: 487–503.

Jacobsen ID, Wilson D, Wächtler B, Brunke S, Naglik JR and Hube B (2012) *Candida albicans* dimorphism as a therapeutic target. *Expert Rev Anti Infect Ther* 10: 85–93.

Jedd G and Chua NH (2000) A new self-assembled peroxisomal vesicle required for efficient resealing of the plasma membrane. *Nat Cell Biol* 2: 226–31.

Lai J, Koh CH, Tjota M, et al. (2012) Intrinsically disordered proteins aggregate at fungal cell-to-cell channels and regulate intercellular connectivity. *Proc Natl Acad Sci USA* 109: 15781–6.

Latgé J-P (2007) The cell wall: a carbohydrate armour for the fungal cell. *Mol Microbiol* 66: 279–90.

Leslie JF and Xu J-R (2010) *Fusarium* genetics and pathogenicity, *in*: KA Borkovich and D Ebbole, eds, *Cellular and Molecular Biology of Filamentous Fungi* (Washington DC: American Society of Microbiology), 607–21.

Lew DJ and Reed SI (1995) Cell cycle control of morphogenesis in budding yeast. *Current Opin Genet Dev* 5: 17–23.

Lew RR (2011) How does a hypha grow? The biophysics of pressurized growth in fungi. *Nat Rev Microbiol* 9: 509–18.

Lin X and Heitman J (2006) The biology of the *Cryptococcus neoformans* species complex. *Annu Rev Microbiol* 60: 69–105.

Lockhart SR, Daniels KJ, Zhao R, Wessels D and Soll DR (2003) Cell biology of mating in *Candida albicans*. *Eukaryot Cell* 2: 49–61.

Lord KM and Read ND (2011) Perithecium morphogenesis in *Sordaria macrospora*. *Fungal Genet Biol* 48: 388–99.

Ma LJ, van der Does HC, Borkovich KA, et al. (2010) Comparative genomics reveals mobile pathogenicity chromosomes in Fusarium. *Nature* 464: 367–73.

Martin SG and Arkowitz RA (2014) Cell polarization in budding and fission yeasts. *FEMS Microbiol Rev* 38: 228–53.

Merlini L, Dudin O and Martin SG (2016) Mate and fuse: how yeast cells do it. *Open Biol* 3: 130008.

Money NP (2015) Spore production, discharge, and dispersal, *in*: S Watkinson, L Boddy and NP Money, eds, *The Fungi* (3rd edn, Amsterdam: Elsevier), 67–97.

Moore D, Robson GD and Trinci APJ (2011) *21st Century Guidebook to Fungi* (Cambridge: CUP).

Moore-Landecker E (2011) Fungal spores. *eLS*. doi: 10.1002/9780470015902.a0000378.pub2

Mourino-Perez RR (2013) Septum development in filamentous ascomycetes. *Fungal Biol Rev* 27: 1–9.

Nimrichter L, de Souza MM, Del Poeta M, et al. (2016) Extracellular vesicle-associated transitory cell wall components and their impact on the interaction of fungi with host cells. *Front Microbiol* 7: 1034.

Nobile SM and Johnson AD (2007) Genetics of *Candida albicans*, a diploid human fungal pathogen. Annu Rev Genet 41: 193–211.

Nobile SM and Johnson AD (2015) Candida albicans biofilms and human disease. *Annu Rev Microbiol* 69: 71–92.

O'Meara TR and Alspaugh JA (2012) The *Cryptococcus neoformans* capsule: a sword and a shield. *Clin Microbiol Rev* 25: 387–408.

Osherov N and Yarden O (2010) The cell wall of filamentous fungi, *in*: KA Borkovich and D Ebbole, eds, *Cellular and Molecular Biology of Filamentous Fungi* (Washington DC: American Society of Microbiology), 2224–37.

Pantazopoulou A, Pinar M, Xiang M and Peñalva M (2014) Maturation of late Golgi cisternae into RabE^{RAB11} exocytic post-Golgi carriers visualized in vivo. *Mol Biol Cell* 25: 2428–43.

Park H-S and Yu J-H (2012) Genetic control of asexual sporulation in filamentous fungi. *Curr Opin Microbiol* 15: 669–77.

Pieuchot L, Lai J, Loh RA, et al. (2015) Cellular subcompartments through cytoplasmic streaming. *Dev Cell* 34: 410–20.

Read ND (1991) Low-temperature scanning electron microscopy of fungi and fungus-plant interactions, *in*: K Mendgen and D-E Lesemann, eds, *Electron Microscopy of Plant Pathogens* (Berlin: Springer-Verlag), 17–29.

Read ND (1994) Cellular nature and multicellular morphogenesis of higher fungi, *in*: D Ingram and A Hudson, eds, *Shape and Form in Plants and Fungi* (London: Academic Press), 254–71.

Read ND (2007) Environmental sensing and the filamentous fungal lifestyle, *in*: GM Gadd, SC Watkinson and PS Dyer, eds, *Fungi and their Environment* (Cambridge: CUP), 38–57.

Read ND (2011) Hyphal growth and exocytosis do *not* only occur at hyphal tips. *Mol Microbiol* 81: 4–7.

Read ND, Fleißner A, Roca GM and Glass NL (2010) Hyphal fusion, *in*: KA Borkovich and D Ebbole, eds, *Cellular and Molecular Biology of Filamentous Fungi* (Washington DC: American Society of Microbiology), 260–73.

Read ND, Goryachev AB and Lichius A (2012) The mechanistic basis of self-fusion between conidial anastomosis tubes during fungal colony initiation. *Fungal Biol Rev* 26: 1–11.

Reiss E, Shadomy HJ and Lyon GM (2012) *Fundamental Medical Mycology* (Hoboken, NJ: Wiley-Blackwell).

Riquelme M (2013) Tip growth in filamentous fungi: a road trip to the apex. *Annu Rev Microbiol* 67: 587–609.

Riquelme M, Bredeweg EL, Callejas O, et al. (2014) The *Neurospora crassa* exocyst complex tethers Spitzenkörper vesicles to the apical plasma membrane during polarized growth. *Mol Biol Cell* 25: 1312–26.

Riquelme M and Sanchez-Leon E (2014) The Spitzenkörper: a choreographer of fungal growth and morphogenesis. *Curr Opin Microbiol* 20: 27–33.

Riquelme M and Sanchez-Leon E (2015) Live imaging of b-1,3-glucan synthase FKS-1 in *Neurospora crassa* hyphae. *Fungal Genet Biol* 82: 104–7.

Roberson RW, Abril M, Blackwell M, et al. (2010) Hyphal structure, *in*: KA Borkovich and D Ebbole, eds, *Cellular and Molecular Biology of Filamentous Fungi* (Washington DC: American Society of Microbiology), 8–24.

Roca MG, Kuo H-C, Lichius A, Freitag M and Read ND (2010) Nuclear dynamics, mitosis and the cytoskeleton during the early stages of colony initiation in *Neurospora crassa*. *Eukaryot Cell* 9: 1171–83.

Rodrigues ML, Godinho RMC, Zamith-Miranda D and Nimrichter L (2015) Traveling into outer space: unanswered questions about fungal extracellular vesicles. *PLoS Pathog* 11: e1005240.

Rodrigues ML, Nimrichter L, Oliveira DL, et al. (2007) Vesicular polysaccharide export in *Cryptococcus neoformans* is a eukaryotic solution to the problem of fungal trans-cell wall transport. *Eukaryot Cell* 6: 48–59.

Roper M, Ellison C, Taylor JW and Glass NL (2011) Nuclear and genome dynamics in multinucleate ascomycete fungi. *Curr Biol* 21: R786–93.

Roper M, Simonin A, Hickey PC, Leeder A and Glass NL (2013) Nuclear dynamics in a fungal chimera. *Proc Natl Acad Sci USA* 110: 12875–80.

Ruiz-Roldán MC, Köhli M, Roncero MI, Philippsen P, Di Pietro A and Espeso EA (2010) Nuclear dynamics during germination, conidiation, and hyphal fusion of *Fusarium oxysporum*. *Eukaryot Cell* 9: 1216–24.

Salogiannis J, Egan MJ and Reck-Peterson SL (2016) Peroxisomes move by hitchhiking on early endosomes using the novel linker protein PxdA. *J Cell Biol* 212: 289–96.

Schultzhaus ZS and Shaw BD (2015) Endocytosis and exocytosis in hyphal growth. *Fungal Biol Rev* 29: 43–53.

Schultzhaus ZS, Quintanilla L, Hilton A and Shaw BD (2016) Live cell imaging of actin dynamics in the filamentous fungus *Aspergillus nidulans*. *Microsc Microanal* 22: 264–74.

Schuster M, Martin-Urdiroz M, Higuchi Y, et al. (2016) Co-delivery of cell-wall-forming enzymes in the same vesicle for coordinated fungal cell wall formation. *Nat Microbiol* 1: 16149.

Shahi S, Beerens B, Manders EMM and Rep M (2015) Dynamics of the establishment of multinucleate compartments in *Fusarium oxysporum*. *Eukaryot Cell* 14: 78–85.

Shoji J-Y and Craven K (2011) Autophagy in basal hyphal compartments: a green strategy of great recyclers. *Fungal Biol Rev* 25: 79–83.

Soll DR and Daniels KJ (2016) Plasticity of *Candida* biofilms. *Microbiol Mol Biol Rev* 80: 565–95.

Staib P and Mourschäuser J (2006) Chlamydospore formation in *Candida albicans* and *Candida dublinensis*—an enigmatic developmental programme. *Mycoses* 50: 1–12.

Steinberg G (2014) Endocytosis and early endosome motility in filamentous fungi. *Curr Opin Microbiol* 20: 10–18.

Sudbery PE (2011) Growth of Candida albicans hyphae. *Nat Rev Microbiol* 9: 737–748.

Takeshita N, Manck R, Grün N, de Vega SH and Fischer R (2014) Interdependence of the actin and the microtubule cytoskeleton during fungal growth. *Curr Opin Microbiol* 20: 34–41.

Thomson DD, Berman J and Brand A (2016) High frame-rate resolution of cell division during *Candida albicans* filamentation. *Fungal Genet Biol* 88: 54–8.

Thomson DD, Wehmeier S, Byfield FJ, et al. (2015) Contact-induced apical symmetry drives the thigmotropic responses of *Candida albicans* hyphae. *Cell Microbiol* 17: 342–54.

Ugalde U and Rodriguez-Urra AB (2014) The mycelium blueprint: insights into the cues that shape the filamentous fungal colony. *Appl Microbiol Biotechnol* 98: 8809–19.

Veses V and Gow NAR (2009) Pseudohypha budding patterns of *Candida albicans*. *Med Mycol* 47: 268–75.

Veses V, Richards A and Gow NAR (2008) Vacuoles and fungal biology. *Curr Opin Microbiol* 11: 503–10.

Webster J and Weber R (2007) *Introduction to Fungi* (3rd edn, Cambridge: CUP).

Xiang X and Oakley B (2010) The cytoskeleton in filamentous fungi, *in*: KA Borkovich and D Ebbole, eds, *Cellular and Molecular Biology of Filamentous Fungi* (Washington DC: American Society of Microbiology), 209–23.

Zaragoza O and Nielsen K (2013) Titan cells in *Cryptococcus neoformans*: cells with a giant impact. *Curr Opin Microbiol* 16: 409–13.

Zaragoza O, Rodrigues ML, De Jesus M, Frases S, Dadachova E and Casadevall A (2009) The capsule of the fungal pathogen *Cryptococcus neoformans*. *Adv Appl Microbiol* 68: 133–216.

CHAPTER 5

Fungal genetics

Paul S. Dyer, Carol A. Munro, and Rosie E. Bradshaw

Introduction to fungal genetics

A key factor in the success of fungi is their remarkable genetic properties. Fungi can occur naturally as haploid, diploid, or higher ploidy forms, i.e. with one, two, or more sets of chromosomes. Certain species can rearrange or even lose whole chromosomes, and some species have several hundred different sexes. The fact that fungi are so interesting from a genetic viewpoint, together with the ease with which many of them can be easily grown and manipulated under laboratory conditions, has meant that fungi have long been used as model eukaryotic organisms to study genetic and cellular processes, with Nobel prizes having been awarded for research involving fungal genetics (see 'Mutagenesis').

Although there is much variation in the genetic make-up of fungi, some general features are observed. Firstly, most groups of fungi are normally haploid when in the hyphal form, reproduce asexually, and only briefly become diploid during sexual reproduction before reverting back to the haploid state (Figure 5.1). The fact that most fungi are haploid simplifies genetic analysis, as there is no masking of phenotypes due to dominance of alleles at a gene locus (as seen in diploid higher eukaryotes such as mammals). Instead, the haploid genotype of the fungus normally directly determines the phenotype, such as whether a fungus is sensitive or resistant to a particular antifungal drug. However, there are exceptions. For example, fungi from the Basidiomycota usually have an extended period of growth in a dikaryotic state, following cellular fusion of different mating partners, before karyogamy (nuclear fusion) and sexual reproduction take place (Figure 5.1). Some yeasts, including the medically important *Candida albicans*, occur as diploids in nature and reproduce by budding asexually (Figure 5.1).

A second general feature is that almost all fungi share the same genetic code, gene structure, and regulatory features as other eukaryotic organisms. Thus, fungal genes have upstream promoter elements, open reading frames composed of exons and introns, and downstream terminator regions (Figure 5.2) (Gurr et al. 1987; Archer et al. 2006). Fungal DNA is packaged into chromatin, containing hundreds of origins of replication and comprised of condensed heterochromatin and less condensed euchromatin, with gene expression mainly from the latter (Brosch et al. 2008; Bi 2014). Most fungi have relatively small genomes of 10–45 Mb in size, encoding between 5,000 and 15,000 proteins which are generally spread over 7–20 chromosomes, and—compared with higher eukaryotic genomes—most fungal genomes have relatively little repetitive DNA (Coleman et al. 2009; Mohanta and Bae 2015). A variety of mechanisms control gene expression. These include either constitutive or inducible expression under the control of transcription factors, but there is also evidence for the roles of RNA modifying systems (e.g. antisense RNA), alternative splicing (albeit to a lesser extent than many higher eukaryotes), upstream open reading frames, and epigenetic modification in mediating gene expression (Brosch et al. 2008; Hood et al. 2009). There is also evidence for prion proteins in fungi, which might provide models for human amyloid diseases (Wickner et al. 2015). However, there are again exceptions to these general rules. Members of a *Candida* clade of yeasts deviate from the standard genetic code, translating CUG codons as serine instead of leucine (Miranda et al. 2006). Meanwhile, many fungal species have developed specialized mechanisms to inactivate and prevent the spread of repetitive DNA (such as transposable elements); repeat-induced point mutation (RIP) and methylation-induced premeiotically (MIP) processes occurring during the sexual cycles of *Neurospora, Ascobolus*, and *Coprinus* species (Irelan and Selker 1996) are examples of such mechanisms.

This chapter outlines key aspects of fungal genetics. It illustrates the genetic tools that are available to gain an understanding of gene function in filamentous fungi and yeasts as might be applied in a medical mycology context and beyond. By necessity, coverage of techniques is limited to those most commonly used, and the reader is referred elsewhere to the texts of Burnett (2003) and Zhan and McDonald (2005) for details of the complementary area of fungal population genetics. Nevertheless, this chapter should provide a working framework for modern fungal genetics.

Classical genetics

Many insights into how fungi function at a genetic level have been gained using classical microbiological experimental techniques, and this knowledge has been used to develop methods for genetic analysis of fungi.

Gene flow in fungal populations by sexual recombination

Most fungal species are able to reproduce sexually, forming haploid spores via meiosis (Figure 5.1). However, there is tremendous diversity in breeding systems. Some fungi are heterothallic, requiring the presence of compatible 'mating types' for sexual reproduction to occur. In the Ascomycotina fungi there are normally just two sexes. The compatible mating types are by convention termed *MAT1-1* and *MAT1-2*, as for example with the opportunistic pathogen *Aspergillus fumigatus* (O'Gorman et al. 2009), but for some species older terminology may be used, such as the alpha (α) and **a** mating types in *Saccharomyces cerevisiae*, and the MATA and MATa in

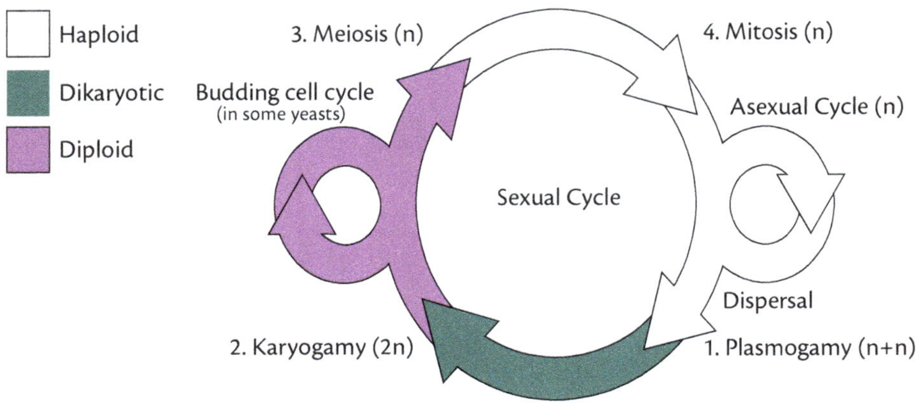

Figure 5.1 Fungal life cycles. Different ploidy levels (haploid 'n' and diploid '2n') are indicated during fungal vegetative growth and asexual and sexual reproduction. Image reproduced courtesy of George Ashton.

N. crassa. Isolates of complementary mating type are morphologically indistinguishable but produce different types of peptide pheromone to attract sexual partners of opposite mating type (Dyer et al. 2016). Mating can result in considerable genetic diversity in the offspring owing to crossing over and independent assortment of chromosomes during meiosis, which can be important for the evolution of species and the occurrence, for example, of increased resistance to antifungals. By contrast, other fungi are homothallic, being self-fertile and able to complete the sexual cycle without the need for a mating partner. This can lead to clonality in the offspring. But many homothallic fungi retain the ability to outcross under suitable conditions and therefore are not restricted to self-fertility (Burnett 2003; Dyer et al. 2016). Intriguingly, there are recent reports that some fungi, notably pathogenic *Candida* and *Cryptococcus* species, can undergo unisexual mating between partners of the same mating type. It remains unclear how widespread this process might be in nature (Heitman et al. 2014). Indeed, *C. albicans* features a very unusual form of sexual mating, involving fusion of compatible diploid cells to form a tetraploid state (Figure 5.3a). Rather than regular meiosis, nuclei then undergo stochastic chromosome loss to return to the diploid state via a parasexual process (Heitman et al. 2014). Sexual crossing in filamentous fungi results in the development of sexual spores within specialized fruiting bodies (Figure 5.3b). The sexual spores normally have a different morphology from asexual spores (Figure 5.3c) and can be highly resistant to environmental stressors such as high temperature and UV exposure. Methods have been described to induce the sexual stages of many fungi under laboratory conditions (Houbraken and Dyer 2015).

Where a sexual cycle has been described and induced *in vitro*, it can be exploited using classical genetic approaches (Moore and Novak Frazer 2002; Ashton and Dyer 2016) to obtain genetic maps with phenotypic and molecular markers (Foulongne-Oriol 2012). In crosses with a reference strain, the segregation of a trait(s) of interest is determined in the progeny relative to known markers. Co-segregation of markers thus enables the position of a gene to be determined relative to known markers on a genetic map (Moore and Frazer 2002; Snustad and Simmons 2010). Further analysis by chromosome walking and sequence analysis allows identification

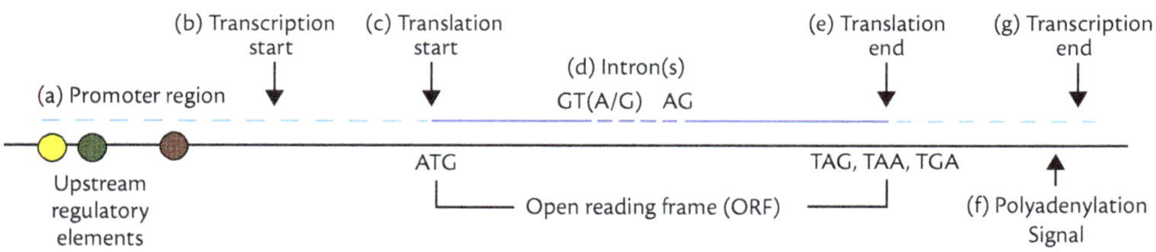

Figure 5.2 Structure of a typical fungal gene (not to scale).

a The 5′ upstream promoter region is often less than 1,000 bp but can extend to 2,000 bp or more. It can include TATA and CCAAT boxes and other promoter elements, upstream activation or repression sequences, binding sites for transcription factors, and upstream open reading frames (uORFs).

b mRNA transcription begins up to 300 bp or more upstream of the ORF, and many genes do not have a unique initiation site.

c The ORF and translation of mRNA begins with an ATG (methionine) codon, with a purine base almost always present three bases upstream (the 'Kozak rule').

d A variable number of introns can be present which range in size from around 50 bp to over 200 bp, with introns more common in filamentous fungi than in *S. cerevisiae* and *C. albicans*.

e Standard stop codon—a wide diversity of different protein sizes are produced, many composed of 100–500 amino acids.

f A polyadenylation site is required for later mRNA processing.

g mRNA transcription stops several hundred base pairs beyond the stop codon, with many genes not having a unique termination site, and the 3′ untranslated region can include introns.

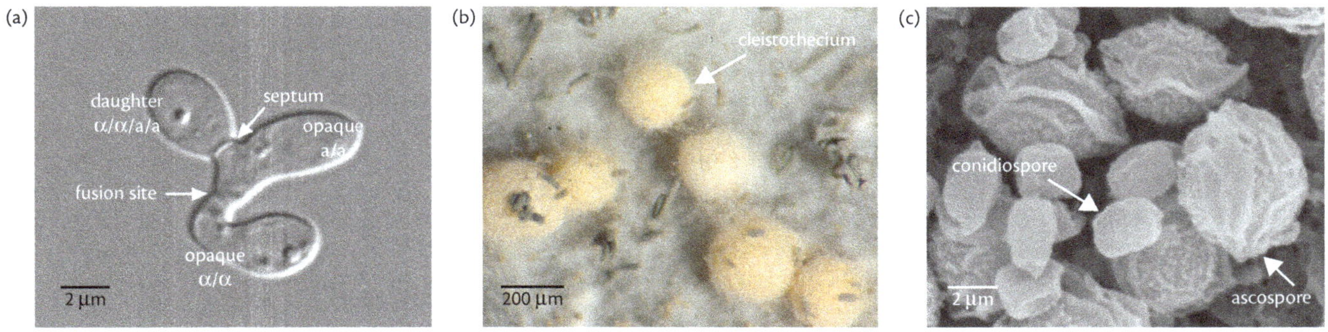

Figure 5.3 Mating and sexual reproduction in fungi.

a Mating in *C. albicans* showing fusion of two opaque cells of opposite a and α mating type to produce a tetraploid daughter.

b Formation of yellow-gold fruiting bodies (cleistothecia) during sexual reproduction of the opportunistic pathogen *Aspergillus lentulus*, a close relative of *A. fumigatus*.

c Scanning electron micrograph of meiotically derived sexual ascospores of *A. lentulus* compared with mitotically derived asexual conidiospores.

a reproduced courtesy of Karla J. Daniels and David R. Soll.

b and **c** reproduced from Swilaiman S. S. et al., 'Discovery of a sexual cycle in *Aspergillus lentulus*, a close relative of *A. fumigatus*,' *Eukaryotic Cell*, Volume 12, Issue 7 pp. 962–69, Copyright © 2013 Swilaiman et al. Reproduced under the terms of the Creative Commons Attribution 3.0 Unported license, https://creativecommons.org/licenses/by/3.0/

of a gene of interest within that region of the genome (Foulongne-Oriol 2012). Such mapping approaches were extensively used before the widespread availability of whole fungal genome sequences. A related form of classical genetic mapping is known as 'tetrad analysis'. This applies to members of the Ascomycotina that produce all four products (the tetrad) of a single meiotic event in a sac-like structure called an ascus. For some species the individual progeny can be dissected out of an ascus, grown, and characterized, to help detect gene linkage and mapping. Furthermore, some *Neurospora*, *Sordaria*, and *Ascobolus* species produce 'ordered tetrads', with the individual haploid products forming sexual ascospores in a linear tube-like ascus in the order in which they are produced during meiosis. Genetic analysis of progeny from ordered fungal tetrads provides a demonstration of first- and second-division segregation during meiosis and can be used to map the positions of both centromeres and genes on chromosomes (Moore and Novak Frazer 2002; Snustad and Simmons 2010). Tetrad analysis was used to show the phenomenon of 'gene conversion', whereby non-reciprocal recombination between closely linked genetic markers is observed (Snustad and Simmons 2010); this provided key insights into general cellular mechanisms of DNA crossing over and recombination.

Gene flow by asexual means

The genetic flexibility of fungi is illustrated by the fact that many species have evolved methods to allow gene exchange and recombination independent of sexual reproduction. As described in Chapter 4, fungal hyphae of the same individual can intermingle and fuse (anastomose) together. By contrast, when fungi of different strains or species meet, an incompatibility reaction involving cell death can occur as a result of non-self recognition. Despite this, certain strains are able to fuse together to form a heterokaryon composed of two nuclear types (Figure 5.4). (The phenomenon of heterokaryon compatibility (also known as vegetative incompatibility) is determined by at least 7–11 so-called *het* gene loci.) For isolates to be vegetatively compatible, they must be genetically identical at all of the *het* loci. Thus, heterokaryon formation is limited to very closely related strains. But where it occurs, it allows mingling of complementary genetic information, which can be important in survival. Furthermore, there can be spontaneous formation of diploid nuclei in such a heterokaryon, and the possibility for mitotic recombination (albeit at a far lower rate than in meiosis). Such diploid nuclei can then spontaneously return to the haploid state by non-disjunction and loss of chromosomes during nuclear division. The overall effect is to enable gene recombination through asexual means; this process is known as the parasexual cycle (Figure 5.4). Although the significance of parasexuality in nature is unclear, it has provided a valuable laboratory genetic tool for the fusion and

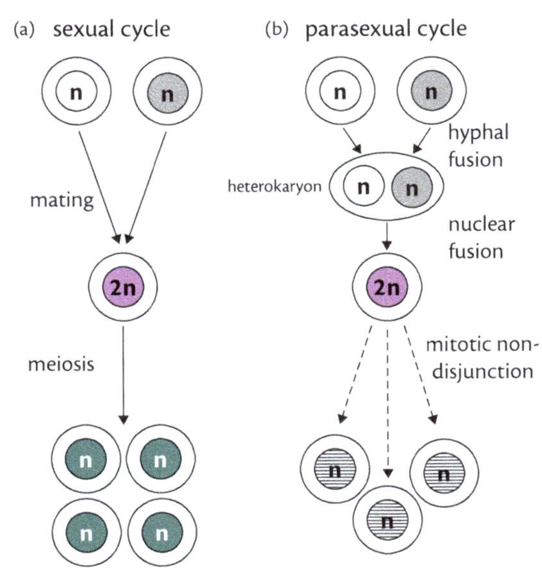

Figure 5.4 Sexual and parasexual cycles in fungi. Fungal cells (indicated by large circles), containing nuclei (smaller circles), are shown as haploid (n) or diploid (2n).

a In the sexual cycle, mating between compatible mating types, followed by meiosis, leads to recombinant progeny by crossover and chromosome reassortment.

b In the parasexual cycle, a series of random events occur that can result in progeny with different genotypes to the parents, with hyphal fusion (anastomosis), nuclear fusion (karyogamy), and mitotic non-disjunction leading to random chromosome loss and the eventual formation of stable haploid cells.

recombination of asexual fungi, particularly those of industrial significance. There is also evidence of horizontal gene transfer in the fungal kingdom, whereby fungi have incorporated DNA from other fungal, or even bacterial, species into their own genomes. The way in which DNA is transferred is unknown, but some important secondary metabolite gene clusters, such as those involved with toxin and penicillin production, may have been transferred by this process (Fitzpatrick 2012).

Such alternative methods to sex to enable gene flow can be particularly important given the fact that about 20% of fungi are only known to reproduce asexually. However, recent discoveries suggest that many of these species might have the potential for sexual reproduction (O'Gorman et al. 2009; Swilaiman et al. 2013; Houbraken and Dyer 2015). Thus, the absence of a reported sexual cycle should not be taken as evidence for obligate asexuality; such species may instead undergo clandestine sexual activity (Gow 2005).

Mutagenesis

Fungi are able to generate genetic diversity by mutations that arise as a result of errors in DNA replication and exposure to environmental mutagens, at a rate of 1×10^{-6} to 1×10^{-8} per gene (Burnett 2003). Mutations can also be induced under laboratory conditions at higher rates—for example, by exposing fungal spores to UV light or X-rays, or to a wide variety of chemical mutagens (Harris 2001). Different types of treatment result in various forms of mutation, including point, frameshift, and larger gross chromosomal rearrangements (Moore and Novak Frazer 2002). Mutant phenotypes include: auxotrophy (where the ability to synthesize particular nutrients is lost), increased production of metabolites of interest (such as penicillin), resistance to antifungal drugs, and even different spore colours. The mutant phenotypes generally arise owing to damage in genes that are either directly responsible for a certain process, or that control (induce or repress) that process. Mutagenesis is an extremely valuable genetic tool and has been widely used to investigate many different fungal activities. In the 1940s, George Beadle and Edward Tatum used X-ray mutagenesis to produce nutritional auxotrophs of *N. crassa*, and by using supplementation growth experiments and sexual crosses were able to demonstrate that genetic mutations affect individual metabolic pathways. They were subsequently awarded a Nobel prize in 1958 for their 'one-gene, one-enzyme' hypothesis.

Mutagenesis also forms the basis of the 'forward-genetics' experimental approach, where a phenotype is first identified via a mutational screen and then genetic analysis 'moves forward' to identify the gene(s) responsible, i.e. phenotype to genotype. This differs from the 'reverse-genetics' approach, where a known gene is disrupted and the phenotype of the consequent mutant analyzed to determine the gene function, i.e. genotype to phenotype. Leland Hartwell and Paul Nurse were awarded a Nobel prize in 2001 for their work in identifying genes controlling the eukaryotic cell cycle, based on a forward-genetics approach involving mutation of the yeasts *S. cerevisiae* and *Schizosaccharomyces pombe*. Most recently, Randy Schekman was awarded a Nobel prize in 2013 for research into cellular vesicle transport, which utilized genetic screens of yeast secretory mutants to identify the corresponding regulatory genes. Further clever variations of the mutational screening approach include the deployment of enhancer screens, whereby a mutant with a phenotype of interest generated from a first round of mutagenesis is subjected to further mutagenesis to identify additional mutations which enhance the original phenotype. Likewise, suppressor screens are used to select for new mutations resulting in reversion of a mutant to the original phenotype. Both of these latter screens can provide insights into pathway control. Temperature-sensitive screens can be used to select for mutations that result in a mutant phenotype at a higher restrictive temperature but allow normal growth at a lower permissive temperature. Such mutations usually lead to an unstable non-functional protein product at the higher temperature. Finally, synthetic lethal screens can be used to identify situations where a combination of mutations in separate genes results in death, whilst cells remain viable with mutation in one gene alone (albeit perhaps with reduced growth). Synthetic lethal screens are useful as they indicate functional relationships between gene products (Griffiths et al. 2015).

Many molecular biology tools are now available to add complementary insights into how fungi function at a genetic level, with a range of techniques available for the molecular-genetic analysis of fungi, as will be described in the following sections.

Molecular genetics: DNA manipulation tools

General principles of transformation

The development of methods to stably transform foreign DNA into fungal cells was arguably the most important advance in fungal genetics in the last decades of the twentieth century. It enabled the addition, deletion, or mutation of specific genes, providing an unprecedented level of genetic dissection for determining gene function. Pioneering work in the production of protoplasts (fungal cells lacking cell walls) (Peberdy 1979) underpinned the development of fungal transformation methods (Fincham 1989), and many laboratories today use protoplasts as hosts for transforming DNA. A key component in the transformation process is the use of a selectable marker gene that enables transformed cells (cells that have taken up the DNA) to be identified amongst the background of non-transformed cells. Different types of selectable marker genes are used—amongst them genes for resistance to antibiotics such as hygromycin, or genes that complement a nutritional deficiency in the host strain such as uridine auxotrophs (Riach and Kinghorn 1996; Bowyer 2001; Archer et al. 2006; Osmani et al. 2008). For transformation, a foreign gene is usually combined in a plasmid along with the selectable marker (although linear DNA fragments are now increasingly being used) and delivered into protoplasts using a fusion agent (polyethylene glycol) or by electroporation (Riach and Kinghorn 1996; Archer et al. 2006). Alternatively, plasmid DNA can be delivered into fungal cells using methods originally developed for plant transformation with the bacterium *Agrobacterium tumefaciens* (Bowyer 2001; Michielse et al. 2005). Sometimes co-transformation is conducted, whereby a fungus is transformed simultaneously with two separate DNA constructs, with the anticipation that the DNA of interest will be taken up by the host at the same time as the DNA encoding a selectable marker. In filamentous fungi, transforming DNA is generally stably integrated into chromosomes, whilst autonomously replicating vectors are also used in yeasts such as *S. cerevisiae*. Depending on the aim of the experiment, the DNA can be integrated at random locations (known as heterologous integration) or targeted to particular loci in the genome by inclusion of homologous DNA in the transformation vector (homologous recombination). In yeasts such as *S. cerevisiae* most gene targeting is efficient, but in filamentous fungi, targeted integration is inefficient and off-target (ectopic) integration often occurs (see 'Reverse genetics').

Forward genetics by transformation

The availability of transformation tools has modernized forward genetics approaches for genetic dissection. Transformation with foreign DNA such as transposons or 'transferred DNA' (T-DNA) (from an *A. tumefaciens* plasmid) can cause random mutagenesis following insertion into chromosomes. Within a population of transformants, different individuals will have mutations in different genes; thus the population can be screened for phenotypes of interest without any prior assumptions about gene identity. The advantage of this method over classical mutagenesis is that sites of mutation are tagged by the presence of the transforming DNA, allowing for subsequent recovery and characterization of a mutated gene. Mutagenesis by T-DNA tagging has been used to identify candidate virulence genes in dimorphic fungal pathogens (Rappleye and Goldman 2006). Large-scale transposon mutagenesis of the model yeast *Saccharomyces cerevisiae* led to the development of a mutant collection comprising over 3,500 tagged genes, each associated with phenotypic, cellular localization and expression data (Kumar et al. 2002), providing a valuable community resource to explore gene function on a genome scale. Insertional mutagenesis based on restriction-enzyme-mediated insertions, where a linearized plasmid is transformed in the presence of the restriction enzyme used for cutting, has also been applied successfully to filamentous fungi (Bowyer 2001).

Reverse genetics

The ability to mutate or delete specific genes to study their function has led to widespread use of the reverse genetics approach as a tool for genetic dissection. Knowledge of the DNA sequence of a specific gene allows transforming DNA to be designed in such a way that it can affect gene function, such as by deletion (gene knockout) or a reduction in gene expression (silencing) by RNA interference (Kück and Hoff 2010). The most commonly used gene knockout method is to transform the fungus with a recombinant DNA molecule consisting of a selectable marker gene, flanked by DNA from either side of the gene of interest, to guide targeted gene-specific integration by homologous recombination. Such transforming DNA can be constructed in a plasmid vector, or linear DNA fragments can be assembled by PCR (polymerase chain reaction) methodology such as fusion (overlap) PCR (Osmani et al. 2008) or Gibson assembly® (New England Biolabs). The outcome is a replacement of the target gene in the chromosome with the selectable marker gene (Osmani et al. 2008) (Figure 5.5a). Because the recombinant DNA can also integrate at non-target (ectopic) locations in the chromosome, transformants are screened to check for correct integration at the targeted gene. This can be achieved using positional PCR with primers designed to target regions flanking the gene of interest, allowing distinction between wild-type and knockout mutants by size. Southern hybridization is also commonly used to check for 'clean' knockouts that do not have a cryptic additional ectopic integration (Osmani et al. 2008). Once a knockout phenotype has been demonstrated, a functional copy of the gene can be transformed back into the knockout mutant to complement the phenotype; this confirms that the phenotype resulted from the gene knockout and not from other off-target effects (Ashton and Dyer 2016). Using genome sequence data, it has been possible to prepare gene knockout libraries of mutants representative of all the genes in a genome for the yeast *S. cerevisiae* (Scherens and Goffeau 2004) as well as for subsets of genes in the medically important *Candida albicans, Candida glabrata,* and *Cryptococcus neoformans* (Roemer et al. 2003; Noble et al. 2010; Goranov and Madhani 2014; Schwarzmüller et al. 2014). Gene deletion libraries are also available for the filamentous fungus *N. crassa*, and work is ongoing to establish a similar resource for the opportunistic pathogen *Aspergillus fumigatus*.

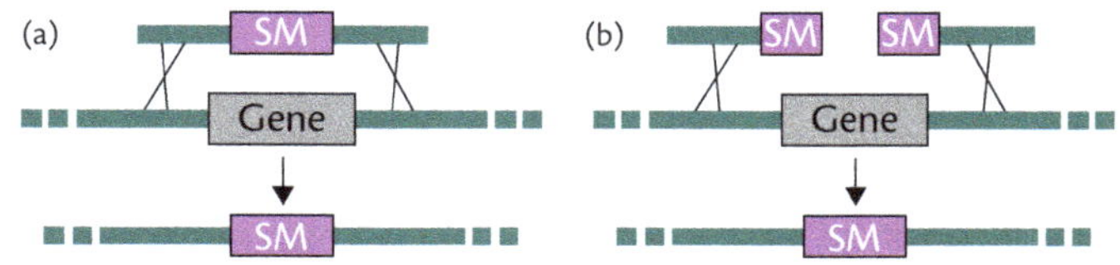

Figure 5.5 Targeted gene knockouts in fungi.

a A selectable marker gene (SM), flanked by DNA matching regions either side of the targeted gene, is transformed into the fungal cell. Recombination with DNA in the chromosome leads to replacement of the target gene with the SM.

b In the split marker method, two overlapping sections of the SM are transformed along with the target gene-matching regions as shown. Most transformants selected on the basis of SM function will be targeted gene knockouts in which recombination has occurred between both sides of the gene, as well as between sections of the SM.

In contrast to a gene knockout, gene silencing does not involve altering the DNA of the gene of interest; instead, double-stranded (ds) RNA molecules corresponding to the gene of interest are expressed in the cells by one of several techniques, leading to a reduction in expression of that gene by the RNA silencing pathway (Kück and Hoff 2010; Cairns et al. 2016). This method is particularly useful when complete deletion of a gene would be lethal, or when there are multiple members of a gene family with functional redundancy, as all members can be targeted by a common dsRNA.

Improving gene targeting

In yeasts such as *S. cerevisiae* and *C. albicans*, homologous recombination leads to efficient gene targeting with even short (<100 base pair, bp) regions of homology with the gene of interest. In contrast, gene targeting is much less efficient in most filamentous fungi because of off-target (ectopic) integration of DNA that occurs in most transformants because of illegitimate recombination by components of the non-homologous end-joining (NHEJ) mechanism, even if larger flanking regions of homology (such as 1,000 bp regions) are included (Krappmann 2007). Many methods have been developed to improve the targeting efficiency in filamentous fungi (Osmani et al. 2008; Kück and Hoff 2010). One is a 'split marker' method in which the two gene-flanking regions used to guide integration are each joined to a truncated fragment of the selectable marker gene; only transformants in which both fragments have integrated adjacent to one another at the correct locus will have a functional complete copy of the selectable marker gene (Figure 5.5b) (Kück and Hoff 2010). Another method involves prior mutation of a gene encoding one of the components of the NHEJ recombination mechanism in the host strain, such as DNA-binding proteins Ku80 and Ku70, or DNA ligase Lig4. In these mutants, the alternative homologous recombination mechanism results in a substantial increase in gene targeting efficiency (Krappmann 2007; Kück and Hoff 2010).

Gene editing technologies

A detailed study of gene function often benefits from the availability of specific types of mutations, such as those that impair function of a specific domain of the encoded protein or confer a different property. The ability to make specific mutations has been revolutionised by the development of new gene editing methods based on the bacterial immune system CRISPR-Cas9 (Doudna and Charpentier 2014). Homing in on the gene of interest by an RNA guide molecule, the Cas9 nuclease induces a double-strand break in the target gene, which can lead to mutations either by error-prone repair or by insertion of a co-transformed marker gene or edited gene. Many variations of this method have been developed (Cairns et al. 2016; Nødvig et al. 2015) and this elegant system has been used successfully to edit specific genes in *A. fumigatus* (Fuller et al. 2015) and *C. albicans* (Vyas et al. 2015). Major benefits of this technology include the ability to make homozygous disruptions in diploids in a single step, as well as multiple gene edits in a single step (Vyas et al. 2015).

Molecular Genetics: Investigating gene products

Inducible expression and overexpression

As well as investigating gene function by knockout, silencing, or mutation, it is valuable to be able to regulate levels of gene expression, even to the extent of overexpressing genes beyond normal levels. Such analyses can provide important information about the functions of the proteins they encode, as well as the interactions of these proteins with other cellular components (Prelich 2012). Inducible gene expression can be achieved by introducing transforming DNA with a gene under the control of promoter elements from genes whose expression can be triggered by external factors such as ethanol (e.g. *alcA*) or an antibiotic (e.g. the Tet-On system) (Osmani et al. 2008). Constitutive gene overexpression can be achieved by placing a gene under the control of promoter elements from strongly expressed housekeeping genes (e.g. *gpd*). Analysis of gene function by overexpression is particularly useful for diploid systems such as *C. albicans* in which knockouts of both copies of a gene pose special challenges (Chauvel et al. 2012; Shahana et al. 2014).

In some cases the protein itself, or the product of a biosynthetic pathway, is the focus of scientific investigation or the basis for a pharmaceutical product. In this case overexpression in heterologous (foreign) host cells such as the yeast *Pichia pastoris* can be used to obtain large amounts of a product (Ahmad et al. 2014). Depending on the product, one or more genes may have to be transformed into the heterologous host using promoters known to work in that host (Anyaogu and Mortensen 2015). Secondary metabolites with immunosuppressive, antibiotic, or other pharmaceutical properties are produced by filamentous fungi, and sets of genes required for their production are often clustered. Transfer of whole sets of genes into the well-characterized heterologous fungal host *Aspergillus oryzae* has allowed the production of specific secondary metabolites in what has been coined a 'synthetic biology' approach (Wiemann and Keller 2014; Anyaogu and Mortensen 2015).

Cellular expression levels and localization

It is often of interest to monitor changes in gene expression under different conditions. Gene transcription can be determined using end-point or real-time reverse transcriptase (RT-) PCR methodology, but does not necessarily represent actual levels of translated proteins. Instead, recombinant DNA constructs can be made with the regulatory promoter region of the target gene driving expression of a reporter gene, such as the green fluorescent protein (GFP) or a colour variant (Oakley and Xiang 2008). After transformation into the fungus, expression of the reporter gene can then be assessed, for example by intensity of fluorescence of GFP, to indicate levels of gene expression.

Fluorescent reporter genes also enable localization of protein gene products within cells or hyphae (Oakley and Xiang 2008). DNA constructs are made where a reporter gene, for example GFP, is fused with the gene to be analyzed and then transformed into the cell. Transcription and translation result in the formation of a hybrid protein that includes the original gene product and the fluorescent GFP moiety. Fluorescent microscopy can then be used to indicate the location of the protein within the cell/hyphae. Classical *in-situ* hybridization methods using labelled antibodies provide an alternative to this approach. Bioluminescent strains of *A. fumigatus* and *C. albicans* have been developed that constitutively express a luciferase gene; these have been used to visualize invasive fungal material in a mouse model (Ibrahim-Granet et al. 2010; Jacobsen et al. 2014). A broad range of other fluorescent reporters with different spectral properties, such as yellow (YFP), cyan (CFP), and a range of red fluorescent protein (RFP) derivatives such as mCherry and DsRed, are also available (Shcherbakova and Verkhusha 2014), along with an increasingly sophisticated set of techniques for tagging proteins and other molecules in cells (Chen et al. 2013).

Protein–protein interactions

Gene products function in complex biological systems, so an important set of tools for determining gene function are those used to determine how proteins interact with other proteins. A large number of increasingly sophisticated genetic methods have been developed to explore these interactions (Phizicky and Fields 1995; Rao et al. 2014; Feng et al. 2015). The most widely used method to determine whether two proteins interact with each other is the yeast two-hybrid system, which involves introducing two recombinant DNA molecules into yeast cells. Genes encoding the two proteins in question ('bait' and 'prey') are fused to sequences encoding yeast transcription factor DNA-binding or activation domains, respectively. When expressed together in yeast cells, if the bait and prey molecules interact with each other, then a functioning transcription factor will form to induce expression of a reporter gene (Feng et al. 2015). This methodology has been adapted for use with *C. albicans* (Stynen et al. 2010). Alternative methods include the addition of one or more affinity tags to the proteins by the creation of recombinant DNA molecules that are introduced into cells, enabling recovery of interacting proteins from the cells by affinity purification (Feng et al. 2015) or use of mass spectrometry to identify the interacting partners.

Conclusion

The use of fungal genetic approaches in medical mycology has, and continues to provide, valuable insights into areas such as the molecular-genetic basis of pathogenicity, resistance to antifungals, and invasive dimorphism. The 'omics' technologies and next-generation sequencing revolutions are impacting greatly on fungal genetic studies, offering new opportunities. For example, changes in gene expression during infection and other developmental processes can be studied using high-throughput sequencing of RNA (RNA-Seq), and genome-wide binding sites of transcription factors controlling gene expression can be identified by chromatin immunoprecipitation sequencing (ChIP-Seq). Such 'omics' approaches will be discussed in Chapter 6. Finally, it is noted that the Fungal Genetics Stock Center (http://www.fgsc.net/) in the USA has become an invaluable repository for fungal genetic resources, with reference stocks of mutant strains of *Aspergillus, Candida, Cryptococcus, Neurospora, Saccharomyces*, and several other fungi available.

Acknowledgements

The authors are funded by grants from the BBSRC, EU, MRC, Wellcome Trust, and Massey University, New Zealand. We thank G. Ashton (University of Nottingham, UK), K.J. Daniels and D.R. Soll (University of Iowa, USA) for providing images.

References

Ahmad M, Hirz M, Pichler H and Schwab H (2014) Protein expression in *Pichia pastoris*: recent achievements and perspectives for heterologous protein production. *Appl Microbiol Biotechnol* 98: 5301–17.

Anyaogu DC and Mortensen UH (2015) Heterologous production of fungal secondary metabolites in *Aspergilli*. *Front Microbiol* 6: 1–6.

Archer DB, MacKenzie DA and Jeenes DJ (2006) Genetic engineering: yeasts and filamentous fungi, *in*: C Ratledge and B Kristiansen, eds, *Basic Biotechnology* (Cambridge: CUP), 119–54.

Ashton G and Dyer PS (2016) Sexual development in fungi and its uses in gene expression systems, *in*: M Schmoll and C Dattenböck, eds, *Gene Expression Systems of Fungi: Applications and Advancements* (Switzerland: Springer International Publishing), 335–50.

Bi X (2014) Heterochromatin structure: lessons from the budding yeast. *IUBMB Life* 66: 657–66.

Bowyer P (2001) DNA-mediated transformation of fungi, *in*: N Talbot, ed., *Molecular and Cellular Biology of Filamentous Fungi* (Oxford: OUP), 33–46.

Brosch G, Loidl P and Graessle S (2008) Histone modifications and chromatin dynamics: a focus on filamentous fungi. *FEMS Microbiol Rev* 32: 409–39.

Burnett J (2003) *Fungal Populations and Species* (Oxford: OUP).

Cairns TC, Studholme DJ, Talbot NJ and Haynes K (2016) New and improved techniques for the study of pathogenic fungi. *Trends Microbiol* 24: 35–50.

Chauvel M, Nesseir A, Cabral V, et al. (2012) A versatile overexpression strategy in the pathogenic yeast *Candida albicans*: identification of regulators of morphogenesis and fitness. *PLoS One* 7: e45912.

Chen Z, Cornish VW and Min W (2013) Chemical tags: inspiration for advanced imaging techniques. *Curr Opin Chem Biol* 17: 637–43.

Coleman JJ, Rounsley SD, Rodriguez-Carres M, et al. (2009) The genome of *Nectria haematococca*: contribution of supernumerary chromosomes to gene expansion. *PLoS Genet* 5: e1000618.

Doudna JA and Charpentier E (2014) The new frontier of genome engineering with CRISPR-Cas9. *Science* 346: 1258096.

Dyer PS, Inderbitzin P and Debuchy R (2016) Mating-type structure, function, regulation and evolution in the Pezizomycotina, *in*: J Wendland, ed., *Growth, Differentiation and Sexuality*, The Mycota I (3rd edn, Switzerland: Springer International Publishing), 351–85.

Feng S, Zhou L, Huang C, Xie K and Nice EC (2015) Interactomics: toward protein function and regulation. *Expert Rev Proteomics* 12: 37–60.

Fincham JR (1989) Transformation in fungi. *Microbiol Rev* 53: 148–70.

Fitzpatrick DA (2012) Horizontal gene transfer in fungi. *FEMS Microbiol Lett* 329: 1–8.

Foulongne-Oriol M (2012) Genetic linkage mapping in fungi: current state, applications, and future trends. *Appl Microbiol Biotechnol* 95: 891–904.

Fuller KK, Chen S, Loros JJ and Dunlap JC (2015) Development of the CRISPR/Cas9 system for targeted gene disruption in *Aspergillus fumigatus*. *Eukaryot Cell* 14: 1073–80.

Goranov AI and Madhani HD (2014) Functional profiling of human fungal pathogen genomes. *Cold Spring Harb Perspect Med* 5: a019596.

Gow NAR (2005) Fungal genomics: forensic evidence of sexual activity. *Curr Biol* 15: R509–11.

Griffiths AJF, Wessler SR, Carroll SB and Doebley J (2015) *An Introduction to Genetic Analysis* (11th edn, New York: W.H. Freeman and Company).

Gurr SJ, Unkles SE and Kinghorn JR (1987) The structure and organization of nuclear genes of filamentous fungi, *in*: JR Kinghorn, ed., *Gene Structure in Eukaryotic Microbes* (Oxford: IRL Press), 93–99.

Harris SD (2001). Genetic analysis of ascomycete fungi, *in*: N Talbot, ed., *Molecular and Cellular Biology of Filamentous Fungi* (Oxford: OUP), 47–58.

Heitman J, Carter DA, Dyer PS and Soll DR (2014) Sexual reproduction of human fungal pathogens. *Cold Spring Harb Perspect Med* 4: a019281.

Hood HM, Neafsey DE, Galagan J and Sachs MS (2009) Evolutionary roles of upstream open reading frames in mediating gene regulation in fungi. *Annu Rev Microbiol* 63: 385–409.

Houbraken J and Dyer PS (2015) Induction of the sexual cycle in filamentous ascomycetes, *in*: M van den Berg and K Maruthachalam, eds, *Genetic Transformation Systems in Fungi*, 2: Fungal Biology (Switzerland: Springer International Publishing), 23–46.

Ibrahim-Granet O, Jouvion G, Hohl TM, et al. (2010) In vivo bioluminescence imaging and histopathopathologic analysis reveal distinct roles for resident and recruited immune effector cells in defense against invasive aspergillosis. *BMC Microbiol* 10: 105.

Irelan JT and Selker EU (1996) Gene silencing in filamentous fungi: RIP, MIP and quelling. *J Genet* 75: 313–24.

Jacobsen ID, Lüttich A, Kurzai O, Hube B and Brock M (2014) *In vivo* imaging of disseminated murine *Candida albicans* infection reveals unexpected host sites of fungal persistence during antifungal therapy. *J Antimicrob Chemother* 69: 2785–96.

Krappmann S (2007) Gene targeting in filamentous fungi: the benefits of impaired repair. *Fungal Biol Rev* 21: 25–9.

Kück U and Hoff B (2010) New tools for the genetic manipulation of filamentous fungi. *Appl Microbiol Biotechnol* 86: 51–62.

Kumar A, Cheung KH, Tosches N, et al. (2002) The TRIPLES database: a community resource for yeast molecular biology. *Nucleic Acids Res* 30: 73–5.

Michielse CB, Hooykaas PJ, van den Hondel CA and Ram AF (2005) *Agrobacterium*-mediated transformation as a tool for functional genomics in fungi. *Curr Genet* 48: 1–17.

Miranda I, Silva R and Santos MA (2006) Evolution of the genetic code in yeasts. *Yeast* 23: 203–13.

Mohanta TK and Bae H (2015) The diversity of fungal genome. *Biol Proced Online* 17: 8.

Moore D and Novak Frazer LAN (2002) *Essential Fungal Genetics* (New York: Springer).

Noble SM, French S, Kohn LA, Chen V and Johnson AD (2010) Systematic screens of a *Candida albicans* homozygous deletion library decouple morphogenetic switching and pathogenicity. *Nat Genet* 42: 590–8.

Nødvig CS, Nielsen JB, Kogle ME and Mortensen UH (2015) A CRISPR-Cas9 system for genetic engineering of filamentous fungi. *PloS One* 10: e0133085.

Oakley BR and Xiang X (2008) Fluorescent labels for intracellular structures and organelles, *in*: GH Goldman and SA Osmani, eds, *The Aspergilli. Genomics, Medical Aspects, Biotechnology and Research Methods* (Boca Raton: CRC Press), 513–25.

O'Gorman CM, Fuller HT and Dyer PS (2009) Discovery of a sexual cycle in the opportunistic fungal pathogen *Aspergillus fumigatus*. *Nature* 457: 471–74.

Osmani SA, Liu H-L, Hynes MJ and Oakley BR (2008) Advances in gene manipulations using *Aspergillus nidulans*, in: GH Goldman and SA

Osmani, eds, *The Aspergilli. Genomics, Medical Aspects, Biotechnology and Research Methods* (Boca Raton: CRC Press) 493–511.

Peberdy JF (1979) Fungal protoplasts: isolation, reversion, and fusion. *Annu Rev Microbiol* 33: 21–39.

Phizicky EM and Fields S (1995) Protein-protein interactions: methods for detection and analysis. *Microbiol Rev* 59: 94–123.

Prelich G (2012) Gene overexpression: uses, mechanisms, and interpretation. *Genetics* 190: 841–54.

Rao VS, Srinivas K, Sujini GN and Kumar GN (2014) Protein-protein interaction detection: methods and analysis. *Int J Proteomics* 2014: 147648.

Rappleye CA and Goldman WE (2006) Defining virulence genes in the dimorphic fungi. *Annu Rev Microbiol* 60: 281–303.

Riach MBR and Kinghorn JR (1996) Genetic transformation and vector developments in filamentous fungi, *in* CJ Bos, ed., *Fungal Genetics: Principles and Practice* (New York: Marcel Dekker), 209–34.

Roemer T, Jiang B, Davison J, et al. (2003) Large-scale essential gene identification in *Candida albicans* and applications to antifungal drug discovery. *Mol Microbiol* 50: 167–81.

Scherens B and Goffeau A (2004) The uses of genome-wide yeast mutant collections. *Genome Biol* 5: 229.

Schwarzmüller T, Ma B, Hiller E, et al. (2014) Systematic phenotyping of a large-scale *Candida glabrata* deletion collection reveals novel antifungal tolerance genes. *PLoS Pathog* 10: e1004211.

Shahana S, Childers DS, Ballou ER, et al. (2014) New Clox systems for rapid and efficient gene disruption in *Candida albicans*. *PLoS One* 9: e100390.

Shcherbakova DM and Verkhusha VV (2014) Chromophore chemistry of fluorescent proteins controlled by light. *Curr Opin Chem Biol* 20: 60–8.

Snustad DP and Simmons MJ (2010) *Principles of Genetics* (5th edn, Asia: John Wiley).

Stynen B, Van Dijck P and Tournu H (2010) A CUG codon adapted two-hybrid system for the pathogenic fungus *Candida albicans*. *Nucleic Acids Res* 38: e184.

Swilaiman SS, O'Gorman CM, Balajee SA and Dyer PS (2013) Discovery of a sexual cycle in *Aspergillus lentulus*, a close relative of *A. fumigatus*. *Eukaryot Cell* 12: 962–9.

Vyas VK, Barrasa MI and Fink GR (2015) A *Candida albicans* CRISPR system permits genetic engineering of essential genes and gene families. *Sci Adv* 1: e1500248.

Wickner RB, Shewmaker FP, Bateman DA, et al. (2015) Yeast prions: structure, biology, and prion-handling systems. *Microbiol Mol Biol Rev* 79: 1–17.

Wiemann P and Keller NP (2014) Strategies for mining fungal natural products. *J Ind Microbiol Biotechnol* 41: 301–13.

Zhan J and McDonald BA (2005) Analytical and experimental methods for estimating population genetic structure of fungi, *in*: J Dighton, JF White and P Oudemans, eds, *The Fungal Community: Its organization and role in the ecosystem* (Boca Raton: Taylor and Francis), 241–63.

CHAPTER 6

Fungal genomics and transcriptomics

Carol A. Munro and Duncan Wilson

Introduction to fungal genomics

Sequencing of fungal genomes over the last decade has provided a wealth of information regarding the genetic blueprints of different species. The yeast *Saccharomyces cerevisiae* was the first eukaryote to have its genome sequenced, and still remains a widely used reference genome (Goffeau et al. 1996). Genome sequences are openly available at a number of curated websites, providing researchers with sequences (DNA, intergenic and coding sequences, and predicted protein) and chromosomal position of genes, as well as information on predicted or proven gene function and the accompanying literature. Tools are also available to identify genes that are similar to each other using alignment software, and to allow searches to be performed on short sequences of bases. One example is the *Candida* Genome Database (http://www.candidagenome.org/) (Inglis et al. 2012). *C. albicans* was the first *Candida* species to have its genome sequenced (Braun et al. 2005), and this information provided insights into the differences in the genetic repertoire of a human pathogen versus the largely benign yeast *S. cerevisiae*. Researchers are investigating how these genetic differences confer diverse phenotypic attributes to different fungal species. The genome sequence information provides clues as to how the fungi have evolved to survive in different habitats: one in the environment—on trees and grapes—and the other on the mucosal surfaces and gastrointestinal tract of humans.

Comparative genomics of fungal pathogens

Genome sequences are available for the species that occupy the CTG clade of the fungal tree of life, species that are mostly related to *C. albicans* (Butler et al. 2009). This clade, which, in the vast majority of cases, translates the CTG codon as serine rather than leucine, includes species with a range of abilities to cause infection in susceptible hosts, as well as the halo-tolerant marine species *Debaryomyces hansenii,* which is a rare pathogen. Elucidation of the genome sequences of these species identified large variations in their overall genome sizes and variability in the composition of gene families, with the most successful pathogens having larger gene families encoding cell wall associated proteins, transporters, and secreted proteins (Butler et al. 2009). It is also important to note that the variation in genome sequences resulting in altered virulence profiles is not the entire story. It has become clear that the most successful pathogen, *C. albicans*, has a highly flexible genome, with genome rearrangements conferring important virulence-related attributes such as drug resistance (Selmecki et al. 2006; Selmecki et al. 2010; Hirakawa et al. 2015). This topic—as well as the contribution of loss of heterozygosity to fitness of a diploid organism such as *C. albicans* (Forche et al. 2011)—will not be covered in this chapter.

Genome sequence information is also available for the major filamentous fungal pathogen *Aspergillus fumigatus* within the database FungiDB (http://fungidb.org/fungidb/) (Fedorova et al. 2008). Sequencing of the genomes of the related species *Neosartorya fischeri* and *Aspergillus clavatus*, which are rare pathogens, highlighted genes that were unique to each species and identified gene clusters that function in the production of, for example, secondary metabolites. The *A. fumigatus*-specific subset of genes has been found to be enriched in genes related to transport, secondary metabolite production, and chitin and carbohydrate metabolism.

The third major group of fungal pathogenic species to be considered here are *Cryptococcus* species, members of the basidiomycetes. These include *Cryptococcus neoformans* (with two serotypes, A and D), represented as two varieties—var. *grubii* and var. *neoformans,* respectively—which cause cryptococcal meningitis in immunocompromised species, and *Cryptococcus gattii*, which was responsible for the Vancouver Island outbreak that began in 1999 and affected healthy individuals. The genomes of both *C. neoformans* varieties are available (Loftus et al. 2005; Janbon et al. 2014). Of particular interest has been the comparison of the genome sequences of a *C. gattii* strain, responsible for infections in immunocompetent hosts, in western North America, and the more typical global *C. gattii* strain (D'Souza et al. 2011). Chromosomal arrangements of the two strains were similar and co-linear, but extensive differences were found at the sequence level, making it difficult to pinpoint the traits that altered the virulence of the two strains towards immunocompetent individuals. A recurring theme when comparing isolates of the same species has been altered ploidy and chromosomal copy number, indicating that large genome variations exist within the same species, as observed with *C. albicans*. Comparative genome analysis of three *Pneumocystis* species—intracellular obligate lung pathogens—with fission yeast *Schizosaccharomyces pombe* has also shed light on important differences, suggesting that these *Pneumocystis* species are inositol auxotrophs that need to acquire exogenous inositol from their mammalian hosts (Porollo et al. 2014).

Table 6.1 Fungal pathogen mutant libraries

Species	Mutant library description	Reference
Candida albicans	Tn homozygous insertion mutants	Davis et al. 2002
	Haploinsufficiency	Uhl et al. 2003; Oh et al. 2010
	Tet-Off conditional gene depletion	Roemer et al. 2003
	Null mutants	Noble et al. 2010
	Transcription factor null mutants	Homann et al. 2009; Vandeputte et al. 2011
	Tet-On conditional overexpression	Cabral et al. 2014
Candida glabrata	Null mutants	Schwarzmuller et al. 2014
Cryptococcus neoformans	Insertional and replacement mutants	Ianiri and Idnurm 2015
	Transcription factor gene deletions	Jung et al. 2015
	Gene knockout mutants	Liu et al. 2008
	Signature tagged mutagenesis	Nelson et al. 2001
Aspergillus fumigatus	Conditional promoter replacement	Hu et al. 2007
	Transposon insertion	Firon et al. 2003
	Signature-tagged mutagenesis	Brown et al. 2000

The wealth of genome sequencing information has highlighted important inter- and intra-species (Hirakawa et al. 2015) differences based on predicted functions of the divergent sequences. This knowledge has provided insights that have enabled researchers to formulate new hypotheses regarding the relevance of specific genetic features to fungal pathogenicity. Experimental investigations to prove or disprove these hypotheses are dependent upon the ability to genetically manipulate fungi in order to determine gene functions. In recent decades, significant advances have been made in fungal functional genomics, but we are still lacking genome-wide libraries of mutants to facilitate high-throughput phenotyping in order to assign functions to gene products. A number of partial mutant libraries do exist for *Candida albicans, Candida glabrata, Aspergillus fumigatus*, and *Cryptococcus neoformans* (Table 6.1) and have been utilized in a number of informative screening procedures.

Mutant libraries

Access to mutant libraries has facilitated high-throughput screening assays of individual mutants to test, for example, for morphogenesis (Uhl et al. 2003; O'Meara et al. 2015) and strain fitness under different growth conditions (Homann et al. 2009), in the presence of different stressing agents including antifungal drugs (Schwarzmuller et al. 2014) and novel compounds (Oh et al. 2010; Brown et al. 2014). Current approaches use mutant strains that carry individual, unique molecular barcodes which enable pools of mutants to be assessed at the same time. Abundance of strains within the pools can be quantified by hybridizing to DNA microarrays, but more recently a next-generation sequencing approach, so-called 'Bar-seq', has been used. This approach has been used with *C. albicans* to assess biofilm formation (Cabral et al. 2014) and virulence in mice systemic infection models, and in the mini-host *Galleria mellonella* (Becker et al. 2010; Noble et al. 2010; Amorim-Vaz et al. 2015). These library screens are not only providing valuable insights into factors that are important for fungal pathogenesis, stress resistance, and host interactions, but are also improving the annotation of fungal genomes by assigning functions to uncharacterized ORFan genes.

Essential genes of *A. fumigatus* (Hu et al. 2007; Firon et al. 2003), *C. albicans* (Roemer et al. 2003), and *C. neoformans* (Ianiri and Idnurm 2015) have also been identified in mutant library screens. Approaches include using collections of strains, with each strain carrying a specific gene placed under the control of a regulatable promoter, or making use of parasexual genetics or meiosis and sporulation. Essential genes that are fungal-specific or sufficiently different to their mammalian counterparts provide potential targets for the development of antifungal drugs. Therefore, the construction of mutant libraries is also facilitating antifungal drug development.

Application of sequencing technologies

The advent of advanced sequencing technologies has provided researchers with the ability to rapidly sequence the genomes of strains under investigation in a cost-effective manner. This has greatly helped evolution studies and allowed researchers to track individual genetic changes in the genomes of fungi that have evolved in certain environments. Two such examples are the identification of new mutations conferring echinocandin drug resistance in *Candida glabrata* by sequencing sequential isolates from the same patient (Singh-Babak et al. 2012), and the identification of a single nucleotide change which results in the restoration of filamentous growth in a non-filamentous mutant that has evolved in the macrophage environment (Wartenberg et al. 2014).

Sequencing approaches used for metagenomics (the investigation of microbial DNA recovered directly from environmental samples) have also been applied to the study of the human mycobiome. This is a burgeoning and rapidly advancing field, with studies investigating the mycobiome of the lung (Nguyen et al. 2015), gastrointestinal tract (Tang et al. 2015), oral cavity (Mukherjee et al. 2014), and skin (Findley et al. 2013).

Transcriptomics

Following the genome, the transcriptome represents the next level of hierarchical complexity in a fungal cell. Transcriptomics describes investigation of the total RNA transcript content of a cell under a particular environmental condition, time, or developmental stage. Unlike the genome, which is relatively static within the timeframe of most laboratory experiments, the transcriptome is highly dynamic, and the expression levels of many genes are rapidly upregulated or repressed in response to exogenous or endogenous signals. In the context of human fungal pathogens, transcriptomics has mainly been applied to the measurement of global changes in gene expression in response to specific environmental conditions, or to investigating adaptation to infection-mimicking conditions, either *in vitro, ex vivo*, or *in vivo*.

The transcriptome of a fungal cell can be measured using a variety of technologies. More recently, RNA-sequencing (RNA-seq) technologies have become popular owing to their sensitivity and capacity to quantify most of the RNA species within a cell, and have already been applied to the study of gene expression in pathogenic fungi (e.g. in the study by Bruno et al. 2010). RNA-seq offers a number of advantages, such as the ability to detect novel transcripts and splicing events (Wang et al. 2010). RNA-seq is also well-suited to the simultaneous determination of the transcriptional response of multiple species, and can be used to measure co-culture-dependent changes in gene expression of both the fungal pathogen and its host during their interactions (Tierney et al. 2012; Liu et al. 2015).

NanoString is another recent technology which has been applied to the study of *C. albicans* biology. The NanoString platform is extremely sensitive as it directly measures individual RNA molecules. However, the number of target genes under investigation is limited and must be selected during the experimental design, and thus (current) NanoString datasets do not represent unbiased transcriptomics. Nevertheless, a series of recent studies from The Mitchell Group have successfully used the NanoString platform to probe the transcriptional responses of *C. albicans* during *in vivo* infections (Finkel et al. 2012; Xu et al. 2015).

Whilst improvements in transcriptomics technology, such as RNA-seq, continue, at the time of publication, studies using microarray hybridization technology have dominated the exploration of fungal transcriptomes. Earlier investigations focused on the response of human fungal pathogens to distinct laboratory growth conditions, such as changes in pH, the presence of antifungal drugs, or other environmental stimuli. These pioneering studies yielded a wealth of data on the transcriptional response of fungi to these environments, identifying genes and transcriptional signatures associated with the condition of interest. One early such example is the study conducted by Barker and co-workers, where *C. albicans* cells were exposed to increasing concentrations of the antifungal drug amphotericin B, resulting in enhanced drug tolerance, and then, using genome-wide microarray analysis, transcriptional upregulation of multiple genes involved in the ergosterol biosynthetic pathway was identified (Barker et al. 2004).

Transcriptomics to study host–pathogen interactions

From the perspective of medical mycology, the application of transcriptomics to the study of fungal pathogens during interactions with host cells or tissues has provided unparalleled insight into the processes that occur during fungal infections. This is because the

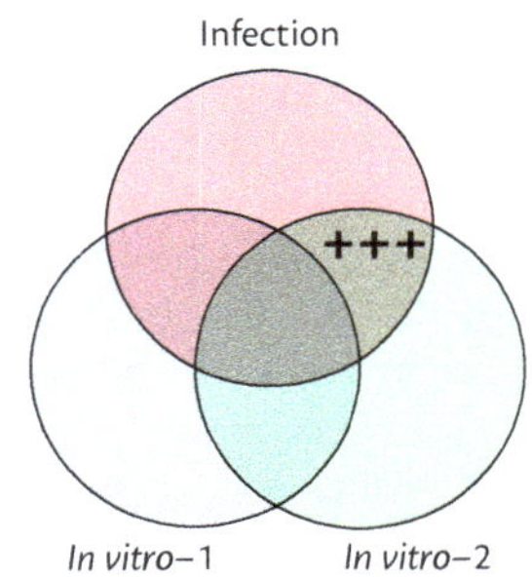

Figure 6.1 Principle of using the fungal transcriptome as a signature to probe the nature of an infected niche. By comparing the transcriptional response of an infecting fungal pathogen to the transcriptome under defined *in vitro* conditions, researchers can use the biological output of the microbe (i.e. the transcriptome) to gain insight into the nature of the infected niche.

actual physical and chemical environment which fungal pathogens encounter during infection is often difficult to measure. That is, although the physiology of particular anatomical sites may be well understood under conditions of homeostasis, the disease state and presence of the infecting fungus can have a major impact on local physiology. For example, fungi can modify the chemical environment of infected host niches via the action of secreted hydrolytic enzymes.

By utilizing marker genes (i.e. a transcriptional signature which reflects a particular environmental condition), the transcriptome of the infecting fungi can be used as a biological probe, or 'fingerprint', to investigate the physiological properties of the microenvironment of interest (Figure 6.1). In this section, case studies are provided where such 'transcriptomic detective work' has been employed to gain greater insight into the nature of the infected host niche and the biology of the infecting fungus.

Lorenz et al. (2004) used microarray analysis to probe the response of *C. albicans* to macrophage phagocytosis. The authors found that, within this type of immune cell, *C. albicans* upregulated multiple genes associated with alternative carbon metabolism, including isocitrate lyase and malate synthase, indicating that *C. albicans* cells within macrophages face acute carbon starvation. Rubin-Bejerano et al. (2003) used a similar approach to study the response of *C. albicans* to neutrophils, this time identifying wholesale upregulation of arginine and methionine biosynthetic pathways following phagocytosis. Whilst these are excellent examples of transcriptomics yielding biological insight into the fate of phagocytosed fungi, conserved processes such as alternative carbon metabolism and amino acid biosynthesis are relatively simple to identify because the associated genes can be easily inferred by comparative genomics (i.e. by sequence similarity with model organisms, such as *S. cerevisiae*). But what about situations where the transcriptional signature of a fungus to a particular environment is not known?

McDonagh et al. (2008) used an integrated transcriptomic approach to dissect the environmental conditions faced by *A. fumigatus* during adaptation to pulmonary aspergillosis. Here, the authors defined the transcriptome of *A. fumigatus* during growth in the mouse lung and directly compared that transcriptional signature to that of fungi adapting to multiple defined *in vitro* conditions, including iron limitation, oxidative stress, alkaline *vs* acidic pH, and nitrogen starvation. By then directly comparing the sets of genes induced *in vivo* with the different *in vitro* conditions, the authors were able to conclude that the dominant environmental stimulus faced by *A. fumigatus* during the initial stages of infection was an adaptation to alkaline pH. Such an *in vitro*/*in vivo* approach is particularly powerful, as many genes which are differentially regulated during infection by pathogenic fungi are uncharacterized, or of unknown function (Wilson et al. 2009). By utilizing comparative transcriptomics such as this, even the expression of unknown function genes can, in principle, be employed to probe infection-relevant conditions (Figure 6.1).

Transcriptional regulatory networks

Another powerful application of global expression profiling is the identification of transcription factor targets and transcriptional networks. In this context, the transcriptome of a transcription factor deletion mutant is simply compared with that of the parental wild-type strain, typically under relevant environmental conditions. The resulting sets of differentially expressed genes then indicate potential regulatory targets of the transcription factor in question—that is, genes which are upregulated in the wild-type strain, but not the transcription factor mutant, can be inferred to be positively regulated by the transcription factor in question, under the conditions tested (Figure 6.2).

An excellent example of such an approach was the study conducted by Bensen et al. (2004), who investigated the role of *C. albicans* Rim101 in fungal pH adaptation (*RIM101* encodes the master regulator of pH responsiveness in fungi). As *C. albicans* is capable of infecting niches of widely varying pH, from the acidic environment of the vaginal mucosa to the neutral-alkaline pH of the bloodstream and internal organs such as the liver, the ability to respond appropriately to changes in local pH is critical for pathogenicity. In fact, coordinated adaptation to local pH appears to be essential for the pathogenicity of many, if not all, human fungal pathogens.

In this study, Bensen et al. used microarrays to measure the relative gene expression in wild-type and *rim101Δ* cells at both pH 4 and pH 8. The authors found little difference in the transcriptional regulons of wild-type and *rim101Δ* at acidic pH, but a large number of differentially expressed genes at pH 8. These included a group of genes (such as *PHR2*) which were alkaline-downregulated in the wild type, but upregulated in *rim101Δ*, and another group of genes which were alkaline-upregulated in the wild type, but exhibited reduced expression in *rim101Δ*. From these types of observations, the authors could conclude that Rim101 exerts very little regulatory influence in acidic environments, and that, in response to alkaline pH, Rim101 simultaneously represses the

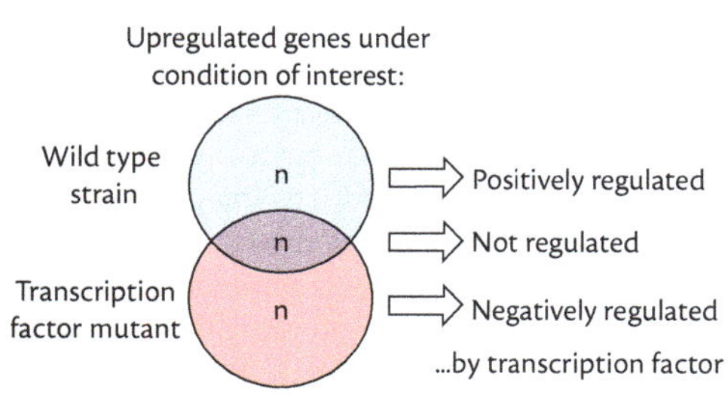

Figure 6.2 Utilising transcriptomics to identify transcription factor target genes. By comparing the transcriptomes of wild-type and transcription factor mutant strains, it is possible to infer potential targets of the transcriptional regulator in question.

expression of acidic-expressed genes and induces the expression of alkaline-expressed genes.

A novel finding of this study was that Rim101 was required for the alkaline-induced expression of numerous genes involved in high-affinity iron assimilation. So the authors went on to examine the growth behaviour of the *rim101Δ* mutant under conditions of iron depletion. In line with their observed transcriptomic data, they found that *rim101Δ* grew close to wild-type levels under iron depletion at acidic pH, but did not grow under simultaneous iron depletion and alkaline pH: an excellent example of translating global transcriptomic observations to the novel functionality of an important transcription factor in a pathogenic fungus.

One limitation of studies such as this is that they do not demonstrate a direct link between the transcription factor of interest and their presumed target genes. That is, alterations in gene expression in a transcription factor mutant may be due to secondary effects (compare Figure 6.3a and b). However, several of the predicted Rim101 target genes were found to contain Rim101 binding consensus sequences in their promoters, indicative of direct regulation.

Combining transcriptomics with chromatin immunoprecipitation in order to directly link transcription factor activity (gene activation/repression) to function (DNA binding), simply measuring changes in gene expression between wild-type fungi and transcription factor mutants, is insufficient (see, for example, Figure 6.3). To overcome this issue, the study by Nobile et al. (2009) combined expression profiling with full-genome chromatin immunoprecipitation. These authors were interested in exploring the transcriptional control of extracellular matrix production within *C. albicans* biofilms. They identified a transcription factor deletion mutant (*zap1Δ*) which produced elevated levels of the biofilm extracellular material β-glucan.

To identify potential Zap1 targets, they first performed microarray analysis of *C. albicans* wild type *vs* the *zap1Δ* mutant growing under biofilm conditions. They identified 232 upregulated genes in the *zap1Δ* mutant and 272 downregulated genes (including genes involved in zinc uptake), representing Zap1-repressed and -induced genes, respectively. They then used full-genome chromatin immunoprecipitation to directly assess the capacity of the transcription factor (Zap1) to bind to the promoter regions of potential target genes. This technology is based on tagging the protein of interest (in this case the transcription factor), followed by expression within the cell. The transcription factor will bind to the promoter regions of its target genes under the relevant conditions and is then artificially crosslinked to the DNA. Following antibody-mediated pull down (immunoprecipitation) of the transcription factor, the associated DNA can be sequenced to identify which promoter regions are directly bound by the transcription factor.

Using full-genome chromatin immunoprecipitation, Nobile et al. went on to show that Zap1 directly binds to the promoters of several genes which were downregulated in the *zap1Δ* compared with the wild type; these included the zinc transporters *ZRT1*, *ZRT2*, and *ZRT3*. Therefore, by measuring both expression profiles (microarrays) and DNA-binding activity (immunoprecipitation), the authors were able to provide compelling evidence that Zap1 acts as a direct activator of genes involved in zinc uptake in *C. albicans*. In contrast, those genes which were more highly expressed in the *zap1Δ* mutant compared with the wild type ('Zap1-repressed genes') did not exhibit direct Zap1 binding to their promoter regions, indicating that Zap1 repression may be indirect

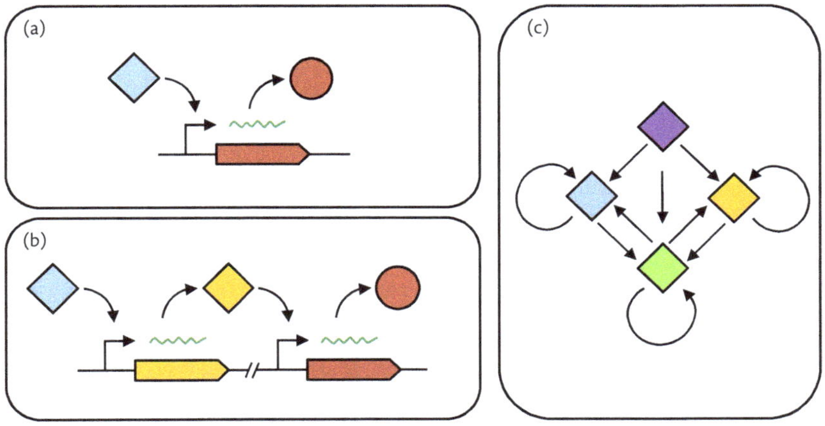

Figure 6.3 Increasing complexity in transcriptional networks. Diamonds represent transcriptional regulators, and circles represent target genes.

a A simple transcriptional circuit where the transcription factor of interest directly regulates the target gene; here, comparing the regulons of wild type *vs* transcription factor mutant strains would identify the target gene (see Figure 6.2).

b The transcription factor of interest regulates expression of a second transcription factor, which regulates a target gene; here, transcriptomics alone might suggest that the primary transcription factor regulates the target gene, but chromatin immunoprecipitation would reveal that the primary transcription factor does not directly bind the promoter of the target gene.

c A tightly knit regulatory circuit here, multiple transcription factors regulate their own, and each others' expression, and different transcription factors within the circuit may regulate the expression of the same targets. This complex form of regulation appears to dominate during *C. albicans* growth within a mammalian host (Pérez and Johnson 2013).

c Adapted courtesy of J. Christian Pérez.

(for example, via the regulation of another transcriptional regulator—compare Figure 6.3a and b).

Such combined 'omics' approaches represent powerful methods for dissecting fungal biology and have been applied to the study of how transcription factors interact and form regulatory networks. It is becoming increasingly apparent that transcriptional regulation within the cell is far more complex than the simple unidirectional events illustrated in Figure 6.3a and b *vs* Figure 6.3c (Pérez and Johnson 2013). A recent study by Pérez et al. (2013) used a combination of transcription factor mutant phenotypic analysis and genome-wide chromatin immunoprecipitation to explore the transcriptional networks operating during *C. albicans* colonization and infection. The authors first screened the library of transcriptional regulator mutants for their ability to colonize the gastrointestinal tracts (commensalism) and kidneys (systemic candidiasis) of mice. They identified three sets of transcriptional regulator-encoding genes: those required for gastrointestinal colonization (orf19.3625, *LYS144*, and *TYE7*); those required for systemic candidiasis (*ZCF21* [*zcf21Δ* also displayed a moderate defect in gastrointestinal colonization] and *LYS14*); and a set of genes which were required for both kidney and gastrointestinal colonization (*RTG1*, *RTG3*, and *HMS1*). Next, they used chromatin immunoprecipitation to identify the intergenic regions of DNA bound by the different transcription factors.

What they found was interesting. Many target gene promoters were bound by more than one transcriptional regulator (including the promoter regions of the transcriptional regulators themselves), and there was no obvious segregation in target gene binding and transcriptional regulator function. For example, although *LYS14* was solely required for systemic infection, and *LYS144* for gastrointestinal colonization, the transcription factors bound several shared target genes. This suggests that the regulatory network governing *C. albicans* commensalism is related to that controlling systemic candidiasis.

Next, the authors compared those genes that were targeted by the transcriptional regulators (which were required for mouse colonisation) with a whole genome transcriptomic dataset of genes upregulated during colonization of the mouse gastrointestinal tract (Rosenbach et al. 2010). Reassuringly, they found a highly significant overlap in the targets of the transcriptional regulators required for mouse colonization and those genes which were transcriptionally upregulated during mouse gastrointestinal colonization. Finally, the authors selected a subgroup of genes which were both transcriptional regulator targets (as defined by chromatin immunoprecipitation) and upregulated during colonization (as defined by genome-wide microarray transcriptomics), deleted the genes in *C. albicans*, and assessed the ability of the resultant mutants to colonize the gastrointestinal tracts of mice. Of the tested mutants, 20% (3/15) exhibited a strongly reduced colonization potential. Therefore, the simultaneous use of multiple 'omics' technologies to study the biology of *C. albicans* during growth within a host represents an extremely powerful approach: from *in vivo* screening of a transcription factor mutant library, immunoprecipitation-based identification of direct transcription factor–DNA interactions, and transcriptomics, to final validation of target gene function via the functional analysis of identified genes.

Summary

In this chapter we provide an overview of the impact of global genome-wide DNA and RNA studies and how they have advanced our knowledge and understanding of fungal pathogenesis. Investigations can now encompass the entire or partial genome, resulting in much more detailed, in-depth, holistic analyses of fungal biology that would have taken decades to achieve if genes were analyzed and studied one at a time. As technologies advance and become miniaturized, cheaper, and more accessible, and applicable to single cells, these 'omics' approaches will continue to provide important insights in the field of medical mycology. Ultimately, this knowledge can be applied to improving diagnostics relating to invading pathogens and improving therapeutics to combat these life-threatening infections.

Acknowledgements

The authors are funded by grants from The Wellcome Trust, BBSRC, and MRC.

References

Amorim-Vaz S, Delarze E, Ischer F, Sanglard D and Coste AT (2015) Examining the virulence of *Candida albicans* transcription factor mutants using *Galleria mellonella* and mouse infection models. *Front Microbiol* 6: 367.

Barker KS, Crisp S, Wiederhold N, et al. (2004) Genome-wide expression profiling reveals genes associated with amphotericin B and fluconazole resistance in experimentally induced antifungal resistant isolates of *Candida albicans*. *J Antimicrob Chemother* 54: 376–85.

Becker JM, Kauffman DJ, Hauser M, et al. (2010) Pathway analysis of *Candida albicans* survival and virulence determinants in a murine infection model. *Proc Natl Acad Sci U S A* 107: 22044–9.

Bensen ES, Martin SJ, Li M, Berman J and Davis DA (2004) Transcriptional profiling in *Candida albicans* reveals new adaptive responses to extracellular pH and functions for Rim101p. *Mol Microbiol* 54: 1335–51.

Braun BR, Van Het Hoog M, D'Enfert C, et al. (2005) A human-curated annotation of the *Candida albicans* genome. *PLoS Genet* 1: 36–57.

Brown JC, Nelson J, Vandersluis B, et al. (2014) Unraveling the biology of a fungal meningitis pathogen using chemical genetics. *Cell* 159: 1168–87.

Brown JS, Aufauvre-Brown A, Brown J, et al. (2000) Signature-tagged and directed mutagenesis identify PABA synthetase as essential for Aspergillus fumigatus pathogenicity. *Mol Microbio* 36: 1371–80.

Bruno VM, Wang Z, Marjani SL, et al. (2010) Comprehensive annotation of the transcriptome of the human fungal pathogen *Candida albicans* using RNA-seq. *Genome Res* 20: 1451–8.

Butler G, Rasmussen MD, Lin MF, et al. (2009) Evolution of pathogenicity and sexual reproduction in eight *Candida genomes*. *Nature* 459: 657–62.

Cabral V, Znaidi S, Walker LA, et al. (2014) Targeted changes of the cell wall proteome influence *Candida albicans* ability to form single- and multi-strain biofilms. *PLoS Pathog* 10: e1004542.

Davis DA, Bruno VM, Loza L, Filler SG and Mitchell AP (2002) Candida albicans Mds3p, a conserved regulator of pH responses and virulence identified through insertional mutagenesis. *Genetics* 162: 1573–81.

D'Souza CA, Kronstad JW, Taylor G, et al. (2011) Genome variation in *Cryptococcus gattii*, an emerging pathogen of immunocompetent hosts. *MBio* 2: e00342-10.

Fedorova ND, Khaldi N, Joardar VS, et al. (2008) Genomic islands in the pathogenic filamentous fungus *Aspergillus fumigatus*. *PLoS Genet* 4: e1000046.

Findley K, Oh J, Yang J, et al. (2013) Topographic diversity of fungal and bacterial communities in human skin. *Nature* 498: 367–70.

Finkel JS, Xu W, Huang D, et al. (2012) Portrait of *Candida albicans* adherence regulators. *PLoS Pathog* 8: e1002525.

Firon A, Villalba F, Beffa R and D'Enfert C (2003) Identification of essential genes in the human fungal pathogen *Aspergillus fumigatus* by transposon mutagenesis. *Eukaryot Cell* 2: 247–55.

Forche A, Abbey D, Pisithkul T, et al. (2011) Stress alters rates and types of loss of heterozygosity in *Candida albicans*. *MBio* 2: e00129-11.

Goffeau A, Barrell BG, Bussey H, et al. (1996) Life with 6000 genes. *Science* 274: 546, 563–7.

Hirakawa MP, Martinez DA, Sakthikumar S, et al. (2015) Genetic and phenotypic intra-species variation in *Candida albicans*. *Genome Res* 25: 413–25.

Homann OR, Dea J, Noble SM and Johnson AD (2009) A phenotypic profile of the *Candida albicans* regulatory network. *PLoS Genet* 5: e1000783.

Hu W, Sillaots S, Lemieux S, et al. (2007) Essential gene identification and drug target prioritization in *Aspergillus fumigatus*. *PLoS Pathog* 3: e24.

Ianiri G and Idnurm A (2015) Essential gene discovery in the basidiomycete *Cryptococcus neoformans* for antifungal drug target prioritization. *MBio* 6: e02334-14.

Inglis DO, Arnaud MB, Binkley J, et al. (2012) The *Candida* genome database incorporates multiple *Candida* species: multispecies search and analysis tools with curated gene and protein information for *Candida albicans* and *Candida glabrata*. *Nucleic Acids Res* 40: D667–74.

Janbon G, Ormerod KL, Paulet D, et al. (2014) Analysis of the genome and transcriptome of *Cryptococcus neoformans* var. *grubii* reveals complex RNA expression and microevolution leading to virulence attenuation. *PLoS Genet* 10: e1004261.

Jung KW, Yang DH, Maeng S, et al. (2015) Systematic functional profiling of transcription factor networks in Cryptococcus neoformans. *Nat Commun* 6: 6757.

Liu OW, Chun CD, Chow ED, et al. (2008) Systematic genetic analysis of virulence in the human fungal pathogen Cryptococcus neoformans. *Cell* 135: 174–88.

Liu Y, Shetty AC, Schwartz JA, et al. (2015) New signaling pathways govern the host response to *C. albicans* infection in various niches. *Genome Res* 25: 679–89.

Loftus BJ, Fung E, Roncaglia P, et al. (2005) The genome of the basidiomycetous yeast and human pathogen *Cryptococcus neoformans*. *Science* 307: 1321–4.

Lorenz MC, Bender JA and Fink GR (2004) Transcriptional response of *Candida albicans* upon internalization by macrophages. *Eukaryot Cell* 3: 1076–87.

McDonagh A, Fedorova ND, Crabtree J, et al. (2008) Sub-telomere directed gene expression during initiation of invasive aspergillosis. *PLoS Pathog* 4: e1000154.

Mukherjee PK, Chandra J, Retuerto M, et al. (2014) Oral mycobiome analysis of HIV-infected patients: identification of Pichia as an antagonist of opportunistic fungi. *PLoS Pathog* 10: e1003996.

Nelson RT, Hua J, Pryor B and Lodge JK (2001) Identification of virulence mutants of the fungal pathogen Cryptococcus neoformans using signature-tagged mutagenesis. *Genetics* 157: 935–47.

Nguyen LD, Viscogliosi E and Delhaes L (2015) The lung mycobiome: an emerging field of the human respiratory microbiome. *Front Microbiol* 6: 89.

Nobile CJ, Nett JE, Hernday AD, et al. (2009) Biofilm matrix regulation by *Candida albicans* Zap1. *PLoS Biol* 7: e1000133.

Noble SM, French S, Kohn LA, Chen V and Johnson AD (2010) Systematic screens of a *Candida albicans* homozygous deletion library decouple morphogenetic switching and pathogenicity. *Nat Genet* 42: 590–8.

Oh J, Fung E, Schlecht U, et al. (2010) Gene annotation and drug target discovery in *Candida albicans* with a tagged transposon mutant collection. *PLoS Pathog* 6: e1001140.

O'Meara TR, Veri AO, Ketela T, Jiang B, Roemer T and Cowen LE (2015) Global analysis of fungal morphology exposes mechanisms of host cell escape. *Nat Commun* 6: 6741.

Pérez JC and Johnson AD (2013) Regulatory circuits that enable proliferation of the fungus *Candida albicans* in a mammalian host. *Plos Pathog* 9: e1003780.

Pérez JC, Kumamoto CA and Johnson AD (2013) *Candida albicans* commensalism and pathogenicity are intertwined traits directed by a tightly knit transcriptional regulatory circuit. *PLoS Biol* 11: e1001510.

Porollo A, Sesterhenn TM, Collins MS, Welge JA and Cushion MT (2014) Comparative genomics of *Pneumocystis* species suggests the absence of

genes for myo-inositol synthesis and reliance on inositol transport and metabolism. *MBio* 5: e01834.
Roemer T, Jiang B, Davison J, et al. (2003) Large-scale essential gene identification in *Candida albicans* and applications to antifungal drug discovery. *Mol Microbiol* 50: 167–81.
Rosenbach A, Dignard D, Pierce JV, Whiteway M and Kumamoto CA (2010) Adaptations of *Candida albicans* for growth in the mammalian intestinal tract. *Eukaryot Cell* 9: 1075–86.
Rubin-Bejerano I, Fraser I, Grisafi P and Fink GR (2003) Phagocytosis by neutrophils induces an amino acid deprivation response in *Saccharomyces cerevisiae* and *Candida albicans*. *Proc Natl Acad Sci U S A* 100: 11007–12.
Schwarzmuller T, Ma B, Hiller E, et al. (2014) Systematic phenotyping of a large-scale *Candida glabrata* deletion collection reveals novel antifungal tolerance genes. *PLoS Pathog* 10: e1004211.
Selmecki A, Forche A and Berman J (2006) Aneuploidy and isochromosome formation in drug-resistant *Candida albicans*. *Science* 313: 367–70.
Selmecki A, Forche A and Berman J (2010) Genomic plasticity of the human fungal pathogen *Candida albicans*. *Eukaryot Cell* 9: 991–1008.
Singh-Babak SD, Babak T, Diezmann S, et al. (2012) Global analysis of the evolution and mechanism of echinocandin resistance in *Candida glabrata*. *PLoS Pathog* 8: e1002718.
Tang J, Iliev ID, Brown J, et al. (2015) Mycobiome: approaches to analysis of intestinal fungi. *J Immunol Methods* 421: 112–21.
Tierney L, Linde J, Muller S, et al. (2012) An interspecies regulatory network inferred from simultaneous RNA-seq of *Candida albicans* invading innate immune cells. *Front Microbiol* 3: 85.
Uhl MA, Biery M, Craig N and Johnson AD (2003) Haploinsufficiency-based large-scale forward genetic analysis of filamentous growth in the diploid human fungal pathogen *C. albicans*. *EMBO J* 22: 2668–78.
Vandeputte P, Ischer F, Sanglard D and Coste AT (2011) In vivo systematic analysis of Candida albicans Zn2-Cys6 transcription factors mutants for mice organ colonization. *PLoS One* 6: e26962.
Wang B, Guo G, Wang C, et al. (2010) Survey of the transcriptome of *Aspergillus oryzae* via massively parallel mRNA sequencing. *Nucleic Acids Res* 38: 5075–87.
Wartenberg A, Linde J, Martin R, et al. (2014) Microevolution of *Candida albicans* in macrophages restores filamentation in a nonfilamentous mutant. *PLoS Genet* 10: e1004824.
Wilson D, Thewes S, Zakikhany K, et al. (2009) Identifying infection-associated genes of *Candida albicans* in the postgenomic era. *FEMS Yeast Res* 9: 688–700.
Xu W, Solis NV, Ehrlich RL, Woolford CA, Filler SG and Mitchell AP (2015) Activation and alliance of regulatory pathways in *C. albicans* during mammalian infection. *PLoS Biol* 13: e1002076.

CHAPTER 7

Epidemiology of fungal disease

Rajal K. Mody, Angela Ahlquist Cleveland, Shawn R. Lockhart, and Mary E. Brandt

Surveillance

Infectious disease surveillance is the practice of monitoring the number of infections over time in a given population to inform and evaluate infection control measures, and to identify questions that require further study (Figure 7.1).

Most large-scale and long-term infectious disease monitoring coordinated by public health agencies is done through passive surveillance, which relies on clinical providers and laboratories to submit information about reportable infections to health authorities. One of a few fungal disease examples of this passive form of surveillance is national surveillance for coccidioidomycosis (commonly known as Valley fever) in the United States. Coccidioidomycosis is associated with considerable morbidity and economic repercussions from costs of care and treatment, and lost productivity. The disease is caused by inhalation of arthroconidia of *Coccidioides immitis* and *C. posadasii*, soil-dwelling fungi endemic to states in the American Southwest (Arizona, Texas, Utah, New Mexico, Nevada) and the Central Valley of California, and recently identified in Washington state. Cases also occur among patients residing in non-endemic states following travel to endemic areas. Clinical providers and laboratories in 20 US states report cases of laboratory-diagnosed coccidioidomycosis to local and state health departments. These health departments then submit data electronically to the Centers for Disease Control and Prevention (CDC) through the National Notifiable Diseases Surveillance System, which compiles and reports data in the weekly *Morbidity and Mortality Weekly Report* (http://www.cdc.gov/mmwr). A steady increase in cases from 1998 to 2011 compelled public health authorities to prioritize efforts to address this disease (CDC 2013). Passive reporting by clinical providers and laboratories is prone to incomplete data collection because of reliance on reporting by providers who may have little time or incentive to report cases.

Compared with passive surveillance, active surveillance better captures cases of disease in a population by including regular review and audits of medical and laboratory information to ensure more complete case ascertainment. Active surveillance is also better able to collect fungal isolates, which allows scientists to characterize the strains causing illness more precisely, including antifungal susceptibility testing. However, because active surveillance is also more resource intensive, many of the examples of active surveillance projects we will describe were conducted for limited durations of time, or were only conducted in selected geographic areas.

Active population-based surveillance projects have been conducted to assess the epidemiology of candidaemia. Surveillance has revealed notable variation in the epidemiology of candidaemia in different parts of the world. These likely result from a combination of factors, including ecological factors that influence the predominant *Candida* species, predisposing host conditions, antifungal use, and infection control practices (Guinea 2014). For example, in 2010–2011, the highest incidence observed from nationwide surveillance of candidaemia in Denmark occurred among adults aged 70–89 years (nearly 40 cases per 100,000 inhabitants), whereas surveillance in five cities in Spain during these same years identified infants aged <1 year as having the highest incidence (96.4 cases per 100,000 inhabitants). This difference in risk groups was accompanied by differences in species distribution and antifungal drug susceptibility. As in most countries, *C. albicans* was the most frequently isolated species in both countries. However, the second most common species differed: *C. glabrata* in Denmark and *C. parapsilosis* in Spain (Arendrup et al. 2013; Puig-Asensio et al. 2014). *C. glabrata* is frequently resistant to azole antifungals and is more common among older patients, especially those with conditions requiring antifungal prophylaxis such as stem cell and organ transplant recipients. In contrast, the incidence of *C. parapsilosis* infection reportedly decreases with increasing patient age. This species is often carried on the hands of healthcare workers and can easily colonize central venous catheters. *C. parapsilosis* is a particular problem in neonatal intensive care units, given the high proportion of patients with central catheters (Guinea 2014).

In the United States, CDC has coordinated active population-based surveillance for candidaemia in two metropolitan areas periodically since 1992. Although the percentage of fluconazole-resistant infections has remained relatively stable since 2008 (at ~7–8%), this system documented the emergence of echinocandin-resistant infections during 2008–2013, increasing in frequency by 147% in Georgia (2.9% of all cases in 2013) and by 77% in Maryland (3.5% of all cases in 2013); most (74%) echinocandin-resistant infections were caused by *C. glabrata*. Furthermore, the emergence of multi-drug resistance (resistance to both azoles and echinocandins) among *C. glabrata* infections rose from 1.8% to 2.6% (Cleveland et al. 2015). Analysis of surveillance data revealed that most patients with echinocandin-resistant *C. glabrata* infections had no prior exposures to echinocandins, suggesting that these resistant strains are circulating in community or hospital environments (Vallabhaneni et al. 2015).

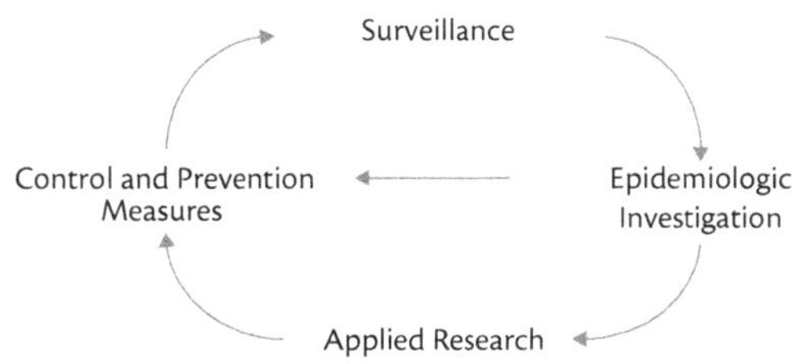

Figure 7.1 Public health cycle of disease control. The cycle starts with disease surveillance. Surveillance findings help direct further epidemiological investigations aimed at studying the determinants of disease. Insights into the causes of infections can directly inform control measures or identify areas of applied research that, in turn, influence prevention and control measures. Effectiveness of control measures is assessed through ongoing surveillance. Copyright © Centers for Disease Control and Prevention, U.S. Department of Health & Human Services.

Another emerging threat is azole-resistant aspergillosis. Active surveillance of all clinical *Aspergillus* spp. isolates from seven medical centres in the Netherlands, for the occurrence of azole resistance between June 2007 and January 2009, found that 5.3% of the isolates were azole-resistant. Most patients with resistant isolates had no prior azole exposure, and nearly all azole-resistant isolates harboured the TR/L98H resistance mechanism believed to be associated with agricultural fungicide use. Given the widespread use of fungicides and the high mortality rate (88%) reported among patients with invasive-aspergillosis caused by azole-resistant strains, this serious public health concern has spawned surveillance in medical centres throughout the world (van der Linden et al. 2011, 2015).

Several surveillance projects have been established to monitor the frequency of invasive fungal infections (IFIs) among higher risk groups, especially persons undergoing solid organ and stem cell transplants. The Transplant-Associated Infection Surveillance Network (TRANSNET) was a sentinel surveillance system for IFIs used in 23 transplant centres in the United States between 2001 and 2006. TRANSNET identified a large number of IFIs occurring >1 year after organ transplant, and suggested the need for updated treatment strategies that take into account the risk of late-occurring infections (Pappas et al. 2010).

Surveillance challenges

Surveilling for fungal infections involves many challenges (Ellis et al. 2000).

Perhaps most importantly, fungal infections are rarely deemed notifiable. In the United States, the only nationally notifiable fungal disease is coccidioidomycosis, and only a few fungal diseases, such as cryptococcosis, blastomycosis, and histoplasmosis, are reportable to health officials in select states. The limited number of notifiable mycoses prevents passive government-coordinated surveillance for many common and clinically important infections, including candidiasis, invasive aspergillosis, and many other less common invasive mould infections. Surveillance, therefore, often takes the form of time-limited, resource-intensive active surveillance projects in select locations, which limits the ability to assess trends over time or over larger geographic areas. Dedicated clinical research networks, such as the European Confederation of Medical Mycology (ECMM), can facilitate these types of surveillance projects across a broader geographic area than could be accomplished within a single country. The ECMM has published a diverse array of studies, including surveys of fusariosis, mucormycosis, and IFI among patients in intensive care units.

In the absence of surveillance, some investigators have used administrative healthcare data, such as hospital discharge and cause of death data, in which diseases are classified according to International Classification of Diseases (ICD) codes to retrospectively assess long-term trends in fungal infections, such as IFI in France (Bitar et al. 2014). However, ICD coding is prone to inaccuracies in the identification of fungal infections.

Methods for diagnosing fungal infections pose a challenge to the thorough detection of fungal infections by surveillance. First, it can be difficult to distinguish colonization from infection. Doing so often requires a combination of microbiological, radiological, and histopathological findings, as well as consistent clinical findings. Second, serological tests used to detect infections with dimorphic fungi such as *Histoplasma* and *Coccidioides* often lack optimal sensitivity or specificity and may require repeat testing to make a diagnosis.

Limited clinical suspicion for fungal infections reduces ascertainment of cases. For example, even in Arizona—an area highly endemic for coccidioidomycosis—one study found that only 2–13% of patients with community-acquired pneumonia are tested for this infection, despite the fact that 15% of those tested had coccidioidomycosis (Chang et al. 2008). In addition, many fungal infections have a diverse array of clinical presentations, making it challenging for clinicians to know when to test for these infections. Similarly, invasive fungal infections in immunocompromised persons may go undetected because they may not be routinely considered, especially when symptoms are similar to more common aetiologies.

Outbreak investigations

Outbreaks are infections clustered in time, space, or both that share a common source. Typically, outbreaks result in an increase in the expected number of cases of a particular infection within a given group of people. Although a small fraction of fungal infections occur as part of recognized outbreaks, the number of fungal outbreaks is likely underestimated.

A timely investigation may truncate an outbreak by preventing additional illnesses if the source of infections is identified and controlled. The rapid response to a large outbreak of fungal meningitis cases resulted in a recall of contaminated steroid injections produced by a compounding pharmacy, and was estimated to avert 153 infections and 124 deaths (Smith et al. 2015). However, sometimes outbreaks are not detected until after they are over. These events are still worth investigating because they can identify routes of exposure and clinical risk factors that inform measures to prevent future infections, and can also provide important descriptions of the natural history of rare or emerging infections.

In the absence of widespread surveillance of fungal infections, most fungal outbreaks are detected by astute clinicians and infection preventionists who recognize an increase in a certain type of illness, by laboratorians who detect an increase in recovery of a particular organism, or by patients themselves if multiple acquaintances fall ill with similar symptoms. Once a cluster of illnesses is identified, important steps in an investigation include the following: 1) confirm the diagnosis; 2) establish a case definition; 3) determine the background rate of the infection; 4) search for additional cases; 5) generate hypotheses regarding the source(s); 6) test hypotheses through epidemiological studies and possibly environmental sampling; and 7) implement control measures and disseminate information (Reingold 1998).

It is important to assess early on whether clusters identified by laboratory testing correlate with true disease. Given the ubiquitous nature of fungi, pseudo-outbreaks caused by environmental contamination of clinical specimens, with no signs or symptoms of fungal infection in the patients, are not uncommon (Davoudi et al. 2015). Identifying the source of contamination leading to these pseudo-outbreaks is still necessary to restore confidence in microbiological test interpretation and to prevent true infection if the source of contamination could be putting immunocompromised patients at risk, such as contaminated ice used to control bleeding in patients undergoing endoscopies (Blake et al. 2015).

Outbreak case definitions and case finding

Establishing investigation-specific case definitions is essential. Case definitions are used to find additional cases and to help ensure that illnesses being investigated may be related in some way, minimizing the chances of erroneously including illnesses that are not part of the outbreak, which could lead investigators down the wrong paths or obscure epidemiological clues pointing to the source of outbreak. Case definitions can include several elements, including laboratory or radiological findings, symptoms, timing of infections, and specification of the patient group at risk. While a highly specific definition can aid in finding commonalities among patients, it runs the risk of identifying too few cases to investigate. Therefore, it is often appropriate to use multiple case definitions that differ by level of certainty (e.g. confirmed, probable, suspected). When investigating a cluster of suspected hospital-acquired infections, especially invasive mould infections, it is important to develop case definitions designed to exclude illnesses acquired outside of the hospital. This is challenging because the incubation periods of many fungal infections are not well characterized and likely vary by dose and route of exposure and by the immune status of the patient (Davoudi et al. 2015).

To assess whether an outbreak is truly occurring, it is helpful to compare the number of cases in the cluster to an estimated background rate of the disease. If the suspected outbreak is occurring among hospitalized patients, it is helpful to review several years of microbiology, histopathology, and hospital discharge records to estimate how many cases of the infection typically occur among patients in the facility. Because most healthcare-associated outbreaks tend to be small and span several weeks to months (Vonberg and Gastmeier 2006; Repetto et al. 2012), it is not always obvious whether the number of cases in the cluster under investigation represents a true increase over baseline, especially for rare infections for which the baseline itself is unstable and when the number of hospital admissions has varied over time. When the pathogen is very rare, the occurrence of just two cases that occur close in time should prompt an outbreak investigation irrespective of baseline rates (Repetto et al. 2012). Outbreaks occurring among persons in the community are often obvious, characterized by a high illness attack rate among a group of people who share a common exposure.

Generating hypotheses

If an outbreak is likely present, a thorough description of cases by person, place, and time is essential to generate hypotheses regarding the source(s) of infections. By describing factors relating to the people affected (e.g. demographic characteristics, recent leisure or occupational activities, pre-existing medical conditions or medical procedures, contact with specific healthcare workers), where cases are occurring (e.g. widely dispersed through a country, in a specific community, in patients admitted to a particular hospital ward), and when they are occurring (e.g. soon after a natural disaster, during hospital construction activities), important clues to shared exposures are often revealed.

There are several other sources of information that can aid in hypothesis generation. First, review of the medical literature can reveal established associations between certain infections and exposures. Examples include *Candida parapsilosis* fungaemia and contaminated healthcare workers' hands, histoplasmosis and disturbed bird roosts or bat guano, *Saccharomyces cerevisiae* fungaemia and probiotics, invasive aspergillosis and hospital construction or renovation, and sporotrichosis and contact with sphagnum moss, hay, or cat scratches. Second, interviews with case-patients or their care-givers may reveal commonalities among patients. Third, molecular subtyping of fungal pathogens provides important insights into the nature of the cluster. This is because in common source outbreaks caused by a contaminated product, at least some clinical isolates would be expected to be genetically indistinguishable. In contrast, identification of multiple species or strains is often seen in outbreaks caused by environmental exposures such as natural disaster or construction-related environmental disruptions (Kanamori et al. 2015; Litvintseva et al. 2015).

Molecular epidemiology

The increasing importance of molecular subtyping in outbreak investigations highlights the importance of collaboration between laboratory and epidemiology teams. Molecular epidemiology, often called strain typing or DNA fingerprinting, is used to determine the relatedness among isolates. Relatedness can be used to show that isolates are identical (clonal) or non-identical (non-clonal). There are many methods for typing isolates but not all are suitable for fungi. Random amplified polymorphic DNA (RAPD) and amplified fragment length polymorphism (AFLP) are easy to perform and can be accomplished without any prior knowledge about the organism, but their poor discriminatory power (RAPD) and lack of reproducibility (RAPD and AFLP) make them unsuitable for outbreak investigation and can often result in misleading interpretations.

Highly reproducible methodologies include multi-locus sequence typing (MLST) and microsatellite typing (sometimes referred to as 'variable number tandem repeats' [VNTR]). However, genomic sequence information must be available in order to perform MLST or VNTR. The discriminatory power of MLST is dependent upon the sequences used, and ranges from identifying large clonal groups—as seen for *Candida glabrata* (Lott et al. 2010) and *Cryptococcus neoformans* (Litvintseva et al. 2006)—to identification at the individual isolate—as seen for *Bipolaris spicifera* (Pham et al. 2015). Microsatellite typing is discriminatory but is time-consuming and expensive and is subject to homoplasy (shared traits not derived from a common ancestor) (Reiss et al. 2012). The most discriminatory typing tool is whole-genome sequence (WGS) analysis. No prior knowledge of the organism is necessary. It can distinguish between each individual isolate, but it is time-consuming and expensive, and requires specialized equipment, software, and a skilled bioinformatician. WGS analysis is most likely the molecular epidemiological tool of the future (Etienne et al. 2012).

One of the shortcomings of molecular epidemiological analysis is that validated sub-species typing systems are available for use in an outbreak situation for only a few taxa, and species-level identification is often the only available tool. The other consideration is that appropriate control isolates (unrelated to the outbreak) may not be available. Showing that all of the isolates in an investigation have the same typing pattern may not be useful unless control isolates can be shown to have a different pattern. The best controls are isolates from the same hospital or immediate geographic area as the outbreak, so that it can be determined that the population structure (the relatedness of a group of isolates within a given area) of the tested isolates is not clonal.

Testing hypotheses

After investigators identify suspicious exposures, unless the source of infection is obvious, it is important to test the leading hypotheses through case-control or retrospective cohort studies. These studies may also identify clinical factors that influence susceptibility to infection and can guide control measures even if an exact source of infection is not identified. However, because of the small size of many fungal disease outbreaks, these studies often lack statistical power.

Given the ubiquitous nature of many fungi, environmental sampling should be limited to epidemiologically guided hypotheses. Isolating the causative organism from a suspected source of infection adds further evidence implicating that source, such as isolation of *Rhizopus delemar* from bed linens during an outbreak of cutaneous mucormycosis (Duffy et al. 2014). However, failure to isolate the organism does not exonerate that source because fungi can be difficult to isolate, environmental conditions may have changed from the time of the outbreak to sampling, and the sampling may have been inadequate.

Prevention

Control measures identified through individual outbreak investigations have collectively provided the evidence base needed for best practices for the ongoing prevention of fungal infections such as those associated with hospital construction projects, nosocomially acquired candidaemia, and occupationally acquired histoplasmosis (Ellis et al. 2000; Kanamori et al. 2015).

More recently investigated fungal outbreaks provide highlight areas for continued infection control efforts (Table 7.1). Large outbreaks caused by contaminated compounded injectable medications indicate important gaps that must be addressed to assure the safety of compounded medications. Emergency medical responders should be aware of the increasing reports of fungal infections

Table 7.1 Selected recent fungal outbreak investigations

Infection	Agent	Source	Typing method	Description	Reference
Outbreaks caused by contaminated compounded medications:					
Meningitis and other infections	*Exserohilum rostratum*	Methylprednisolone acetate	Whole genome sequencing	753 cases with 54 deaths from injection of a contaminated steroid; 14,000 injections and rapid patient notification saved countless lives	Smith et al. 2013
Endophthalmitis	*Fusarium incarnatum-equiseti, Bipolaris hawaiiensis*	Brilliant Blue G, triamcinolone	Multi-locus sequence typing	47 cases caused by two different contaminated products from the same compounding pharmacy were injected into the eyes of patients	Mikosz et al. 2014
Outbreaks caused by natural disasters:					
Meningitis	*Aspergillus fumigatus*	Contaminated needles	None	5 cases with 3 deaths; needles used for spinal anaesthesia were contaminated with mould, possibly because of suboptimal storage conditions following nnna large tsunami	Gunaratne et al. 2007
Cutaneous mucormycosis	*Apophysomyces trapeziformis*	Tornado debris	Whole genome sequencing	13 people were infected and 5 people died following traumatic implantation of debris following a devastating tornado; the number of puncture wounds was a risk factor for infection	Etienne et al. 2012; Neblett Fanfair et al. 2012
Outbreaks caused by solid organ transplantation:					
Coccidioidomycosis	*Coccidioides immitis*	Infected organ donor	Whole genome sequencing	3 patients were infected following organ transplantation with infected organs; donor was not screened for Coccidioides despite neurological symptoms	Engelthaler et al. 2011; Blodget et al. 2012
Outbreaks or disease clusters caused by environmental exposures in healthcare settings:					
Cutaneous mucormycosis	*Rhizopus delemar*	Hospital linens	None	5 infants infected with 5 deaths; hospital linens were not stored in a sterile environment before use	Duffy et al. 2014

(continued)

Table 7.1 (Continued)

Infection	Agent	Source	Typing method	Description	Reference
Aspergillosis	*Aspergillus fumigatus*	Unknown	Microsatellite	7 cases with 6 deaths among patients in an intensive care unit; abnormally high spore counts were detected in the air inside the unit and coincided with extensive building construction	Pelaez et al. 2012
Outbreaks caused by outdoor environmental exposures:					
Blastomycosis	*Blastomyces dermatitidis*	Environmental exposure	Random amplified polymorphic DNA	21 cases in non-rural residents; case-control study suggested that proximity to a yard waste collection site was the predominant risk factor	Pfister et al. 2011
Histoplasmosis	*Histoplasma capsulatum*	Cave	None	4 cases among 8 biologists studying *Histoplasma* levels in a cave before allowing tourism. Brief break in protective equipment protocol during investigation led to infection	Rocha-Silva et al. 2014
Outbreaks likely caused by person-to-person spread:					
Fungaemia	*Candida guilliermondii*	Being cared for by a specific private care attendant (non-hospital staff) while hospitalized	None	13 cases and 7 deaths of hospitalized patients attended by a single external care attendant while hospitalized; no controls used by this attendant	Asensio et al. 2015
Unsolved outbreaks:					
Fungaemia and other infections	*Saprochaete clavata*	Unknown	Whole genome sequencing	26 cases with 22 deaths among immunocompromised patients; a case-case study suggested contaminated medical devices as the source	Vaux et al. 2014

following natural disasters. Additionally, vigilance is needed for donor-derived fungal infections among transplant recipients. With much aging of medical centres throughout the world, we can expect ongoing outbreaks associated with hospital renovation and construction, without better methods to limit the intrusion of mould spores into patient care areas. Investigations of outbreaks of endemic mycoses continue to highlight the importance of personal protective equipment by workers, and also identify novel routes of exposure. Although the outbreaks of *Candida* infection have decreased in frequency, likely because of improved hand-washing and catheter care by hospital staff, outbreaks still occur and serve as a reminder of the importance of basic infection control practices and unrecognized risks, such as care provided by persons external to the hospital staff. Finally, the fact that some deadly fungal outbreaks go unsolved, despite rigorous epidemiological investigation aided by whole-genome sequencing, attests to the continued challenges posed by fungal outbreaks.

Disclaimer

The findings and conclusions in this chapter are those of the authors and do not necessarily represent the official position of the Centers for Disease Control and Prevention.

References

Arendrup MC, Dzajic E, Jensen RH, et al. (2013) Epidemiological changes with potential implication for antifungal prescription recommendations for fungaemia: data from a nationwide fungaemia surveillance programme. *Clin Microbiol Infect* 19: E343–53.

Asensio A, Munez E, Cantero M and Ramos A (2015) Candida guilliermondii fungemia in hospitalized patients epidemiologically linked to a patient care attendant. *Am J Infect Control* 43: 1012–14. doi: 10.1016/j.ajic.2015.04.207

Bitar D, Lortholary O, Le Strat Y, et al. (2014) Population-based analysis of invasive fungal infections, France, 2001-2010. *Emerg Infect Dis* 20: 1149–55.

Blake M, Embil JM, Trepman E, Adam H, Myers R and Mutcher P (2015) Pseudo-outbreak of Phaeoacremonium parasiticum from a hospital ice dispenser. *Infect Control Hosp Epidemiol* 35: 1063–5.

Blodget E, Geiseler PJ, Larsen RA, Stapfer M, Qazi Y and Petrovic LM (2012) Donor-derived Coccidioides immitis fungemia in solid organ transplant recipients. *Transpl Infect Dis* 14: 305–10.

Centers for Disease Control and Prevention (2013) Increase in reported coccidioidomycosis—United States, 1998–2011. *MMWR* 62: 217–21.

Chang DC, Anderson S, Wannemuehler K, et al. (2008) Testing for coccidioidomycosis among patients with community-acquired pneumonia. *Emerg Infect Dis* 14: 1053–9.

Cleveland AA, Harrison LH, Farley MM, et al. (2015) Declining incidence of candidemia and the shifting epidemiology of candida resistance in two US metropolitan areas, 2008-2013: results from population-based surveillance. *PLoS One* 10: e0120452.

Davoudi S, Graviss LS and Kontoyiannis DP (2015) Healthcare-associated outbreaks due to Mucorales and other uncommon fungi. *Eur J Clin Invest* 45: 767–73.

Duffy J, Harris J, Gade L, et al. (2014) Mucormycosis outbreak associated with hospital linens. *Pediatr Infect Dis J* 33: 472–6.

Ellis D, Marriott D, Hajjeh RA, Warnock D, Meyer W and Barton R (2000) Epidemiology: surveillance of fungal infections. *Med Mycol* 38, Suppl 1: 173–82.

Engelthaler DM, Chiller T, Schupp JA, et al. (2011) Next-generation sequencing of Coccidioides immitis isolated during cluster investigation. *Emerg Infect Dis* 17: 227–32.

Etienne KA, Gillece J, Hilsabeck R, et al. (2012) Whole genome sequence typing to investigate the Apophysomyces outbreak following a tornado in Joplin, Missouri, 2011. *PLoS One* 7: e49989.

Guinea J (2014) Global trends in the distribution of Candida species causing candidemia. *Clin Microbiol Infect* 20, Suppl 6: 5–10.

Gunaratne PS, Wijeyaratne CN and Seneviratne HR (2007) Aspergillus meningitis in Sri Lanka—a post-tsunami effect? *N Engl J Med* 356: 754–6.

Kanamori H, Rutala WA, Sickbert-Bennett EE and Weber DJ (2015) Review of fungal outbreaks and infection prevention in healthcare settings during construction and renovation. *Clin Infect Dis* 61: 433–44.

Litvintseva AP, Brandt ME, Mody RK and Lockhart SR (2015) Investigating fungal outbreaks in the 21st century. *PLoS Pathog* 11: e1004804.

Litvintseva AP, Thakur R, Vilgalys R and Mitchell TG (2006) Multilocus sequence typing reveals three genetic subpopulations of Cryptococcus neoformans var. grubii (serotype A), including a unique population in Botswana. *Genetics* 172: 2223–38.

Lott TJ, Frade JP and Lockhart SR (2010) Multilocus sequence type analysis reveals both clonality and recombination in populations of Candida glabrata bloodstream isolates from U.S. surveillance studies. *Eukaryot Cell* 9: 619–25.

Mikosz CA, Smith RM, Kim M, et al. (2014) Fungal endophthalmitis associated with compounded products. *Emerg Infect Dis* 20: 248–56.

Neblett Fanfair R, Benedict K, Bos J, et al. (2012) Necrotizing cutaneous mucormycosis after a tornado in Joplin, Missouri, in 2011. *N Engl J Med* 367: 2214–25.

Pappas PG, Alexander BD, Andes DR, et al. (2010) Invasive fungal infections among organ transplant recipients: results of the Transplant-Associated Infection Surveillance Network (TRANSNET). *Clin Infect Dis* 50: 1101–11.

Pelaez T, Munoz P, Guinea J, et al. (2012) Outbreak of invasive aspergillosis after major heart surgery caused by spores in the air of the intensive care unit. *Clin Infect Dis* 54: e24–31.

Pfister JR, Archer JR, Hersil S, et al. (2011) Non-rural point source blastomycosis outbreak near a yard waste collection site. *Clin Med Res* 9: 57–65.

Pham CD, Purfield AE, Fader R, Pascoe N and Lockhart SR (2015) Development of a multi-locus sequence typing system for medically relevant bipolaris species. *J Clin Microbiol* 53: 3239–46.

Puig-Asensio M, Padilla B, Garnacho-Montero J, et al. (2014) Epidemiology and predictive factors for early and late mortality in Candida bloodstream infections: a population-based surveillance in Spain. *Clin Microbiol Infect* 20: O245–54.

Reingold AL (1998) Outbreak investigations—a perspective. *Emerg Infect Dis* 4: 21–7.

Reiss E, Lasker BA, Lott TJ, et al. (2012) Genotyping of Candida parapsilosis from three neonatal intensive care units (NICUs) using a panel of five multilocus microsatellite markers: broad genetic diversity and a cluster of related strains in one NICU. *Infect Genet Evol* 12: 1654–60.

Repetto EC, Giacomazzi CG and Castelli F (2012) Hospital-related outbreaks due to rare fungal pathogens: a review of the literature from 1990 to June 2011. *Eur J Clin Microbiol Infect Dis* 31: 2897–904.

Rocha-Silva F, Figueiredo SM, Silveira TT, et al. (2014) Histoplasmosis outbreak in Tamboril cave—Minas Gerais state, Brazil. *Med Mycol Case Rep* 4: 1–4.

Smith RM, Derado G, Wise M, et al. (2015) Estimated deaths and illnesses averted during fungal meningitis outbreak associated with contaminated steroid injections, United States, 2012-2013. *Emerg Infect Dis* 21: 933–40.

Smith RM, Schaefer MK, Kainer MA, et al. (2013) Fungal infections associated with contaminated methylprednisolone injections. *N Engl J Med* 369: 1598–609.

Vallabhaneni S, Cleveland AA, Farley MM, et al. (2015) Epidemiology and risk factors for echinocandin non-susceptible Candida glabrata bloodstream infections: data from a large multi-site population-based Candidemia surveillance program, 2008-2014. *Epidemiol Infect* 2: ovf163.

van der Linden JW, Arendrup MC, Warris A, et al. (2015) Prospective multicenter international surveillance of azole resistance in Aspergillus fumigatus. *Emerg Infect Dis* 21: 1041–4.

van der Linden JW, Snelders E, Kampinga GA, et al. (2011) Clinical implications of azole resistance in Aspergillus fumigatus, The Netherlands, 2007-2009. *Emerg Infect Dis* 17: 1846–54.

Vaux S, Criscuolo A, Desnos-Ollivier M, et al. (2014) Multicenter outbreak of infections by Saprochaete clavata, an unrecognized opportunistic fungal pathogen. *MBio* 5:e02309-14.

Vonberg RP and Gastmeier P (2006) Nosocomial aspergillosis in outbreak settings. *J Hosp Infect* 63: 246–54.

CHAPTER 8

Pathogenesis of fungal disease

Frank C. Odds

Pathogenesis of fungal disease

In common with all infectious processes, the pathogenesis of fungal disease can be envisaged as a battle between the molecular and cellular virulence armaments of the fungus and the molecular and cellular defences of the host. The damage done to the 'battlefield'—host tissue—is the resulting disease. The subsequent chapter, on immunity (Chapter 9), will describe host defence mechanisms in detail. The focus of the present chapter is on fungal virulence attributes.

Only one fungal type, the anthropophilic dermatophytes, routinely invades normal human tissues. These species produce many types of proteolytic enzymes, which enable them to damage keratin in skin, hair, nail, and so on (Achtermann and White 2012). However, dermatophytes appear to lack other virulence factors that might facilitate their penetration to deeper tissues; they also have a maximum growth temperature below 37°C. These limitations restrict their pathogenicity to invasion only of superficial keratinized tissues.

Some other fungi, notably *Coccidioides* spp., *Histoplasma capsulatum, Blastomyces dermatitidis, Cryptococcus neoformans*, and *Cryptococcus gattii*, occasionally infect immunologically intact humans, but—in common with most fungi associated with human disease—they are most likely to cause serious, life-threatening infections in patients who already lack one or more immune defence mechanisms. This situation is known as '*opportunism*', and reflects the relative impotence of fungi as pathogens compared with highly virulent bacteria and viruses. Host defences appear to be well adapted to prevent fungi invading tissues.

The ability of a fungus to develop within the tissues of a human host depends on its microenvironment. A fungal element that is inhaled to the lungs needs to be able to penetrate pulmonary epithelial layers if it is to gain access to the bloodstream, while one that is implanted directly into the bloodstream via, for example, a penetrating wound, does not require its own epithelial penetration mechanisms. In short, the molecular factors of virulence expressed by a fungus will vary according to its location in the body, and the immune defences that are locally mounted against it. In most instances a fungus will need to express different sets of multiple virulence attributes to survive in the many different microenvironments it encounters. Flexibility in expression of multiple virulence factors is a positive property for a fungus that has to survive in a human or other mammalian host. This perspective has been expressed delightfully in a review article that considers how soil-dwelling fungi also act as human pathogens (Casadevall 2006).

Discovery of fungal virulence factors

The earliest investigations into fungal pathogenicity were based on intelligent guesses, partly informed by research into bacterial virulence. The common presumption was that hydrolytic enzymes such as proteinases and phospholipases might damage host tissues, particularly if they were secreted or located at the cell surface, the most likely site of interaction with host immune cells. Surface adhesin molecules might facilitate attachment of fungal cells to host surfaces, and some aspects of fungal morphology, such as the capsule of *Cryptococcus neoformans*, might serve to resist host defence processes such as phagocytosis. Evidence pointing to a particular cellular or molecular attribute as a virulence factor came from a range of types of experiment—for example, demonstration of reduced virulence *in vivo* of strains deficient in the putative virulence factor, demonstration that a possible virulence factor was expressed in infected tissues, and detection of the virulence factor (or antibodies to it) in the circulation of patients suffering from the fungal infection.

In the late twentieth century, the arrival of molecular genetic techniques applicable to pathogenic fungi facilitated discovery of their virulence attributes. It became possible to specifically disrupt or delete the gene encoding a putative virulence factor, then to demonstrate attenuated virulence in the mutant. More recently, the arrival of whole-genome sequencing (genomics) for fungi extended these possibilities by allowing bioinformatic detection of genes that might encode virulence attributes by analogy with other pathogens (see, for example, Achtermann and White 2012). Proteomics (see, for example, Kniemeyer et al. 2011) and RNA transcript profiling of fungi from infected tissues (see, for example, Walker et al. 2009) have also been applied to detect fungal virulence factor candidates.

The philosophy underpinning virulence research is heavily based on the assumption that when expression of a particular gene is arrested without impacting the overall growth of a fungus *in vitro*, but with a demonstrable attenuation of its virulence in an experimental animal, that gene probably encodes a virulence factor. However, this form of evidence does not distinguish genes required for general survival of the fungus *in vivo* from genes encoding molecules that interact *directly* with host surfaces or molecules. More sophisticated additional experimentation is therefore needed to provide a compelling case for a fungal molecule as a virulence factor.

Small rodents, particularly mice, have been, for many years, the preferred experimental hosts for fungal virulence work. The ready availability of mouse strains with specific gene knockouts related to host defence provides valuable tools for fine-scale investigation of the interaction between individual fungal and host molecules.

However, the desire to minimize experimentation with sentient mammals has led to the introduction of several models involving invertebrates or vertebrate embryos with characteristics that can sometimes be used to investigate specific fungus–host interactions. New experimental hosts include the nematode *Caenorhabditis elegans*, larvae of the moth *Galleria mellonella*, and embryos of the zebrafish, *Danio rerio*. Such organisms lack the full range of defence factors found in the mammalian immune system, but can provide useful information in experiments designed to investigate interactions of fungal molecules with the parts of host immunity present in the non-mammalian host. Pathogenesis experiments can also be conducted *ex vivo* in artificial tissues; once again, such models provide useful information but do not necessarily reflect the changeable conditions and time-dependent host defence responses encountered in an intact host.

It is important to maintain restraint in interpreting experiments on fungal pathogenesis. The further the experimentation is removed from a mammalian host, the less the result may be generalizable to the natural infection situation. As others have pointed out (Upadhya et al. 2014), fungi have to overcome fluctuating microenvironments in order to infect human hosts, so that the narrowly defined conditions of many pathogenesis experiments come nowhere near mimicking the medically important situation. For example, the study by Jain et al. (2009) of *Saccharomyces cerevisiae*—essentially a non-pathogen for humans—infecting *C. elegans*—a nematode not normally infected by yeasts—moves virulence investigation a long way from natural mammal–fungus interactions. If the objective is to discover how fuel is delivered from the tank to the engine, investigating the coolant circulation may not produce information of value.

Table 8.1 lists a selection of virulence factors for all the major pathogenic fungal species. The evidence for each factor ranges from robust to tentative. The list will provide the reader with an overview of the sorts of fungal attributes that have been investigated for a role in disease pathogenesis. The majority of fungal virulence factors are of three general types: those related to cell shape; polysaccharides and proteins located at the cell surface; and secreted enzymes. Other factors in the table, e.g. siderophores, are required for full nutrition of the growing fungal cells. Pathogenesis of disease is a consequence of the fungus expressing the necessary combination of virulence factors at the appropriate time within host tissues.

Table 8.1 Selected virulence factors for the major human pathogenic fungal species

Species	Virulence factor	Comment	Reference
A. fumigatus	Biofilm formation	Enhances gliotoxin production—may be important in chronic infections	Kniemeyer et al. 2011
	Secreted proteinases	Probably assist adhesion/penetration/host peptide destruction	Hogan et al. 1996; Sriranganadane et al. 2011
	Methylcitrate synthase	Assimilates amino acids released by proteases	Ibrahim-Granet et al. 2008
	Hydroxamate siderophores	Chelate iron to maintain iron homeostasis	Kniemeyer et al. 2011; Moore 2013
	Gliotoxin	Mycotoxin; may affect phagocytic leucocytes	Hogan et al. 1996; Scharf et al. 2012
B. dermatitidis	Bad1 (adhesin)	Involved in adherence to host cells and in immunomodulation	Wuthrich et al. 2006; Krajaejun et al. 2010
C. albicans	Hypha formation	Important for epithelial penetration	Zheng et al. 2004; Kumamoto and Vinces 2005
	Biofilm formation	Enhances adherence to plastic surfaces, e.g. intravenous catheters	Kniemeyer et al. 2011
	Als family of cell wall proteins	Involved in adherence to host proteins/surfaces and biofilm formation	Klis et al. 2009; Martin et al. 2011
	Hwp1 (hyphal cell wall protein)	Involved in epithelial adherence and biofilm formation	Klis et al. 2009; Martin et al. 2011
	Sap isoenzyme family	Proteinases; probably assist adhesion/penetration/host cell destruction	Schaller et al. 2005; Martin et al. 2011
	Lip isoenzyme family	Lipases; probably assist adhesion/penetration/host cell destruction	Schaller et al. 2005; Martin et al. 2011
	Plb1 (phospholipase B)	Phospholipase; probably assists adhesion/penetration/host cell destruction	Schaller et al. 2005
	Catalases	Deactivate host antimicrobial reactive oxygen species	Kniemeyer et al. 2011
	Sod4, Sod5 (superoxide dismutases)	Help fungi resist oxidative stress responses	Klis et al. 2009
	Phenotypic switching	White and opaque phenotypes differ in virulence for deep tissues and skin	Soll 2014

(continued)

Table 8.1 (Continued)

Species	Virulence factor	Comment	Reference
C. immitis/ C. posadasii	Spherule outer wall glycoprotein (SOWgp)	Modulates host cell-mediated immune response	Hung et al. 2007
	Arginase I	Reduces nitric oxide production	Hung et al. 2007
	Urease	Alkalinizes microenvironment	Hung et al. 2007
C. neoformans/ C. gattii	Polysaccharide capsule	Immunomodulatory; protects against phagocytosis	Hogan et al. 1996; Ma and May 2009; Kronstad et al. 2012
	Melanin in the cell wall	Helps fungi withstand antimicrobial stresses *in vivo*	Hogan et al. 1996; Ma and May 2009; Kronstad et al. 2012
	Proteinases	Damage host proteins, including phagosomal membranes	Ma and May 2009
	Phospholipases	Damage phagosomal membranes	Ma and May 2009
	Urease	Enhances CNS invasion	Ma and May 2009; Kronstad et al. 2012
	Superoxide dismutase	Helps yeasts grow out from macrophages	Kronstad et al. 2012
	MATα mating type	More virulent than type a in mice; far more common among clinical isolates	Hogan et al. 1996; Ma and May 2009
	Phenotypic switching	Affects capsule size and structure	Ma and May 2009
Dermatophytes	Secreted keratinase	Direct evidence for this enzyme in *Microsporum canis*	Viani et al. 2001
Dermatophytes	Secreted proteinases (of many subtypes)	Damage keratin and other proteins in skin, hair, nail, etc.	Monod 2008; Achtermann and White 2012
Dermatophytes	Sulphite secretion	Reduces S-S bonds to make keratin susceptible to proteolysis	Monod 2008
H. capsulatum	Cell wall α-glucan	'Smooth' variants lack α-glucan and are attenuated in mouse virulence	Edwards and Rappleye 2011; Sepúlveda et al. 2014
	Melanin in the cell wall	Helps fungi withstand antimicrobial stresses *in vivo*	Edwards and Rappleye 2011; Mihu and Nosanchuk 2012
	Cell surface Hsp60	Mediates attachment of yeasts to macrophage complement receptors	Edwards and Rappleye 2011; Mihu and Nosanchuk 2012
	Cell surface Hsp82	Helps fungi withstand antimicrobial stresses *in vivo*	Mihu and Nosanchuk 2012
	Secreted Cbp1 (calcium-binding protein)	Aids survival and replication within phagocytic leucocytes	Edwards and Rappleye 2011; Mihu and Nosanchuk 2012
	Secreted Yps3	Putative adhesin: involved in dissemination to spleen and liver	Edwards and Rappleye 2011; Mihu and Nosanchuk 2012
	Sid1 (siderophore)	Maintains iron homeostasis; absence causes mild loss of virulence	Edwards and Rappleye 2011; Mihu and Nosanchuk 2012
	Secreted catalase CatB	Deactivates host antimicrobial reactive oxygen species	Edwards and Rappleye 2011; Holbrook et al. 2011

References cited are mainly review articles, which should be consulted to locate citations for original discoveries.

Growth at 37°C and virulence

Omitted from Table 8.1 is one self-evident, fundamental requirement for virulence in human fungal pathogens. For any fungus to invade deep human tissues it needs to be able to grow at human body temperature (or higher, since infected patients typically develop fever). Fungi that cannot grow at 37°C do not cause disseminated infections. This consideration explains the inability of dermatophytes to invade beyond external surfaces, and why highly thermotolerant fungi such as *Aspergillus fumigatus* are seen far more often as opportunistic pathogens than other *Aspergillus* species that grow and survive only at lower temperatures.

Morphogenesis and virulence

Many of the most important fungal pathogens undergo morphological changes associated with pathogenesis of infection. *Coccidioides* spp., *Histoplasma capsulatum, Blastomyces dermatitidis, Paracoccidioides brasiliensis, Sporothrix schenckii*, and *Talaromyces (Penicillium) marneffei* are all thermally dimorphic fungi: they grow as hyphal mycelia in their natural environmental habitats at 25°C or lower, but convert to single-celled forms when invading tissues in humans at 37°C (the single cells are spherules for *Coccidioides* species, and yeasts for the other dimorphic pathogens). It is unclear whether the morphological change per se contributes to fungal virulence, or whether the switch gratuitously accompanies other gene expression changes that lead to production of the molecules required for virulence.

For the polymorphic yeast *Candida albicans*, the situation concerning the significance of morphology is complicated by the fact that the full range of cell shapes (yeasts, pseudohyphae, and true hyphae) is commonly observed in histopathological sections of infected tissues. The ability of this fungus to form hyphae has been well proven to be a requirement for virulence, but the morphological change to hyphae is associated with the expression of several other genes that encode molecular virulence factors (Mayer et al. 2014) so that the hyphal form itself may not be important for virulence. The study by Zheng et al. (2004) resolved this dilemma. These authors deleted the gene *HGC1*, which encodes a protein essential for the hyphal shape, but this deletion did not alter the expression of hypha-associated virulence factors; the mutant was nevertheless attenuated in virulence for mice, thus showing that the hyphal shape is required for normal pathogenetic processes. The review by Kumamoto and Vinces (2005) updates and details the role of hyphae in the virulence of *C. albicans*.

The yeast species *Candida glabrata* is an opportunistic pathogen that forms, at best, only rudimentary pseudohyphae. A recent study described a spontaneous mutant of *C. glabrata* which had gained the ability to form pseudohyphae: the mutant was *hyper*virulent in a mouse model, once again indicating a role for filamentous forms in the pathogenesis of disease (Brunke et al. 2014). By contrast, in *B. dermatitidis*, a mutant that formed both pseudohyphae and yeast forms *in vivo* showed no alteration in virulence for mice (Krajaejun et al. 2010). Formation of elongated cell shapes cannot therefore be required as an inevitable virulence factor. For fungi such as those *Candida* species that can freely form both filaments and single yeast cells, the advantage of morphological flexibility is that their filamentous forms are probably superior for penetrating epithelial and endothelial surfaces (Kumamoto and Vinces 2005), while their yeast forms allow for easy dissemination in the bloodstream and other fluids.

Cell surface adhesins and other external structures in fungal pathogenesis

For a fungal cell to interact with a mammalian host, it needs to be capable of anchoring itself to host cells and/or intercellular matrices. Conversely, for host leucocytes to be able to effectively remove fungal cells, they need to recognize fungal surface structures (epitopes) and attach themselves to the fungi. Fungal pathogens have evolved a diverse variety of surface properties that play a role in the pathogenesis of disease.

Perhaps the most obvious and striking example of a surface structure involved in pathogenesis is the polysaccharide capsule surrounding yeast cells of *C. neoformans* and *C. gattii*. This variably sized, but sometimes huge, outer layer surrounding the infecting yeast cells protects the fungus against phagocytosis by host leucocytes. The cryptococcal capsule is a complex structure, whose biosynthesis is encoded and regulated by a very large number of genes (Ma and May 2009; Kronstad et al. 2012). Capsular polysaccharides are the antigens detected in the standard latex antigen test for cryptococcal infection; they can alter the osmolarity of cerebrospinal fluid, thus contributing to several of the symptoms associated with cryptococcal meningitis (Ma and May 2009).

Melanin is a common component of many fungal cell walls. It is the source of the colour of the dematiaceous (dark) fungi, many of which are occasional pathogens of immunocompromised patients. In *C. neoformans* (Ma and May 2009) and *H. capsulatum* (Mihu and Nosanchuk 2012), melanin in the cell wall has been shown to protect the fungi against host oxidative stresses and antimicrobial peptides; melanized cells also show lower susceptibility to some antifungal drugs. Alpha-1,3-glucan, a major component of the cell wall of *H. capsulatum*, has been shown to be required for virulence of this fungus (Edwards and Rappleye 2011; Sepúlveda et al. 2014), although details of its role remain to be elucidated.

Several cell wall proteins and glycoproteins help fungi adhere to host surfaces, including epithelia, endothelia, and leucocyte membranes. These include Bad1 in *B. dermatitidis*, SOWgp in *Coccidioides* species, and the heat-shock proteins Hsp60 and Hsp82 in *H. capsulatum*. *C. albicans* has been studied for surface adhesins over very many years. This species expresses a family of glycoprotein 'agglutinin-like sequences', Als1–Als9, in its cell wall, among which Als3 plays a prominent role in adhesion to host surfaces (Hoyer et al. 2008). It also expresses adhesin Hwp1 in its cell wall, which is recognized by human transglutaminases and becomes covalently linked to epithelial cell layers (Martin et al. 2011). Many other cell wall-associated molecules in *C. albicans* probably contribute to adhesion and host resistance, though their details are less well studied than those of the Als and Hwp1 glycoproteins.

It is not only molecules bound to the cell surface that contribute to fungal adhesion: several secreted enzymes also appear to play a role in the process. For example, in *H. capsulatum*, a secreted calcium-binding protein and a secreted adhesin, Yps3, contribute to the pathogenesis of histoplasmosis (Edwards and Rappleye 2011; Mihu and Nosanchuk 2012). Secreted hydrolytic enzymes can also play a role in fungal adhesion (see 'Hydrolytic enzymes and virulence' below).

Hydrolytic enzymes and virulence

Fungi commonly secrete proteins into their environment, or house proteins within their cell walls, attached to structural wall polysaccharides. Among fungal pathogens, a number of secreted and surface proteins are hydrolytic enzymes, some of which have been associated with pathogenicity. These include secreted catalases in *H. capsulatum* (Holbrook et al. 2011) and *C. albicans* (Kusch et al. 2007), which may help the fungus deal with host antimicrobial reactive oxygen species, lipases in *C. albicans* (Schaller et al. 2005; Martin et al. 2011), and phospholipases in *C. albicans* (Leidich et al. 1998; Schaller et al. 2005) and *C. neoformans* (Ma and May 2009), which probably contribute to pathogenetic processes such as host surface adhesion and damage. Urease enzymes contribute (in different ways) to the virulence of *Coccidioides* species and of *C. neoformans* and *C. gattii* (Table 8.1). The latter yeasts, and *C. albicans,* also produce superoxide dismutases, which help resist phagocytic destruction (Klis et al. 2009; Kronstad et al. 2012). Arginase 1 in *Coccidioides* species has been shown to be a virulence factor (Hung et al. 2007).

By far the most commonly encountered 'virulence hydrolases' are surface and secreted proteinase enzymes, of virtually every biochemical type. These have been implicated in the pathogenesis of *Aspergillus, Candida, Cryptococcus*, and dermatophyte infections (Table 8.1). Dermatophyte proteinases can degrade the highly crosslinked protein keratin (Viani et al. 2001), assisted by secretion of sulphite ions which denature disulphide bonds (Monod 2008). *A. fumigatus* secretes a methylcitrate synthase that allows the fungus to assimilate amino acids released by fungal enzymes degrading host proteins (Ibrahim-Granet et al. 2008)—a second instance where two fungal molecules are required for optimal pathogenic effect.

The secreted aspartyl proteinases (Saps) of *C. albicans* are among the most thoroughly studied of fungal virulence factors, and can serve as adhesins as well as protein destroyers. Proteolytic activity by *C. albicans* was initially discovered in the 1960s (Staib 1965), and until the early 1990s the fungus was assumed to produce a single proteolytic enzyme (Ruchel et al. 1992). Molecular genetic approaches finally revealed a family of ten Saps, whose members are differentially expressed by yeast and hyphal forms and differentially expressed between and within types of superficial and deep-seated *Candida* infections (Schaller et al. 2005).

Biofilm formation and virulence

For many infections, the formation of microbial biofilms on host surfaces constitutes an important part of pathogenesis. Biofilms, comprising tightly packed microbial cells bonded by an intercellular matrix, are generally more adhesive, more resistant to host defences, and more resistant to the action of antimicrobial drugs than free-swimming (planktonic) microbes.

Among pathogenic fungi, biofilm formation has been specifically implicated in the virulence of *A. fumigatus* (Kniemeyer et al. 2011) and *C. albicans* (Kniemeyer et al. 2011). It is usually proposed that biofilms are important when fungi adhere to foreign bodies such as intravenous catheter plastic, but the complex changes in gene regulation and expression associated with biofilm formation in both species may also play a role in the organization of fungal 'tissues' that can be seen to develop in deep organs as well. *A. fumigatus* produces gliotoxin, a typical fungal toxin. In chronically infected patients, biofilm formation appears to be associated with an increase in gliotoxin levels (Kniemeyer et al. 2011).

Phenotypic switching and virulence

The phenomenon whereby an organism undergoes detectable phenotypic changes en masse as a result of differential gene regulation rather than mutation is a common event for many microbes. In *Candida albicans, Cryptococcus neoformans*, and *Cryptococcus gattii*, particular phenotypic switches have been shown to play significant roles in virulence. The switching process in the *Cryptococcus* species affects the size and structure of the capsule, thus altering the ability of the fungus to evade host immune defences (Ma and May 2009). In *C. albicans*, the white–opaque (cell) switch is particularly associated with processes such as mating, but white and opaque cells also differ in virulence, with white cells more invasive for deep tissues, and opaque cells more invasive for skin (Soll 2014).

Iron homeostasis and virulence

Among trace metals essential for fungal growth, iron is relatively scarce in human tissues. Several fungal pathogens, including *A. fumigatus* and *H. capsulatum* (Table 8.1) produce siderophores that enhance the ability of the fungi to take up iron. Demonstration of the significance of such siderophores in pathogenesis is experimentally difficult, since very small changes in iron homeostasis may not be reflected in gross shifts in virulence (Edwards and Rappleye 2011; Mihu and Nosanchuk 2012).

Other virulence factors

C. neoformans cells of mating type MATα are considerably more mouse-virulent than MATa strains, and they are isolated far more often from clinical samples of *C. neoformans* than are MATa types (Hogan et al. 1996; Ma and May 2009). This evidence strongly suggests a role for mating type in pathogenesis, but it remains for future research to reveal how the association functions.

Strain variations in virulence

From the earliest days of research into fungal infections, it has been self-evident that different natural isolates of a pathogenic species vary in virulence for experimental hosts. The differences arise, of course, because each fungal strain possesses its own complement of genes encoding virulence factors, and some strains will therefore be better adapted than others to invade and damage a mammalian host (discussion of whether or not causing damage offers the fungus a selective advantage is beyond the scope of this chapter).

One of the best studied examples of strain variation in virulence concerns the capsule of *C. neoformans*. Spontaneous and engineered mutants deficient in capsule formation are considerably attenuated in virulence (Hogan et al. 1996). A very large number of genes are involved in the biosynthesis and regulation of the cryptococcal capsule, and deletion of individual capsule genes often leads to measurable changes in virulence (Kronstad et al. 2012; O'Meara and Alspaugh 2012). The species *C. gattii*, for many years regarded as a subtype of *C. neoformans*, can be subtyped by multi-locus gene sequencing. *C. gattii* subtypes VGIIa/major and VGIIb/minor have been shown to be responsible for an epidemic outbreak of cryptococcal disease still spreading in the north-west of the American continent. VGIIa/major, in particular, is able to cause symptomatic infections in healthy humans: the reasons for its enhanced virulence are still under investigation (Byrnes et al. 2011).

C. albicans can be subtyped by a number of DNA-based methods, among which multi-locus sequence typing and microsatellite length polymorphism analysis have been the most widely used (Garcia-Hermoso et al. 2007). No clear relationships between strain type and virulence have been established for this species (MacCallum et al. 2009). However, the observation that approximately one-third of all *C. albicans* clinical isolates belong to a clade of closely related strains (Odds 2010) hints that members of this clade may be better adapted to survive as human commensals and are therefore more often available to cause disease when their host becomes immunocompromised.

H. capsulatum isolates can be divided into seven phylogenetically based clades. Detailed characterization of some isolates from different clades has revealed large differences in the complements of virulence factors used by different strains to cause experimental infections (Edwards and Rappleye 2011). Two strain chemotypes commonly isolated from infected patients in the USA, NAm1 and NAm2, differ in virulence. NAm1 strains are deficient in cell wall alpha-1,3-glucan and typically infect immunocompromised patients, particularly those infected with human immunodeficiency virus, while NAm2 strains can infect immunologically intact hosts. In animal models, both types are virulent when injected at a high dose to cause an acute infection, although concentrations of the fungi in infected lungs differ; when mice are infected with lower doses, leading to slowly evolving infections, the virulence differences between the fungal strain types are much less apparent (Sepúlveda et al. 2014). These findings emphasize the complexity of the pathogenesis of fungal disease. Multiple interactions between fungal virulence factors and the host responses described in Chapter 9, combined with specific locations and quantities of fungal cells within a host and the passage of time, serve to determine the types, symptoms, and severity of each individual case of fungal infection.

References

Achtermann RR and White TC (2012) Dermatophyte virulence factors: identifying and analyzing genes that may contribute to chronic or acute skin infections. *Int J Microbiol* 2012: 358305.

Brunke SKS, Fischer D, Jacobsen ID, et al. (2014) One small step for a yeast—microevolution within macrophages renders *Candida glabrata* hypervirulent due to a single point mutation *PloS Pathog* 10: e1004478.

Byrnes EJI, Bartlett KH, Perfect JR, et al. (2011) *Cryptococcus gattii*: an emerging fungal pathogen infecting humans and animals. *Microbes Infect* 13: 895–907.

Casadevall A (2006) Cards of virulence and the global virulome for humans. *Microbe* 1: 359–64.

Edwards JA and Rappleye CA (2011) *Histoplasma* mechanisms of pathogenesis—one portfolio doesn't fit all. *FEMS Microbiol Lett* 324: 1–9.

Garcia-Hermoso D, Cabaret O, Lecellier G, et al. (2007) Comparison of microsatellite length polymorphism and multilocus sequence typing for DNA-based typing of *Candida albicans*. *J Clin Microbiol* 45: 3958–63.

Hogan LH, Klein BS and Levitz SM (1996) Virulence factors of medically important fungi. *Clin Microbiol Rev* 9: 469.

Holbrook ED, Edwards JA, Youseff BH, et al. (2011) Definition of the extracellular proteome of pathogenic-phase *Histoplasma capsulatum*. *J Proteome Res* 10: 1929–43.

Hoyer LL, Green CB, Oh SH, et al. (2008) Discovering the secrets of the *Candida albicans* agglutinin-like sequence (ALS) gene family—a sticky pursuit. *Med Mycol* 46: 1–15.

Hung CY, Xue JM and Cole GT (2007) Virulence mechanisms of *Coccidioides*. *Ann N Y Acad Sci* 1111: 225–35.

Ibrahim-Granet O, Dubourdeau M, Latgé J-P, et al. (2008) Methylcitrate synthase from *Aspergillus fumigatus* is essential for manifestation of invasive aspergillosis. *Cell Microbiol* 10: 134–48.

Jain C, Yun M, Politz SM, et al. (2009) A pathogenesis assay using *Saccharomyces cerevisiae* and *Caenorhabditis elegans* reveals novel roles for yeast AP-1, Yap1, and host dual oxidase BLI-3 in fungal pathogenesis. *Eukaryot Cell* 8: 1218–27.

Klis FM, Sosinska GJ, De Groot PWJ, et al. (2009) Covalently linked cell wall proteins of *Candida albicans* and their role in fitness and virulence. *FEMS Yeast Res* 9: 1013–28.

Kniemeyer O, Schmidt AD, Vödisch M, et al. (2011) Identification of virulence determinants of the human pathogenic fungi *Aspergillus fumigatus* and *Candida albicans* by proteomics. *Int J Med Microbiol* 301: 368–77.

Krajaejun T, Wuthrich M, Gauthier GM, et al. (2010) Discordant influence of *Blastomyces dermatitidis* yeast-phase-specific gene *BYS1* on morphogenesis and virulence *Infect Immun* 78: 2522–8.

Kronstad J, Saikia S, Nielson ED, et al. (2012) Adaptation of *Cryptococcus neoformans* to mammalian hosts: integrated regulation of metabolism and virulence. *Eukaryot Cell* 11: 109–18.

Kumamoto CA and Vinces MD (2005) Contributions of hyphae and hypha-co-regulated genes to *Candida albicans* virulence. *Cell Microbiol* 7: 1546–54.

Kusch H, Engelmann S, Albrecht D, et al. (2007) Proteomic analysis of the oxidative stress responses in *Candida albicans*. *Proteomics* 7: 686–97.

Leidich SD, Ibrahim AS, Fu Y, et al. (1998) Cloning and disruption of ca*PLB1*, a phospholipase B gene involved in the pathogenicity of *Candida albicans*. *J Biol Chem* 273: 26078–86.

Ma HS and May RC (2009) Virulence in *Cryptococcus* species. *Adv Appl Microbiol* 67: 131–90.

MacCallum DM, Castillo L, Nather K, et al. (2009) Property differences among the four major *Candida albicans* strain clades. *Eukaryot Cell* 8: 373–87.

Martin R, Wächtler B, Schaller M, et al. (2011) Host–pathogen interactions and virulence-associated genes during *Candida albicans* oral infections. *Int J Med Microbiol* 301: 417–22.

Mayer FL, Wilson D and Hube B (2014) *Candida albicans* pathogenicity mechanisms. *Virulence* 4: 119–28.

Mihu MR and Nosanchuk JD (2012) *Histoplasma* virulence and host responses. *Int J Microbiol* 2012: 268123.

Monod M (2008) Secreted proteases from dermatophytes. *Mycopathologia* 166: 285–94.

Moore MM (2013) The crucial role of iron uptake in *Aspergillus fumigatus* virulence. *Curr Opin Microbiol* 16: 692–9.

Odds FC (2010) Molecular phylogenetics and epidemiology of *Candida albicans*. *Future Microbiol* 5: 67–79.

O'Meara TR and Alspaugh JA (2012) The *Cryptococcus neoformans* capsule: a sword and a shield. *Clin Microbiol Rev* 25: 387–408.

Ruchel R, De Bernardis F, Ray TL, et al. (1992) *Candida* acid proteinases. *J Med Vet Mycol* 30 (suppl. 1): 123–32.

Schaller M, Borelli C, Korting HC, et al. (2005) Hydrolytic enzymes as virulence factors of *Candida albicans*. *Mycoses* 48: 365–77.

Scharf HD, Heinekamp T, Remme N, et al. (2012) Biosynthesis and function of gliotoxin in *Aspergillus fumigatus*. *Appl Microbiol Biotechnol* 93: 467–72.

Sepúlveda VE, Williams CL and Goldman WE (2014) Comparison of phylogenetically distinct *Histoplasma* strains reveals evolutionarily divergent virulence strategies *MBio* 5: e01376-14.

Soll DR (2014) The role of phenotypic switching in the basic biology and pathogenesis of *Candida albicans*. *J Oral Microbiol* 6: 22993.

Sriranganadane D, Reichard U, Salamin K, et al. (2011) Secreted glutamic protease rescues aspartic protease Pep deficiency in *Aspergillus fumigatus* during growth in acidic protein medium. *Microbiology* 157: 1541–50.

Staib F (1965) Serum-proteins as nitrogen source for yeast-like fungi. *Sabouraudia* 4: 187–93.

Upadhya R, Donlin MJ and Lodge JK (2014) *Cryptococcus* at work: gene expression during human infection. *MBio* 5: 1–2.

Viani FC, Dos Santos JI, Paula CR, et al. (2001) Production of extracellular enzymes by *Microsporum canis* and their role in its virulence. *Med Mycol* 39: 463–68.

Walker LA, MacCallum DM, Bertram G, et al. (2009) Genome-wide analysis of *Candida albicans* gene expression patterns during infection of the mammalian kidney. *Fungal Genet Biol* 46: 210–19.

Wuthrich M, Finkel-Jimenez B, Brandhorst TT, et al. (2006) Analysis of non-adhesive pathogenic mechanisms of *BAD1* on *Blastomyces dermatitidis*. *Med Mycol* 44: 41–9.

Zheng XD, Wang YM and Wang Y (2004) Hgc1, a novel hypha-specific G1 cyclin-related protein regulates *Candida albicans* hyphal morphogenesis. *EMBO J* 23: 1845–56.

CHAPTER 9

Immunology of fungal disease

Ivy M. Dambuza*, Jeanette Wagener*,
Gordon D. Brown, and Neil A.R. Gow

Introduction to immunology of fungal infections

The mammalian immune system is characterized by its ability to distinguish between self and non-self and to eliminate the non-self. Immune defence mechanisms range from physical barriers, such as skin and mucosal membranes, to mechanisms developed early during evolution, such as innate and trained immunity, and more sophisticated adaptive immune mechanisms (Table 9.1).

Fungi are associated with a wide spectrum of diseases in humans. In immunocompetent individuals, fungi cause acute self-limiting cutaneous lesions and pulmonary manifestations, whereas in immunocompromised patients they are associated with inflammatory diseases and severe life-threatening infections. Fungi are part of our natural environment, inhabiting soil and rotten vegetation and materials. Humans are constantly exposed to fungi by inhaling spores or by ingesting contaminated food. Examples of common disease-causing fungi acquired from the environment include *Aspergillus fumigatus, Cryptococcus neoformans, Histoplasma capsulatum, Blastomyces dermatitidis, Paracoccidioides brasiliensis*, and *Coccidioides immitis*. Other medically important fungi such as *Candida* and *Malassezia* yeast, on the other side, have co-evolved with their mammalian host over millions of years. These fungi colonize the human skin and mucosal surfaces (oral, gastrointestinal, and urinary tract) without causing an infection. The occurrence of infections therefore reflects a disturbance in the health of the immune surveillance of the host. This demonstrates the complexity of the human immune system and its ability to distinguish between self and non-self, and moreover, between commensalism and pathogenicity. The host immune response to fungi comprises two main components: resistance to fungal infections by limiting fungal burden, and tolerance to fungal presence by limiting self-damaging inflammatory host responses.

Innate immunity

Innate immunity is defined as non-specific host defence against invading pathogens. Innate defence mechanisms are constitutive to the host and do not require time for induction as specific adaptive immune responses—discussed later in this chapter. We distinguish between non-cellular innate defence mechanisms, such as anatomical barriers, the sequestration of essential nutrients (nutritional immunity), intact commensal microbiome and host defence molecules (enzymes and antimicrobial peptides) including complement, and cell-mediated innate immunity, the ability to undergo inflammatory and phagocytic responses.

* These authors contributed equally.

Constitutive non-cellular innate defence mechanisms

Anatomical defences

Mechanical and chemical resistance are the main contributors to anatomical defence. The physical barrier of skin and mucosae protects the body against the invasion of pathogenic fungi. Although the skin is a hostile barrier, covered with oily and acidic (pH 3–5) secretions from sebaceous and sweat glands, *Malassezia* yeasts have successfully adapted to this harsh environment.

Microbial antagonism

The human microbiome of skin and mucosae antagonizes the colonization and overgrowth of pathogenic microbes through the restriction of adherence sites, the production of bacteriocins and metabolites, and nutrient limitation. The human body engages in symbiotic associations with commensal microbiota, and it has been demonstrated that symbiotic factors produced by commensal microbes beneficially modulate the host immune system (Gallo and Nakatsuji 2011). Changes in the commensal microbiota (dysbiosis) due to antibiotic treatment, for example, can lead to fungal overgrowth and dissemination (Koh 2013).

Host defence peptides

Host defence peptides (HDPs), or as initially termed 'antimicrobial peptides', are a key element of innate immunity against fungal pathogens. These peptides are found in epithelial layers throughout the body, such as skin and mucosal surfaces, including the airway, oral cavity, and digestive tract, but also in phagocytic cells and body fluids (e.g. sweat, saliva, tears, and mucus) (Bahar and Ren 2013). Some HDPs are constitutively produced, while others are induced in response to infection and inflammation. The predominantly cationic oligopeptides kill microbes by disrupting the cell membrane integrity, by inhibiting the production of DNA and RNA, or by interacting with other intracellular targets. Antifungal HDPs either interfere with intracellular components,

Table 9.1 Host immune defence mechanisms

Innate/natural immunity (non-specific responses)		Adaptive/acquired immunity (specific responses)
1st line	**2nd line**	**3rd line**
Non-cellular defence	Cellular defence	Specialized lymphocytes
Anatomical/physical barriers (e.g. skin, mucous membranes) Secretions (e.g. mucus, sweat) Microbial antagonism (e.g. commensal flora)	Innate immune cells (e.g. neutrophils, monocytes, macrophages) Inflammation (e.g. cytokines) Phagocytic cells Host defence peptides Complement system Nutritional immunity	Humoral response (e.g. B cells, antibodies) Cell-mediated response (e.g. T cells) Memory response

or bind to fungal cell wall components (e.g. chitin), or disrupt the cell membrane integrity by increasing the permeability or formation of pores (Bahar and Ren 2013). Human HDPs with known antifungal activity are the β-defensins, histatins, calprotectins, and cathelicidins (Mehra et al. 2012). Besides their antimicrobial activity, recent advances in the field have expanded the repertoire of activities for HDPs to include immunostimulatory and immunomodulatory capacities, such as immune cell chemotaxis and maturation, and the enhancement of adaptive immune responses (Ganz 2003; Guani-Guerra et al. 2010).

Complement system

The complement system comprises a large number of distinct plasma proteins that mark foreign cells for ingestion and elimination by phagocytes—a process called opsonization. Activated complement proteins act in three ways: first, they covalently bind to pathogens to initiate the opsonization process; second, they attract and activate phagocytic cells at the site of infection; and third, they create membrane pores, directly damaging the pathogen. All three known pathways of complement activation—the antibody-activated classical pathway, the mannose-binding lectin (MBL)-activated pathway, and the alternative pathway, triggered by pathogen surface structures—have the same consequences: the opsonization of pathogens, the recruitment of inflammatory cells, and the direct killing of pathogens. Several medically prominent fungal species, such as *C. albicans*, *A. fumigatus*, and *C. neoformans*, employ various strategies to inactivate complement. These are: binding to complement regulatory factors, the secretion of proteins that bind to complement receptors on phagocytes, and the degradation of complement proteins through secreted proteases (Collette and Lorenz 2011; Luo et al. 2013).

Cell-mediated innate immunity

The main cells of the host innate immune response (an overview is given in Figure 9.1) that recognize invading pathogens are blood-circulating monocytes and neutrophils, together with macrophages and dendritic cells (DCs) in tissues. Other immune cells, such as eosinophils and mast cells, and even non-classical immune cells such as epithelial and endothelial cells, contribute to pathogen recognition and defence by producing inflammatory mediators, such as cytokines and chemokines, that activate and modulate immune responses after encountering pathogenic microorganisms.

Neutrophils

Neutrophils are the most abundant (40–75%) type of white blood cell. During the acute phase of an infection, neutrophils are the first inflammatory cells recruited to the site of infection. Neutrophils play a key role in innate defence as they directly attack the invading pathogen, utilizing three different methods: (1) phagocytosis—the uptake, intracellular killing and digestion of microbes; (2) degranulation—the release of granule-stored antimicrobial proteins (e.g. myeloperoxidase, defensins, cathepsins, and cathelicidin) into the environment; and (3) neutrophil extracellular traps (NETs) or 'NETosis'—the release of traps composed of decondensed chromatin, histones, and granule proteins (Brinkmann et al. 2004). Neutrophils further secrete chemokines and cytokines to orchestrate an ongoing inflammatory and adaptive immune response (Underhill and Goodridge 2012). Recent research has shown the ability of neutrophils to deploy their antimicrobial strategies in a way that is selectively tailored to the encountered pathogen. Fungal yeast cells are rapidly phagocytosed by neutrophils, whereas hyphae—the filamentous growth form of *Aspergillus* and *Candida*, for example—are too large to be phagocytosed and trigger NETosis instead (Branzk et al. 2014). The importance of neutrophils in antifungal immune defence is highlighted by the increased risk of individuals with abnormally low numbers of neutrophils (neutropenia) developing systemic fungal infections and fungal septicaemia. Furthermore, use of neutrophils as adjunctive immune therapy in these patients has been shown to be beneficial for treating invasive and disseminated fungal infections (Casadevall and Pirofski 2001).

Monocytes

Monocytes are a subset of white blood cells that can differentiate into macrophages and DCs after migration into the tissue. Human monocytes are divided into three subsets on the basis of cell surface marker and chemokine receptor expression: classical, intermediate, and non-classical monocytes. In the steady state, monocytes replenish tissue macrophages and DCs, but in cases of infection, they are recruited into the infected tissue where they mediate direct antimicrobial activity (Serbina et al. 2008). Moreover, inflammatory monocytes have been shown to mediate an appropriate adaptive immune response in the lung towards *A. fumigatus*, *B. dermatitidis*, and *C. neoformans* (Shi and Pamer 2011; Espinosa et al. 2014). Recent developments in the field of innate immunity

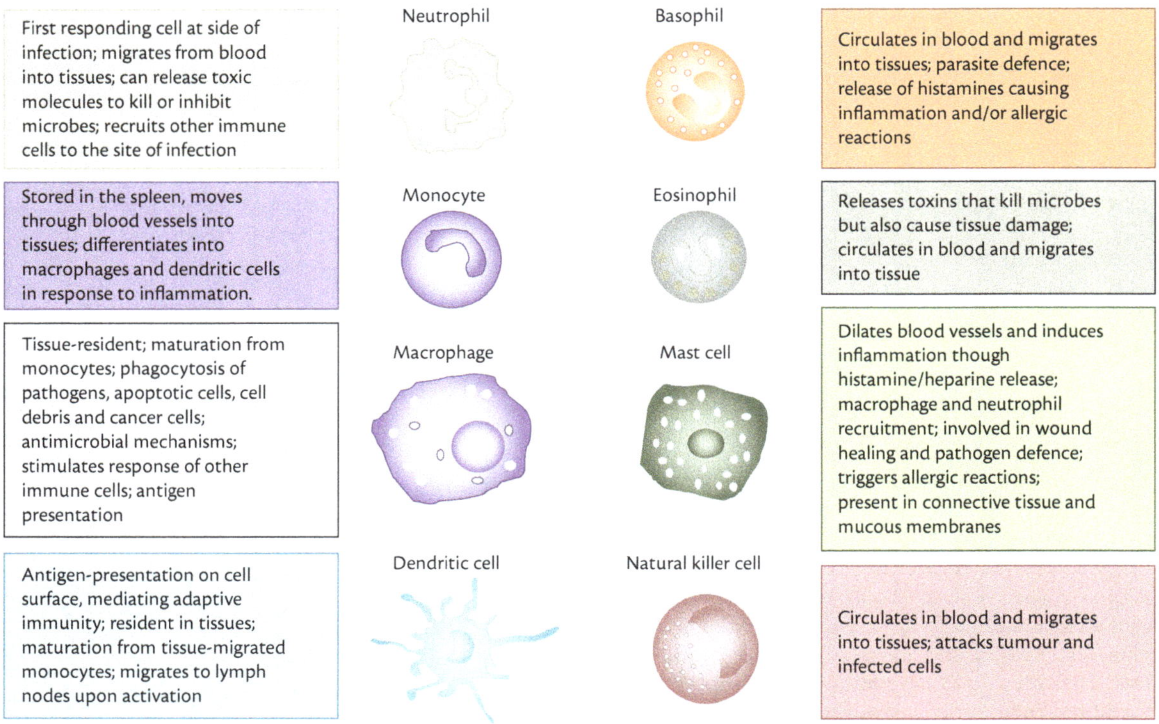

Figure 9.1 Primary functions of innate immune cells.

have demonstrated a short-term immunological memory in monocytes, named 'trained immunity' (Netea et al. 2011). Monocytes stimulated with low amounts of the fungal cell wall component β-glucan *in vitro* have been shown to mediate protection against subsequent lethal systemic candidiasis in mice, deficient in an adaptive immune system, demonstrating that the innate system, like the adaptive immune system, can be primed by pre-exposure to fungal cell components and has some capacity to remember previous encounters with pathogens (Quintin et al. 2012, 2014).

Macrophages

Macrophages are present in virtually all body tissues and are characterized by the ability to engulf and digest apoptotic cells, cellular debris, cancer cells, and microbes. Macrophages emerge from blood-circulating monocytes, migrating into the tissue, where they mature into inflammatory or long-living tissue-specific macrophages. Macrophages display a remarkable plasticity in response to environmental cues, which gives rise to a spectrum of activated macrophages with distinct functions (Mosser and Edwards 2008; Murray and Wynn 2011). These functions are host defence, immune regulation, and wound healing. The immune response of macrophages triggered by infection comprises four interrelated phases: (1) pathogen recognition; (2) macrophage enrichment in infected tissue by recruitment of monocytes and/or *in-situ* proliferation; (2) microbicidal activity and conversion to an anti-inflammatory phenotype, terminating anti-infectious responses; and (4) promotion of tissue repair. During an infection, macrophages engulf microbes and contain them in vesicles called phagosomes. These phagosomes undergo a series of fusion events, leading to the formation of phagolysosomes—which creates a degradative and microbicidal environment with a reduced pH, enriched with hydrolytic enzymes, defensins, and toxic oxidative compounds to kill the microbes. Nonetheless, several pathogenic fungi have evolved efficient strategies to avoid and overcome the killing by macrophages (Seider et al. 2010). These are the avoidance of immune recognition, the prevention of engulfment by phagocytes, the interference with phagosome maturation, and the escape from phagocytes. The human pathogenic fungus *C. neoformans*, for example, can reside intracellularly in phagosomes, thereby avoiding immune recognition. *C. neoformans* replicates inside the phagosome and exits without damaging the host cell in a process called 'vomocytosis' (Johnston and May 2013). Interestingly, it is believed that *C. neoformans* has evolved this sophisticated intracellular adaptation to resist its natural phagocytic predator in the soil, the amoeba (Coelho et al. 2014).

Dendritic cells

Dendritic cells are the major link between the innate and the adaptive immune system. They are strategically positioned throughout the body tissues, where they comprise a dense surveillance network. DCs sample antigenic material in the environment, and through complex processing and presentation of the antigen to T cells, they shape and instruct T-cell responses. Several DC subsets have been described, based on phenotype, anatomical location, and other functional characteristics. Initiation of a proper adaptive immune response via DCs is important in antifungal immunity, and DC activation and maturation depend on the 'right' signals derived from the interactions with the fungi itself (Ramirez-Ortiz and Means 2012). Phagocytosis of *Aspergillus* conidia by DCs, for example, leads to a protective Th1 (type-1 T helper cell) response, whereas interactions with hyphae result in a non-protective Th2 response (Bozza et al. 2002).

Recognition of fungi by innate immune cells

Pathogen-associated molecular patterns

In addition to the constitutive defence mechanisms of the human body, host cells express a variety of germ-line encoded pattern recognition receptors (PRRs) that sense pathogen-associated molecular patterns (PAMPs). PRR activation initiates downstream, cell type specific, intracellular signalling events that promote activation of other immune cells and further induce adaptive immune responses such as the induction of protective T-helper cells, which result in the clearance of an infection. PAMPs are conserved, invariant molecular structures, shared by large groups of pathogens. Carbohydrate components of the fungal cell wall are the main PAMPs recognized by PRRs on mammalian cells (Netea et al. 2008). The composition of the cell wall varies between fungal species, and further depends on the fungal environment, growth stage, and morphology, and so is a moving target for the immune system (Gow et al. 2012; Brown et al. 2014). The three main cell wall components shared by all fungal species are: mannans (chains of mannose molecules attached to cell wall proteins via *N*- or *O*-linkages), β-glucans (β-(1,3)-linked polymers of glucose with various β-(1,6)-linked branches), and chitin (a polymer of *N*-acetylglucosamine). Additional species-specific components with immunomodulatory capacity can be found in the fungal cell wall, such as galactomannans and galactosaminogalactan in the cell wall of *Aspergillus*, or galactoxylomannan and glucoronoxylomannan in the extracellular polysaccharide capsule of *Cryptococcus* (Barreto-Bergter and Figueiredo 2014). Several PRR families are involved in antifungal immunity and the recognition of one or more fungal PAMPs. These are toll-like receptors (TLRs), C-type lectin receptors (CLRs), NOD-like receptors (NLRs), and the galectin family of proteins; a summary of these is provided in Figure 9.2.

C-type lectins

CLRs comprise a large family of receptors with one or more carbohydrate recognition domains (Dambuza and Brown 2015). Dectin-1 is the best-described receptor of the family and has been intensively studied in antifungal immunity (Plato et al. 2015). Dectin-1 recognizes β-glucans in the cell walls of numerous fungi, including *C. albicans, A. fumigatus*, and *Pneumocystis jirovecii* (Drummond and Brown 2011). Innate recognition and downstream signalling of Dectin-1 have significant functional consequences to *in vivo* antifungal immunity. Studies in Dectin-1-deficient mice have revealed an increased mortality in systemic *C. albicans* and *A. fumigatus* infections, and increased fungal burden in *P. carinii* and *C. immitis* infections. In humans, single-nucleotide proteins in Dectin-1 and its signalling adapter protein, Card9, are highly associated with mucosal candidiasis and deep dermatophytosis (Ferwerda et al. 2009; Lanternier et al. 2013). Dectin-1 signalling leads to several cellular responses, including phagocytosis, cytokine production, respiratory burst, and inflammasome activation (Drummond and Brown 2011; Plato et al. 2015). Another recently described downstream function of Dectin-1 is the modulation of the autophagy

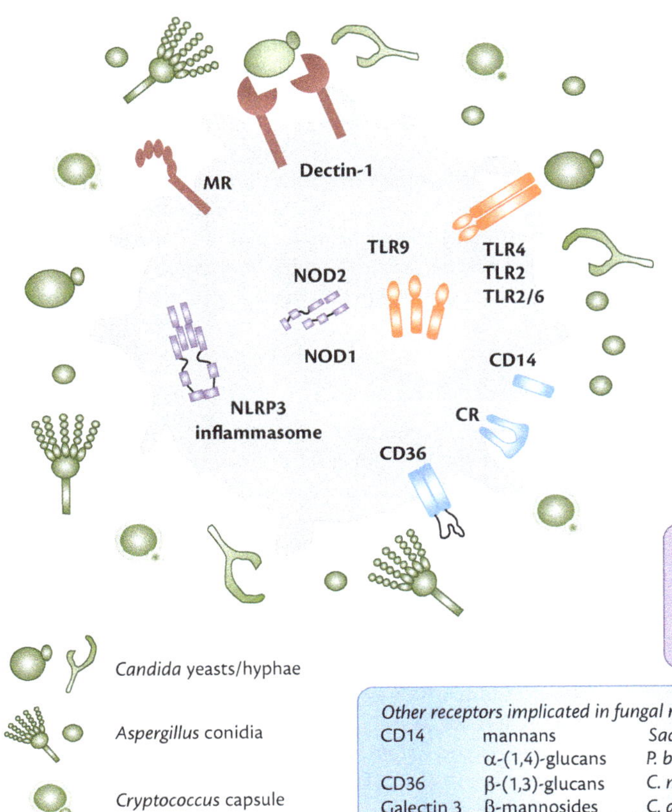

C-type lectin receptors (CLRs)

MR	*N*-linked mannans	*C. albicans*
	mannans	*P. carinii*
	mannoproteins	*C. neoformans*
DC-SIGN	galactomannans	*A. fumigatus*
	mannans	*C. albicans*
Dectin-1	β-(1,3)-glucans	*A. fumigatus, C. albicans*, others
Dectin-2	α-mannans	*C. albicans*
Mincle	α-mannosylation	*C. albicans, Malassezia* spp.

TLRs

TLR2	a-(1,4)-glucans	*P. boydii*
TLR2/TLR1	glucuronoxylomannans	*C. neoformans*
TLR2/TLR6	phospholipomannans	*C. albicans*
	glucuronoxylomannans	*C. neoformans*
TLR4	*O*-linked mannans	*C. albicans*
	rhamnomannans	*P. boydii*
	phospholipomannans	*C. albicans*
TLR9	unmethylated DNA	*C. albicans, A. fumigatus*

NLRs

NOD1	unknown	*A. fumigatus*
NOD2	chitin	*C. albicans*
	unknown	*A. fumigatus*
NLRP3	β-(1,3)-glucans	*A. fumigatus, C. albicans*

Other receptors implicated in fungal recognition

CD14	mannans	*Saccharomyces* spp.
	α-(1,4)-glucans	*P. boydii*
CD36	β-(1,3)-glucans	*C. neoformans*
Galectin 3	β-mannosides	*C. albicans*

Figure 9.2 Selected pattern recognition receptors and fungal PAMPs (pathogen-associated molecular patterns) recognized.

pathway to promote antigen presentation (Ma and Underhill 2013). Other CLRs that recognize fungal PAMPs and shape innate and adaptive host responses are Dectin-2, Mincle (macrophage-inducible C-type lectin), and the mannose receptor (reviewed in Vautier et al. 2012).

Toll-like receptors

The importance of toll-like receptors in antifungal defence was discovered in *Drosophila* flies nearly 20 years ago (Lemaitre et al. 1996). Since then, intensive studies on the homologues in mammals have confirmed a crucial role for TLRs in innate defence against fungi. Moreover, single-nucleotide polymorphisms (SNPs) in human TLRs (e.g. TLR1, TLR4, TLR6, and TLR9) have been determined that are associated with increased susceptibility to chronic and invasive fungal infections (Carvalho et al. 2010). After sensing various fungal components—such as *O*- and *N*-linked mannans phospholipomannan and glucuronoxylomannan, DNA, and RNA—TLRs initiate intracellular signalling pathways which activate antifungal immunity through the production of type I interferons (IFNs), the release of pro-inflammatory cytokines (e.g. Tumor necrosis factor [TNF]-α and interleukin-12 [IL-12]), and the promotion of an adaptive immune response. Interestingly, TLRs, such as TLR2, have been shown to collaborate with CLRs (e.g. Dectin-1) to trigger cytokine responses upon recognition of *C. albicans*, or mediate phagocytic uptake of *A. fumigatus*.

Nod-like receptors and the inflammasome

Inflammasomes have been shown to be central mediators of host defence to a wide range of pathogens. These large, cytoplasmic multiprotein signalling complexes are formed by proteins of the NLR family, which lead to caspase-1 activation and maturation of pro-inflammatory cytokines IL-1β and IL-18 (Schroder and Tschopp 2010; Lamkanfi and Dixit 2014). Although best studied in bacterial infections, recent research is highlighting the importance of NLRs and inflammasome activation in antifungal immunity. *C. albicans, A. fumigatus*, and *Malassezia* spp. have been shown to activate the NLRP3 inflammasome (Ganesan et al. 2014; Kistowska et al. 2014; Gabrielli et al. 2015), and moreover, gain-of-function mutation in NLRP3, resulting in reduced IL-1β production in humans, has been linked to increased susceptibility to developing recurrent vulvovaginal candidiasis (Lev-Sagie et al. 2009).

Adaptive immunity

In all jawed vertebrates that have been investigated, conventional adaptive (acquired) immunity is mediated by B-cell receptors (BCRs) or immunoglobulins (Igs) and T-cell receptors (TCRs). These antigen receptors are generated by an evolutionary conserved DNA breakage and repair process that involves recombination of the variable (V), diversity (D), and joining (J) gene segments within the BCR and TCR loci (Tonegawa 1983). During development of T (thymus-derived) and B (bursal-derived [or bone marrow derived, for human equivalent]) lymphocytes, *V(D)J recombination* generates TCRs and BCRs with the potential to recognize an unlimited number of antigens, generating *clonal diversity*, a hallmark feature of adaptive immunity. Mature immunocompetent lymphocytes exit the thymus or bone marrow into the circulation and migrate to secondary lymphoid tissues (e.g. spleen and lymph nodes). Upon antigen encounter, *clonal selection* is initiated, whereby only T and B cells bearing receptors with specificity to the antigen are "selected" to expand, differentiate, and develop into *memory cells* providing lifelong resistance to re-infection with the same pathogen.

B cells

B cells are the precursors of antibody-secreting plasma cells, the products of which are Ig molecules constructed from several units (Paul 2013), each comprising two heavy (H) and two light (L) polypeptide chains with antigen recognition sites. The H chains of Ig molecules comprise several types, including the μ, δ, γ (which has several subclasses), α, and ε types; thus there are IgM, IgD, IgG, IgA, and IgE antibodies based on the H chain they possess. These antibodies exist as membrane-bound B-cell receptors or secreted products. Of fundamental importance in the immune system is that an individual B cell can "switch" the Ig class that it produces—that is, a cell that expresses receptors of the IgM and IgD classes can differentiate into IgA- (or IgG- or IgE-) producing plasma cells through a process known as *Ig class switching*. Ig class switching is regulated by the action of T cells partly via the type of lymphokines they produce. Each antibody class mediates the following non-redundant biological functions: (1) complement system activation (IgM), (2) mucosal immunity (IgA), (3) allergic-type phenomena (IgE), (4) membrane-bound antigen receptors (IgD), and (5) cross-placental protection (IgG).

T cells

T cells, similar to B cells, derive from precursor stem cells that inhabit haematopoietic tissues. They undergo maturation within the thymus; upon exit, they populate the peripheral lymphoid tissues and form part of the recirculating pool of lymphocytes. T cells can be divided into two main classes based on cell surface expression of the CD4 or CD8 molecules. Unlike B-cell receptors, T-cell receptors do not bind free antigens (with the exception of γδTCRs). Instead, the T-cell receptor interacts with a complex expressed on the surfaces of antigen-presenting cells that consists of an antigenic determinant coupled to a class I (CD8 cell restricted) or a class II (CD4 cell restricted) major histocompatibility complex (MHC) protein. Antigen-experienced T cells have both regulatory and effector roles that are critical in shaping the outcome of the immune response.

Antifungal T- and B-cell immunity

Neutrophils, macrophages, and monocytes (all innate immune cells) are fundamentally important antifungal effector cells that effectively phagocytose and clear yeast and fungal spores. However, for reasons still under vigorous debate, the innate immune system is not always sufficient to resolve certain fungal infections. For instance, larger size hyphae interfere with uptake by phagocytes, and some fungi have adapted to life inside the very hostile micro-environment of phagocytes. Transition from innate to adaptive immunity is mediated by dendritic cells (DCs), which process and present fungal antigens for perusal by naïve CD4 and CD8 T cells (bearing αβTCRs). DC/T-cell interaction initiates activation of the effector fungi-specific helper CD4 T cell subsets, cytotoxic CD8 T cells, and regulatory T cells facilitating induction of cell-mediated immunity. Although B-cell activation does not require MHC-presentation of fungal antigens by DCs, the production of high-affinity neutralizing immunoglobulins requires help from CD4

T cells. Thus, an appropriate finely tuned immune response requires extensive 'crosstalk' between innate and adaptive immune cells.

Helper T-cell subsets and mechanisms of fungal resistance or susceptibility

A critical contribution of T cells to host defence against fungal pathogens (Figure 9.3) is illustrated by the high susceptibility of patients with acquired immune deficiency syndrome (AIDS) to fungal infections with, for example, *Cryptococcus, Aspergillus, Candida, Pneumocystis*, and *Histoplasma* spp. (Shoham and Levitz 2005). In mice, depletion of CD4 T cells also leads to uncontrolled fungal growth, while CD8 T cells have been shown to mediate protection against *B. dermatitidis* and *H. capsulatum* (Rivera 2014).

Th1 immunity

The role of Th1 cells in protective immunity against most fungal pathogens in both experimental mouse models and in man is well established. Interleukin 12 (IL-12) produced by innate immune cells, as well as natural killer (NK) cell-derived interferon gamma (IFN-γ), skews naïve cells towards a Th1 differentiation programme driven by STAT4 (signal transducer and activator of transcription 4), STAT1, and the T-box transcription factor T-bet. Th1 cells are primarily defined by production of mainly IFN-γ, but also produce other important pro-inflammatory cytokines such as TNF and granulocyte-macrophage colony-stimulating factor (GM-CSF). Several studies have shown that IFN-γ and TNF stimulate macrophages to release nitric oxide and reactive oxygen species (ROS), causing intracellular growth arrest of fungi, including *H. capsulatum, B. dermatitidis, P. brasiliensis*, and *Coccidioides immitis* (Beaman 1987; Brummer and Stevens 1995; Sugar et al. 1995; Calvi et al. 2003; Novak and Koh 2013). In both mice and man, defects in Th1 polarization or expression of the effector cytokines results in increased susceptibility to a myriad of fungal infections. In contrast, patients on IFN-γ immunotherapy show augmented protection against aspergillosis, cryptococcosis, and coccidioidomycosis (Verma et al. 2015a). Subramanian Vignesh et al. (2013) recently elucidated the role of GM-CSF in fungal immunity, showing that GM-CSF mediates antifungal responses in macrophages by sequestering intracellular zinc (a micronutrient required by yeast cells) as well as stimulating ROS. Of clinical significance is that GM-CSF immunotherapy, in combination with IFN-γ, has been shown to improve the outcome of invasive fungal diseases (Safdar 2013).

Th2 immunity

Differentiation towards the Th2 subset requires IL-4, STAT6, and the transcription factor GATA3. Th2 cells primarily express IL-4, IL-5, and IL-13, which are considered to promote alternatively

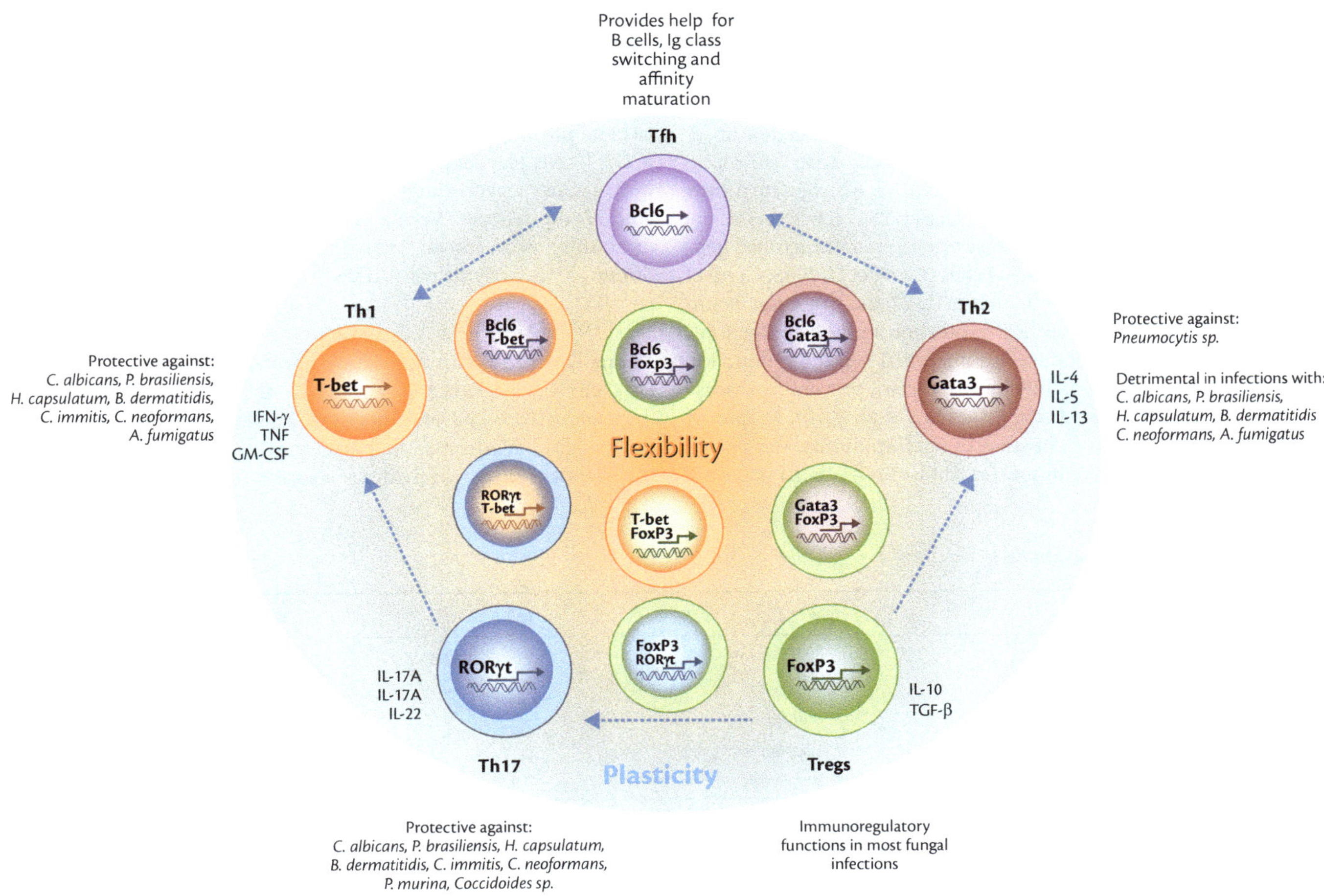

Figure 9.3 Role of different helper CD4 T-cell subsets in mycoses.

activated macrophages. These macrophages have reduced nitric oxide and fail to restrain intracellular growth of fungi (Davis et al. 2013). A case in point is a switch from Th1 to the detrimental Th2 response observed in progressive fungal infections such as those due to *Cryptococcus neoformans, H. capsulatum, Coccidioides immitis*, and *Coccidioides posadasii* (Wuthrich et al. 2012). Th2-derived IL-4 is also thought to promote intracellular growth of fungi by modulating the availability of micronutrients such as iron and zinc in macrophages (Weiss et al. 1997; Winters et al. 2010). Conversely, other investigators have suggested that Th2 immunity can confer protection against fungal infections. For instance, macrophage activation with IL-13 has been shown to protect mice from *Pneumocystis murina* (Nelson et al. 2011). The fungicidal activities of IL-13-activated macrophages are still under investigation.

Th17 immunity

Th17 cells are the newest subset of helper CD4 T cells to be discovered, and their biology is still not well understood. Differentiation and commitment to Th17 polarization require STAT3 activation by IL-6, IL-21, and IL-23 as well as TGF-β induction of retinoid-related orphan receptor γt. Th17 cells produce IL-17A, IL-17F, and IL-22. Increasing evidence shows that Th17 plays a very significant role in clearance of fungi, particularly at the mucosa. Individuals with STAT3 loss-of-function mutations, or lacking IL-17 signalling, are susceptible to a wide range of fungal infections. In addition, defects in the autoimmune regulator gene that result in autoantibodies against Th17 cytokines predispose individuals with APECED (autoimmune polyendocrinopathy with candidiasis and ectodermal dystrophy) to chronic and recurrent mucocutaneous candidiasis (Verma et al. 2015a). To date, two distinct mechanisms of Th17-mediated antifungal responses have been described. In systemic *Candida* infection models, Th17 cells drive neutrophil recruitment via expression of CXC chemokines, which in turn clear the infection (Hernandez-Santos and Gaffen 2012), whereas at the mucosae, IL-17A promotes the release of various antimicrobial peptides by keratinocytes and epithelial cells (Liang et al. 2006; Conti et al. 2011). Other Th17 cytokines, such as IL-22 and to a lesser extent IL-17F, are also implicated in host protection to fungal infections. IL-22 has been shown to induce antimicrobial peptide production by epithelial cells and maintain barrier integrity, preventing disease dissemination (Eyerich et al. 2009; De Luca et al. 2010). In spite of significant contributions to host antifungal immunity, the potential of Th17 to cause severe immunopathologies has been noted. In mouse models of gastric candidiasis and aspergillosis, Th17-mediated inflammation exaggerated disease (Zelante et al. 2007).

It is important to note that the described subsets of T cells are not fixed lineages. Recent evidence shows that there is considerable plasticity and flexibility in T-cell differentiation. This new T-cell paradigm has implications for the way we consider antifungal T-cell immunity and provides opportunities for tailoring desirable immune responses for specific fungal pathogens.

Regulatory T cells

Regulatory T cells, or 'Tregs', play an essential role in restraining excessive immune responses, and thus limit collateral damage to the host. Mechanisms of action mediated by Tregs include the secretion of anti-inflammatory cytokines such as IL-10, TGF-β, or IL-35, the sequestration of IL-2, and many more (Verma et al. 2015a). In many scenarios, Tregs represent a double-edged sword. Fewer Treg numbers, as observed in mice lacking toll-like receptor TLR2 and the chemokine receptor CCR5, efficiently clear infections with *C. albicans, P. brasiliensis*, and *H. capsulatum*. In contrast, the inhibition of immune responses by Tregs allows the persistence of fungus, promoting induction of a more robust secondary immune response. An interesting clinical observation is that humans with defects in Treg development suffer from chronic mucocutaneous candidiasis (Kekalainen et al. 2007).

Cytotoxic CD8 T cells

The function of CD8 T cells in fungal immunity has been eclipsed by the comprehensive studies focused on CD4 cells. Recent findings suggest that in the absence of CD4 T cells, cytotoxic CD8 T cells suppress fungal infections by lysing infected macrophages, and secrete pro-inflammatory cytokines IFN-γ and IL-17. In addition, CD8 T cells play an important role in vaccination-induced immunity against several fungi, including *A. fumigatus, B. dermatitidis*, and *H. capsulatum* (Verma et al. 2015a). Antifungal CD8-driven immunity provides an attractive strategy for cellular-mediated immunity in patients with AIDS.

Immunoglobulins

Clonally derived antibodies confer protection to fungi (Table 9.2). The clinical relevance of antibodies in mycoses is apparent in humans with B-cell abnormalities, such as those with X-linked hyper-IgM syndrome, hypogammaglobulinaemia, and IgG2 deficiency. These individuals display high susceptibility to

Table 9.2 Role of immunoglobulins in mycoses

	IgD	IgM	IgA	IgE	IgD
Protects against	*C. neoformans* *C. albicans* *A. fumigatus* *H. capsulatum* *P. brasiliensis*	*C. neoformans* *C. albicans* *P. murina* *H. capsulatum* *P. brasiliensis*	Protects against *C. albicans*	Not yet characterized	Not yet characterized
Mode of action	Opsonization Ab-mediated cellular toxicity Modifies inflammatory responses Direct fungicidal activity	Opsonization Complement activation Modifies inflammatory responses Direct fungicidal activity	Direct fungicidal activity in systemic infection Possible role at mucosa		

cryptococcosis and pneumocystosis (Gupta et al. 1987; Wahab et al. 1995; Neto et al. 2000; Winkelstein et al. 2003; de Gorgolas et al. 2005).

To date, antibodies that mediate protection target cell-wall antigens such as β-glucan of *A. fumigatus* and *C. albicans*, the capsule of *Cryptococcus*, mannotriose, heat shock protein 60 and histones from *H. capsulatum*, and kexin and glycoprotein 120 from *P. murina* (Wuthrich et al. 2012). The effector functions mediated by these antibodies range from inhibition of growth, fungicidal activity, suppression of virulence factors, antibody-mediated induction of microbicidal activity of effector cells, opsonization, and activation of complement pathway, to antibody-directed cell toxicity (Verma et al. 2015a). Antibodies also shape the immune response to fungi through the induction of cytokines; for example, the antibody to histone-like protein H2B, from *H. capsulatum*, promotes IFN-γ-regulated macrophage fungicidal activities. In contrast, the adoptive transfer of anticapsular IgG1 limits inflammation by upregulating IL-10 in mice infected with *Cryptococcus*.

Summary

Consensus themes are emerging about the types of effector mechanisms that confer protection and those that mediate host susceptibility, bolstering endeavours for designing immune-based therapies in the form of passive immunity or vaccine immunity. This is particularly urgent for individuals with immune suppression, in whom fungal infections could be fatal.

Acknowledgements

The authors are funded by grants from The Wellcome Trust and the Medical Research Council, UK.

References

Bahar AA and Ren D (2013) Antimicrobial peptides. *Pharmaceuticals (Basel)* 6: 1543–75.

Barreto-Bergter E and Figueiredo RT (2014) Fungal glycans and the innate immune recognition. *Front Cell Infect Microbiol* 4: 145.

Beaman L (1987) Fungicidal activation of murine macrophages by recombinant gamma interferon. *Infect Immun* 55: 2951–5.

Bozza S, Gaziano R, Spreca A, et al. (2002) Dendritic cells transport conidia and hyphae of *Aspergillus fumigatus* from the airways to the draining lymph nodes and initiate disparate Th responses to the fungus. *J Immunol* 168: 1362–71.

Branzk N, Lubojemska A, Hardison SE, et al. (2014) Neutrophils sense microbe size and selectively release neutrophil extracellular traps in response to large pathogens. *Nat Immunol* 15: 1017–25.

Brinkmann V, Reichard U, Goosmann C, et al. (2004) Neutrophil extracellular traps kill bacteria. *Science* 303: 1532–5.

Brown AJ, Brown GD, Netea MG and Gow NA (2014) Metabolism impacts upon *Candida* immunogenicity and pathogenicity at multiple levels. *Trends Microbiol* 22: 614–22.

Brummer E and Stevens DA (1995) Antifungal mechanisms of activated murine bronchoalveolar or peritoneal macrophages for *Histoplasma capsulatum*. *Clin Exp Immunol* 102: 65–70.

Calvi SA, Peracoli MT, Mendes RP, et al. (2003) Effect of cytokines on the in vitro fungicidal activity of monocytes from paracoccidioidomycosis patients. *Microbes Infect* 5: 107–13.

Carvalho A, Cunha C, Pasqualotto AC, Pitzurra L, Denning DW and Romani L (2010) Genetic variability of innate immunity impacts human susceptibility to fungal diseases. *Int J Infect Dis* 14: e460–8.

Casadevall A and Pirofski LA (2001) Adjunctive immune therapy for fungal infections. *Clin Infect Dis* 33: 1048–56.

Coelho C, Bocca AL and Casadevall A (2014) The intracellular life of *Cryptococcus neoformans*. *Annu Rev Pathol* 9: 219–38.

Collette JR and Lorenz MC (2011) Mechanisms of immune evasion in fungal pathogens. *Curr Opin Microbiol* 14: 668–75.

Conti HR, Baker O, Freeman AF, et al. (2011) New mechanism of oral immunity to mucosal candidiasis in hyper-IgE syndrome. *Mucosal Immunol* 4: 448–55.

Dambuza IM and Brown GD (2015) C-type lectins in immunity: recent developments. *Curr Opin Immunol* 32: 21–7.

Davis MJ, Tsang TM, Qiu Y, et al. (2013) Macrophage M1/M2 polarization dynamically adapts to changes in cytokine microenvironments in Cryptococcus neoformans infection. *MBio* 4: e00264-13. doi:10.1128/mBio.00264-13

De Gorgolas M, Erice A, Gil A, et al. (2005) *Cryptococcal* meningitis in a patient with X-linked hyper-IgM1 syndrome. *Scand J Infect Dis* 37: 526–8.

De Luca A, Zelante T, D'angelo C, et al. (2010) IL-22 defines a novel immune pathway of antifungal resistance. *Mucosal Immunol* 3: 361–73.

Drummond RA and Brown GD (2011) The role of Dectin-1 in the host defence against fungal infections. *Curr Opin Microbiol* 14: 392–9.

Espinosa V, Jhingran A, Dutta O, et al. (2014) Inflammatory monocytes orchestrate innate antifungal immunity in the lung. *PLoS Pathog* 10: e1003940.

Eyerich S, Eyerich K, Pennino D, et al. (2009) Th22 cells represent a distinct human T cell subset involved in epidermal immunity and remodeling. *J Clin Invest* 119: 3573–85.

Ferwerda B, Ferwerda G, Plantinga TS, et al. (2009) Human dectin-1 deficiency and mucocutaneous fungal infections. *N Engl J Med* 361: 1760–7.

Gabrielli E, Pericolini E, Luciano E, et al. (2015) Induction of caspase-11 by aspartyl proteinases of *Candida albicans* and implication in promoting inflammatory response. *Infect Immun* 83: 1940–8.

Gallo RL and Nakatsuji T (2011) Microbial symbiosis with the innate immune defense system of the skin. *J Invest Dermatol* 131: 1974–80.

Ganesan S, Rathinam VA, Bossaller L, et al. (2014) Caspase-8 modulates dectin-1 and complement receptor 3-driven IL-1beta production in response to beta-glucans and the fungal pathogen, *Candida albicans*. *J Immunol* 193: 2519–30.

Ganz T (2003) The role of antimicrobial peptides in innate immunity. *Integr Comp Biol* 43: 300–4.

Gow NA, Van De Veerdonk FL, Brown AJ and Netea MG (2012) *Candida albicans* morphogenesis and host defence: discriminating invasion from colonization. *Nat Rev Microbiol* 10: 112–22.

Guani-Guerra E, Santos-Mendoza T, Lugo-Reyes SO and Teran LM (2010) Antimicrobial peptides: general overview and clinical implications in human health and disease. *Clin Immunol* 135: 1–11.

Gupta S, Ellis M, Cesario T, Ruhling M and Vayuvegula B (1987) Disseminated cryptococcal infection in a patient with hypogammaglobulinemia and normal T cell functions. *Am J Med* 82: 129–31.

Hernandez-Santos N and Gaffen SL (2012) Th17 cells in immunity to *Candida albicans*. *Cell Host Microbe* 11: 425–35.

Johnston SA and May RC (2013) *Cryptococcus* interactions with macrophages: evasion and manipulation of the phagosome by a fungal pathogen. *Cell Microbiol* 15: 403–11.

Kekalainen E, Tuovinen H, Joensuu J, et al. (2007) A defect of regulatory T cells in patients with autoimmune polyendocrinopathy-candidiasis-ectodermal dystrophy. *J Immunol* 178: 1208–15.

Kistowska M, Fenini G, Jankovic D, et al. (2014) *Malassezia* yeasts activate the NLRP3 inflammasome in antigen-presenting cells via Syk-kinase signalling. *Exp Dermatol* 23: 884–9.

Koh AY (2013) Murine models of *Candida* gastrointestinal colonization and dissemination. *Eukaryot Cell* 12: 1416–22.

Lamkanfi M and Dixit VM (2014) Mechanisms and functions of inflammasomes. *Cell* 157: 1013–22.

Lanternier F, Pathan S, Vincent QB, et al. (2013) Deep dermatophytosis and inherited CARD9 deficiency. *N Engl J Med* 369: 1704–14.
Lemaitre B, Nicolas E, Michaut L, Reichhart JM and Hoffmann JA (1996) The dorsoventral regulatory gene cassette spätzle/Toll/cactus controls the potent antifungal response in Drosophila adults. *Cell* 86: 973–83.
Lev-Sagie A, Prus D, Linhares IM, Lavy Y, Ledger WJ and Witkin SS (2009) Polymorphism in a gene coding for the inflammasome component NALP3 and recurrent vulvovaginal candidiasis in women with vulvar vestibulitis syndrome. *Am J Obstet Gynecol* 200: 303.e1–6.
Liang W, Huang Y, Yang X, et al. (2006) Oral immunization of mice with plant-derived fimbrial adhesin FaeG induces systemic and mucosal K88ad enterotoxigenic *Escherichia coli*-specific immune responses. *FEMS Immunol Med Microbiol* 46: 393–9.
Luo S, Skerka C, Kurzai O and Zipfel PF (2013) Complement and innate immune evasion strategies of the human pathogenic fungus *Candida albicans*. *Mol Immunol* 56: 161–9.
Ma J and Underhill DM (2013) beta-Glucan signaling connects phagocytosis to autophagy. *Glycobiology* 23: 1047–51.
Mehra T, Koberle M, Braunsdorf C, Mailander-Sanchez D, Borelli C and Schaller M (2012) Alternative approaches to antifungal therapies. *Exp Dermatol* 21: 778–82.
Mosser DM and Edwards JP (2008) Exploring the full spectrum of macrophage activation. *Nat Rev Immunol* 8: 958–69.
Murray PJ and Wynn TA (2011) Protective and pathogenic functions of macrophage subsets. *Nat Rev Immunol* 11: 723–37.
Nelson MP, Christmann BS, Werner JL, et al. (2011) IL-33 and M2a alveolar macrophages promote lung defense against the atypical fungal pathogen *Pneumocystis murina*. *J Immunol* 186: 2372–81.
Netea MG, Brown GD, Kullberg BJ and Gow NA (2008) An integrated model of the recognition of *Candida albicans* by the innate immune system. *Nat Rev Microbiol* 6: 67–78.
Netea MG, Quintin J and Van Der Meer JW (2011) Trained immunity: a memory for innate host defense. *Cell Host Microbe* 9: 355–61.
Neto R, Guimaraes MC, Moya MJ, Oliveira FR, Louzada PL Jr and Martinez R (2000) Hypogammaglobulinemia as risk factor for *Cryptococcus neoformans* infection: report of 2 cases. *Rev Soc Bras Med Trop* 33: 603–8.
Novak ML and Koh TJ (2013) Phenotypic transitions of macrophages orchestrate tissue repair. *Am J Pathol* 183: 1352–63.
Paul WE (2013) *Fundamental Immunology* (Philadelphia: Wolters Kluwer Health/Lippincott Williams & Wilkins).
Plato A, Hardison SE and Brown GD (2015) Pattern recognition receptors in antifungal immunity. *Semin Immunopathol* 37: 97–106.
Quintin J, Cheng SC, Van Der Meer JW and Netea MG (2014) Innate immune memory: towards a better understanding of host defense mechanisms. *Curr Opin Immunol* 29: 1–7.
Quintin J, Saeed S, Martens JH, et al. (2012) *Candida albicans* infection affords protection against reinfection via functional reprogramming of monocytes. *Cell Host Microbe* 12: 223–32.
Ramirez-Ortiz ZG and Means TK (2012) The role of dendritic cells in the innate recognition of pathogenic fungi (*A. fumigatus, C. neoformans* and *C. albicans*). *Virulence* 3: 635–46.
Rivera A (2014) Protective immune responses to fungal infections. *Parasite Immunol* 36: 453–62.
Safdar A (2013) Immunotherapy for invasive mold disease in severely immunosuppressed patients. *Clin Infect Dis* 57: 94–100.
Schroder K and Tschopp J (2010) The inflammasomes. *Cell* 140: 821–32.
Seider K, Heyken A, Luttich A, Miramon P and Hube B (2010) Interaction of pathogenic yeasts with phagocytes: survival, persistence and escape. *Curr Opin Microbiol* 13: 392–400.
Serbina NV, Jia T, Hohl TM and Pamer EG (2008) Monocyte-mediated defense against microbial pathogens. *Annu Rev Immunol* 26: 421–52.
Shi C and Pamer EG (2011) Monocyte recruitment during infection and inflammation. *Nat Rev Immunol* 11: 762–74.
Shoham S and Levitz SM (2005) The immune response to fungal infections. *Br J Haematol* 129: 569–82.
Subramanian Vignesh K, Landero Figueroa JA, Porollo A, Caruso JA and Deepe GS Jr (2013) Granulocyte macrophage-colony stimulating factor induced Zn sequestration enhances macrophage superoxide and limits intracellular pathogen survival. *Immunity* 39: 697–710.
Sugar AM, Picard M, Wagner R and Kornfeld H (1995) Interactions between human bronchoalveolar macrophages and *Blastomyces dermatitidis* conidia: demonstration of fungicidal and fungistatic effects. *J Infect Dis* 171: 1559–62.
Tonegawa S (1983) Somatic generation of antibody diversity. *Nature* 302: 575–81.
Underhill DM and Goodridge HS (2012) Information processing during phagocytosis. *Nat Rev Immunol* 12: 492–502.
Vautier S, Maccallum DM and Brown GD (2012) C-type lectin receptors and cytokines in fungal immunity. *Cytokine* 58: 89–99.
Verma A, Kroetz DN, Tweedle JL and Deepe GS Jr (2015a) Type II cytokines impair host defense against an intracellular fungal pathogen by amplifying macrophage generation of IL-33. *Mucosal Immunol* 8: 380–9.
Verma A, Wuthrich M, Deepe G and Klein B (2015b) Adaptive immunity to fungi. *Cold Spring Harb Perspect Med* 5: a019612.
Wahab JA, Hanifah MJ and Choo KE (1995) Bruton's agammaglobulinaemia in a child presenting with *cryptococcal* empyema thoracis and periauricular pyogenic abscess. *Singapore Med J* 36: 686–9.
Weiss G, Bogdan C and Hentze MW (1997) Pathways for the regulation of macrophage iron metabolism by the anti-inflammatory cytokines IL-4 and IL-13. *J Immunol* 158: 420–5.
Winkelstein JA, Marino MC, Ochs H, et al. (2003) The X-linked hyper-IgM syndrome: clinical and immunologic features of 79 patients. *Medicine (Baltimore)* 82: 373–84.
Winters MS, Chan Q, Caruso JA and Deepe GS Jr (2010) Metallomic analysis of macrophages infected with *Histoplasma capsulatum* reveals a fundamental role for zinc in host defenses. *J Infect Dis* 202: 1136–45.
Wuthrich M, Deepe GS Jr and Klein B (2012) Adaptive immunity to fungi. *Annu Rev Immunol* 30: 115–48.
Zelante T, De Luca A, Bonifazi P, et al. (2007) IL-23 and the Th17 pathway promote inflammation and impair antifungal immune resistance. *Eur J Immunol* 37: 2695–706.

SECTION 2

Medically important fungi

CHAPTER 10

Aspergillus species

Stephanie J. Smith, Rohini J. Manuel, and Christopher C. Kibbler

Introduction

Aspergillus species are some of the most ubiquitous fungi (Anderson et al. 2011). There are more than 200 *Aspergillus* species, with more than 30 known to be human pathogens.

The fungus is also commercially important. *A. niger* is the source of enzymes such as amylases, lipases, and proteases and is used to produce the majority of the world's citric acid. *A. oryzae* is important in the fermentation processes responsible for the production of sake and soy products.

Genomic sequencing data are now available for many species, with whole genomes varying from 29.3 Mb for *A. fumigatus*, to 37.1 Mb for *A. oryzae*. The latter is predicted to contain more than 12,000 genes (Machida et al. 2005; Nierman et al. 2005).

Taxonomy

Genus name

Aspergillus

First described by Micheli in 1729, these are moulds which are characterized by a typical asexual spore-forming structure (the aspergillum). Many *Aspergillus* species now have an identified sexual (teleomorph) stage (e.g. *Neosartorya, Emericella, Eurotium*). To maintain consistency with the 'one fungus: one name' nomenclature of the revised International Botanical Code and to avoid confusion, it was decided in 2012 to keep the name *Aspergillus* for all species, except where the teleomorph name has a particular meaning, when it should be used alongside the anamorph name (International Commission of Penicillium and Aspergillus 2012).

Significant species

A. fumigatus, A. flavus, A. terreus, A. nidulans, A. niger, A. clavatus, and A. versicolor

Genomic analysis has revealed a large number of cryptic species in recent years. For example, *Aspergillus fumigatus sensu stricto* is now included in the section *Fumigati* along with more than 40 other species. Hence, unless complex molecular identification methods are used, it is preferable to designate an isolate of *A. fumigatus* as within the '*A. fumigatus* complex' group.

Epidemiology/patient risk factors

Humans are exposed to multiple conidia, from different *Aspergillus* species, on a daily basis. The patient groups at high risk of invasive aspergillosis are listed in Chapter 30. *A. fumigatus* is the most common species isolated, followed by *A. flavus* and *A. niger*. The incidence of invasive aspergillosis varies both between, and within, high-risk patient groups. Approximately 12% of allogeneic, and 1% of autologous, HSCT (haematopoietic stem cell transplantation) recipients will develop invasive *Aspergillus* infection. Heart–lung transplant recipients are more likely to develop infections (11%) compared with heart or kidney transplant recipients (<2%). The risk is lower for AIDS patients and those with hereditary immunodeficiencies (<1%) (Cornet et al. 2002).

Chronic pulmonary aspergillosis is being increasingly recognized and is linked with previous mycobacterial infection and other chronic lung conditions, such as sarcoidosis.

Allergic disease has been estimated to occur in 16% of patients with bronchial asthma (Kumar and Gaur 2000), but rates vary worldwide. Allergic bronchopulmonary aspergillosis has been estimated to affect several million individuals globally (see Chapter 37).

Routes of transmission

The fungus is found in soil, rotting vegetation, damp grain, and water, but may be found anywhere where there is moisture and some basic substrate. In the built environment *Aspergillus* has been isolated from damp wallpaper, plaster, concrete, pipe lagging, air conditioning equipment, carpets, fireproofing, and food and water supplies (Manuel and Kibbler 1998; Anderson et al. 2011).

Transmission is mainly by the airborne route through inhalation of air contaminated with *Aspergillus* conidia. Conidia can also be directly inoculated through skin wounds and indwelling devices, such as intravascular catheters.

There is an association between hospital building work and outbreaks of *Aspergillus* infection in high-risk patients through aerosolization of conidia. It is essential that building works are carefully planned in advance (Manuel and Kibbler 1998).

Pathogenesis

Aspergillus conidia pass through the respiratory tract and into the alveoli. In an immunocompetent individual, the innate and adaptive immune systems recognize the cell constituents of the fungi (particularly cell-wall glucans, chitin, and galactomannans) and prevent further invasive sequelae by removing the conidia via ciliary clearance and neutrophil/macrophage responses. These actions are hampered in immunocompromised individuals, particularly those with impaired neutrophil activity (reduced numbers or function), or macrophage and T-cell dysfunction, allowing conidia to germinate, with hyphae invading blood vessels and tissues. Angio-invasion results in endothelial damage, pro-inflammatory cytokine activation, and initiation of the coagulation cascade. Consequent thrombosis causes local infarction followed by tissue necrosis (Denning 1998) (see Chapter 9).

Allergic diseases are triggered via a number of hypersensitivity responses which govern both the nature of the condition and the location of the disease (see Chapters 9, 30, and 37).

Aspergillus species produce a large number of mycotoxins; their role in toxin-mediated disease is discussed in Chapter 31.

Clinical presentation

Diseases caused by *Aspergillus* species can vary widely, from superficial colonization to invasive disease. The disease spectrum is often separated into three categories: non-invasive, invasive, and chronic (Denning 1998).

Non-invasive aspergillosis

Aspergillus species can cause otomycosis, with *A. niger* being the most common causative species. *Aspergillus* species (e.g. *A. versicolor*) are infrequent causes of onychomycosis (see Chapter 23). Chronic allergic rhinosinusitis is a non-invasive *Aspergillus* infection that may be accompanied by nasal polyps.

Allergic bronchopulmonary aspergillosis (ABPA) is a hypersensitivity reaction to *Aspergillus* antigens, occurring particularly in individuals with history of atopy, asthma, or cystic fibrosis. It is characterized by airway inflammation, bronchoconstriction, and mucus production. Diagnosis is based on criteria such as symptoms, imaging, and serology (see Chapters 30 and 37).

Other allergic diseases include extrinsic allergic alveolitis, which may be occupational (e.g. with *A. clavatus* causing 'malt worker's lung'), and severe asthma with fungal sensitization.

Acute invasive aspergillosis

Invasive aspergillosis can involve any organ system, including the lungs, sinuses, central nervous system, eyes, bone, kidneys, and liver. Pulmonary disease is the most common form, presenting as dyspnoea, pleuritic chest pain, and fever. Symptoms may be vague, and dependent on the organ affected. Hence the clinician needs to maintain a low threshold of suspicion.

Chronic pulmonary aspergillosis

Chronic pulmonary aspergillosis (CPA) (Schweer et al. 2014) most commonly occurs in individuals with pre-existing lung disease such as tuberculosis, chronic obstructive pulmonary disease (Guinea et al. 2010), bronchiectasis, and sarcoidosis. *A. fumigatus* is the most common isolate. The spectrum of disease, from aspergilloma to cavitary and fibrosing disease, is discussed in Chapters 30 and 37.

Diagnosis

Microscopy and culture

Aspergillus species can be identified by their gross macroscopic and microscopic features (Table 10.1). Colonies grow on selective agar (Sabouraud agar, corn meal agar) usually within 48–90 hours. Staining of clinical specimens (Calcofluor White, periodic acid-Schiff [PAS], methenamine silver) may show hyphae consistent with *Aspergillus* species.

Distinguishing microscopic features of all *Aspergillus* species include septate hyphae with hyaline, 45-degree angle dichotomous branching. Foot cells are located at the base of the conidiophore. The conidial head is a vesicle with uniserate or biserate rows of phialides/metulae and attached conidia that resemble chains. Species are distinguished morphologically by the size of the conidial head, distribution of phialides (Figure 10.1), and colony colour and texture (Figure 10.2).

Non-culture-based diagnosis

Serum *Aspergillus* precipitins may assist in the diagnosis of ABPA or chronic pulmonary aspergillosis.

The use of biomarkers and molecular techniques can reduce the time to diagnosis of *Aspergillus* infections, thus allowing for early pre-emptive therapy or use of a diagnostic-driven management strategy.

The galactomannan antigen is a component of the *Aspergillus* cell wall. A double-sandwich ELISA (enzyme-linked immuno-sorbent assay) has a good negative predictive value. False-positive results caused by cross-reactivity with beta-lactam antibiotics—e.g. with piperacillin-tazobactam, and with other fungi, such as *Penicillium, Histoplasma*, and *Blastomyces*—have been reported. The lateral-flow device, which utilizes a monoclonal antibody targeting a particular glycoprotein specific to *Aspergillus* species, has similar performance characteristics.

(1→3) β-D-glucan is abundant in all fungal cell walls except those of *Cryptococcus* and Mucoromycotina species. Hence the (1→3) β-D-glucan test is pan-fungal, and not specific for *Aspergillus* species.

Use of molecular methods such as the polymerase chain reaction (PCR) to look for *Aspergillus* DNA in clinical samples such as blood or tissue can provide a rapid and more specific diagnosis (White et al. 2013).

The use of multiple diagnostic modalities has been used to increase sensitivity, particularly in the haemato-oncology setting (Hoenigl et al. 2014; Johnson et al. 2015), and form part of the EORTC (European Organisation for Research and Treatment of Cancer) diagnostic guidelines for aspergillosis (de Pauw et al. 2008).

Clinical investigations

Microscopy and culture of sputum samples may show evidence of hyphae. However, clinical correlation is essential to distinguish colonization from disease.

Non-specific signs on chest radiographs include nodules or evidence of an aspergilloma in a pre-existing pulmonary cavity.

Radiological investigations such as a high-resolution computed tomography scan or magnetic resonance imaging are key to investigating invasive/disseminated disease. Findings are dependent on the type of infection—for example, macronodules with ground glass shadowing (halo sign) in invasive pulmonary aspergillosis, or pre-existing cavitatory lesions with a nodule within (aspergilloma) or clusters of nodules.

If the patient is stable and it is clinically indicated, bronchoscopy with bronchoalveolar lavage and/or a biopsy can be performed.

Other investigations, such as a lumbar puncture or obtaining tissue samples from the nasal sinuses, may be indicated depending on the site of infection.

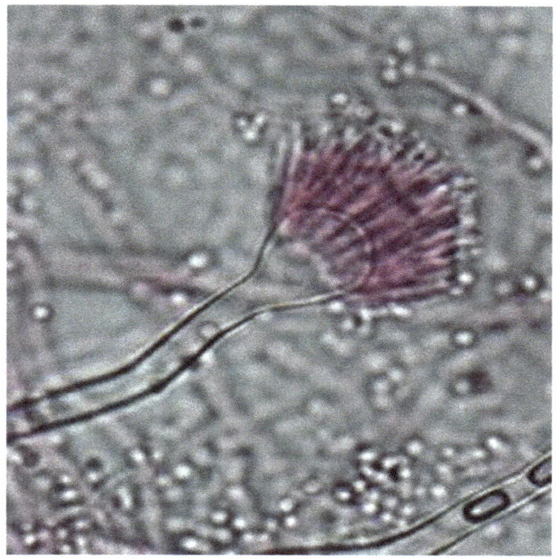

Figure 10.1 Conidiophore of *Aspergillus terreus* with fan shaped vesicle and biseriate phialides attached to the upper surface.
Reproduced courtesy of UK NEQAS, Public Health England

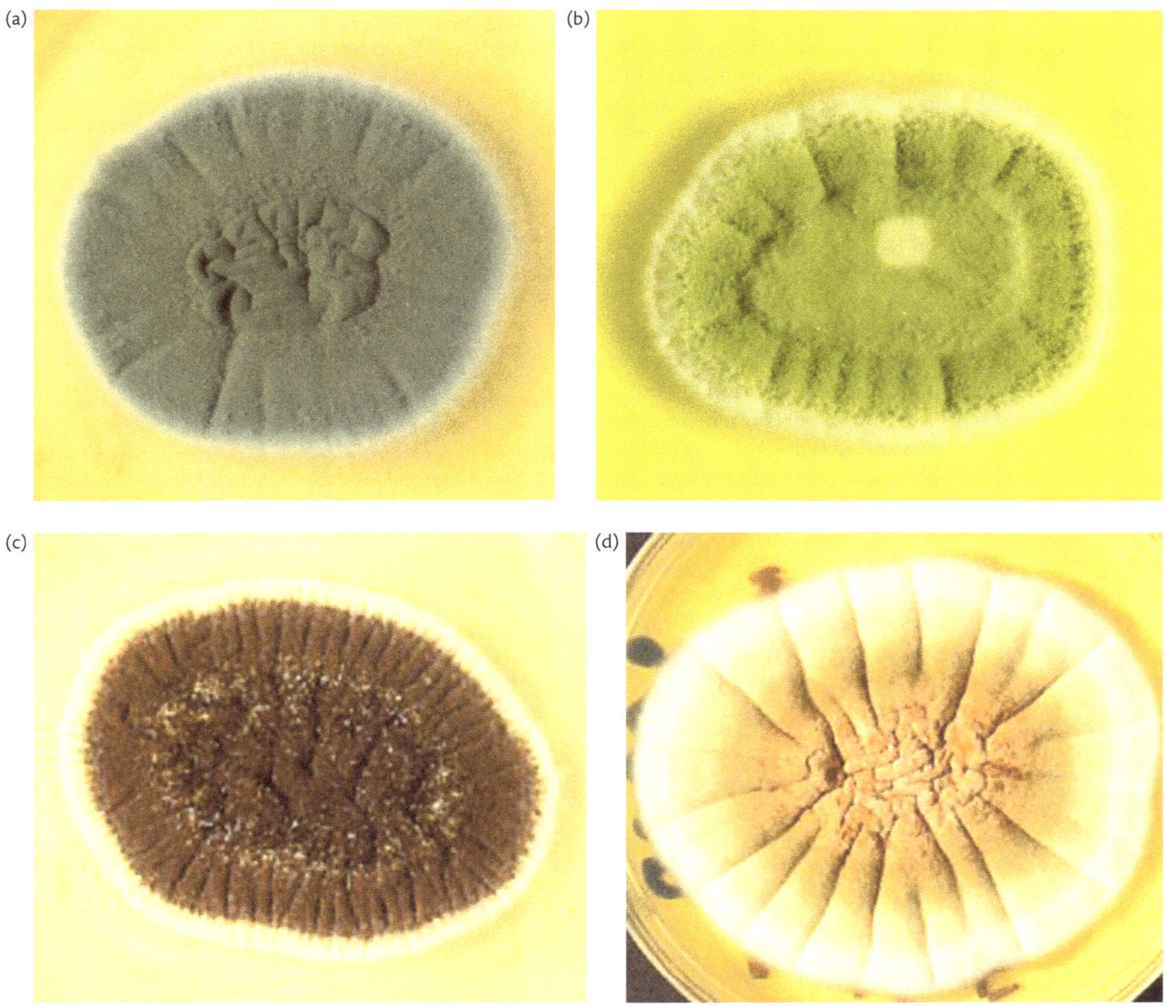

Figure 10.2 Typical colonial appearances of the four commonest causes of invasive aspergillosis. **a** *Aspergillus fumigatus* complex, **b** *Aspergillus flavus* complex, **c** *Aspergillus niger* complex, **d** *Aspergillus terreus* complex.

Table 10.1 Microscopic and cultural characteristics of *Aspergillus* species

Aspergillus species	Macroscopic appearance	Optimum growth temperature	Microscopic appearance	Clinical manifestations and comment
A. fumigatus	Surface green-blue with white outer edge, reverse yellow	37°C Range 12–65°C	Conidial heads columnar, uniseriate; conidia smooth to roughened	Invasive pulmonary aspergillosis, ABPA, CPA, and disseminated aspergillosis
A. flavus	Surface green/yellow, reverse cream/white	37°C Range 12–48°C	Radiate, uni- or biseriate conidial head with rough conidiophores; smooth conidia	Sinusitis, onychomycosis, skin, invasive infections; produces an aflatoxin
A. terreus	Surface beige, reverse brown/yellow	25–40°C	Conidial heads are columnar and biseriate; conidiophores are hyaline and smooth-walled; accessory conidia can be present	Produce ochratoxins
A. nidulans	Surface green colony with red-brown cleistothecia. Reverse green to brown.	37°C Range 2–48°C	Short brown, smooth conidiophores; subglobose vesicles, metulae, and phialides bearing slightly roughened globose conidia	Invasive aspergillosis
A. niger	Black with yellow on the reverse	37°C	Radiate, biseriate conidial head	Otitis externa, dermatitis
A. versicolor	Surface initially white changing to yellow, orange, or green	Optimal growth 22–26°C Up to 40°C	Biseriate conidial head with small vesicle; penicillium-like conidiophores present	Onychomycosis Produces sterigmatocystin

Management

The resistance of *A. fumigatus* to azoles is increasing, mainly in Europe. This could, in part, be due to long-term antifungal prophylaxis and treatment, or the use of agricultural azoles. *A. terreus* and *A. nidulans* are inherently resistant to amphotericin B. Hence, all invasive isolates of *Aspergillus* species should undergo susceptibility testing.

The choice of drugs for therapy depends largely on the condition, with colonization requiring no treatment. Use of topical antifungal agents, such as clotrimazole, may be required for otomycosis. Onychomycosis may require months of topical and oral treatment with an azole.

ABPA treatment aims to reduce airway inflammation and limit lung damage. It typically consists of tapering courses of oral steroids for exacerbations, with or without antifungals. Empirical antifungal therapy and investigations for invasive fungal infections in immunocompromised patients should be considered if the patient is pyrexial with no clear source, despite having broad-spectrum antibiotics.

The recommended first-line antifungal treatment for invasive aspergillosis is voriconazole (Walsh et al. 2008). An alternative agent is liposomal amphotericin B (AmBisome). Salvage therapy for treatment failure or intolerance includes the echinocandins and other triazoles such as itraconazole/posaconazole. In 2015, a novel triazole, isavuconazole (Maertens et al. 2016), was approved by both the FDA and the European Commission for invasive aspergillosis therapy.

Prognosis

The mortality from invasive aspergillosis depends on the underlying condition, use of prophylaxis, rapid diagnosis, and prompt treatment. It can range from 50–60% in patients undergoing organ transplantation, to 70–85% in other immunosuppressed patients.

References

Anderson B, Frisvad JC, Sondergaard I, Rasmussen I and Larsen LS (2011) Associations between fungal species and water-damaged building materials. *Appl Environ Microbiol* 77: 4180–8.

Cornet M, Fleury L, Maslo C, Bernard JF and Brücker G (2002) Invasive Aspergillosis Surveillance Network of the Assistance Publique-Hôpitaux de Paris. Epidemiology of invasive aspergillosis in France: a six-year multicentric survey in the Greater Paris area. *J Hosp Infect* 51: 288–96.

Denning DW (1998) Invasive aspergillosis. *Clin Infect Dis* 26: 781–803.

de Pauw B, Walsh TJ, Donnelly JP, et al. (2008) Revised definitions of invasive fungal disease from the European Organization for Research and Treatment of Cancer/Invasive Fungal Infections Cooperative Group and the National Institute of Allergy and Infectious Diseases Mycoses Study Group (EORTC/MSG) Consensus Group. *Clin Infect Dis* 46: 1813–21.

Guinea J, Torres-Narbona M and Gijón P, et al. (2010) Pulmonary aspergillosis in patients with chronic obstructive pulmonary disease: incidence, risk factors, and outcome. *Clin Microbiol Infect* 16: 870–7.

Hoenigl M, Prattes J, Spiess B, et al. (2014) Performance of galactomannan, beta-D-glucan, *Aspergillus* lateral-flow device, conventional culture, and PCR tests with bronchoalveolar lavage fluid for diagnosis of invasive pulmonary aspergillosis. *J Clin Microbiol* 52: 2039–45.

International Commission of *Penicillium* and *Aspergillus*, http://www.aspergilluspenicillium.org/, accessed 04 May 2017.

Johnson GL, Sarker SJ, Nannini F, et al. (2015) Aspergillus-specific lateral-flow device and real-time PCR testing of bronchoalveolar lavage fluid: a combination biomarker approach for clinical diagnosis of invasive pulmonary aspergillosis. J Clin Microbiol 2015; 53:2103–8.

Kumar R and Gaur SN (2000) Prevalence of allergic bronchopulmonary aspergillosis in patients with bronchial asthma. *Asian Pac J Allergy Immunol* 18: 181–5.

Machida M, Asai K, Sano M, et al. (2005) Genome sequencing and analysis of *Aspergillus oryzae*. *Nature* 438: 1157–61.

Maertens JA, Raad II, Marr KA, et al. (2016) Isavuconazole versus voriconazole for primary treatment of invasive mould disease caused by *Aspergillus* and other filamentous fungi (SECURE): a phase 3, randomised-controlled, non-inferiority trial. *Lancet* 387: 760–9.

Manuel RJ and Kibbler CC (1998) The epidemiology and prevention of invasive aspergillosis. *J Hosp Infect* 39: 95–109.

Nierman WC, Pain A, Anderson MJ, et al. (2005) Genomic sequence of the pathogenic and allergenic filamentous fungus, *Aspergillus fumigatus*. *Nature* 438: 1151–6.

Schweer KE, Bangard C, Hekmat K and Cornely OA (2014) Chronic pulmonary aspergillosis. *Mycoses* 57: 257–70.

Walsh TJ, Anaissie EJ, Denning DW, et al. (2008) Treatment of aspergillosis: clinical practice guidelines of the Infectious Diseases Society of America. *Clin Infect Dis* 46: 327–60.

White PL, Parr C, Thornton C and Barnes RA (2013) Evaluation of real-time PCR, galactomannan enzyme-linked immunosorbent assay (ELISA), and a novel lateral-flow device for diagnosis of invasive aspergillosis. *J Clin Microbiol* 51: 1510–16.

CHAPTER 11

Candida species

Bernhard Hube and Oliver Kurzai

Introduction to *Candida*

Candida species are the most common human fungal pathogens, as the majority of the human population are carriers of *Candida* yeasts, and mucosal *Candida* infections are extremely frequent.

Significant species

Although the genus consists of approximately 150 disparately related species (Moran et al. 2012), the vast majority (>90%) of all *Candida* infections are caused by only four species: *Candida albicans, C. glabrata, C. parapsilosis*, and *C. tropicalis*. Less frequent pathogenic *Candida* species include *C. dubliniensis, C. lusitaniae, C. krusei, C. guilliermondii, C. rugosa, C. orthopsilosis*, and *C. metapsilosis*, and further rare species have been reported as infectious agents. Recently, *C. auris* has emerged as a cause of outbreaks of candidaemia, wound infection, and otitis in Asia, the Americas, the Middle East, and Europe (Satoh et al. 2009; Lee et al. 2011; Chowdhary et al. 2013; Magobo et al. 2014; Emara et al. 2015).

Taxonomy

The genus *Candida* is diverse, as its taxonomy was histologically based on physical traits, such as morphology and sexual reproduction (Moran et al. 2012). Recent DNA-based taxonomy has demonstrated broad evolutionary relationships between *Candida* species. This new data has: confirmed that *Candida* species are ascomycetes, identified new species (e.g. *C. dubliniensis, C. orthopsilosis*, and *C. metapsilosis*) and the genes required for sexual reproduction, revealed the existence of parasexual cycles and a haploid form of *C. albicans* (Hickman et al. 2013), and demonstrated that *C. glabrata* is a closer relative of *S. cerevisiae* than *C. albicans, C. parapsilosis*, or *C. tropicalis* (Brunke and Hube 2013).

Cell biology

Owing to its medical importance, *C. albicans* is the most studied yeast of this genus. Although traditionally described as dimorphic, *C. albicans* is, rather, a polymorphic fungus which can have several morphologies: yeast, pseudohyphal, hyphal, and several 'switching' morphologies such as white/opaque, which is related to mating competence.

The cell wall of *C. albicans* has key functions in pathogenesis, in particular in adhesion, invasion, and host recognition. Key components are mannoproteins (glycoproteins), glucan (β-1,3- and β-1,6-glucan), and chitin.

The metabolism of *C. albicans* is highly flexible, facilitating growth in multiple niches within the host. Of particular importance are metal acquisition (Almeida et al. 2009; Wilson et al. 2012), adaptation to stresses such as reactive oxygen species or pH (Brown et al. 2014), and the active manipulation of the environmental pH (Vylkova and Lorenz 2014).

Pathogenesis

Most common pathogenic *Candida* species are commensals and natural members of the microbiota of mucosal surfaces (*C. albicans, C. parapsilosis*, and *C. glabrata*) (Seed 2015) and the skin (*C. parapsilosis*), while *C. tropicalis* is also an environmental fungus. Therefore, pathogenicity includes a commensal-to-pathogen shift associated with an overgrowth on superficial tissues and/or an invasion into deeper tissue (Figure 11.1).

Pathogenicity mechanisms differ between superficial and invasive infections, but share common stages (Figure 11.2): attachment to epithelial cells mediated by cell surface adhesins such as Hwp1 and Als3 from *C. albicans* (linked to hyphal morphology) or the Epa proteins from *C. glabrata* (yeast form). The invasion mechanisms of *C. albicans* are well described (Sheppard and Filler 2015) and include two different routes: induced endocytosis, where mostly the hyphal-associated invasin Als3 triggers up-take by epithelial cells, and active penetration requiring hyphal formation. Invasion is not necessarily linked to damage. Epithelial cell damage is due to hyphal extension, physical forces, and destructive activities such as proteolysis and toxin production (Moyes et al. 2016). If the fungus invades into deeper tissues, it may reach the bloodstream and can disseminate and infect almost all organs (Mavor et al. 2005). Of note, the most common cause of such invasive and systemic *Candida* infections is breakage of physical barriers, often due to iatrogenic factors (surgery, catheters). Adaptation to the different host niches—from mucosal surfaces to deeper tissue, blood, and organs—together with immune evasion strategies, are crucial for *Candida* pathogenicity. For example, *Candida* cells can survive phagocytosis by macrophages, proliferate intracellularly, and escape (Seider et al. 2010). Another way of immune evasion, and also a drug resistance strategy, is the production of biofilms, often on medical devices such as catheters.

See Chapter 8 for further details of pathogenicity.

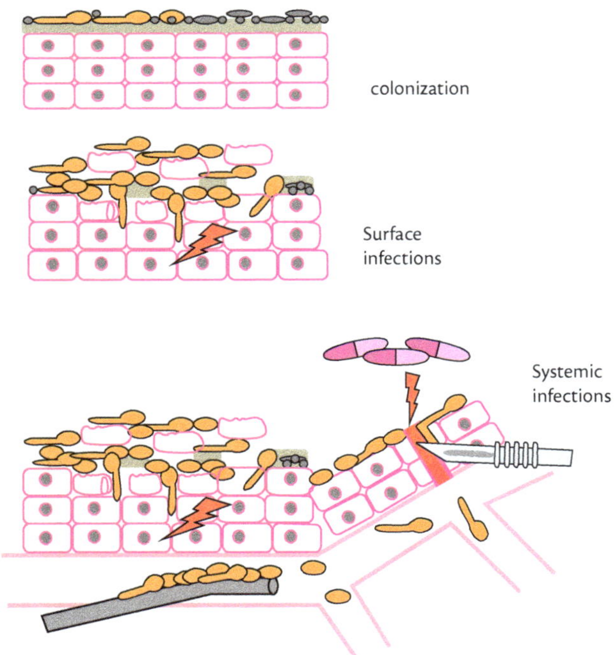

Figure 11.1 Stages of *Candida albicans* infections from colonization to systemic infections: colonization in the commensal phase within the microbiota; surface infections with inflammation; and systemic infection via translocation from the gut due to invasive growth/drug treatment/surgery/trauma causing damaged barriers or from biofilms.

Reproduced courtesy of Bernhard Hube. Adapted from Mavor A. L. et al., (2005) 'Systemic Fungal Infections Caused by *Candida* Species: Epidemiology, Infection Process and Virulence Attributes', *Current Drug Targets*, Volume 6, Issue 8, pp. 863–74, Figure 1, Copyright © Bentham Science Publishers Ltd. DOI: 10.2174/1389450057749127 35

Epidemiology—routes of transmission, patient populations, risk factors, incidence

Data from a murine intestinal colonization model, as well as clinical evidence, suggests that disturbance of the mucosal barrier together with compromised cellular immunity enable *Candida* to invade the human bloodstream and cause invasive infection. In addition, *Candida* species can efficiently colonize implanted materials, resulting in biofilm-associated infections (Cuellar-Cruz et al. 2012). *Candida* species are responsible for 10–20% of healthcare-associated infections (Delaloye and Calandra 2014) and account for 5–15% of bloodstream infections (Perlroth et al. 2007). There is a range of incidences—from 2.0 cases per 10,000 hospital admissions in France in 1997–1999 (Tortorano et al. 2006), to 24.9 cases per 10,000 admissions in Brazil in 2003–2004 (Colombo et al. 2006), and a recent French population-based study has found an incidence of 2.5 per 100,000 for candidaemia (Bitar et al. 2014). Even with antifungal therapy, disseminated candidiasis has a mortality of 40–50% (Tortorano et al. 2006).

Clinical presentations

Superficial infections

Superficial infections involve skin, nail, and mucous membranes. Oral candidiasis risk factors include local factors such as inhaled steroids, or reduction of bacterial flora due to antibiotics (Moyes and Naglik 2011), or systemic (e.g. HIV, human immunodeficiency virus) immunosuppression. Oesophageal candidiasis is a more invasive manifestation typically seen in AIDS. *Candida* vulvovaginitis may be recurrent in as many as 5–8% of cases, with chronic episodes requiring antifungal maintenance therapy (Peters et al. 2014). Rare cases of chronic mucocutaneous candidiasis have been linked to defects in mucosal immunology often affecting IL-17 signalling pathways (Smeekens et al. 2013).

Invasive infections

Invasive *Candida* infections can manifest as:

a. *acute disseminated candidiasis*:
   referring to candidaemia in addition to organ manifestation. Manifestation can take many forms (affecting multiple sites in the human body): endophthalmitis; endocarditis; infection of the liver, kidney, and spleen; cutaneous foci; arthritis; osteomyelitis; and meningitis/meningoencephalitis.
b. *chronically disseminated candidiasis*:
   typically occurring as a late (~2 weeks after candidaemia) consequence of candidaemia in neutropenic patients and mainly affecting the liver and spleen ('hepatosplenic candidiasis')
c. *candidaemia without evidence of organ manifestation*
d. *invasive candidiasis without detectable candidaemia*:
   e.g. in cases of isolated endophthalmitis or peritonitis

See Chapter 25 for further details.

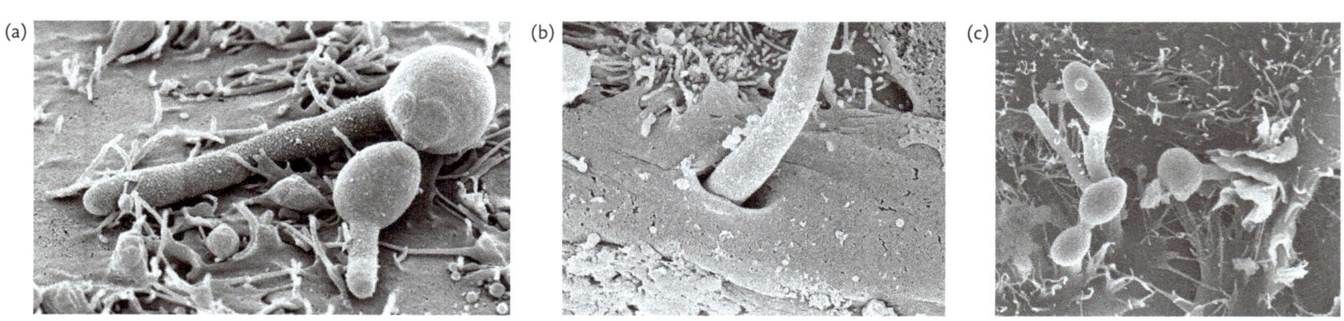

Figure 11.2 Adhesion (**a**) and invasion, due to active penetration (**b**) or induced endocytosis (**c**), of *Candida albicans* during interaction with epithelial cells.

Adapted with permission from Wilson D. et al., (2009) 'Identifying Infection-Associated Genes of *Candida albicans* in the Postgenomic Era', *FEMS Yeast Research*, Volume 9, Issue 5, pp. 688–700, Copyright © 2009 Federation of European Microbiological Societies. DOI: 10.1111/j.1567-1364.2009.00524.x. Published by Blackwell Publishing Ltd. All rights reserved.

Diagnosis

Microscopy

Several stains may be used for diagnosis, including the optical brightener Calcofluor White or Grocott-Gomori's silver stain. *C. albicans* differs from most other species as it can form extensive filamentous forms *in vivo* and may therefore be confused with a hyphomycete. In contrast, *C. glabrata* and *C. parapsilosis* occur exclusively in the yeast form during infection (Willinger et al. 2014).

Culture

Candida species generally grow well in diagnostic culture media and commercial blood culture systems. Owing to frequent colonization, only their detection in primarily sterile samples provides evidence for invasive infection. Species identification can be achieved by MALDI/TOF (matrix-assisted laser desorption/ionization–time-of-flight) mass spectrometry or biochemical profiling (Willinger et al. 2014).

Serology

The detection of antigens (mannoproteins, other antigens) and antibodies, alone or in combination, has been used to improve the diagnosis of candidaemia with variable results, and is not unequivocally recommended by guidelines. The detection of β-glucan can aid in the diagnosis of *Candida* infection (Willinger et al. 2014).

Molecular biology

The detection of nucleic acids has been used in multiple in-house assays to improve diagnostic sensitivity. Several studies have shown that commercially available molecular multiplex kits for sepsis (e.g. Septifast [Roche], Sepsitest [Molzym]) more frequently detect *Candida* species than the conventional blood culture system, thus suggesting that molecular detection can increase sensitivity. However, currently there is insufficient data to support the routine use of molecular detection tools (Willinger et al. 2014).

Treatment

Antifungal strategies have to take into account primary resistance of some species to antifungals. Most notably, *C. krusei* is resistant to fluconazole and *C. glabrata* shows reduced susceptibility against this drug. There is some evidence that species such as *C. parapsilosis* and *C. guilliermondii* are less susceptible to echinocandins. Acquired resistance is rare but can occur against azoles and echinocandins. Recently, the emergence of echinocandin-resistant strains (especially *C. glabrata*) has been reported in several studies (Arendrup and Perlin 2014).

References

Almeida RS, Wilson D and Hube B (2009) *Candida albicans* iron acquisition within the host. *FEMS Yeast Res* 9: 1000–12.

Arendrup, MC and Perlin DS (2014) Echinocandin resistance: an emerging clinical problem? *Curr Opin Infect Dis* 27: 484–92.

Bitar D, Lortholary O, Le Strat Y, et al. (2014) Population-based analysis of invasive fungal infections, France, 2001-2010. *Emerg Infect Dis* 20: 1149–55.

Brown AJ, Budge S, Kaloriti D, et al. (2014) Stress adaptation in a pathogenic fungus. *J Exp Biol* 217: 144–55.

Brunke S and Hube B (2013) Two unlike cousins: *Candida albicans* and *C. glabrata* infection strategies. *Cell Microbiol* 15: 701–8.

Chowdhary A, Sharma C, Duggal S, et al. (2013) New clonal strain of *Candida auris*, Delhi, India. *Emerg Infect Dis*19: 1670–3.

Colombo AL, Nucci M, Park BJ, et al. (2006) Epidemiology of candidemia in Brazil: a nationwide sentinel surveillance of candidemia in eleven medical centers. *J Clin Microbiol* 44: 2816–23.

Cuellar-Cruz M, Lopez-Romero E, Villagomez-Castro JC, et al. (2012) *Candida* species: new insights into biofilm formation. *Future Microbiol* 7: 755–71.

Delaloye J and Calandra T (2014) Invasive candidiasis as a cause of sepsis in the critically ill patient. *Virulence* 5: 161–9.

Emara M, Ahmad S, Khan Z, et al. (2015) *Candida auris* candidemia in Kuwait. *Emerg Infect Dis* 21: 1091–2.

Hickman MA, Zeng G, Forche A, et al. (2013) The 'obligate diploid' *Candida albicans* forms mating-competent haploids. *Nature* 494: 55–9.

Lee WG, Shin JH, Uh Y, et al. (2011) First three reported cases of nosocomial fungemia caused by Candida auris. *J Clin Microbiol* 49: 3139–42.

Magobo RE, Corcoran C, Seetharam S and Govender NP (2014) *Candida auris*-associated candidemia, South Africa. *Emerg Infect Dis* 20: 1250–1.

Mavor AL, Thewes S and Hube B (2005) Systemic fungal infections caused by *Candida* species: epidemiology, infection process and virulence attributes. *Curr Drug Targets* 6: 863–74.

Moran GP, Coleman DC and Sullivan D (2012) An introduction to the medically important *Candida* species, *in*: RA Calderone and CJ Clancy, eds, *Candida and Candidiasis* (Washington DC: ASM Press), 11–25.

Moyes DL and Naglik JR (2011) Mucosal immunity and *Candida albicans* infection. *Clin Dev Immunol* 2011, 346307. doi: 10.1155/2011/346307

Moyes DL, Wilson D, Richardson JP, et al. (2016) Candidalysin is a fungal peptide toxin critical for mucosal infection. *Nature* 532: 64–8.

Perlroth J, Choi B and Spellberg B (2007) Nosocomial fungal infections: epidemiology, diagnosis, and treatment. *Med Mycol* 45: 321–46.

Peters BM, Yano J, Noverr MC, et al. (2014) *Candida* vaginitis: when opportunism knocks, the host responds. *PLoS Pathog* 10: e1003965.

Satoh K, Makimura K, Hasumi Y, Nishiyama Y, Uchida K and Yamaguchi H (2009) *Candida auris* sp. nov., a novel ascomycetous yeast isolated from the external ear canal of an inpatient in a Japanese hospital. *Microbiol Immunol* 53: 41–4.

Seed PC (2015) The human mycobiome. *Cold Spring Harb Perspect Med* 5: a019810.

Seider K, Heyken A, Luttich A, et al. (2010). Interaction of pathogenic yeasts with phagocytes: survival, persistence and escape. *Curr Opin Microbiol* 13: 392–400.

Sheppard DC and Filler SG (2015) Host cell invasion by medically important fungi. *Cold Spring Harb Perspect Med* 5: a019687.

Smeekens SP, van de Veerdonk FL, Kullberg BJ, et al. (2013) Genetic susceptibility to *Candida* infections. *EMBO Mol Med* 5: 805–13.

Tortorano AM, Kibbler C, Peman J, et al. (2006) Candidaemia in Europe: epidemiology and resistance. *Int J Antimicrob Agents* 27: 359–66.

Vylkova S and Lorenz MC (2014) Modulation of phagosomal pH by *Candida albicans* promotes hyphal morphogenesis and requires Stp2p, a regulator of amino acid transport. *PLoS Pathog* 10: e1003995.

Willinger B, Kienzl D and Kurzai O (2014) Diagnostics of fungal infections, *in*: O Kurzai, ed., *The Mycota*, XII (2nd edn, Berlin, Heidelberg: Springer-Verlag), 229–59.

Wilson D, Citiulo F and Hube B (2012) Zinc exploitation by pathogenic fungi. *PLoS Pathog* 8: e1003034.

Wilson D, Thewes S, Zakikhany K, et al. (2009) Identifying infection-associated genes of Candida albicans in the postgenomic era. *FEMS Yeast Res* 9: 688–700.

CHAPTER 12

Cryptococcus species

Catriona L. Halliday and Sarah E. Kidd

Introduction to *Cryptococcus*

The basidiomycete genus *Cryptococcus* comprises a diverse range of over 70 species characterized by round or oval yeast-like cells that reproduce by narrow-necked budding. Cultures are generally mucoid on solid media and most species are encapsulated. All species produce urease and are non-fermentative (Howell et al. 2015).

Taxonomy

Cryptococcus neoformans and *Cryptococcus gattii* are the principal pathogenic species and the causative agents of cryptococcosis. *C. neoformans* is currently recognized as a species complex comprising the two varieties var. *grubii* (serotype A) and var. *neoformans* (serotype D). *C. gattii* has two serotypes, B and C, and was recognized as a distinct species from *C. neoformans* in 2002 (Kwon-Chung et al. 2002). Other cryptococcal species, such as *C. adeliensis, C. albidus, C. curvatus, C. flavescens, C. laurentii*, and *C. uniguttulatus*, were traditionally considered to be non-pathogenic, but occasionally cause invasive infections in humans (Khawcharoenporn et al. 2007).

Pathogenesis

Irrespective of the species, cryptococcal infections are acquired following inhalation of the infectious propagule from the environment. In most cases, symptoms do not develop, indicating that most immunocompetent people clear the infection. Infections may be localized or disseminate, often to the central nervous system (CNS). Dissemination may follow reactivation of dormant infection, particularly during immunosuppression. Disease severity is dependent on both fungal virulence factors and the host's immune response. Although not as comprehensively studied, transmission, virulence factors, and immune response to other species of *Cryptococcus* resemble those of *C. neoformans* and *C. gattii* (Table 12.1) (Ma and May 2009).

(See Chapter 8 for further details of the virulence factors of *Cryptococcus*.)

Epidemiology

Cryptococcosis occurs in both humans and animals, including domestic dogs and cats, and native Australian animals such as the koala. Animal-to-human and human-to-human transmission has been documented rarely. The disease is uncommon in children, with a prevalence of 1% in children with AIDS (Pfaller and Diekema 2010).

C. neoformans

C. neoformans var. *grubii* has a worldwide distribution and causes 95% of all *C. neoformans* infections (Ma and May 2009). It has been isolated from a variety of environmental sources, including avian excreta (particularly pigeons), soil, and decaying wood from trees. *C. neoformans* var. *neoformans* infections are most prevalent in Europe, where it accounts for 30% of isolates (Ma and May 2009).

The overwhelming majority of symptomatic *C. neoformans* infections occur in patients with impaired cell-mediated immunity, including those with advanced HIV (human immunodeficiency virus) infection, organ transplantation, haematological malignancies, and diabetes mellitus; infections among those with intact immune systems are rare. Meningitis is the predominant clinical presentation, with an estimated incidence of 1 million cases per year, with most cases occurring in sub-Saharan Africa (Park et al. 2009). After candidiasis and aspergillosis, cryptococcosis is the third most common invasive fungal infection in patients who undergo solid organ transplantation, particularly kidney and liver transplant recipients (Pfaller and Diekema 2010).

C. gattii

C. gattii has a comparatively restricted geographical distribution, occurring predominantly in tropical and subtropical climates such as Australia. Its prevalence in temperate climates is uncommon, although an emergence on Vancouver Island, Canada, was identified in 2002, with subsequent expansion to the Pacific Northwest and other areas of the USA (Pfaller and Diekema 2010). *C. gattii* has a specific ecological association with numerous species of Eucalyptus trees, which although native to Australia, have been extensively exported to other tropical climates. The Canadian isolates are associated with a range of native non-Eucalyptus species such as the Coastal Douglas Fir (Kidd et al. 2007).

Historically considered a pathogen in persons with apparently normal immune systems, a recent review in Australia noted an increase in HIV-negative immunocompromised patients due to cancer, idiopathic CD4 lymphopenia, and long-term immunosuppressive therapies (Chen et al. 2012). Similarly, the emergence in Canada and the Pacific Northwest, USA, identified new risk factors for infection, including HIV/AIDS, cancer, and smoking (Harris et al. 2011).

C. gattii causes only 1% of cryptococcosis cases worldwide. In Australia's Northern Territory, where *C. gattii* infection is endemic, the annual incidence is 6.5 cases per million (Chen et al. 2012); however, in the recent Pacific Northwest outbreak the annual incidence

Table 12.1 Virulence factors of *Cryptococcus* species

Virulence factor	Role
Polysaccharide capsule: glucuronoxylomannan (GXM) and glucuronoxylomannogalactan (GXMGal)	Inhibits phagocytosis and protects against dehydration
Melanin	Protects from UV light and environmental conditions; an antioxidant protecting against immune response and antifungal drugs
Laccase	Catalyses production of melanin; helps to establish an ecological niche in rotting wood. Activity lower in non-*neoformans/gattii* species
Proteinases and phospholipases	Degrades host cell membrane and lyses cells, providing nutrients for the organism and protection from the host
Urease	Catalyses hydrolysis of urea to ammonia and carbamate; facilitates blood-to-brain transmission
α mating type	More prevalent and more virulent than a mating type

was as high as 35 cases per million (Pfaller and Diekema 2010), and in northern Brazil, *C. gattii* accounts for 62% of all cryptococcosis cases (Ma and May 2009). Cryptococcosis caused by this species is characterized by the development of cryptococcomas (large mass lesions) in the lung and brain. Morbidity from neurological disease is high, although mortality rates are lower compared with *C. neoformans* infections.

Other *Cryptococcus* species

Non-*neoformans/gattii* species are widely distributed geographically and have been identified from air, soil, water, pigeon droppings, and food. Some species, such as *C. laurentii* and *C. uniguttulatus*, can colonize humans (Khawcharoenporn et al. 2007). Eighty per cent of the non-*neoformans/gattii* infections are due to *C. albidus* and *C. laurentii*. Impaired cellular immunity is the most common risk factor, with HIV infection and low CD4 counts a common comorbidity. For *C. laurentii* infection, invasive devices are an additional risk factor (Khawcharoenporn et al. 2007; Arendrup et al. 2013).

Clinical presentation

Cryptococcal infections may present acutely or chronically, with clinical presentations varying depending on the stage of disease rather than the causative species. The most common clinical manifestations involve CNS, bloodstream, and pulmonary infections (Khawcharoenporn et al. 2007; Ma and May 2009) (see Chapters 22, 25, and 30).

Diagnosis

Within tissue sections, mucicarmine or Alcian blue stains the capsule of *Cryptococcus* species to distinguish it from other yeasts with similar morphologies. Cryptococcal cells are typically rounder than the cells of *Candida* species and reproduce by narrow-necked budding. Immunohistochemical staining allows identification and discrimination of *C. neoformans* var. *grubii* from var. *neoformans* and *C. gattii* in formalin-fixed tissues (Krockenberger et al. 2001).

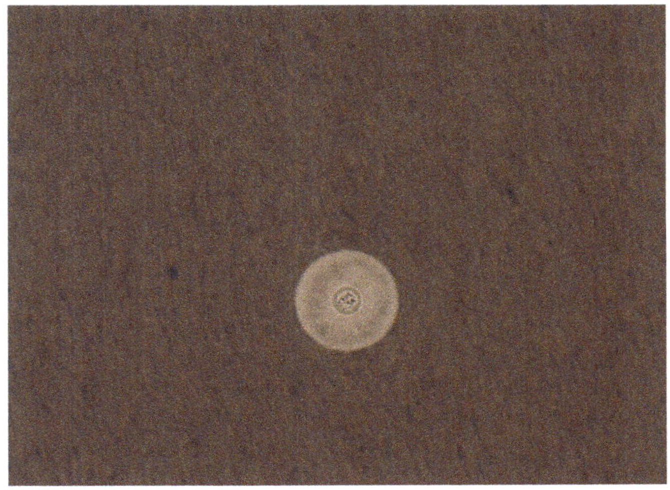

Figure 12.1 India ink stain of *Cryptococcus gattii* cell in cerebrospinal fluid. Approximate ×400 magnification.
Image reproduced courtesy of Catriona Halliday.

For direct examination of cerebrospinal fluid (CSF), urine, and other body fluids, the India ink stain can be used to visualize the capsule, demonstrating a clear halo around the yeast under bright field illumination (Figure 12.1).

Several commercial cryptococcal antigen tests are available to detect capsular proteins of *C. neoformans* and *C. gattii* in serum and CSF with high sensitivity and specificity. False positives have been reported, and they are not a reliable diagnostic test for non-*neoformans/gattii* species, despite having capsular antigens in common (Howell et al. 2015). The IMMY Cryptococcal Lateral Flow assay (Immuno-Mycologics, Inc., OK, USA) is a point-of-care test developed for the early diagnosis of cryptococcosis from serum, CSF, and urine samples, which has replaced conventional antigen techniques in many diagnostic laboratories. Its performance has not been evaluated for the detection of non-*neoformans/gattii* infections.

Cultures of *C. gattii* can be differentiated from *C. neoformans* by growth on CGB (canavanine-glycine-bromothymol blue) agar, turning the medium blue. *C. neoformans* does not grow on this medium.

Commercially available carbohydrate assimilation kits used to be the mainstay of yeast identification; however, reliable species-level identification, particularly of unusual species, increasingly requires rDNA sequencing of the internal transcribed spacer regions and/or D1/D2 domains of the large subunit. MALDI-TOF-MS (matrix-assisted laser desorption/ionization–time-of-flight mass spectrometry) can provide reliable species- and subspecies-level identification of *Cryptococcus* species, but its accuracy depends on database quality (Arendrup et al. 2013).

Treatment

All *Cryptococcus* species are intrinsically resistant to echinocandins. Infections due to *C. neoformans* and *C. gattii* are initially treated with amphotericin B, with or without flucytosine (5-fluorocytosine), followed by maintenance therapy with fluconazole, sometimes for life (see Chapters 33 and 49). The emergence of resistance to amphotericin B, flucytosine, fluconazole, or itraconazole has been reported, particularly after prolonged treatment or prophylaxis with fluconazole. Untreated cryptococcal meningitis is fatal. However, appropriate antifungal treatment, coupled with highly active antiretroviral therapy, has greatly improved the prognosis of AIDS-associated CNS cryptococcosis (Pfaller and Diekema 2010) (see Chapter 33).

Optimal treatment strategies for infections due to other *Cryptococcus* species have not been determined, but depend on the site of infection. *In vitro* susceptibility testing indicates that *C. albidus, C. curvatus*, and *C. laurentii* are susceptible to amphotericin B, but less susceptible to flucytosine, fluconazole, and other azoles than *C. neoformans*. Initial induction therapy with amphotericin B until evidence of clinical improvement—followed by step-down to fluconazole therapy if the isolate is susceptible—is considered an appropriate treatment regimen (Arendrup et al. 2013). Spontaneous recovery in less severe cases of non-*neoformans*/*gattii* infections with non-CNS involvement may occur, usually as a result of catheter or infected-tissue removal (Khawcharoenporn et al. 2007).

References

Arendrup MC, Boekhout T, Akova M, et al. (2013) ESCMID and ECMM joint clinical guidelines for the diagnosis and management of rare invasive yeast infections. *Clin Microbiol Infect* 20 (Suppl. 3): 76–98.

Chen SC, Slavin MA, Heath CH, et al. (2012) Clinical manifestations of *Cryptococcus gattii* infection: determinants of neurological sequelae and death. *Clin Infect Dis* 55: 789–98.

Harris JR, Lockhart SR, Debess E, et al. (2011) *Cryptococcus gattii* in the United States: clinical aspects of infection with an emerging pathogen. *Clin Infect Dis* 53: 1185–95.

Howell SA, Hazen KC and Brandt ME (2015) *Candida, Cryptococcus*, and other yeasts of medical importance, *in*: J Jorgensen, M Pfaller, K Carroll, et al., eds, *Manual of Clinical Microbiology* (11th edn, Washington DC: ASM Press), 1984–2014.

Khawcharoenporn T, Apisarnthanarak A and Mundy LM (2007) *Non-neoformans* cryptococcal infections: a systematic review. *Infection* 35: 51–8.

Kidd SE, Chow Y, Mak S, et al. (2007) Characterization of environmental sources of the human and animal pathogen *Cryptococcus gattii* in British Columbia, Canada, and the Pacific Northwest of the United States. *Appl Environ Microbiol* 73: 1433–43.

Krockenberger MB, Canfield PJ, Kozel TR, et al. (2001) An immunohistochemical method that differentiates *Cryptococcus neoformans* varieties and serotypes in formalin-fixed paraffin-embedded tissues. *Med Mycol* 39: 523–33.

Kwon-Chung KJ, Boekhout T, Fell JW and Diaz M (2002) Proposal to conserve the name *Cryptococcus gattii* against *C. hondurianus* and *C. bacillisporus* (Basidiomycota, Hymenomycetes, Tremellomycetidae). *Taxon* 51: 804–6.

Ma H and May RC (2009) Virulence in *Cryptococcus* species. *Adv Appl Microbiol* 67: 131–90.

Park BJ, Wannemuehler KA, Marston BJ, Govender N, Pappas PG and Chiller TM (2009) Estimation of the current global burden of cryptococcal meningitis among persons living with HIV/AIDS. *AIDS* 23: 525–30.

Pfaller MA and Diekema DJ (2010) Epidemiology of invasive mycoses in North America. *Crit Rev Microbiol* 36: 1–53.

CHAPTER 13

Other yeasts

Chris Linton and Susan Howell

Introduction to other yeasts

The yeasts described in this section are in general rare causes of serious human infection. Many are commonly found in the environment or as human commensals and are therefore opportunistic pathogens.

Diagnosis

Traditional microscopy and culture techniques remain the best methods for isolating these yeast species from a variety of clinical specimens. Many of these yeasts also grow in blood culture medium. Macroscopic and microscopic features, together with fermentation and assimilation tests (e.g. API 20 AUX [bioMérieux] AuxaColor 2 [Bio-Rad], work well for the more common species. Molecular methods have superseded these, and include DNA sequencing (D1-D2 region of the large ribosomal subunit, internal transcribed spacer regions 1 and 2, or the intergenomic spacer region 1), and MALDI-TOF (matrix-assisted laser desorption/ionization–time-of-flight) mass spectrometry, which is continually improving as the protein profile database expands.

Malassezia

All but *M. pachydermatis* require lipid supplementation of the growth media. The colonies are cream to beige, and smooth to deeply folded, and some have a brittle texture that is frequently difficult to suspend. Microscopic features include round, oval-to-elongated, thick-walled blastospores and a prominent broad monopolar bud scar (Figure 13.1). Pseudohyphae are only produced in skin in pityriasis versicolor.

Significant species

M. pachydermatis, M. furfur, M. globosa, M. sympodialis, M. dermatis, M. japonica, M. obtusa, M. restricta, and *M. slooffiae*.

Taxonomy

Approximately 18 *Malassezia* species are currently recognized (http://www.indexfungorum.org, 2015).

Pathogenesis

As commensals, *Malassezia* species become pathogenic when the immune or environmental balance changes. The high lipid content of the cell wall may aid adhesion to host cells, protect from phagocytosis, and cause a reduction in the host immune response. These yeasts can also form biofilms on the skin and indwelling medical devices.

Epidemiology

Malassezia numbers and species vary with age, body site, and geographic location. Superficial infections are therefore endogenous, but examples of exogenous spread exist.

Clinical presentation

Malassezia species cause skin infections, and occasionally systemic infections, in immunocompromised patients (Table 13.1).

Treatment

Superficial infections are treated with topical azoles, selenium sulphide, or oral itraconazole. For systemic infections, fluconazole or amphotericin B are most commonly used, and sometimes voriconazole. However, as lipid supplementation is required for growth, there are no standardized methods for susceptibility testing. Significant variations in minimum inhibitory concentration (MIC) values have been reported, but resistance to flucytosine (5-fluorocytosine) and the echinocandins is a consistent finding.

Rhodotorula

These encapsulated yeasts grow on Sabouraud's glucose–peptone agar (SAB) as red-to-orange colonies which are smooth and shiny, sometimes mucoid, and occasionally dull/rough and wrinkly. Microscopic features include large round-to-elongated blastospores, rarely forming true or pseudo-hyphae (Figure 13.2).

Significant species

R. mucilaginosa (most common), *R. glutinis*, and *R. minuta*.

Taxonomy

Over 170 species have been described, and approximately 80 species are currently accepted (http://www.indexfungorum.org, 2015).

Pathogenesis

Rhodotorula species are opportunistic pathogens with low virulence capable of causing localized or disseminated infection.

Epidemiology

These species are widespread in nature and can be found in, soil, water, fruit/fruit juice, shower curtains, and toothbrushes, and are sometimes found as airborne culture contaminants in the laboratory. They can be part of the commensal flora of human skin, nail, and the respiratory and digestive tracts.

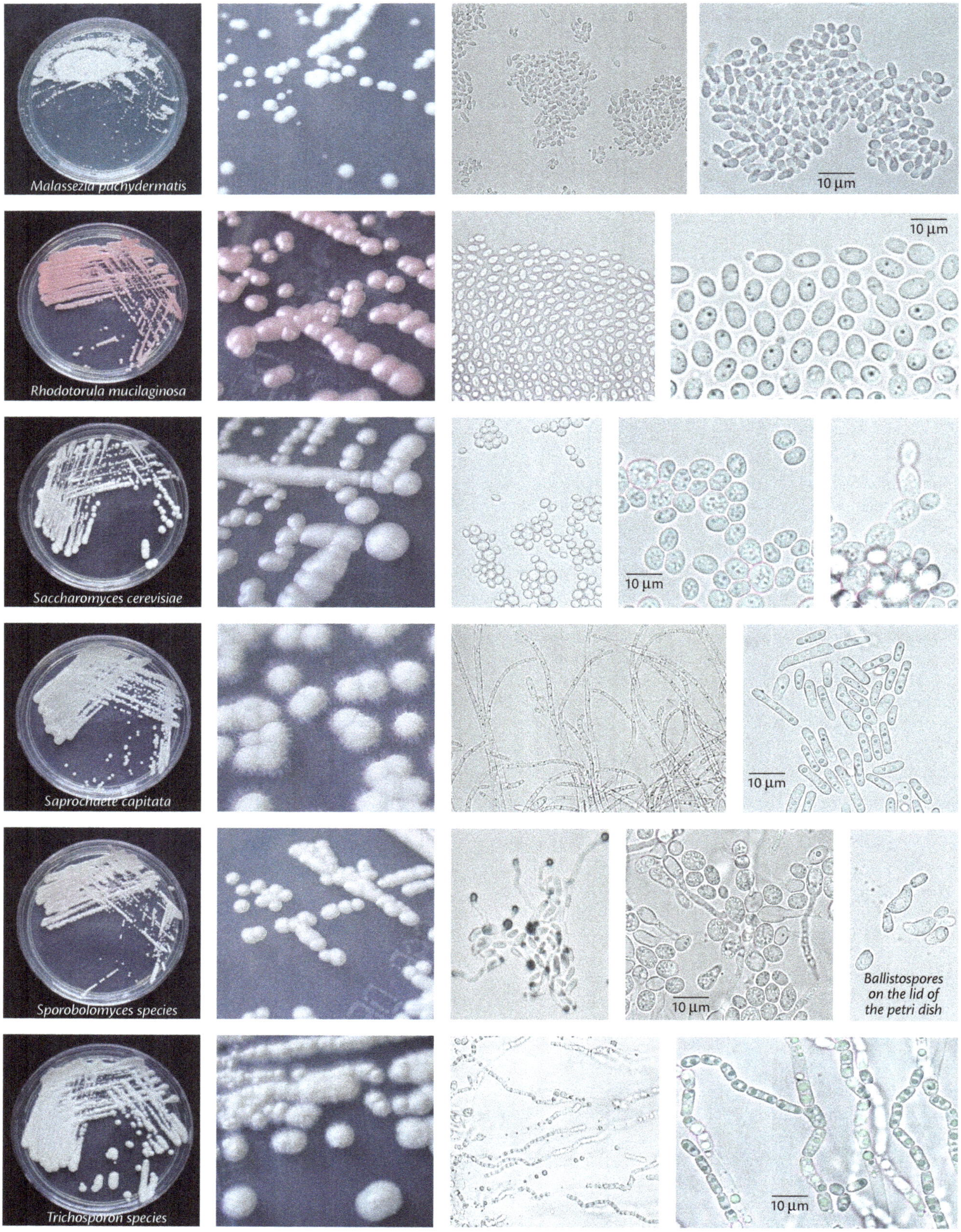

Figure 13.1 Yeast colonial morphologies and microscopic features—grown on Sabouraud's dextrose agar at 30°C.

Table 13.1 Clinical presentations and associated risk factors

Organism	Infections	Risk factors
Malassezia furfur, M .globosa, M. sympodialis, M. dermatis, M. japonica, M. obtusa, M. restricta, M. slooffiae *M. pachydermatis, M. furfur, M. sympodialis* (Many of the lipophilic *Malassezia* species have been reported as *M. furfur*.)	*Superficial infections:* Pityriasis versicolor, atopic dermatitis, eczema, dandruff Folliculitis, seborrhoeic dermatitis *Invasive infections:* Systemic infections, fungaemia (Arendrup et al. 2013; Pedrosa et al. 2014)	Age, underlying skin disease Immune suppression, AIDS, Parkinson's disease Immunosuppression, central venous catheters (CVCs), parenteral nutrition in neonates
Rhodotorula mucilaginosa, R. minuta, R. glutinis	*Superficial infections:* Possible onychomycosis *Invasive infections:* Fungaemia, septicaemia, meningitis, peritonitis, endocarditis, endophthalmitis, systemic infection, sepsis (Forés et al. 2012; Arendrup et al. 2013; Zhou et al. 2014)	CVCs, steroids, peritoneal dialysis, AIDS, immunosuppression, extensive burns, intra-abdominal surgery, intravenous drug abuse, broad-spectrum antibacterial use, breakthrough infections during fluconazole or echinocandin treatment
Saccharomyces cerevisiae	*Superficial infections:* Mucosal infections, vaginitis, *Invasive infections:* Fungaemia, oesophageal ulcer, endocarditis, aortic graft infection, liver abscess, peritonitis, urinary tract infection, disseminated infection (Muñoz et al. 2005; Savini et al. 2008; Arendrup et al. 2013)	Fluconazole exposure CVCs, broad-spectrum antibacterial use, immunosuppression, bone marrow or solid organ transplant, *S. boulardii* probiotic use
Saprochaete capitata	*Superficial infections:* Onychomycosis, skin lesions *Invasive infections:* Respiratory disease, brain and liver abscess, severe sepsis, multi-organ failure, nodular lesions in liver/spleen, spondylodiscitis, osteomyelitis (Arendrup et al. 2013; García-Ruiza et al. 2013; Mazzocato et al. 2015)	Immunocompromised, haematological malignancy, prolonged neutropenia, aggressive chemotherapy, broad-spectrum antibiotics, CVCs, breakdown of skin and mucosa, chronic obstructive pulmonary disorder, diabetes mellitus, endocarditis, solid tumours, solid organ transplant
Sporobolomyces salmonicolor, S. roseus, S. holsaticus	*Superficial infections:* Dermatitis *Invasive infections:* Endophthalmitis, lymphadenitis, cerebral infection, meningitis, central-line associated bloodstream infections, fungaemia (Sharma et al. 2005; Arendrup et al. 2013; Tang et al. 2015)	Immunocompromised, corticosteroid therapy, AIDS, poorly controlled diabetes mellitus
Trichosporon cutaneum, T. inkin, T. loubieri *T. ovoides*	*Superficial infections:* White piedra—hair, scalp, beard, eyebrows, genital tinea pedis, onychomycosis, skin lesions, foot ulcer *Allergic reactions:* Hypersensitivity and pneumonitis (Colombo et al. 2011; Arendrup et al. 2013; Rastogi et al. 2013)	Frequent use of a hairband inhalation of arthrospores present in patients' homes
Trichosporon asahii, T. asteroides, T. inkin, T. loubieri, T. mucoides	*Invasive infections:* Fungaemia, pneumonia, pulmonary involvement, soft tissue lesions, liver, spleen, brain abscesses, peritonitis, endocarditis, meningitis, disseminated infection, endophthalmitis (Colombo et al. 2011; Arendrup et al. 2013; Roman et al. 2014)	Immunocompromised, haematological malignancy, AIDS, solid organ transplant recipients, extensive burns, CVCs, corticosteroids, heart valve surgery, hepatic/renal failure, diabetes, cystic fibrosis Breakthrough infections during amphotericin B or echinocandin treatment

Clinical presentation

These commensal yeasts are capable of causing fungaemia in immunocompromised patients. Superficial infections are rare (Table 13.1).

Treatment

Amphotericin B appears to be the treatment of choice, with the possible addition of flucytosine. *Rhodotorula* species show reduced susceptibilities to most azoles and are resistant to fluconazole and the echinocandins.

Saccharomyces

These yeasts grow on SAB as cream-coloured, smooth, shiny colonies. Microscopic features include large oval blastospores, sometimes with poorly formed pseudohyphae and ascospores (Figure 13.3).

Significant species

S. cerevisiae

Taxonomy

Although over 500 species have been described, only 12 species are currently accepted, with approximately 100 awaiting re-evaluation/reassignment (http://www.indexfungorum.org, 2015).

Pathogenesis

Saccharomyces species are opportunistic pathogens with low virulence.

Epidemiology

These species are widespread in nature and can be isolated from soil, plants, and fruit. *S. cerevisiae* is very important in the baking and brewing industries, *S. boulardii* (a variant of *S. cerevisiae*) is included in some diet and health foods. They are occasional commensals of the human digestive tract.

Clinical presentation

Saccharomyces species can cause mucosal and systemic infections (Table 13.1).

Treatment

Clinical experience suggests favourable outcomes with fluconazole or amphotericin B; however, *S. cerevisiae* often exhibits elevated azole MICs. Amphotericin B in combination with flucytosine has been used in severe or recurrent cases. Vaginal infections may respond to miconazole, nystatin, or amphotericin B-flucytosine cream.

Saprochaete

These yeasts grow on SAB as white to off-white colonies which can be shiny, dull (with low aerial mycelium), heaped, or folded. Microscopic features include true-branching hyphae, arthrospores, and annelloconidia. The lateral hyphae curve away from the main hyphal stem (Figure 13.4).

Significant species

S. capitata (previously *Blastoschizomyces capitatus*)

Taxonomy

Magnusiomyces is the teleomorph name; eight of these species are currently accepted. *Saprochaete* is the anamorph name; over ten of these species are currently accepted (http://www.indexfungorum.org, 2015).

Pathogenesis

S. capitata is an opportunistic pathogen.

Epidemiology

This species is ubiquitous and can be isolated from soil, sand, plants, wood, dairy products, and poultry faeces. This species can be part of the commensal flora of human skin and the respiratory and digestive tracts.

Clinical presentation

S. capitata is a rare cause of invasive human infection, usually in patients with haematological malignancy (Table 13.1).

Treatment

There are no clear recommendations for primary treatment, but recent publications suggest voriconazole with or without amphotericin B. Amphotericin B alone or in combination with flucytosine has also been successful. *In vitro*, this yeast is susceptible to flucytosine, itraconazole, voriconazole, and posaconazole, but resistant to fluconazole and the echinocandins. Amphotericin B resistance has been reported.

Sporobolomyces

Sporobolomyces yeasts grow on SAB as bright red, pink, or orange mucoid colonies. Microscopic features include oval-to-ellipsoidal blastospores, true and pseudo- hyphae, and ballistospores produced on sterigmata. These ballistospores are launched from the sterigmata and can be seen on the underside of the lid of a petri dish (Figure 13.5). This feature helps to distinguish these yeasts from species of *Rhodotorula*.

Significant species

S. salmonicolor (most common), *S. roseus*, and *S. holsaticus*

Taxonomy

Almost 100 species have been described, with just under 60 species currently accepted (http://www.indexfungorum.org, 2015). They are basidiomycetes of uncertain taxonomy.

Pathogenesis

Sporobolomyces species are rare opportunistic pathogens.

Epidemiology

These species are commonly isolated from soil, plant leaves, water, and fruit (orange peel).

Clinical presentation

Rarely, *Sporobolomyces* species cause human infection (Table 13.1).

Treatment

Voriconazole or amphotericin B is an appropriate first-line treatment. Limited data suggests that *S. salmonicolor* is resistant to fluconazole and the echinocandins, although some isolated species may also show resistance to amphotericin B and itraconazole.

Trichosporon

These yeasts have cream colonies when grown on SAB, though different species demonstrate quite different colonial appearances (e.g. shiny, dull, dry, moist, folded). Microscopic features include true hyphae; often branching, cylindrical arthrospores; and budding blastospores (Figure 13.6).

Significant species

At least 16 species are associated with deep infections, of which the most common are: *T. asahii, T. asteroides, T. cutaneum, T. inkin, T. loubieri, T. mucoides*, and *T. ovoides*.

Current taxonomy

These are basidiomycetes. Approximately 120 species have been described; of these, over 50 species are currently accepted and a further 20 require confirmation (http://www.indexfungorum.org, 2015).

Pathogenesis

Trichosporon species are opportunistic pathogens. Some can express glucuronoxylomannan in their cell walls, similarly to *Cryptococcus neoformans*, which may affect the phagocytic capability of neutrophils. *T. asahii* is able to produce biofilms which enable it to adhere to implanted devices such as catheters and resist antifungal treatment.

Epidemiology

These species are widespread in the environment and can be isolated from soil, plants, insects, bird droppings, cattle, water, and food. They can be transient colonizers of the skin and respiratory tract, and occasional commensals of the oral cavity and gastrointestinal tract, which together may act as an endogenous reservoir.

Clinical presentation

Trichosporon species may cause superficial, mucosal-associated, or invasive infections in humans (Table 13.1).

Treatment

The triazoles are used as primary therapy for trichosporonosis in immunocompromised patients. Amphotericin B often shows reduced activity against many *Trichosporon* species, and most species are resistant to flucytosine and echinocandins.

References

Arendrup MC, Boekhout T, Akova M, Meis JF, Cornely OA and Lortholary O (2013) ESCMID and ECMM joint clinical guidelines for the diagnosis and management of rare invasive yeast infections. *Clin Microbiol Infect* 20 (Suppl. 3): 76–98.

Colombo AL, Padovan ACB and Chaves GM (2011) Current knowledge of *Trichosporon* spp. and trichosporonosis. *Clin Microbiol Rev* 24: 682–700.

Forés R, Ramos A, Orden B, et al. (2012) *Rhodotorula* species fungaemia causes low mortality in haematopoietic stem-cell transplantation. A case report and review. *Mycoses* 55: e158–62.

García-Ruiza JC, López-Soria L, Olazábal I, et al. (2013) Invasive infections caused by *Saprochaete capitata* in patients with haematological malignancies: report of five cases and review of the antifungal therapy. *Rev Iberoam Micol* 30: 248–55.

Mazzocato S, Marchionni E, Fothergill AW, et al. (2015) Epidemiology and outcome of systemic infections due to *Saprochaete capitata*: case report and review of the literature. *Infection* 43: 211–5.

Muñoz P, Bouza E, Cuenca-Estrella M, et al. 2005. *Saccharomyces cerevisiae* fungaemia: an emerging infectious disease. *Clin Infect Dis* 40: 1625–34.

Pedrosa AF, Lisboa C and Rodrigues AG (2014) *Malassezia* infections: a medical conundrum. *J Am Acad Dermatol* 71: 170–6.

Rastogi V, Rudramurthy SM, Maheshwari M, Nirwan PS, Chakrabarti A and Batra S (2013) Non-healing ulcer due to *Trichosporon loubieri* in an immunocompetent host and review of published reports. *Mycopathologia* 176: 107–11.

Roman ADE, Salvaña EMT, De Guzman-Peñamora MAJ, Roxas EA, Leyritana KT and Saniel MC (2014) Invasive trichosporonosis in an AIDS patient: case report and review of the literature. *Int J STD AIDS* 25: 70–5.

Savini V, Catavitello C, Manna A, et al. (2008) Two cases of vaginitis caused by itraconazole-resistant *Saccharomyces cerevisiae* and a review of recently published studies. *Mycopathologia* 166: 47–50.

Sharma V, Shankar J and Kotamarthi V (2005) Endogeneous endophthalmitis caused by *Sporobolomyces salmonicolor*. *Eye* 20: 945–6.

Tang HJ, Lai CC and Chao CM (2015) Central-line–associated bloodstream infection caused by *Sporobolomyces salmonicolor. Infect Control Hosp Epidemiol* 36: 1111–12, http://dx.doi.org/10.1017/ice.2015.158

www.indexfungorum.org, The Royal Botanic Gardens Kew, Landcare Research-NZ and the Institute of Microbiology, Chinese Academy of Science (the custodians), June 2015.

Zhou J, Chen M, Chen H, Pan W and Liao W (2014) *Rhodotorula minuta* as onychomycosis agent in a Chinese patient: first report and literature review. *Mycoses* 57: 191–5.

CHAPTER 14

Dematiaceous fungi

Sarah E. Kidd and Catriona L. Halliday

Introduction to dematiaceous fungi

The dematiaceous fungi are classified by their dark olivaceous, brown, and black morphologies, arising from their melanized cell walls. They are phylogenetically diverse, encompassing hyphomycetes, coelomycetes, and yeast-like fungi, and their taxonomy is continually being refined. The majority are plant pathogens and saprophytes; however, the number of species being documented as mammalian pathogens is increasing.

Genera

Documented dematiaceous pathogens of humans include more than 150 species from more than 70 genera (Revankar and Sutton 2010); the most common are summarized in Table 14.1.

Recently, many species names have changed as part of a rationalization of the dual nomenclature applied to teleomorph and anamorph forms, e.g. *Lomentospora* (*Scedosporium*) *prolificans* and *Verruconis* (*Ochroconis*) *gallopava*. Additionally, molecular characterization of morphological species, including that of *Scedosporium apiospermum, Exophiala jeanselmei,* and *Sporothrix schenckii,* has led to the recognition of species complexes.

Pathogenesis

Dihydroxynaphthalene melanin is common to the cell wall of all dematiaceous fungi, and a likely virulence factor. Melanin appears to prevent phagocytosis and killing by neutrophils and macrophages, and reduce susceptibility to antifungals, free radicals, ionizing radiation, toxic metals, and desiccation (Revankar and Sutton 2010).

Chromoblastomycoses are characterized by the formation of muriform sclerotic bodies. These represent a parasitic stage with spherical, multiseptate structures (Figure 14.1), following the introduction of saprophytic conidia or hyphae into subcutaneous tissue.

Several dematiaceous species, e.g. *Cladophialophora bantiana*, appear to be neurotropic, causing central nervous system (CNS) infection, often in patients with no known predisposing factors or immunodeficiency. The molecular basis for neurotropism has not been elucidated.

Epidemiology

Dematiaceous fungal infections have been documented in all regions of the world, but are concentrated in the tropics or specific geographic regions and climatic zones. *Hortaea werneckii* infection is associated with tropical saline environments.

Both immunocompromised and immunocompetent hosts can be infected. From 2001 to 2006, phaeohyphomycoses made up 2.5% of invasive fungal diseases among solid organ and stem cell transplant recipients in the USA, with the most common genera being *Alternaria* spp. (32%), *Exophiala* spp. (11%), *Scopulariopsis*/*Microascus* spp. (12%), and *Cladophialophora* spp. (9%) (McCarty et al. 2015). Approximately half of CNS infections are associated with no underlying illness or risk factors, but 40% are associated with some degree of immune dysfunction, and 10% with haematological or solid malignancy. In developing countries, risk factors include lower socioeconomic status, and rural labour. Disseminated infections are uncommon but almost always occur in immunocompromised individuals (Revankar and Sutton 2010). A noted incidental increase over time may be due to changing risk factors, as well as improved diagnosis (Ben-Ami et al. 2009).

While pulmonary infections are acquired via inhalation of fungal spores, the route of transmission for CNS infections is unclear. This may occur via haematogenous dissemination following inhalation, or transfer from colonized sinuses, or by direct inoculation during neurosurgery. Subcutaneous infections are acquired through traumatic inoculation or following minor abrasions that breach skin integrity. *Aureobasidium pullulans* is an occasional cause of deep infection, including fungaemia due to biofilm formation on implanted or indwelling medical devices.

Clinical presentations

Phaeohyphomycoses present as a wide spectrum of syndromes, but are characterized by the presence of the mycelial form of the pathogen in tissue. These infections may be superficial, subcutaneous, allergic, localized, or disseminated. CNS infections are predominantly caused by *Cladophialophora bantiana*, but may also be caused by *Rhinocladiella mackenziei, Verruconis gallopava, Bipolaris spicifera, Fonsecaea pedrosoi, Fonsecaea monophora, Lomentospora prolificans, and Exophiala dermatitidis* (Revankar et al. 2004, 2010).

Chromoblastomycoses are chronic subcutaneous infections characterized by the presence of muriform sclerotic bodies. They have global distribution but occur more frequently in tropical/subtropical regions. Species most commonly causing chromoblastomycoses are *C. carrionii, F. compacta, F. pedrosoi*, and *Phialophora verrucosa,* and the route of transmission is typically through traumatic inoculation.

Mycetoma is a chronic subcutaneous infection characterized by draining sinuses, granules, and tumefaction, usually of the foot or hand. Sinuses discharge serosanguinous fluid containing characteristic granules. Granules vary in size, colour, and degree of

Table 14.1 Predominant species, distribution, and clinical presentations of dematiaceous fungal pathogens

Genus	Predominant species	Distribution	Predominant clinical presentations
Alternaria	*A. alternata* *A. infectoria* *A. tenuissima*	Worldwide	Cutaneous, subcutaneous, onychomycosis, oculomycosis, allergic rhinosinusitis
Aureobasidium	*A. pullulans*	Worldwide	Localized cutaneous or deep infections, oculomycosis, fungaemia
Bipolaris	*B. australiensis* *B. hawaiiensis* *B. spicifera*[a]	Worldwide	Disseminated infection, cerebral infection and meningoencephalitis, cutaneous lesions, oculomycosis, rhinosinusitis
Cladophialophora	*C. arxii* *C. bantiana*[a] *C. boppii* *C. carrionii* *C. devriesii*	Worldwide; *C. bantiana* is concentrated in India	Chromoblastomycosis, cerebral abscess, cutaneous lesions, pulmonary and disseminated infection
Curvularia	*C. clavata* *C. geniculata* *C. lunata* *C. pallescens*	Worldwide	Oculomycosis, allergic rhinosinusitis, cutaneous lesions, cerebral infection, mycetoma
Exophiala	*E. dermatitidis*[a] *E. jeanselmei* complex *E. spinifera*	Worldwide	Cerebral abscess, systemic infection, mycetoma, subcutaneous lesions, rhinosinusitis
Exserohilum	*E. rostratum*	Worldwide	Rhinosinusitis, oculomycosis, subcutaneous, invasive infections; USA meningitis outbreak due to contaminated epidurally administered steroid
Fonsecaea	*F. compacta* *F. monophora*[a] *F. nubica* *F. pedrosoi*	Tropical South America, East Asia	Chromoblastomycosis, cutaneous and subcutaneous lesions, cerebral abscess, occasional disseminated infection
Hortaea	*H. werneckii*	Tropical, subtropical	Tinea nigra of hands or soles of feet
Leptosphaeria	*L. senegalensis* *L. tompkinsii*	Tropical, subtropical, esp. Africa	Black grain mycetoma
Madurella	*M. mycetomatis*	Arid zones of India and East Africa	Black grain mycetoma
Scedosporium/ Lomentospora	*S. apiospermum* complex *S. aurantiacum* *L. prolificans*[a]	Worldwide; Australia, Spain (*S. aurantiacum, L. prolificans*)	Otitis externa, cutaneous, subcutaneous, cerebral abscess, osteomyelitis, disseminated infection
Neoscytalidium	*N. dimidiatum*	Tropical, subtropical	Onychomycosis; cutaneous, subcutaneous, and disseminated infection
Verruconis	*V. gallopava*[a]	Worldwide	Pulmonary and cerebral
Piedraia	*P. hortae*	Tropical, esp. South America	Black piedra of scalp hair
Phaeoacremonium	*P. parasiticum* *P. alvesii* *P. krajdenii*	Worldwide	Cutaneous, subcutaneous, osteomyelitis, oculomycosis, disseminated infection
Phialophora	*P. verrucosa* *P. richardsiae*	Tropical, subtropical, esp. South America and Japan	Subcutaneous, chromoblastomycosis
Phoma	*P. exigua* *P. minutella*	Worldwide	Subcutaneous, oculomycosis, deep infection
Rhinocladiella	*R. mackenziei*[a] *R. aquaspersa*	Middle East (*R. mackenziei*) South America (*R. aquaspersa*)	Cerebral abscess, chromoblastomycosis

(continued)

Table 14.1 (Continued)

Genus	Predominant species	Distribution	Predominant clinical presentations
Scopulariopsis/ Microascus	*S. brevicaulis* *S. brumptii* *M. cinerea*	Worldwide	Onychomycosis, disseminated infection, endocarditis
Sporothrix	*S. schenckii* complex	Tropical, subtropical	Cutaneous, subcutaneous, osteomyelitis, pulmonary and disseminated infection
Trematosphaeria	*T. grisea*	South America	Black grain mycetoma
Veronaea	*V. botryosa*	Tropical, subtropical, esp. China.	Chromoblastomycosis; cutaneous, subcutaneous, and disseminated infection

[a] neurotropic species

hardness, depending on the species. Distribution is world-wide but most common in bare-footed populations living in tropical or subtropical regions. Aetiological agents include *Madurella, Exophiala, Trematosphaeria, Leptosphaeria,* and *Curvularia* spp. (see Chapters 20 and 23).

Diagnosis

Diagnosis requires a high degree of clinical suspicion and a multifaceted approach to diagnosis, including direct microscopy, culture, histopathology, and radiology. Collection of specimens from the site of infection is critical for differentiating fungal pathogens from environmental contaminants.

Direct microscopy of fresh specimen should include digestion with 10% KOH (potassium hydroxide); melanized structures can be visualized with KOH alone, or in combination with Parker Ink. For tissue sections, the haematoxylin & eosin (H&E) and Fontana-Masson stains are useful for detecting melanized hyphae and sclerotic bodies (Revankar and Sutton 2010; Chowdhary et al. 2014).

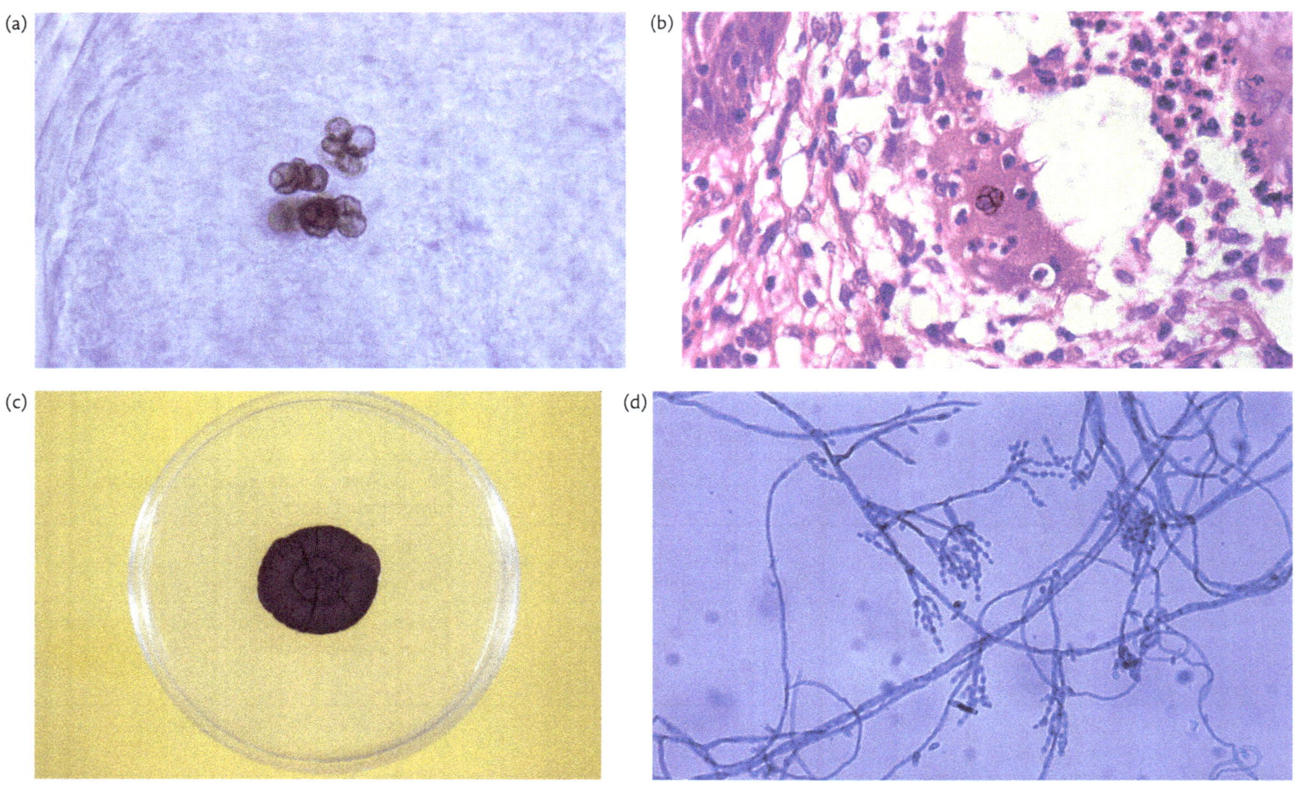

Figure 14.1 Skin scrapings mounted in 10% potassium hydroxide and Parker ink (**a**) and haematoxylin & eosin (**b**) revealing sclerotic bodies associated with chromoblastomycosis. *Cladophialophora carrionii* morphology on Sabouraud's dextrose agar (**c**) and on slide culture stained with lactophenol cotton blue (approx. ×400 magnification) (**d**).

Reproduced with permission from Associate Professor David H. Ellis and Dr. Sarah Kidd, University of Adelaide.

Primary culture media must specifically support fungal growth and inhibit bacteria owing to the slow growth of many dematiaceous fungi; cultures should be incubated for a minimum of three weeks (Revankar and Sutton 2010). Minimal media to stimulate sporulation, and temperature tests, are important for morphological identification; *C. bantiana* may be differentiated from other *Cladophialophora* species by its growth at 42°C, and *V. gallopava* grows at ≤48°C. In the case of the *Sporothrix schenckii* complex, mycelial-to-yeast phase conversion on brain heart infusion agar at 37°C is important for species confirmation. Accurate identification to species level is essential to differentiate contaminants from the pathogenic agent. DNA sequencing can potentially reduce time to identification, particularly when sporulation or other features are limited (Halliday et al. 2015).

Antigenic and molecular detection assays are currently not well-developed for dematiaceous fungi, although panfungal PCR (polymerase chain reaction) with sequencing may assist in genus or species identification where tissue is unavailable for culture or culture is slow (Halliday et al. 2015). However, given that the vast majority of cultured dematiaceous fungi represent contaminants, clinical utility is dependent on specimen selection from normally sterile sites, or where pigmented fungal elements are observed on direct microscopy.

Treatment

In the absence of treatment standards, the management of dematiaceous fungal infections is largely guided by case reports and antifungal susceptibility testing of individual isolates. Itraconazole, voriconazole, posaconazole, and in some cases amphotericin B, demonstrate the most consistent *in vitro* activity, and are often used in combination. Surgery is often indicated (Chowdhary et al. 2014). Susceptibility testing is recommended in all cases of culture-confirmed infection, although interpretive criteria are lacking. Table 14.2 summarizes documented susceptibility trends of dematiaceous fungal species.

Table 14.2 *In vitro* activity of antifungal drugs against selected dematiaceous fungi

Species	*In vitro* antifungal activity							
	AMB	ITZ	VRZ	PSZ	ISV	TBF	5FC	ECH
Alternaria spp.	+	++	+	++	+	+	–	+
Aureobasidium pullulans	+	++	++	++		–	–	+
Bipolaris spp.	+	++	++	++	+	+	–	+
Chaetomium spp.	+	++	++	++			–	–
Cladophialophora spp.	–	++	++	++	++	+		+
Curvularia spp.	+	++	++	++	+	+	–	+
Exophiala spp.	+	++	++	++	+	+	+	+
Exserohilum rostratum	++	++	++	++	+	++		+
Fonsecaea spp.	++	++	++	++	++	+	+	+
Hortaea werneckii	++	++	++	++	++		–	
Lomentospora prolificans	–	–	–	–	–	–	–	–
Madurella mycetomatis	+	++	++	+	++	+	–	–
Neoscytalidium dimidiatum	++	+	+	+		+	–	–
Phaeoacremonium spp.	+	+	++	+		+	–	–
Phialophora spp.	+	+	++	++	+	+	+	–
Phoma spp.	+	+	+					
Rhinocladiella spp.	+	++	+	+	+			–
Scedosporium spp.	–	+	++	+	+	+	–	–
Scopulariopsis spp.	+	–	+	+		+	–	
Sporothrix spp.	+	+	+	+	–	+	–	–
Verruconis gallopava	++	++	++	++	–	++	–	+
Veronaea botryosa	–	+	+	+	–	+		–

++ Good activity based upon consistently low minimal inhibitory concentrations (MICs); + limited data suggestive of some activity; – no activity based upon consistently high MICs.

AMB = amphotericin B; ITZ = itraconazole; VRZ = voriconazole; PSZ = posaconazole; ISV = isavuconazole; TBF = terbinafine, 5FC = 5-fluorocytosine (flucytosine); ECH = echinocandin.

Adapted with permission from Revankar S. G. and Sutton D. A., 'Melanized Fungi in Human Disease', *Clinical Microbiology Reviews*, Volume 23, Issue 3, pp. 884–928, Copyright © 2010 American Society for Microbiology. DOI: 10.1128/CMR.00019-10

References

Ben-Ami R, Lewis RE, Raad II and Kontoyiannis DP (2009) Phaeohyphomycosis in a tertiary care cancer. *Clin Infect Dis* 48:1033–41.

Chowdhary A, Meis JF, Guarro J, et al. (2014) ESCMID and ECMM joint clinical guidelines for the diagnosis and management of systemic phaeohyphomycosis: diseases caused by black fungi. *Clin Microbiol Infect* 20 (Suppl. 3): 47–75.

Halliday CL, Kidd SE, Sorrell TC and Chen SC (2015) Molecular diagnostic methods for invasive fungal disease: the horizon draws nearer? *Pathology* 47: 257–69.

McCarty TP, Baddley JW, Walsh TJ, et al. (2015) Phaeohyphomycosis in transplant recipients: results from the Transplant Associated Infection Surveillance Network (TRANSNET). *Med Mycol* 53: 440–6.

Revankar SG and Sutton DA (2010) Melanized fungi in human disease. *Clin Microbiol Rev* 23: 884–928.

Revankar SG, Sutton DA and Rinaldi MG (2004) Primary central nervous system phaeohyphomycosis: a review of 101 cases. *Clin Microbiol Rev* 38: 206–16.

CHAPTER 15

The dermatophytes

Susan Howell

Introduction to the dermatophytes

The dermatophyte fungi are the commonest causes of human superficial fungal infection worldwide. They can infect skin, nail, and hair. Species may be anthropophilic, zoophilic, or geophilic. All species grow well at 28–30°C, but many grow poorly at 37°C. Infections with dermatophytes are called tinea, and this is followed by the site, e.g. capitis (scalp), pedis (foot).

Genus names

Arthroderma
Epidermophyton
Microsporum
Nannizia
Trichophyton

Description of genera

Epidermophyton:

Colonies are powdery, may have a wrinkled centre, and are khaki to olive in colour. Microscopic features include club-shaped macroconidia (young cultures) and large chlamydospores (older cultures). No microconidia.

Trichophyton:

Colonies may be white/cream/tan/yellow/red/purple, powdery to granular, floccose, or waxy, and may be flat or domed or have a wrinkled centre. The reverse pigment production is characteristic for *T. rubrum* (red/brown with white border), *T. erinacei* (diffusing yellow) and nodular forms of *T. interdigitale* (bright orange). Most *Trichophyton* species have a tan-to-brown colour on the reverse of the colony. Microscopic features include characteristic microconidia which may be round to clavate. Macroconidia are genus specific and are smooth and pencil-shaped (Campbell et al. 2013). Spiral hyphae may be seen in some species, while reflexive hyphae are a particular feature of *T. soudanense*. Small terminal chlamydospores may be seen in culture plates at room temperature with *T. verrucosum*, and antler hyphae in *T. schoenleinii*. The ability to produce urease and to penetrate hair is commonly used to distinguish *T. rubrum* (negative) from *T. interdigitale* (positive).

Microsporum:

Colonies may be white/cream/beige/tan, powdery to floccose, and flat or with striations. The reverse orange-yellow pigment is characteristic for *M. canis* and a salmon-pink colour for *M. audouinii*; other species have a reverse pigment that is pale tan to brown. Microscopic features include species-characteristic macroconidia which are rough and vary in shape and size. Microconidia may be present, but are not species specific. Other structures may be present too, including spiral hyphae, racket hyphae, and chlamydospores (Campbell et al. 2013). Growth on 1% salt agar promotes the rough appearance on macroconidia, facilitating the distinction between *M. persicolor* and *T. mentagrophytes*.

Arthroderma:

A. benhamiae has a flat, white, powdery-to-soft colony with a feathery edge, occasionally with small grains appearing at the periphery as the culture ages. The reverse pigment is bright yellow but not diffusing. Microscopic features include numerous round-to-clavate microconidia.

Examples of some common species are shown in Figure 15.1.

Significant species

There are over 50 species of dermatophytes. Tables 15.1 to 15.3 list the common, uncommon, and non-pathogenic species isolated from humans, animals, and soil.

Taxonomy

These fungi belong to the phylum *Ascomycota*, order *Onygenales*, along with other fungi able to produce aleuriospores such as *Chrysosporium*, *Histoplasma*, and the family *Arthrodermataceae*. The teleomorph has not been identified for all species, but the genera *Arthroderma* and *Nannizia* were used for species from *Trichophyton* and *Microsporum* when the sexual forms were discovered. However, the anamorphic names are well known clinically and are used in preference.

There is much current revision of species: *M. gypseum* has been renamed *Nannizia gypsea*, *M. fulvum* becomes *N. fulva*, *M. persicolor* becomes *N. persicolor*, *M. nanum* becomes *N. nana*, *M. gallinae* becomes *Lophophyton gallinae*, and *Paraphyton* replaces the genus name for *M. cookei* (see http://www.mycology.adelaide.edu.au for updates and species descriptions).

Pathogenesis

Dermatophytes are unique in their ability to digest keratin, making them the primary pathogen for the keratin-rich substrates skin, hair, and nails (Monod 2008). Species have evolved

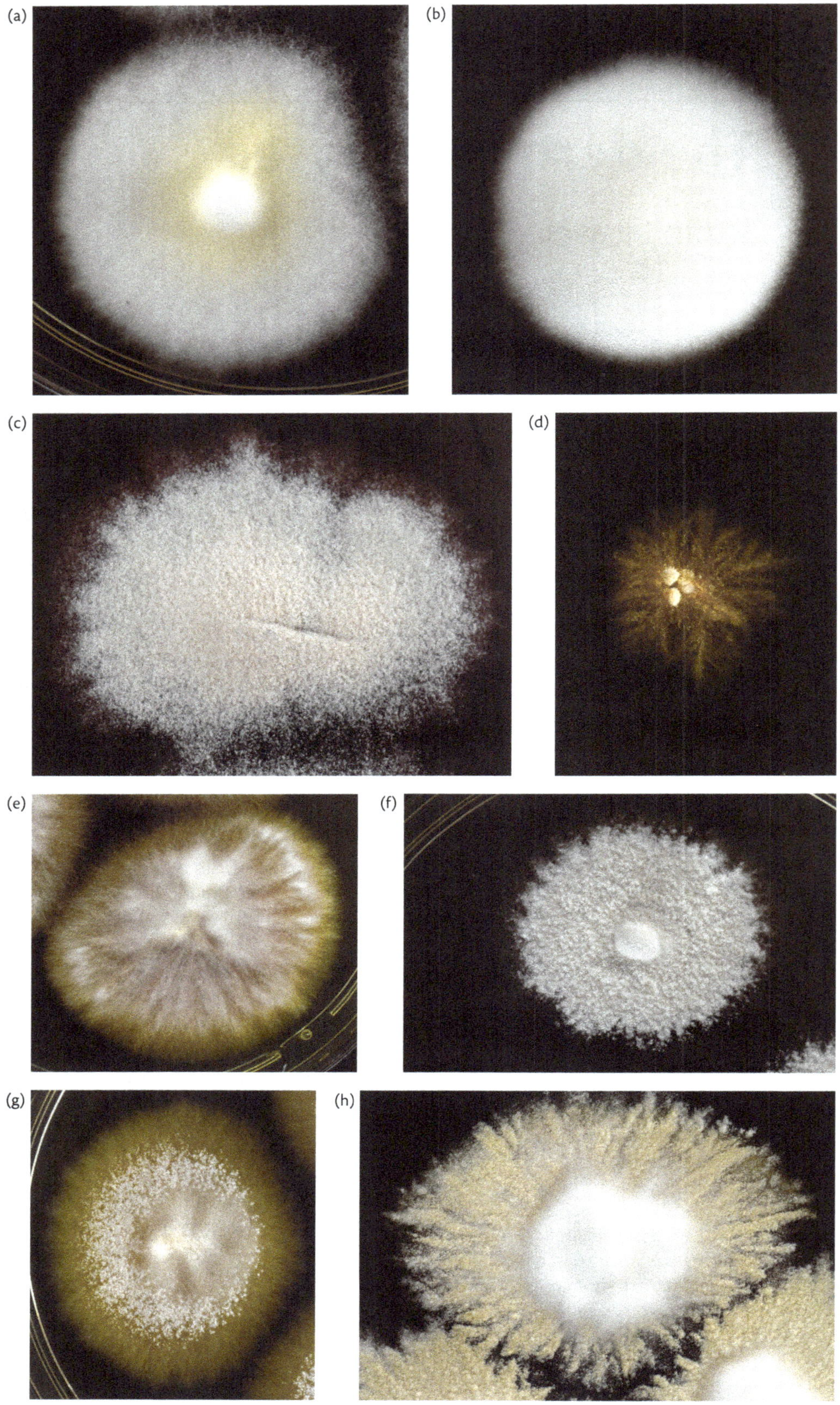

Figure 15.1 Dermatophytes grown on Sabouraud's dextrose agar.

a *Trichophyton interdigitale*; **b** *Trichophyton rubrum*; **c** *Trichophyton tonsurans*; **d** *Epidermophyton floccosum*; **e** *Microsporum canis*; **f** *Trichophyton mentagrophytes*; **g** *Arthroderma benhamiae*; **h** *Microsporum gypseum*.

Reproduced courtesy of Susan Howell.

Table 15.1 The commonest species causing human infection

Genus	Species	Source	Common sites of infection
Epidermophyton	*floccosum*	Humans	Feet, toenails, groin
Trichophyton	*rubrum*	Humans	Hands, feet, nails, groin, body, face
	interdigitale	Humans	Feet, toenails, groin
	tonsurans	Humans	Scalp, body, fingernails
	violaceum	Humans	Scalp, body, fingernails
	soudanense	Humans	Scalp, body, fingernails
	schoenleinii	Humans	Scalp
	erinacei	Hedgehogs	Body, hands
	verrucosum	Cattle, sheep, goats	Body, hands, face, scalp
	mentagrophytes	Rodents, small mammals	Body, hands, scalp
Microsporum	*audouinii*	Humans	Scalp, body
	canis	Cats and dogs	Scalp, body
	persicolor	Voles	Body
	gypseum complex	Soil	Body
Arthroderma	*benhamiae*	Rodents	Scalp

Table 15.2 Less common species causing human infection

Genus	Species	Source	Notes
Microsporum	*ferrugineum*	Humans	Parts of Africa, Asia, and eastern Europe
	gallinae	Chickens	Human infection now rare
	nanum	Pigs	Human infection now rare
Trichophyton	*concentricum*	Humans	Contact with tinea imbricata, found only in the South Pacific islands, parts of Central & South America, and Australia
	equinum	Horses	
	megninii	Humans	Endemic to Portugal and the surrounding regions
	simii	Monkeys, poultry	Endemic to India and Africa

Table 15.3 Species rarely causing human infection

Genus	Species	Source	Notes
Microsporum	*cookei*	Soil	
	praecox	Soil	
	racemosum	Soil	
	vanbreuseghemii	Soil	
Trichophyton	*ajelloi*	Soil	
	terrestre	Soil	
	vanbreuseghemii	Soil	

to live on specific hosts and have been shown to elicit a higher inflammatory reaction when infecting a different host, with zoophilic and geophilic infections usually being more inflammatory than anthropophilic sources (Giddey et al. 2007; Vermout et al. 2008).

The human skin secretes fatty acids that can inhibit the growth of dermatophytes. Tinea capitis is less common after puberty owing to the increase in oily secretions in the scalp. There is evidence to suggest possible suppression of local immune response involving lymphocyte proliferation or immune mediators (Vermout et al. 2008). There is also evidence that some hosts are genetically more susceptible to dermatophyte infection.

Epidemiology

Routes of transmission

The sources of infection are indicated in Tables 15.1 to 15.3. Zoophilic infections require contact with the animal or fomites with which the animal has had contact, e.g. bedding, fencing, cages, burrows. As a result, infections often occur at contact sites, such as hands, arms, and legs. Similarly, infection from geophilic organisms requires contact with soil, and the sites of infection are similar.

Anthropophilic infections may be acquired by direct contact with the infection or by contact with fomites. Scalp infection is easily passed between children in close contact, so siblings of children with this condition should be screened for infection or carriage of the organisms.

Patient populations

Dermatophytes affect normal healthy hosts as well as immune compromised hosts, although the latter group are more likely to develop widespread or florid infections.

Tinea capitis predominantly affects children (from a few weeks old to middle teenage years).

Onychomycosis becomes more likely with age, with infection commonest in middle to old age.

Risk factors

The primary risk factor is contact with a source of infection: animals, fomites in contact with animals, or soil. Anthropophilic species have been isolated from swimming pool areas, gym equipment, household fomites, and clothing.

Infection requires contact and probably mild abrasion of the skin to inoculate fungal elements. Pre-existing damage of nails provides a portal of entry. Occasionally, subcutaneous infections occur such as Majocchi's granuloma (follicular infection) or a kerion on the scalp.

Age is a risk factor. Tinea capitis is a disease of childhood as the fungus does not grow well in the presence of the oily scalp secretions post puberty. Onychomycosis (fungal nail infection) increases in incidence with age.

Peripheral circulatory disease and smoking have been linked to an increase in toenail infection. Other underlying diseases increase risk of infection. Diabetics have an elevated risk of foot infection owing to peripheral neuropathy, and circulatory and biochemical changes, brought on by the disease.

Incidence

The incidence in the literature varies according to population and geographic location. However, approximately 5% of the population may have nail infection, and 10–30% have foot infection most commonly in the toe webs (athlete's foot).

Clinical presentations

Skin manifestations vary from the classic ring-shaped lesion with a raised edge and central clearance, to a diffuse, erythematous rash. There is usually scaling and often itch is reported. Signs of scalp infection are varied and include scaling, folliculitis, patchy alopecia, and kerion. Nail infections may present as superficial white onychomycosis, or with thickening (hyperkeratosis) and discolouration, to total nail dystrophy (destruction) (see Chapter 23).

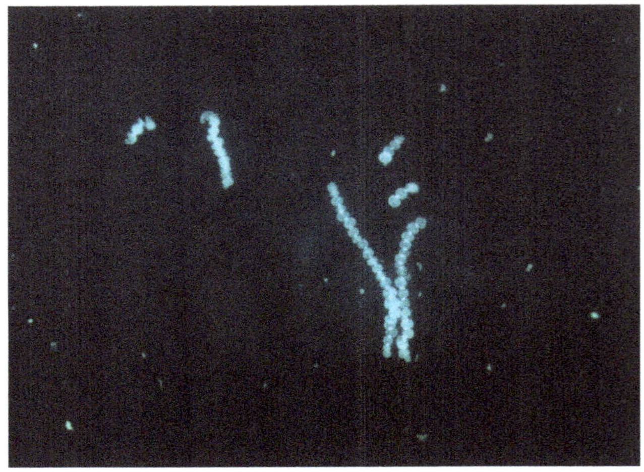

Figure 15.2 Dermatophyte arthroconidia seen in a toenail sample using Calcofluor stain and UV fluorescence microscopy (×400 magnification).

Diagnosis

Microscopy of tissue softened in potassium hydroxide (10–30%), using bright field or Calcofluor White stain with ultraviolet fluorescence, will reveal the presence of fungal elements, even-sided hyphae, and occasionally arthrospores (Figure 15.2). Dermatophytes are cultured on Sabouraud's dextrose agar plates containing actidione (cycloheximide) to inhibit the faster growing environmental moulds, and on chloramphenicol to reduce bacterial growth.

As up to 40% of microscopy positive nail samples may fail to grow a pathogen, PCR (polymerase chain reaction) techniques have been developed to detect *Trichophyton rubrum* (Chandran et al. 2013) as it is the commonest cause of onychomycosis worldwide. PCR has been shown to detect up to 37% more *T. rubrum* infections than culture alone; however, this methodology does not detect other species of dermatophyte or identify non-dermatophyte causes of infection.

Treatment

Systemic treatment is recommended for all but small areas of skin infection. Toenails and fingernails are treated with terbinafine for three months and six weeks respectively. Skin lesions (not scalp) are treated with topical terbinafine for two weeks. Scalp infections with *Trichophyton* species are treated off-licence with terbinafine for at least one month, whereas *Microsporum* species respond better to griseofulvin for six to eight weeks. Scalp treatment should always include a topical shampoo such as ketoconazole to reduce infectivity. Itraconazole is an alternative treatment for all conditions, and for nails it is given as a pulse therapy. Topical azoles may be used instead of topical terbinafine.

Prevention of reinfection is advisable by treating infected pets, preventing children with scalp infection sharing combs/brushes/hats, and washing bedding, towels, and clothing regularly to remove skin scales harbouring spores.

References

Campbell CK, Johnson EM and Warnock DW (2013) *Identification of Pathogenic Fungi* (2nd edn, Wiley-Blackwell).

Chandran NS, Pan J-Y, Pramono ZAD, Tan H-H and Seow C-S (2013) Complementary role of a polymerase chain reaction test in the diagnosis of onychomycosis. *Australas J Dermatol* 54: 105–8.

Giddey K, Favre B, Quandroni M and Momod M (2007) Closely related dermatophyte species produce different patterns of secreted proteins. *FEMS Microbiol Lett* 267: 95–101.

Monod M (2008) Secreted proteases from dermatophytes. *Mycopathologia* 66: 285–94.

Vermout S, Tabart J, Baldo A, Mathy A, Losson B and Mignon B (2008) Pathogenesis of dermatophytosis. *Mycopathologia* 166: 267–75.

CHAPTER 16

Endemic dimorphic fungi

Angela Restrepo, Angel González, and Beatriz L. Gómez

An overview of dimorphic infections caused by species of *Paracoccidioides, Histoplasma, Blastomyces, Coccidioides, Talaromyces,* and *Emmonsia*

The dimorphic fungi are human pathogens that exhibit thermal dimorphism. At 22°C, they grow as conidia-producing moulds, whereas at 37°C they transition to budding yeasts. When inhaled by a mammalian host—either immunocompetent or immunocompromised—conidia convert into virulent yeasts. These fungi, endemic to certain areas of the world (see Chapter 25: Figure 25.1), comprise 10 ascomycete species—namely, *Blastomyces dermatitidis, B. gilchristii, Histoplasma capsulatum, Coccidioides immitis, C. posadasii, Paracoccidioides brasiliensis, P. lutzii, Talaromyces marneffei, Emmonsia* spp., and *Sporothrix schenckii. S. schenckii* is described in Chapter 23 as it does not share the same geographic restrictions as the endemic dimorphics, and the primary mode of infection is not inhalation. The size of the inhaled inoculum and the integrity of the host's immune defences influence the extent and severity of the ensuing infectious process.

Taxonomy

Table 16.1 shows the taxonomic relationships between the endemic dimorphics.

Paracoccidioidomycosis

Significant species

P. brasiliensis and *P. lutzii*

Taxonomy

Since 2009, the Broad Institute has completed and recently updated the sequencing, assembly, and annotation of the genomes of two strains of *P. brasiliensis* and one strain of *P. lutzii* (accession number codes ABHV02/PABG, ABKI02/PADG, and ABKH02/PAAG; Muñoz et al. 2014).

Pathogenesis

The aetiologic agents are the thermally dimorphic fungi *Paracoccidioides brasiliensis* and *P. lutzii*, which grow as moulds below 24°C, while at 37°C they transition into yeasts—a morphotype also observed in patients.

Residents of endemic areas are thought to acquire the infection by inhaling airborne conidia present in nature. However, the disease's long latency period and the lack of reported outbreaks hinder definition of the primary infection (Restrepo et al. 2011; Colombo et al. 2011).

Epidemiology

Paracoccidioidomycosis (PCM) is a systemic, endemic disorder confined to Latin American countries from Mexico to Argentina, with Brazil accounting for most patients. The natural habitat of *Paracoccidioides* has not been identified, but *P. brasiliensis* has occasionally been isolated from soil, while *P. lutzii* has not.

Paracoccidioidomycosis is uncommon in children and young adults, with a predominance of patients aged over 30 years. Gender distribution shows a male-to-female ratio of 13:1 or more, except in children, in whom this difference is absent. The main associated occupational risks are agriculture, followed by masonry work (Colombo et al. 2011; Restrepo et al. 2015); hence, PCM afflicts predominantly adult males engaged in agriculture. Prolonged latency has been demonstrated through reports on non-indigenous PCM cases diagnosed in Europe, the United States, and Asia. All these patients have had previous residence in endemic areas for over ten years prior to overt disease (Restrepo et al. 2015).

Clinical presentation

The following categories are recognized:

1. Subclinical infection

Demonstrated in healthy individuals mainly by reactive paracoccidioidin skin tests;

2. Progressive disease

When the host is unable to contain fungal multiplication, the mycosis disseminates, giving rise to the following clinical presentations:

Acute/subacute or juvenile form is reported in <10% of the cases, mainly in undernourished children, youngsters, and HIV (human immunodeficiency virus)-infected individuals. It preferentially affects the reticuloendothelial system. Bones, skin, and gastrointestinal organs are also involved.

Table 16.1 Taxonomic relationship of the endemic dimorphic fungi

Phylum	*Ascomycota*		
Subphylum	*Pezizomycotina*		
Class	*Eurotiomyces*		
Subclass	*Euromycetidae*		
Order	*Onygenales*	*Onygenales*	*Eurotiales*
Family	*Ajellomycetaceae*	*Onygenaceae*	*Trichocomaceae*
Genera	*Paracoccidioides, Histoplasma, Blastomyces, Emmonsia*	*Coccidioides*	*Talaromyces*

The chronic adult form is the most common presentation (90%), probably resulting from endogenous reactivation of a primary focus, as demonstrated by patients diagnosed in non-endemic areas who had previously lived in Latin America (Pereira et al. 2004; Shikanai-Yasuda et al. 2006; Restrepo et al. 2008, 2012, 2015). Imaging studies show a multi-organ disease afflicting the lungs and other organs; in the former, bilateral, symmetrical, alveolar, and interstitial infiltrates are noticed in lower and central fields (Costa et al. 2013). Lung fibrosis predominates (60%) and is accompanied by emphysema, bullae, and cavities. Oral mucosa lesions in gums, hard palate, oropharynx, and larynx are also observed (35%). Dysphonia, dysphagia, and sialorrhoea are recorded. Neighbouring lymph nodes become hypertrophied (Restrepo et al. 2011, 2012; Abreu-Silva et al. 2012). The skin is another common target (23%). Dissemination to the adrenal glands occurs commonly and is as frequent as 90% in autopsy series (Tobón et al. 2010). Central nervous system involvement occurs in 15% of cases (Hotez et al. 2008; Restrepo et al. 2012). A residual form is also considered, although it is not due to fungal multiplication but to fibrosis of the initially infected organs (Restrepo et al. 2012, 2015).

In endemic areas, healthy individuals reacting to the paracoccidioidin skin test are considered infected by the fungus. They exhibit a predominantly Th1 immune response, accounting for the activation of macrophages, the most important cells in resistance to *P. brasiliensis* infection (Cano et al. 2012; de Castro et al. 2013; Restrepo et al. 2015). The most severe juvenile form is characterized by a Th2/Th9 cell response with increased humoral immune response and augmented eosinophil numbers. The milder inflammatory response characteristic of adult chronic patients has a predominant Th17-cell population with important participation from Th1 cells. The Th17 response in these patients, although contributing to a certain resistance to infection, can induce a significant inflammatory response, leading to tissue destruction and fibrosis (Cano et al. 2012; de Castro et al. 2013; Restrepo et al. 2015).

Diagnosis

Diagnosis is performed by direct examination, culture, and immunodiagnostic tests including antibody testing and antigen detection, as well as molecular tests (Thompson and Gómez 2015). When cultured at room temperature under nutritional deprivation, they produce arthroconidia and other unicellular conidia (3.5–5.0 μm) (Figure 16.1a) capable of converting—in mammalian hosts—into yeast cells of varying sizes (4–40 μm), some characterized by a mother cell with multiple buds—the 'pilot's wheel'—a pathognomonic feature that establishes the diagnosis (Restrepo et al. 2011, 2012, 2015) (Figure 16.1b). Owing to the high risk of infection from inhalation of spores, *Paracoccidioides* spp., and all other species in this chapter, must be handled inside a biosafety cabinet according to biosafety level-3 containment conditions. *P. brasiliensis* can be identified in up to 85% of clinical specimens from oral, pharyngeal, and cutaneous lesions; sputum; bronchoalveolar lavage fluid; lymph nodes; adrenal glands; or biopsy materials from other tissues.

Treatment

Antimicrobial agents from three different classes are currently used to treat PCM, with varying success. They include the sulphonamides, the polyene antimycotic amphotericin B and its lipid formulations and certain triazoles (Restrepo et al. 2015).

(a) (b)

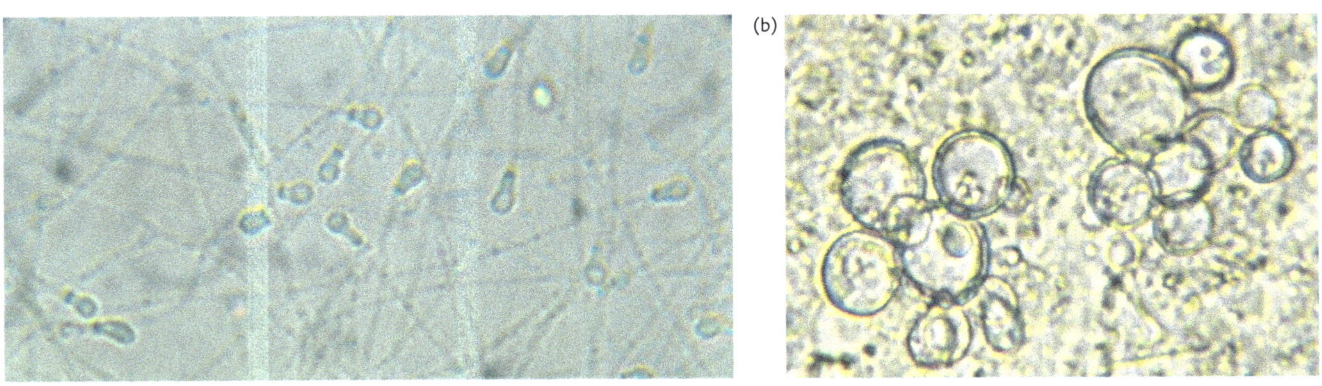

Figure 16.1 **a** Arthroconidia of *Paracoccidioides brasiliensis* from culture at 25°C, ×400 magnification. **b** Wet mount showing blastoconidia of *P. brasiliensis* (×290 magnification).
Reproduced courtesy of Angela Restrepo and Beatriz L. Gómez.

Histoplasmosis

Significant species

H. capsulatum

Taxonomy

Historically, *H. capsulatum* was divided into three varieties: *H. capsulatum* var. *capsulatum*, var. *duboisii*, and var. *farciminosum*. Recent advances in molecular genotyping and phylogenetic studies have defined at least eight clades. Seven of the eight clades may be considered distinct phylogenetic species, but the Eurasian clade contains examples of all three species, and genetically the variety *duboisii* seems to be very similar to var. *capsulatum* (Kasuga et al. 2003).

Teixeira et al. (2016), more recently, using different phylogenetic and population genetic methods, proposed at least six new phylogenetic species in the *Histoplasma* species complex, comprising LAm A1, LAm A2, LAm B1, LAm B2, RJ, and BAC-1 phylogenetic species.

The genome of *H. capsulatum* has an estimated size of between 28 Mbp and 39 Mbp, and currently sequence assemblies and annotations are available for four strains (http://www.broadinstitute.org/fungal-genome-initiative/histoplasma-genome-project).

Pathogenesis

The causative agent of histoplasmosis, *H. capsulatum*, is a temperature-dependent dimorphic fungus, existing as a mould in the environment and a yeast in tissues at 37°C. Infection begins when the microconidia of *H. capsulatum* are inhaled into the alveoli and the main host defence is cell-mediated immunity. The extent of disease is determined by both the number of conidia inhaled and the immune response of the host. A small inoculum can cause severe infection in markedly immunosuppressed hosts. Conversely, healthy individuals, who most commonly have asymptomatic pulmonary infection, can develop life-threatening pneumonia if they inhale a large quantity of conidia.

Epidemiology

H. capsulatum is found primarily in the Ohio and Mississippi River valleys and in Central and South America, but other localized foci also exist in Europe, Africa, and Asia. The environmental niche for *H. capsulatum* is soil that is enriched by the nitrogen contained in bird and bat guano. In the endemic areas, exposure to *H. capsulatum* is common, and most infections are sporadic. Outbreaks have been reported and are associated with spelunking, demolition of buildings, and activities that disrupt contaminated soil (Kauffman 2007; Colombo et al. 2011; Smith and Kauffman 2012).

Clinical presentation

Local lymphatic spread and haematogenous dissemination occur in most persons, but are asymptomatic in most. There are three main presentations of histoplasmosis:

Acute self-limited pneumonia is characterized by fever, dry cough, mild chest discomfort, and fatigue (Wheat et al. 2007; Kauffman 2007).

Chronic cavitary pulmonary histoplasmosis is a disease of older adults with underlying emphysema. Symptoms are present for months and include fever, fatigue, anorexia, weight loss, cough with purulent sputum, and haemoptysis (Kauffman 2007).

Disseminated disease occurs most often in immunosuppressed individuals. Pulmonary manifestations of disseminated histoplasmosis vary, from subtle diffuse nodules noted in the more chronic form of disseminated infection, to life-threatening pneumonia.

Diagnosis

Histoplasmosis is definitively diagnosed by growth of the organism. Sputum, BAL (bronchoalveolar lavage) fluid, lung tissue, or lymph nodes can be cultured. *H. capsulatum* may take as long as four to six weeks to grow at room temperature in the mould form, which may contain two types of conidia: macroconidia that are thick walled with a diameter of 8–15 μm and display characteristic tubercles or projections on their surfaces, and microconidia that are smooth walled with a diameter of 2–4 μm (Figure 16.2a) The yeast phase develops as small, oval, budding cells with a diameter of 2–4 μm, often within macrophages (Figure 16.2b) (Thompson and Gómez 2015).

(a) (b)

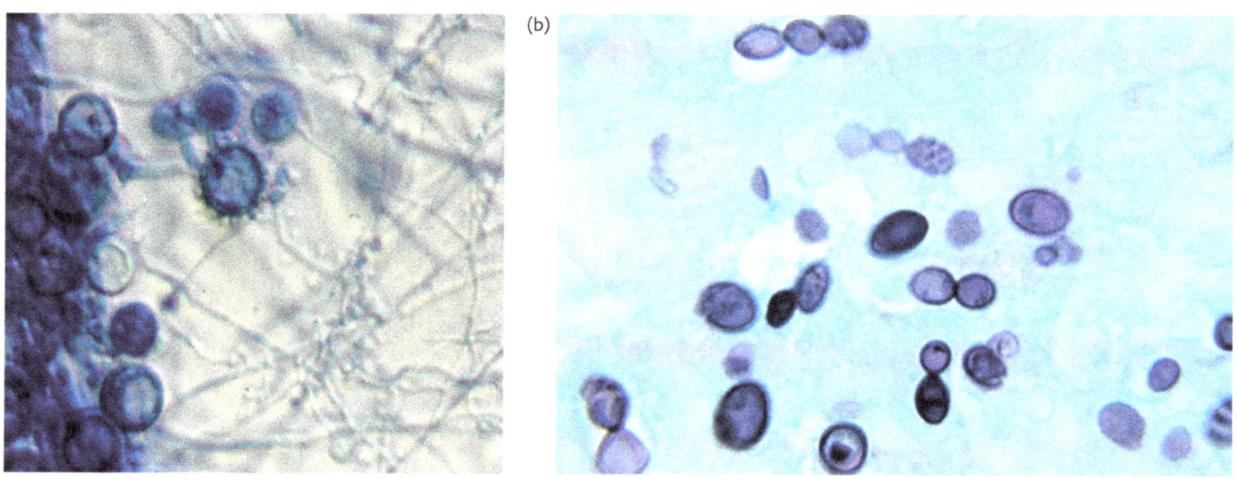

Figure 16.2 **a** Mycelial phase of *H. capsulatum* showing tuberculate macroconidia and microconidia. Lactophenol cotton blue stain (×245 magnification). **b** GMS (Gomori methenamine silver) stain showing blastoconidia of *H. capsulatum* (×100 magnification).

Reproduced courtesy of Angela Restrepo and Beatriz L. Gómez.

Identification of the typical small budding yeasts in tissue or fluid samples allows an early diagnosis while awaiting culture results. Immunodiagnosis plays an important role in the diagnosis, via detection of circulating antigens and also antibody detection. New antigen tests have been developed that aid clinicians in the prompt diagnosis of histoplasmosis (Thompson and Gómez 2015). Molecular tests are also used; however, they are not commercially available.

Treatment

Amphotericin B is recommended for patients with severe pulmonary histoplasmosis and for immunosuppressed patients. The newest IDSA (Infectious Diseases Society of America) recommendations are to use liposomal amphotericin B preferentially over the deoxycholate formulation, based on a controlled trial that showed the superiority of this agent in AIDS patients with severe disseminated histoplasmosis. Azoles are recommended as first-line treatment for patients with mild-to-moderate pulmonary histoplasmosis, and as step-down therapy after a patient with severe disease has responded to initial treatment with amphotericin B. Itraconazole is the drug of choice and is also recommended for patients with chronic cavitary pulmonary histoplasmosis (Wheat et al. 2007).

Blastomycosis

Significant species

Blastomyces dermatitidis, Blastomyces gilchristii

Taxonomy

The genus *Blastomyces* has previously been represented by a single species, *B. dermatitidis,* yet more recent work has suggested that *B. dermatitidis* includes a cryptic subspecies or a separate species (Meece et al. 2011; Thompson and Gómez 2015). Phylogenetic analysis using nuclear loci has placed *Blastomyces* isolates into one of two monophyletic clades: *B. dermatitidis* and the novel species *B. gilchristii* (Brown et al. 2013). Genome sequences and annotations are available for three strains of *B. dermatitidis* (ER-3, ATCC18188, and ATCC26199) and one strain of *B. gilchristii* (SLH14081) (http://www.broadinstitute.org/fungal-genome-initiative/blastomyces-genome-project; Muñoz et al. 2015).

Pathogenesis

Infection begins with inhalation of conidia into the alveoli, at which point the organism converts to the yeast form. It is likely that haematogenous dissemination occurs in most patients, but clinical manifestations of this event, as well as the initial pulmonary infection, are uncommon. Both neutrophils and cell-mediated immunity are important in the response to *Blastomyces* species, and the histopathological picture is a mixed pyogranulomatous process (Smith and Kauffman 2010).

Epidemiology

Most cases occur in states that border the Mississippi River basin, the Great Lakes, and the St. Lawrence Seaway, and in the Canadian provinces of Ontario and Manitoba (Saccente and Woods 2010; Kauffman 2007). The environmental niche for the organism appears to be soil and decaying wood, especially along waterways. Most cases are sporadic, but outbreaks have been reported.

Clinical presentation

There are three main presentations of blastomycosis: acute pulmonary, chronic pulmonary, and disseminated infection.

Acute pulmonary infection in most patients is an asymptomatic or mild illness with fever, dry cough, dyspnoea, and mild chest pain.

Chronic pulmonary infection may present as mass-like lesions that resemble lung cancer or as upper-lobe cavitary lesions that resemble tuberculosis or histoplasmosis.

In **disseminated infection**, cutaneous lesions are the most common manifestation; prostate and osteoarticular involvement is less common. The cutaneous lesions are frequently multiple, usually well circumscribed, and can be verrucous or ulcerated.

Diagnosis

Growth of *Blastomyces* from a tissue biopsy or body fluid sample sent to the laboratory remains the definitive diagnostic test for blastomycosis. The organism takes several weeks to grow. Once growth occurs, a highly specific DNA probe is used for rapid identification. Available rapid tests include histopathological examination of tissues, cytological examination of body fluids, such as sputum or BAL, and antigen detection (Thompson and Gómez 2015). The organisms are larger than most yeasts (8-10 μm) and thick walled, and have a single broad-based bud (Figure 16.3). The newest development in the diagnosis of blastomycosis is an enzyme immunoassay performed on urine or serum that detects a cell-wall galactomannan antigen found in *B. dermatitidis* (Bariola et al. 2011). A real-time PCR assay for *B. dermatitidis* has been reported recently, but no commercial test is available.

Treatment

Patients with severe infection and those who are immunosuppressed are treated initially with amphotericin B until stable and then changed to an oral azole therapy. Guidelines suggest that either amphotericin B deoxycholate or a lipid formulation can be used. The primary azole recommended is itraconazole.

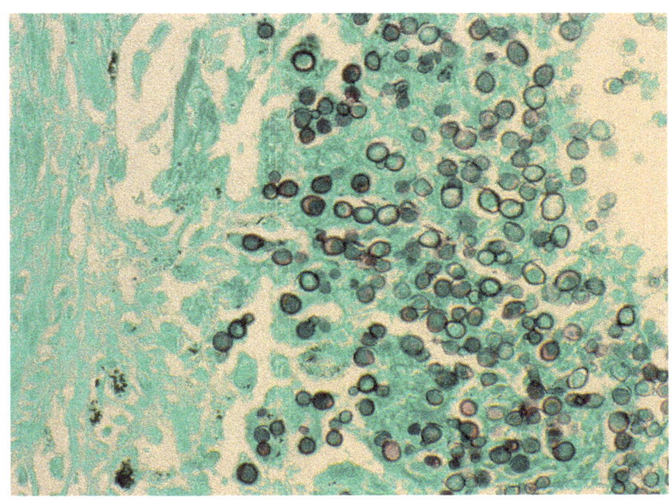

Figure 16.3 Blastoconidia of *B. dermatitidis in human tissue.* GMS (Gomori methenamine silver) stain (×100 magnification).

Reproduced courtesy of Angela Restrepo and Beatriz L. Gómez.

Coccidioidomycosis

Significant species

Coccidioides immitis and *C. posadasii*

Taxonomy

Currently two species are described: *C. immitis* and *C. posadasii* (Hirschmann 2007; Sharpton et al. 2009; Neafsey et al. 2010). Genome sequences of strains from both species are available (http://www.broadinstitute.org/scientific-community/science/projects/fungal-genome-initiative/coccidioides-genomes).

Pathogenesis

Infection occurs primarily after inhalation of arthroconidia; the incubation period is one to three weeks. Once arthroconidia reach the lungs, they interact with several types of host cells and molecules; thus, macrophages and T cells are pivotal for defence against *Coccidioides*. Macrophages are able to internalize fungal cells, and once activated, produce nitric oxide—a molecule with microbicidal activity (Gonzalez et al. 2011). Additionally, T cells secrete cytokines which activate macrophages. Immunity against this fungus is characterized by a mixed Th1-, Th2- and Th17-type immune response (Hung et al. 2011). However, this fungal pathogen is able to produce molecules such as a dominant SOWgp (spherule outer wall glycoprotein), urease, ammonia, metalloproteinases, melanin, and other unknown soluble factors which allow it to survive in the host; these molecules are not only capable of modulating the host immune response, but also contribute to tissue damage at sites of infection (Hung et al. 2007; Gonzalez et al. 2011).

Epidemiology

Coccidioidomycosis is restricted to certain regions of the United States, especially central and southern California, southern Arizona, southern New Mexico, Utah, and western Texas, as well as desert regions of northern Mexico, Argentina, Brazil, and Venezuela (Fisher et al. 2002; Hirschmann 2007).

Infection is associated with soil-disturbing activities in endemic areas. In addition, outbreaks have been associated with natural events such as earthquakes and windstorms (Nguyen et al. 2013, Schneider et al. 1997).

Clinical presentation

The majority of cases of coccidioidomycosis are either asymptomatic or result in self-limited pneumonia. Although this mycosis is rarely life-threatening, most patients who do not recover spontaneously develop extrapulmonary infections (Cole et al. 2006). Disseminated infection is seen more frequently in persons of African, Asian, or Filipino ancestry, as well as in pregnant women in the third trimester. Other immunosuppressed populations, including HIV-infected patients, are at risk of dissemination (Ampel 2007). Involvement of skin, soft tissues, bones, joints, or meninges is frequent (Ampel 2007).

Diagnosis

Diagnosis is confirmed by direct examination, culture techniques, and immunodiagnostic tests including antibody testing and antigen detection, as well as molecular tests (Thompson and Gómez 2015).

The mould morphotype is found in the environment and in cultures at room temperature; this morphotype is characterized by the production of thin and septate hyphae which, in turn, produce the arthroconidia (2–5 μm, barrel-shaped), which are considered to be the infectious propagules (Figure 16.4a). At 37°C and in culture media or in the host, the arthroconidia transform into structures named spherules, a unique structure among the dimorphic fungi. Spherules are characterized by their large size (up to 120 μm) and thick-walled spherical structure containing endospores (Figure 16.4b) (Cole et al. 2006).

Treatment

Treatment of coccidioidomycosis depends on both the clinical form and the severity of the disease. Amphotericin B lipid formulations and azoles are the therapies most commonly used (Nguyen et al. 2013).

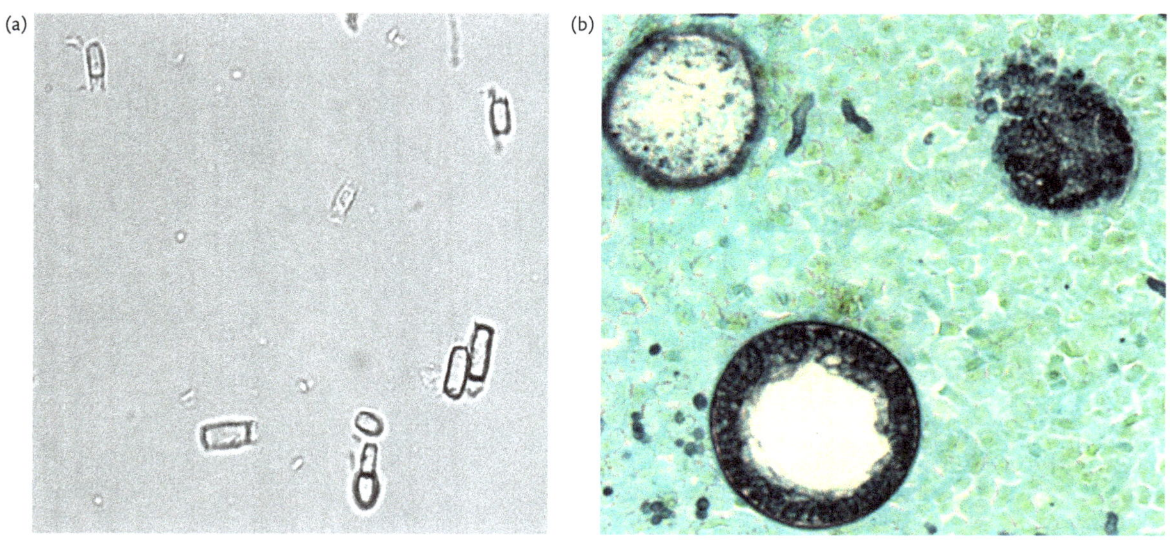

Figure 16.4 **a** Arthroconidia of *Coccidioides* spp. from culture at 25°C (×400 magnification). **b** Spherules and endospores of *Coccidioides* spp. in mouse tissue; GMS (Gomori methenamine silver) stain (×200 magnification).
Reproduced courtesy of Angela Restrepo and Beatriz L. Gómez.

Talaromycosis

Significant species

Talaromyces marneffei (formerly *Penicillium marneffei*)

Taxonomy

Genome sequences of this species are available (e.g. annotated sequences of strain ATCC18224 and the closely related *T. stipitatus* strain ATCC10500 have GenBank accession numbers DS995899/DS996350 and EQ962652/EQ963471, respectively; Nierman et al. 2015).

Pathogenesis

After *T. marneffei* conidia are inhaled, they interact with several types of host cells. Phagocytic cells, including macrophages and neutrophils, are likely to be the primary line of host defence against this fungus; this interaction is mediated through the recognition of extracellular matrix proteins in the host by lectins present on the fungal surface (Hamilton et al. 1998, 1999; Vanittanakamon et al. 2006). Macrophages, once activated by T-cell-derived cytokines, are able to control *T. marneffei* growth through dependent and independent oxidative mechanisms (Vanittanakamon et al. 2006). T cells, mainly CD4+, and the development of a Th1 response are associated with protection (Vanittanakamon et al. 2006). Nonetheless, *T. marneffei* is able to survive and evade the immune response. The evasion mechanisms include the inhibition of reactive oxygen metabolite production and neutralization of inhibitory metabolites produced by the host (Vanittanakamon et al. 2006).

Epidemiology

T. marneffei is the causal agent of a systemic and endemic mycosis restricted to Southeast Asia, including Thailand, Vietnam, Hong Kong, southern China, Taiwan, India, and Laos (Supparatpinyo et al. 1994; Duong 1996; Vanittanakom et al. 2006; Samson et al. 2011).

Talaromycosis occurs as a consequence of an environmental or zoonotic transmission. Bamboo rats are the only known animal host of *T. marneffei*. Four species of bamboo rats (*Rhizomys sinensis, R. pruinosus, R. sumatrensis*, and *Cannomys badius*) are reported to be enzootic reservoirs (Vanittanakom et al. 2006; Cao et al. 2011; Wong and Wong 2011). However, no strong association between bamboo rats and human infection has been found (Vanittanakom et al. 2006).

As is the case for the other endemic and systemic mycoses, infection with *T. marneffei* is acquired after inhalation of the airborne environmental conidia. The incubation period is not known; nonetheless, reports indicate the possibility of a long latency with subsequent reactivation of the infection (Jones and See 1992). Similar to histoplasmosis, talaromycosis is an AIDS-defining illness (Vanittanakom et al. 2006). This mycosis mostly develops in HIV-infected patients with a CD4+ count of less than 100/μL (Supparatpinyo et al. 1994; Wu et al. 2008).

Clinical presentation

Clinical manifestations include pneumonia, cytopenia, skin lesions (mainly subcutaneous abscesses and papule-like ulcers), lymphadenopathy, and hepatosplenomegaly. Additionally, many patients undergo a disseminated disease with rapid progression to multiorgan failure and possible death, determined by the host's immune status (Lee et al. 2012).

Diagnosis

Diagnosis of *T. marneffei* infection is performed via cytological and histological examination, isolation by culture, immunodiagnostic tests (antibody testing and antigen detection) and molecular assays (Wong and Wong 2011).

This dimorphic fungus grows as a mould at 25°C and as yeast at 37°C in culture or in the host. The mould morphotype is typical of *Penicillium* species, with hyaline septated hyphae and fruiting structures composed of branching metulae and phialides which produce conidia (Figure 16.5a); in addition, it

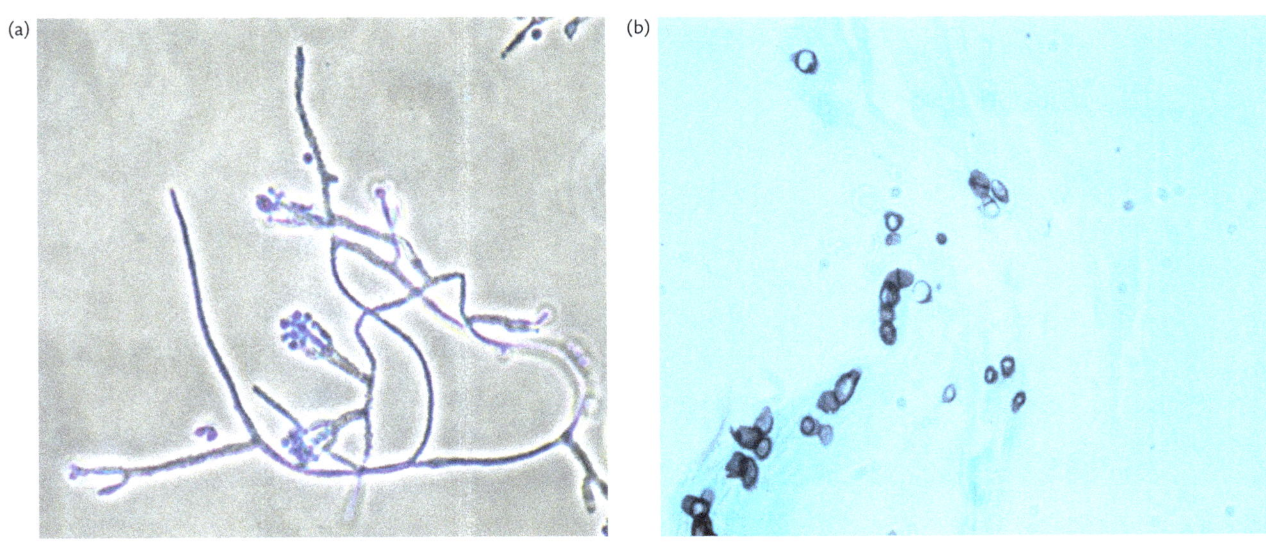

Figure 16.5 **a** Hyphae of *Talaromyces marneffei* from culture at 25°C (×200 magnification). **b** Yeast of *Talaromyces marneffei* from direct examination GMS (Gomori methenamine silver) stain (×100 magnification).

Reproduced courtesy of Susan Howell.

produces a soluble red pigment in culture. Yeast cells exhibit a characteristic central transverse septum which may be sparse and can be found in histiocytes or extracellularly (Figure 16.5b) (Wong and Wong 2011).

Treatment

Treatment is mandatory in HIV patients; the use of amphotericin B followed by itraconazole is the therapy of choice (Kaplan et al. 2009).

Emmonsiosis

Significant species

New strains of *Emmonsia*-like fungi, with phylogenetic and clinical similarities to *Blastomyces* and/or *Histoplasma*, have emerged as causes of systemic human mycoses worldwide. They differ from classical *Emmonsia* species by producing a thermally dependent, yeast-like phase rather than adiaspores, and by causing disseminated infections, predominantly in immunocompromised patients and often with high case-fatality rates. It is likely that these strains will be renamed in the near future.

Taxonomy

Genome sequences for *Emmonsia* species (http://www.ncbi.nlm.nih.gov/bioproject/179100) have been deposited in the public domain (Muñoz et al. 2015). It is expected that the taxonomic relations of these novel species with other genera, such as *Blastomyces*, will become clearer over the next few years.

Pathogenesis

Once the single-celled conidia (Figure 16.6a) have been inhaled, they transform into yeast cells at 37°C (Thompson and Gómez 2015). These replicate and disseminate to skin and other extrapulmonary tissues. Macrophages and T cells play a key role in the pathogenesis of this disease, and it is likely that the mechanisms and pathways involved are similar to those underlying other endemic fungal diseases.

Epidemiology

In contrast with adiaspiromycosis, infection with these novel *Emmonsia* species occurs mostly in immunocompromised individuals. Cases have been described in the HIV population, solid organ transplant recipients, and those receiving corticosteroid therapy, who are residing in South Africa, Canada, Germany, Israel, Italy, and China (Schwartz et al. 2015b).

Clinical presentation

These infections typically mimic histoplasmosis or blastomycosis, and indeed, have been misdiagnosed as such in the past (Kenyon et al. 2013; Schwartz et al. 2015b). The majority of patients have skin lesions, and lower (and upper) respiratory tract symptoms are common. Around a quarter of patients suffer neurological symptoms, including headaches, seizures, and altered mental state (Schwartz et al. 2015a).

Diagnosis

Histopathological appearance may show yeasts which resemble *Histoplasma* or *Blastomyces* species (Figure 16.6b). Any cultured organisms should undergo molecular identification. Sequence analysis of large-subunit ribosomal DNA, internal transcribed spacer (ITS1-2) ribosomal DNA regions, and portions of the genes encoding β-tubulin have been used to differentiate different *Emmonsia* species from infected patients (Kenyon et al. 2013; Thompson and Gómez 2015).

Treatment

As noted, this disease carries a high mortality in immunocompromised patients, and treatment should be mandatory. A number of agents have been used, and in the largest case series, amphotericin B therapy appears to be associated with improved survival compared with azole therapy alone (Kenyon et al. 2013). Hence, an amphotericin B formulation should probably be used in the acute phase of the infection.

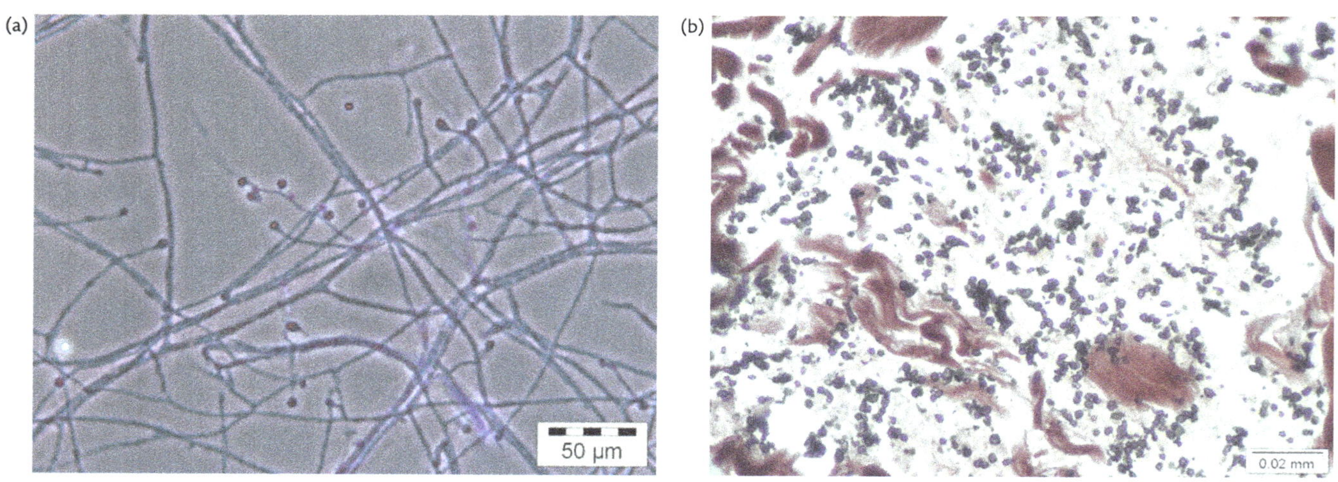

Figure 16.6 **a** Hyphae of *Emmonsia* from culture at 25°C. **b** Yeast of *Emmonsia* from direct examination Gomori methenamine silver (GMS)-stained skin biopsy.
Reproduced courtesy of Nelesh Govender.

Acknowledgements

We are grateful to Nelesh Govender for the images of *Emmonsia* species in Figure 16.6.

References

Abreu-Silva MA, Salum FG, Figuereido MA, Lopes TG, da Silva VD and Cherubini K (2012) Interrelationship of clinical, histomorphometric and immunohistochemical features of oral lesions in chronic paracoccidioidomycosis. *J Oral Pathol Med* 42: 235–42.

Ampel NM (2007) The complex immunology of human coccidioidomycosis. *Ann N Y Acad Sci* 1111: 245–58.

Bariola JR, Hage CA, Durkin M, et al. (2011) Detection of *Blastomyces dermatitidis* antigen in patients with newly diagnosed blastomycosis. *Diagn Microbiol Infect Dis* 69: 187–91.

Brown EM, McTaggart LR, Zhang SX, Low DE, Stevens DA and Richardson SE (2013) Phylogenetic analysis reveals a cryptic species *Blastomyces gilchristii*, sp. nov. within the human pathogenic fungus *Blastomyces dermatitidis*. PLoS One 8: e59237.

Cano LE, González A, Lopera D, Naranjo TW and Restrepo A (2012) Pulmonary paracoccidioidomycosis: clinical, immunological and histopathological aspects, *in*: E Malcolm-Irusen, ed., *Lung Diseases: Selected state of the art reviews* (Rijeka, Croatia: InTech), 359–92. ISBN 978-953-51-0180-2 (online).

Cao C, Liang L, Wang W, et al. (2011) Common reservoirs for *Penicillium marneffei* infection in humans and rodents, China. *Emerg Infect Dis* 17: 209–14.

Cole GT, Xue J, Seshan K, et al. (2006) Virulence mechanisms of *Coccidioides*, *in*: J Heitman, SG Filler and Mitchell AP, eds, *Molecular Principles of Fungal Pathogenesis* (Washington DC: American Society for Microbiology Press), 363–91.

Colombo AL, Tobón A, Restrepo A, Queiroz-Telles F and Nucci M (2011) Epidemiology of endemic systemic fungal infections in Latin America. *Med Mycol* 49: 785–9.

Costa AN, Marchiori E, Benard G, et al. (2013) Lung cysts in chronic paracoccidioidomycosis. *J Bras Pneumol* 39:368–72.

de Castro LF, Ferreira MC, da Silva RMS, Blotta SLM, Longhi LNA and Mamoni RL (2013) Characterization of the immune response in human paracoccidioidomycosis. *J Infect* 67: 470–85.

Duong TA (1996) Infection due to *Penicillium marneffei*, an emerging pathogen: review of 155 reported cases. *Clin Infect Dis* 23: 125–30.

Fisher MC, Koenig GL, White TJ and Taylor JW (2002) Molecular and phenotypic description of *Coccidioides posadasii* sp. nov., previously recognized as the non-California population of *Coccidioides immitis*. *Mycologia* 94: 73–84.

Gonzalez A, Hung CY and Cole GT (2011) *Coccidioides* releases a soluble factor that suppresses nitric oxide production by murine primary macrophages. *Microb Pathog* 50: 100–8.

Hamilton AJ, Jeavons L, Youngchim S and Vanittanakom N (1999) Recognition of fibronectin by *Penicillium marneffei* conidia via a sialic acid dependent process and its relationship to the interaction between conidia and laminin. *Infect Immun* 67: 5200–5.

Hamilton AJ, Jeavons L, Youngchim S, Vanittanakom N and Hay RJ (1998) Sialic-acid dependent recognition of laminin by *Penicillium marneffei* conidia. *Infect Immun* 66: 6024–6.

Hirschmann JV (2007) The early history of coccidioidomycosis: 1892–1945. *Clin Infect Dis* 44: 1202–7.

Hotez PJ, Bottazzi ME, Franco-Paredes C, Ault SK and Periago MR (2008) The neglected tropical diseases of Latin America and the Caribbean: a review of disease burden and distribution and a roadmap for control and elimination. *PLoS Negl Trop Dis* 2: e300. http://journals.plos.org/plosntds/article?id=10.1371/journal.pntd.0000300

Hung CY, Gonzalez A, Wüthrich M, Klein BS and Cole GT (2011) Vaccine immunity to coccidioidomycosis occurs by early activation of three signal pathways of T helper cell response (Th1, Th2, and Th17). *Infect Immun* 79: 4511–22.

Hung CY, Xue J and Cole GT. (2007) Virulence mechanisms of coccidioides. *Ann N Y Acad Sci* 1111: 225–35.

Jones PD and See J (1992) *Penicillium marneffei* infection in patients infected with human immunodeficiency virus: late presentation in an area of nonendemicity. *Clin Infect Dis* 15: 744.

Kaplan JE, Benson C, Holmes KH, Brooks JT, Pau A and Masur H (2009) Guidelines for prevention and treatment of opportunistic infections in HIV-infected adults and adolescents: recommendations from CDC, the National Institutes of Health, and the HIV Medicine Association of the Infectious Diseases Society of America. *MMWR Morb Mortal Wkly Rep* 58: RR.4.

Kasuga T, White TJ, Koenig G, et al. (2003) Phylogeography of the fungal pathogen *Histoplasma capsulatum*. *Mol Ecol* 12: 3383–401.

Kauffman CA (2007) Histoplasmosis: clinical and laboratory update. *Clin Microbiol Rev* 20: 115–32.

Kenyon C, Bonorchis K, Corcoran C, et al. (2013) A dimorphic fungus causing disseminated infection in South Africa. *N Engl J Med* 369: 1416–24.

Lee PP, Chan KW, Lee TL, et al. (2012) Penicilliosis in children without HIV infection—are they immunodeficient? *Clin Infect Dis* 54: e8–19.

Meece JK, Anderson JL, Fisher MC, Henk DA, Sloss BL, Reed KD (2011) Population genetic structure of clinical and environmental isolates of Blastomyces dermatitidis, based on 27 polymorphic microsatellite markers. *Appl Environ Microbiol* 77: 5123–31.

Muñoz JF, Gallo JE, Misas E, et al. (2014) Genome update of the dimorphic human pathogenic fungi causing paracoccidioidomycosis. *PLoS Negl Trop Dis* 8: e3348.

Muñoz JF, Gauthier GM, Desjardins CA, et al. (2015) The dynamic genome and transcriptome of the human fungal pathogen *Blastomyces* and close relative *Emmonsia*. *PLoS Genet* 11: e1005493.

Neafsey DE, Barker BM, Sharpton TJ, et al. (2010) Population genomic sequencing of *Coccidioides* fungi reveals recent hybridization and transposon control. *Genome Res* 20: 938–46.

Nguyen C, Barker BM, Hoover S, et al. (2013) Recent advances in our understanding of the environmental, epidemiological, immunological, and clinical dimensions of coccidioidomycosis. *Clin Microbiol Rev* 26: 505–25.

Nierman WC, Fedorova-Abrams ND and Andrianopoulos A (2015) Genome sequence of the AIDS-associated pathogen *Penicillium marneffei* (ATCC18224) and its near taxonomic relative *Talaromyces stipitatus* (ATCC10500). *Genome Announc* 3: e01559–14.

Pereira R, Bucaretchi F, Barison E, Hessel G and Tresoldi AT (2004) Paracoccidioidomycosis in children: clinical presentation, follow-up and outcome. *Rev Inst Med Trop Sao Paulo* 46: 127–31.

Restrepo A, Gómez BL and Tobón A (2012) Paracoccidioidomycosis: Latin America's own fungal disorder. *Curr Fungal Infect Rep* 6: 303–11. doi 10.1007/s12281-012-0114-x (online)

Restrepo A, Gónzalez A and Agudelo CA (2011) Paracoccidioidomycosis, *in*: W Dismukes, C Kauffman, P Pappas, et al., eds, *Essentials of Medical Mycology*, Chapter 21 (2nd edn, New York: Springer), 367–85.

Restrepo A, Tobón AM, Agudelo CA, et al. (2008) Co-existence of integumentary lesions and lung X-ray abnormalities in patients with paracoccidioidomycosis (PCM). *Am J Trop Med Hyg* 79: 159–63.

Restrepo A, Tobón Orozco AM, Gómez BL and Benard G (2015) Paracoccidioidomycosis, *in*: DR Hospenthal and MG Rinaldi, eds, *Diagnosis and Treatment of Fungal Infections*, Chapter 19 (2nd edn, Switzerland: Springer International Publishing), 225–36.

Saccente M and Woods GL (2010) Clinical and laboratory update on blastomycosis. *Clin Microbiol Rev* 23: 367–81.

Samson RA, Yilmaz N, Houbraken J, et al. (2011) Phylogeny and nomenclature of the genus *Talaromyces* and taxa accommodated in *Penicillium* subgenus *Biverticillium*. *Stud Mycol* 70: 159–83.

Schneider E, Hajjeh RA, Spiegel RA, et al. (1997) A coccidioidomycosis outbreak following the Northridge, Calif., earthquake. *JAMA* 277: 904–8.

Schwartz IS, Govender NP, Corcoran C, et al. (2015a) Clinical characteristics, diagnosis, management, and outcomes of disseminated Emmonsiosis: a retrospective case series. *Clin Infect Dis* 61: 1004–12.

Schwartz IS, Kenyon C, Feng P, et al. (2015b) 50 Years of *Emmonsia* disease in humans: the dramatic emergence of a cluster of novel fungal pathogens. *PLoS Pathog* 11: e1005198.

Sharpton TJ, Stajich JE, Rounsley SD, et al. (2009) Comparative genomic analyses of the human fungal pathogens *Coccidioides* and their relatives. *Genome Res* 19: 1722–31.

Shikanai-Yasuda M, de Queiroz Tellez Filho F, Poncio Mendes R, Colombo AL and Moretti ML (2006) Consenso en paracoccidiodomicosis. *Rev Soc Bras Med Trop* 39: 297–310.

Smith JA and Kauffman CA (2010) Blastomycosis. *Proc Am Thorac Soc* 7: 173–80.

Smith JA and Kauffman CA (2012) Pulmonary fungal infections. *Respirology* 17: 913–26.

Supparatpinyo K, Khamwan C, Baosoung V, Nelson KE and Sirisanthana T (1994) Disseminated *Penicillium marneffei* infection in Southeast Asia. *Lancet* 344: 110–13.

Teixeira M de M, Pataná JSL, Taylor ML, et al. (2016) Worldwide phylogenetic distribution and population dynamics of the genus *histoplasma*. *PLoS Negl Trop Dis* 10: e0004732.

Thompson G III and Gómez BL (2015) *Histoplasma, Blastomyces, Coccidioides*, and other dimorphic fungi causing systemic mycoses, *in*: J Versalovic and D Warnock eds, Manual of Clinical Microbiology, Volume 2, Section VI, Chapter 122 (11th edn, Washington DC: ASM Press), 2109–27.

Tobón AM, Agudelo CA, Restrepo CA, et al. (2010) Adrenal function status in patients with Paracoccidioidomycosis after prolonged post-therapy follow-up. *Am J Trop Med Hyg* 83: 111–14.

Vanittanakom N, Cooper CR Jr and Fisher MC and Sirisanthana T (2006) *Penicillium marneffei* infection and recent advances in the epidemiology and molecular biology aspects. *Clin Microbiol Rev* 19: 95–110.

Wheat LJ, Freifeld AG, Kleiman MB, et al. (2007) Clinical practice guidelines for the management of patients with histoplasmosis: update by the Infectious Diseases Society of America. *Clin Infect Dis* 45: 807–25.

Wong SY and Wong KF (2011) *Penicillium marneffei* infection in AIDS. Patholog Res Int 2011: 764293.

Wu TC, Chan JWM, Ng CK, Tsang DNC, Lee MP and Li PCK (2008) Clinical presentations and outcomes of *Penicillium marneffei* infections: a series from 1994 to 2004. *Hong Kong Med J* 14: 103–9.

CHAPTER 17

Hyaline moulds

Elizabeth M. Johnson

Introduction to hyaline moulds

The term 'hyaline moulds' includes all moulds that have hyaline or non-pigmented hyphae, most of which live as environmental saprobes or plant pathogens, with the exception of the dermatophytes, many of which are obligate human or animal pathogens. Within this group is a small subset of opportunistic pathogenic moulds that cause the invasive fungal infection known as hyalohyphomycosis—infection with a hyaline filamentous fungus adopting a septate hyphal form in tissues—and it is this group that will form the focus of this chapter. The term hyalohyphomycosis was introduced to reduce the proliferation of new disease names every time a new species with pathogenic potential was recognized (Ajello 1982). There are currently at least 75 different species from 30 different genera that are agents of hyalohyphomycosis, and this is increasing in line with the expanding pool of susceptible patients, thus supporting the wisdom of this approach.

Fungi not included as causes of hyalohyphomycosis are the aspergilli, endemic dimorphic fungi, *Sporothrix* species, and mucoraceous moulds as these form distinct disease entities.

Hyaline moulds are frequently implicated in keratitis, otomycosis, onychomycosis, peritonitis, wound infection, cutaneous and subcutaneous infection following traumatic implantation, pulmonary infection, occasional sinusitis, and prosthetic valve endocarditis, and are frequently encountered colonizing the lungs of patients with cystic fibrosis, which may then evolve into invasive disease.

Taxonomy of hyaline moulds most frequently implicated in infection

Table 17.1 lists the clinically most important genera, many of which are polyphyletic (Das et al. 2010; Summerbell et al. 2011; Doyen et al. 2013, Tortorano et al. 2014).

Among the recognized human pathogens are the species complexes encompassing *F. solani* (FSSC), which alone contains at least 49 different species most only discernible by MLST (multi-locus sequence typing) techniques, *F. oxysporum* (FOSC), and *F. fujikuroi* (FFSC), and less commonly *Fusarium dimerum* (FDSC) and other species complexes (van Diepeningen et al. 2015). In contradiction of the rule that the teleomorph name should take precedence, it has been suggested that most *Fusarium* names should be retained (Geiser et al. 2013).

Cell biology of hyaline moulds

The *Fusarium* genus is characterized by floccose colonies ranging from pink to purple and vinaceous shades (Figure 17.1.a) to the orange wet-looking colony of *F. dimerum* (Figure 17.1.c). Enteroblastic microconidia are produced by phialides in wet masses evolved for water dispersal, in addition to multiseptate, crescent-shaped macroconidia (Figure 17.1b)—or in the case of *F. dimerum*, crescent-shaped macroconidia with a single septum (Figure 17.1d). For a full description of the colonial and microscopic morphology of pathogenic fungi in this section, see identification manuals such as those compiled by Campbell et al. (2013) and de Hoog et al. (2000).

Colonies of the human pathogenic *Sarocladium* species often resemble those of *Fusarium*, although they are usually more restricted (Figure 17.1e), but on microscopy only kidney-shaped to cylindrical microconidia are visible in wet masses at the ends of phialides. Rope-like aggregations of hyphae are also a key feature (Figure 17.1f).

Purpureocillium lilacinum has a floccose, lilac-coloured colony (Figure 17.1g) and was at one time classified as *Paecilomyces* as, morphologically, it shares the same branching conidiophores, producing long, flask-shaped phialides with elongated necks; however, the spores are small and globose and produced in long, non-branching chains suited for air dispersal (Figure 17.1h). *Paecilomyces variotii* has powdery-to-granular, khaki-coloured colonies (Figure 17.1i) and long chains of oat-shaped spores produced from the tips of long, delicate phialides (Figure 17.1j). *Rasamsonia argillacea* has a similar colonial and microscopic morphology, but the chains of spores are brick-shaped, and the conidiophore stipes are conspicuously roughened.

Scopulariopsis brevicaulis has granular, sand-coloured colonies (Figure 17.1k) and produces brush-like branching conidiophores and flask-like annellides (Figure 17.1l). The rough-walled, flat-bottomed spores are produced in long, dry chains suited for air dispersal.

Scedosporium apiospermum (Figures 17.1m and 17.1n), *S. aurantiacum*, *S. boydii*, and *S. dehoogii* produce single spores with a flattened end from elongated annellides. *Lomentospora prolificans* (*Scedosporium prolificans*) has a moist-looking colony (Figure 17.1o) and produces dark-coloured flat-ended spores from short, fat annellides with elongated necks, with rings of wall material (annellidic rings) visible at the tip (Figure 17.1p).

Pathogenesis of hyaline moulds

Many of these agents, especially the *Fusarium* species, produce mycotoxins, which might contribute to the virulence of the organism and lead to increased localized damage to the host tissues. *Fusarium*, *Sarocladium*, and *Purpureocillium* spp. are able to

Table 17.1 Taxonomy of common hyaline moulds

Order	Genus	Most significant species
Hypocreales	*Fusarium*	*solani, oxysporum, fujikuroi, dimerum*
Hypocreales	*Acremonium*	
Hypocreales	*Sarocladium (Acremonium)*	*kiliense, strictum*
Hypocreales	*Purpureocillium (Paecilomyces)*	*lilacinus*
Microascales	*Scopulariopsis*	*brevicaulis*
Microascales	*Scedosporium*	*apiospermum, aurantiacum*
Microascales	*Lomentospora (Scedosporium)*	*prolificans*
Euriotales	*Rasamsonia*	*argillaceum*
Euriotales	*Paecilomyces*	*variotii*

Source: data from Doyen et al., 2013; Tortorano et al., 2014; Das, Saha, Dar, Ramachandran, 2010; Summerbell, 2011.

produce adventitious spores *in vivo* and are thus more prone than other filamentous fungi to haematogenous dissemination and proliferation in multiple organs including the skin. *Scedosporium* and *Lomentospora* spp. are neurotropic, so even though the lungs are usually the primary portal of entry, central nervous system involvement is also seen.

Epidemiology of hyaline moulds

The hyaline moulds are opportunistic pathogens usually acquired from an environmental source by inhalation or aspiration of water-borne spores, although they may also gain entry to the body via breaches in the skin or mucous membranes or as corneal infections. There have been reports of infections associated with contamination of fluids and air conditioning systems. The most common pathogens are in the *Fusarium solani* species complex. Invasive infection is most often seen in immunocompromised patients with low neutrophil counts or on long-term corticosteroid therapy for graft-versus-host disease (GvHD). However, *Scedosporium* spp. and *Lomentospora prolificans* can cause pneumonia and subsequent cerebral infection in otherwise healthy individuals following aspiration of spores during near-drowning accidents.

Risk factors and incidence of infection with hyaline moulds

Haematological malignancy and haematopoietic stem cell transplant (HSCT), which lead to prolonged periods of neutropenia, are the major risk factors for invasive disease, although immunosuppression associated with organ transplantation is also a predisposing factor. The highest incidence of invasive disease is amongst recipients of mismatched donor allogeneic HSCT, and may often occur during chronic steroid treatment of GvHD.

Clinical presentation of infection with hyaline moulds

The clinical presentation of hyaline mould infection is dictated largely by the immune status of the host and the organism's portal of entry. Invasive infection is often initially pulmonary or sinonasal, and signs and symptoms resemble those of invasive aspergillosis. Specific features of *Fusarium, Sarocladium,* and *Purpureocillium* infection include cutaneous lesions, and blood culture is frequently positive. The mortality attributable to *Fusarium* infections in immunocompromised patients ranges from 50% to 70%. *Scedosporium and Lomentospora* infections may arise from aspiration pneumonia but are neurotropic and may present as cerebral lesions.

Diagnosis of hyaline mould infection

Diagnosis usually requires isolation and subsequent identification of the infecting pathogen (Borman and Johnson 2014); imaging techniques and clinical manifestations can be suggestive but are not specific. The β-1,3,d-glucan test is usually positive but, again, is non-specific. Sequencing of pan-fungal PCR products from blood, normally sterile fluids and tissues can identify the infecting organism helping to direct appropriate therapy (Borman and Johnson 2013). Blood culture is more likely to be positive than it is in invasive aspergillosis. Other body fluids and tissues, including biopsies of any cutaneous lesions, can be examined microscopically, which can be enhanced by the addition of fluorescent brighteners, and cultured on glucose-peptone agar incubated at 30°C and 37°C. Growth is usually apparent within about 48 hours, although longer incubation may be necessary, and isolates can be identified by microscopic examination of mounts stained with mounting fluid which reveal the size, shape, and ornamentation of spores and the way in which they are produced. Molecular identification methods can be used to confirm the identity of isolates with similar phenotypic appearance or those not producing spores. Although many of these organisms can be culture contaminants, direct microscopic examination of the specimen or histology results can enhance the significance of a subsequent isolate (Borman and Johnson 2014). Pan-fungal PCR (polymerase chain reaction) is possible on wax-embedded fixed tissue, and amplification followed by sequencing of the product can reveal the identity.

Treatment of hyaline mould infection

Reversal of immunosuppression is an important adjunctive treatment. Species differ in their susceptibility to antifungal agents, so specific susceptibility testing may be helpful in directing appropriate therapy (Tortorano et al. 2014). Historically, response to amphotericin treatment has been variable and species may have reduced susceptibility *in vitro*. Currently, voriconazole is the treatment of choice (Perfect et al. 2003; Tortorano et al. 2014); however, some members of the *F. solani* species complex are pan-azole resistant. *Scedosporium* species are often resistant to amphotericin, so voriconazole is usually the first-line treatment. *Lomentospora prolificans* is multi-drug resistant, and this is reflected by frequent failure of therapy. There have been successful outcomes with

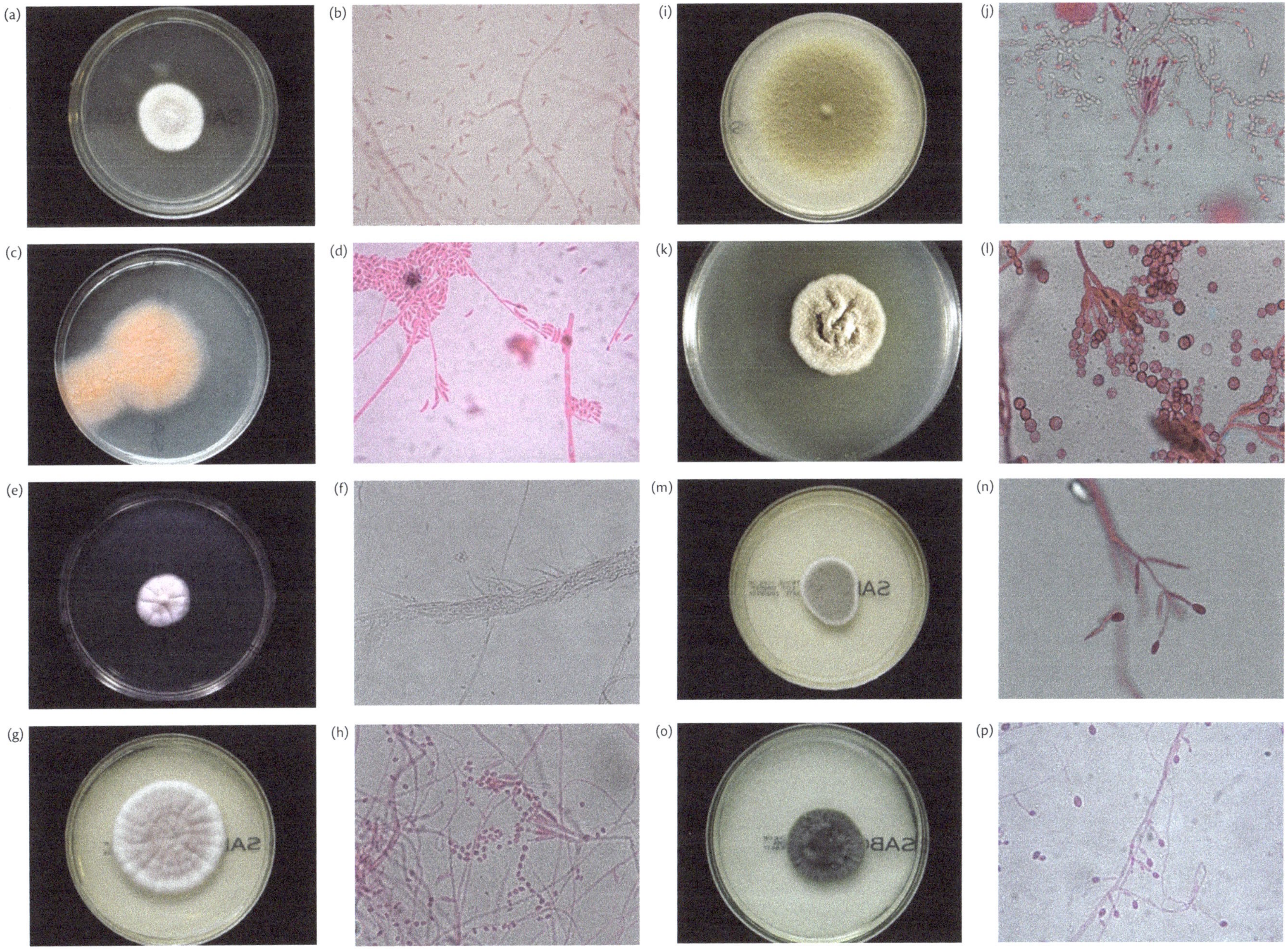

Figure 17.1 Photographs of the phenotypic culture and microscopic features of hyaline moulds frequently implicated in hyalohyphomycosis.

a,b *Fusarium solani*; **c,d** *Fusarium dimerum*; **e,f** *Sarocladium* spp; **g,h** *Purpureocillium lilacinum*; **i,j** *Paecilomyces variotii*; **k,l** *Scopulariopsis brevicaulis*; **m,n** *Scedosporium apiospermum*; **o,p** *Lomentospora prolificans*.

voriconazole and terbinafine in combination (Howden et al. 2003; Bhat et al. 2007).

References

Ajello L (1982) Hyalohyphomycosis: a disease entity whose time has come (Newsletter). *Med Mycol Soc NY* 2: 3–5.

Bhat SV, Paterson DL, Rinaldi MG and Veldkamp PJ (2007) *Scedosporium prolificans* brain abscess in a patient with chronic granulomatous disease: successful combination therapy with voriconazole and terbinafine. *Scand J Infect Dis* 39: 87–90.

Borman AM and Johnson EM (2013) Genomics and proteomics as compared to conventional phenotypic approaches for the identification of the agents of invasive fungal infections. *Curr Fungal Infect Rep* 7: 235–43.

Borman AM and Johnson EM (2014) Interpretation of fungal culture results. *Curr Fungal Infect Rep* 8: 312. doi 10.1007/5 12281-014-0204-2

Campbell CK, Johnson EM and Warnock DW (2013) *Identification of Pathogenic Fungi* (Chichester, UK: Wiley-Blackwell).

Das S, Saha R, Dar SA and Ramachandran VG (2010) *Acremonium* species: a review of the etiological agents of emerging hyalohyphomycosis. *Mycopathologia* 70: 361–75.

de Hoog GS, Guarro J, Gené J and Figueras MJ (eds) (2000) *Atlas of Clinical Fungi* (2nd edn, Centraalbureau voor Schimmelcultures, Baarn, and Universitat Rovira I Virgili, Reus).

Doyen JB, Sutton DA, Theodore P, et al. (2013) *Rasamsonia argillacea* pulmonary and aortic graft infection in an immune-competent patient. *J Clin Microbiol* 51: 719–22.

Geiser DM, Aoki T, Bacon CW, et al. (2013) One fungus, one name: defining the genus *Fusarium* in a scientifically robust way that preserves longstanding use. *Phytopathology* 103: 400–8.

Howden BP, Slavin MA, Schwarer AP and Mijch AM (2003) Successful control of disseminated *Scedosporium prolificans* infection with a combination of voriconazole and terbinafine. *Eur J Clin Microbiol Infect Dis* 22: 111–13.

Perfect JR, Marr KA, Walsh TJ, et al. (2003) Voriconazole treatment for less-common, emerging, or refractory fungal infections. *Clin Infect Dis* 36: 1122–31.

Summerbell RC, Gueidan C, Schroers H-J, et al. (2011) *Acremonium* phylogenetic overview and revision of *Gliomastix, Sarocladium,* and *Trichothecium. Stud Mycol* 68: 139–62.

Tortorano AM, Richardson M, Roilides E, et al. (2014) ESCMID and ECMM joint guidelines on diagnosis and management of hyalohyphomycosis: *Fusarium* spp., *Scedosporium* spp. and others. *Clin Microbiol Infect* 20 (Suppl. 3): 27–46.

van Diepeningen AD, Brankovics B, Iltes J, van der Lee TAJ and Waalwijk C (2015) Diagnosis of *Fusarium* infections: approaches to identification by the Clinical Mycology Laboratory. *Curr Fungal Infect Rep* 9: 135–43.

CHAPTER 18

Mucoraceous moulds

Thomas R. Rogers and Elizabeth M. Johnson

Introduction to mucoraceous moulds

The first description of the microscopic appearance of a *Mucor* sp. (bread mould) was by Robert Hooke in 1665 (Gest 2004), while the first report of a histopathologically proven clinical case was by Arnold Paltauf in 1885 (Cornely et al. 2014). Mucormycosis has been regarded as a relatively rare mould infection, but recent reports suggest that its incidence may be increasing (Binder et al. 2014). Historically, these infections have been seen in immunocompromised hosts—in particular, patients being treated for haematological malignancies, where it is the second most common invasive mould infection after invasive aspergillosis. Because of the small study populations, retrospective nature of many published surveys, and challenging diagnosis, its incidence is difficult to determine, but may approximate to one case per million population in Europe. Delayed diagnosis very likely contributes to the poor outcomes reported in the literature. Treatment of mucormycosis is especially challenging owing to the multifactorial nature of the determinants of outcome; these include reversal of the underlying host risk factors, surgical intervention to stem the progressive angio-invasive infection, and the unpredictable susceptibility of the causative fungal species to the limited number of possible antifungal agents used for therapy (Katragkou et al. 2013).

The occurrence of entomophthoromycosis is due to the fungal genera *Basidiobolus* and *Conidiobolus*. These have as their niche the environment of tropical and subtropical countries, principally in Africa, the Middle East, India, South-East Asia, and Central or South America. They typically cause infections in immunologically competent hosts, although they can also cause opportunistic invasive infections in immunocompromised hosts.

Taxonomy of mucoraceous moulds and genera most frequently implicated in infection

There are two main groups of medically important mucoraceous moulds: those belonging to the order *Mucorales*, and members of the order *Entomophthorales*. Until recently, these would have been classified in the *Zygomycota*. However, it has long been accepted that this phylum is polyphyletic, and a comprehensive study based on multi-gene sequence analyses suggested a redistribution of taxa (Hibbett et al. 2007). There have been further modifications as genotypic relationships are better defined, but the traditional members of the *Zygomycota* were redistributed into *Glomeromycota* and four newly introduced subphyla of uncertain position ('*incertae sedis*'). The subphylum *Mucoromycotina* was proposed to accommodate the *Mucorales*, which includes the most common human pathogens in the genera *Lichtheimia* (formerly *Absidia*), *Mucor, Rhizomucor*, and *Rhizopus*, while the subphylum *Entomophthoromycotina*—more recently elevated to the phylum *Entomophthoromycota*—encompasses the *Entomophthorales*, which includes the genera *Basidiobolus* and *Conidiobolus*, members of which are agents of subcutaneous infection in certain geographically restricted areas (Box 18.1).

Cell biology of mucoraceous moulds

Typically, the opportunistic pathogenic species grow rapidly at 37°C—sometimes also at higher temperatures—on glucose-peptone agar, producing a luxuriant aerial mycelium that occupies all the available airspace in a Petri dish, although *Mucor* and *Rhizomucor* species usually have a more restricted aerial turf (Figure 18.1). Large numbers of asexual sporangiospores of varying size, shape, and ornamentation are produced, in structures known as sporangia formed at the ends of stalks known as sporangiophores (Figure 18.2). Some genera, mainly *Rhizopus* and *Rhizomucor,* produce root-like structures or rhizoids at the base of the sporangiophore to anchor them into the substrate (Figure 18.3). Some members of the *Mucorales*, such as *Cunninghamella* (Figure 18.4), *Syncephalastrum*, and *Cokeromyces*, produce their spores on the outside of the vesicle at the tip of the sporangiophore (see Campbell et al. [2013] for a text on identification).

Another feature shared by many genera in *Mucorales* is the capacity to produce sexual spores known as zygospores (Figure 18.5). These are large, thick-walled spores formed by meiosis, sometimes spontaneously in homothallic strains, but more often by mating of compatible plus/minus heterothallic strains. These spores are very resilient to extreme environmental conditions, so confer a survival advantage.

Basidiobolus and *Conidiobolus* species produce ballistospores, which are forcibly ejected and may aid in their environmental dispersal, and can often be seen adhering to the lid of the Petri dish when they are cultured in the laboratory.

Pathogenesis of mucoraceous moulds

As mucoraceous moulds have few septa in their hyphae, allowing more rapid nutrient transport, they can grow faster than many other moulds. Their speed of growth and angio-invasive potential leads to blocking of blood vessels with associated ischaemia and necrosis, and there may be rapid contiguous spread of infection. Another possible virulence mechanism is their ability to chelate

Box 18.1 Mucoraceous mould species

Order *Mucorales*:

Lichtheimia (Absidia) corymbifera

Mucor circinelloides

Rhizopus arrhizus, R. microsporus

Saksenaea vasiformis

Apophysomyces variabilis, A. elegans

Cunninghamella bertholletiae

Mucor indicus, M. ramosissimus

Rhizomucor pusillus

Syncephalastrum racemosus

Order *Entomophthorales*:

Basidiobolus ranarum

Conidiobolus coronatus, C. incongruous

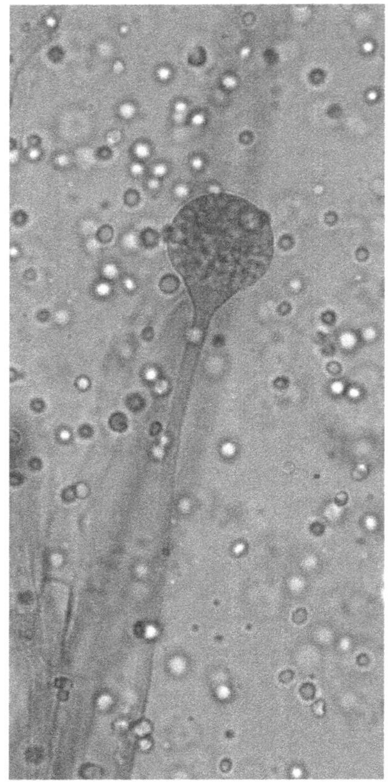

Figure 18.2 Sporangiophore of *Lichtheimia corymbifera* with terminal sporangium containing sporangiospores.
Photo © Crown copyright 2017 Public Health England.

available iron, and iron overload is a risk factor. The comparatively larger size of their spores, relative to those of *Aspergillus,* means that many are trapped in the nasal turbinates, causing rhinocerebral mucormycosis more often than pulmonary infection. For wound infections, an extended area of surgical resection may be required to limit the spread.

Epidemiology of mucoraceous moulds

Many of the mucoraceous moulds are important saprobes on decaying plant material and are usually acquired from an environmental source by inhalation of spores. They may also cause wound infections. Invasive infection is most often seen in uncontrolled diabetic patients with keto-acidosis or in immunocompromised patients with low neutrophil counts or on long-term corticosteroid therapy for graft-versus-host disease (GvHD). Infections usually occur as isolated cases, but there have been instances where contaminated fomites such as dressings or wooden tongue depressors used as splints have caused localized outbreaks (Mitchell et al. 1996). Recent nosocomial outbreaks of mucormycosis have been reported where

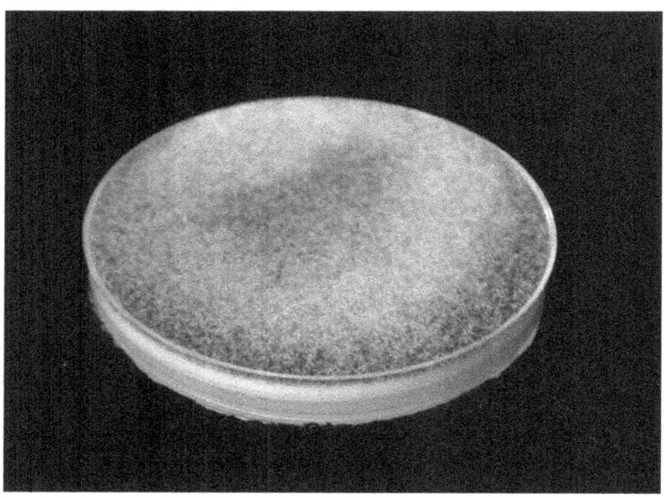

Figure 18.1 Rapidly growing aerial mycelium of *Rhizopus arrhizus* filling the available airspace within 48 hours. Note formation of macroscopically visible sporangia at air interface at edge of plate.
Photo © Crown copyright 2017 Public Health England.

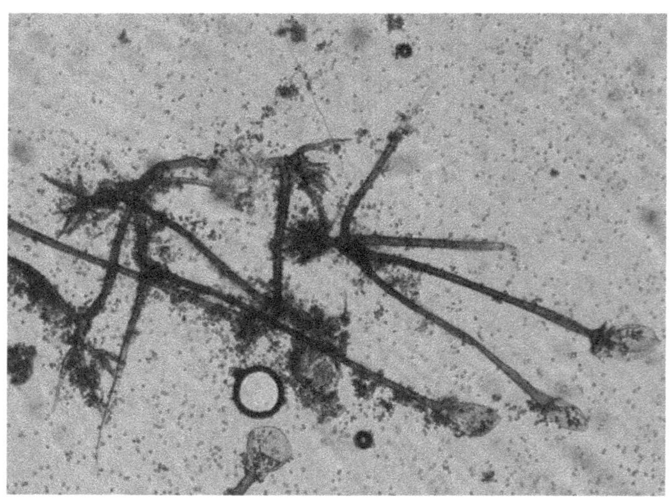

Figure 18.3 Collapsed heads and root-like structures at base of sporangiophores in *Rhizopus microsporus*.
Photo © Crown copyright 2017 Public Health England.

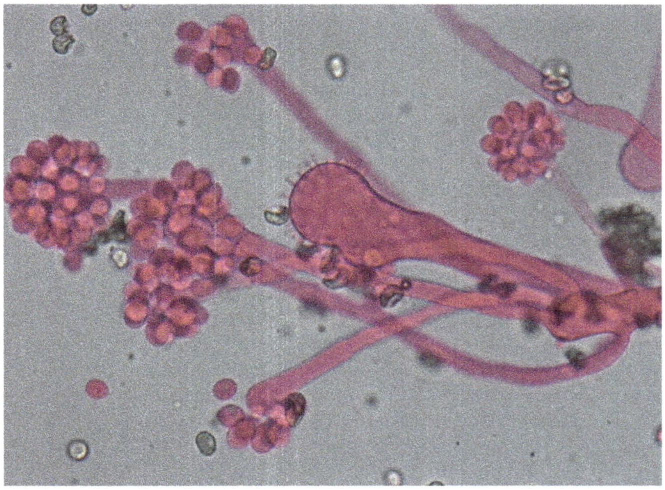

Figure 18.4 Sporangia of *Cunninghamella bertholletiae* showing spore production around the vesicle on little pegs.
Photo © Crown copyright 2017 Public Health England.

contaminated bed linen was, in each case, identified as the source of fungal spores; *Rhizopus microsporus* and *R. delemar* were respectively identified as the species responsible (Duffy et al. 2014; Cheng et al. 2016). *Conidiobolus* and *Basidiobolus* are usually associated with insects or amphibia, and infection arises owing to inoculation of spores under the dermis or in the nasal mucosa by minor trauma.

The commonest cause of mucormycosis is *Rhizopus arrhizus*.

Risk factors and incidence of infection with mucoraceous moulds

In a US review of 929 cases of mucormycosis, Roden et al. (2005) found the most common risk factor was type 2 diabetes mellitus. This was followed by patients with no known risk factor, then those with underlying malignancies. A more recent European review of diseases/conditions predisposing to mucormycosis identified, in descending order of frequency, haematological and non-haematological malignancies, diabetes mellitus (especially with keto-acidosis), and trauma or no risk factors (Petrikkos et al. 2014). Other reported predisposing conditions/factors include: burns (Schaal et al. 2015), lung/heart–lung transplant (Vazquez et al. 2015), alcohol or intravenous drug use (Terry et al. 2016), tornados and flooding (Davies et al. 2015), and iron overload (Boelaert et al. 1993). The incidence of mucormycosis after allogeneic stem cell transplant is estimated to be around 0.3%, (Robin et al. 2014); however, one-year survival from mucormycosis after allogeneic stem cell transplantation is less than 25% (Riches et al. 2016). There are no reliable incidence data for other underlying conditions, and cases are often the subject of limited case report series.

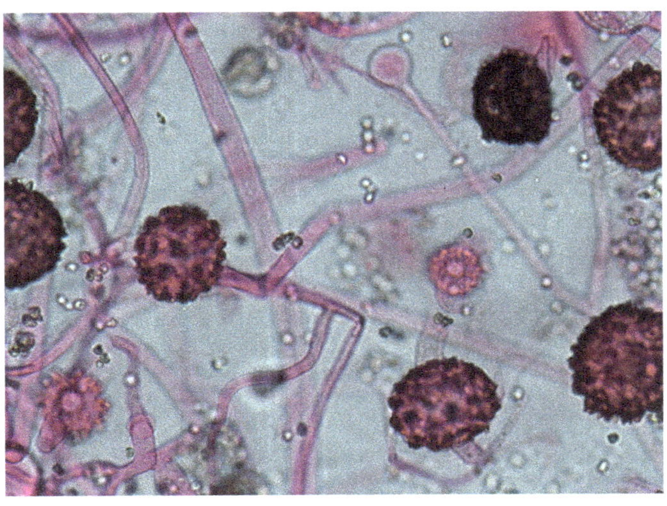

Figure 18.5 Thick-walled zygospore formation in *Mucor* spp.
Photo © Crown copyright 2017 Public Health England.

Clinical presentation of infection with mucoraceous moulds

Initially, mucormycosis may present as paranasal sinusitis. Delayed recognition and diagnosis may result in rapid progression to involve the orbit, retro-orbital tissues, and brain, with devastating consequences. Patients' symptoms may include headache, sinus pain, facial swelling, alteration or loss of vision, and fever. A black eschar may appear on the hard palate or nasal mucosa. Cerebral involvement may result in loss of consciousness, cranial nerve palsies, or features associated with a space-occupying lesion. The clinical presentation of pulmonary disease resembles that of invasive aspergillosis. Cutaneous mucormycosis may result in skin/tissue swelling, necrosis, fasciitis, or the presence of a black eschar. Disseminated mucormycosis, often from a pulmonary origin, may involve any organ and may be associated with skin lesions.

Basidiobolomycosis causes subcutaneous tissue infection involving the trunk or lower limbs, but can affect other parts of the body. It is more common in children and in males. Gastrointestinal infection may result in an abdominal mass which is misdiagnosed because of the relative rarity of this fungal infection. Conidiobolomycosis is most commonly reported in Nigeria, affecting young males. It is acquired by the inhalation of spores or their implantation into the nose on contaminated hands. Initial presentation is of painless facial swelling with sinus involvement and facial disfiguration. Cerebral or disseminated disease is rare except in the immunocompromised (El-Shabrawi et al. 2014).

Diagnosis of mucoraceous mould infection

Diagnosis usually requires isolation and subsequent identification of the infecting pathogen (Borman and Johnson 2014), although the typical appearance of broad, pauci-septate, ribbon-like hyphae branching at 90°—either on direct microscopy of tissue stained with Calcofluor (Figure 18.6), or on histological staining, especially with Grocott's methenamine silver stain—can alert the clinician to the probability of mucoraceous mould infection (Guarner and Brandt 2011). Imaging techniques may reveal the reverse halo phenomenon (Wahba et al. 2008), and clinical manifestations can be highly suggestive, especially with the extent of necrosis often encountered, but are not specific. The (1→3) β-D-glucan test is usually not positive as mucoraceous moulds have reduced β-glucan in the cell wall (Odabasi et al. 2006). There are investigational diagnostic pan-fungal PCR (polymerase chain reaction) tests, which can be conducted on normally sterile fluids and tissues or on wax-embedded fixed tissue, from which the amplified product can be sequenced to provide the identity of the infecting organism (Bialek et al. 2005; Hammond et al. 2011; Cornely et al. 2014).

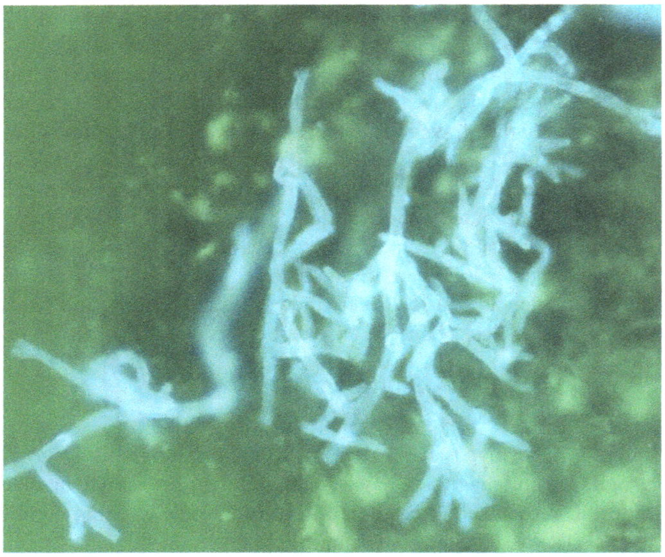

Figure 18.6 Calcofluor staining of hyphae on fluorescence microscopy.
Photo © Crown copyright 2017 Public Health England.

After culture on glucose-peptone agar incubated at 30°C and 37°C, growth is usually apparent within 24 hours, and the fast-growing aerial mycelium typically invades all the air-space in the Petri dish. It is very important that tissue samples sent for culture are not homogenized as that will render the hyphae non-viable. Isolates can be identified by the size, shape, and ornamentation of spores, and the way in which they are produced, as well as the presence or absence of rhizoids (Campbell et al. 2013). Molecular identification methods can be used to confirm the identity of isolates with similar phenotypic appearance or those not producing spores. Although many environmental mucoraceous moulds are also culture contaminants, the ability to grow at 37°C can indicate their pathogenic potential (Cornely et al. 2014). Smears or biopsy samples from affected nasal or other tissues in entomophthoromycosis may reveal hyphal structures with few septae; the Splendore-Hoeppli phenomenon refers to the presence of eosinophilic cells surrounding hyphae.

Treatment of mucoraceous mould infection

Consensus guidelines on the management of mucormycosis recommend a lipid formulation of amphotericin B (+/>5mg/kg/day depending on formulation) and, where indicated, surgical intervention to debride necrotic tissues (Cornely et al. 2014; Vercillo et al. 2015). Alternative agents are posaconazole and the newer triazole isavuconazole (Marty et al. 2016). Epidemiological cut-off MIC (minimal inhibitory concentration) values, do not correlate well with clinical outcome, but they may aid in identifying individual isolates with drug resistance or reduced susceptibility (Espinel-Ingroff et al. 2015). Other potential treatments, albeit with uncertain efficacy, include hyperbaric oxygen, iron chelation, or immunotherapy. Acetic acid has been shown experimentally to have useful efficacy against the agents of mucormycosis (Trzaska et al. 2015). Treatment options for cases of entomophthoromycosis include oral itraconazole, co-trimoxazole, or topical saturated potassium iodide solution.

References

Bialek R, Konrad F, Kern J, et al. (2005). PCR based identification and discrimination of agents of mucormycosis and aspergillosis in paraffin wax embedded tissue. *J Clin Pathol* 58: 1180–4.

Binder, U, Maurer, E and Lass-Florl C (2014) Mucormycosis—from the pathogens to the disease. *Clin Microbiol Infect* 20 (Suppl. 6): 60–6.

Boelaert JR, de Locht M, van Cutsem J, et al. (1993) Mucormycosis during deferoxamine therapy is a siderophore-mediated infection. In vitro and in vivo animal studies. *J Clin Invest* 91: 1979–86.

Borman AM and Johnson EM (2014) Interpretation of fungal culture results. *Curr Fungal Infect Rep* 8: 312. doi 10.1007/5 12281-014-0204-2

Campbell CK, Johnson EM and Warnock DW (2013) *Identification of Pathogenic Fungi* (2nd edn, Oxford: Wiley-Blackwell).

Cheng VCC, Chen JHK, Wong SCY, et al. (2016) Hospital outbreak of pulmonary and cutaneous zygomycosis due to contaminated linen items from substandard laundry. *Clin Infect Dis* 62: 714–21.

Cornely OA, Arikan-Akdagli S, Dannaoui E, et al. (2014) ESCMID and ECMM Joint Clinical Guidelines for the Diagnosis and Management of Mucormycosis 2013. *Clin Microbiol Infect* 20 (Suppl. 3): 5–26.

Davies BW, Smith JM, Hink EM, et al. (2015) Increased incidence of rhino-orbital-cerebral mucormycosis after Colorado flooding. *Ophthal Plast Reconstr Surg* 33 (3S Suppl. 1): S148–151.

Duffy J, Harris J, Gade L, et al. (2014) Mucormycosis outbreak associated with hospital linens. *Pediatr Infect Dis J* 33: 472–6.

El-Shabrawi MHF, Arnaout H, Madkour L, et al. (2014) Entomophthoromycosis: a challenging emerging disease. Mycoses 57 (Suppl. 3): 132–7.

Espinel-Ingroff A, Chakrabarti A, Chowdhary A, et al. (2015) Multicenter evaluation of MIC distributions for epidemiological cutoff value definition to detect amphotericin B, posaconazole, and itraconazole resistance among the most clinically relevant species of *Mucorales*. *Antimicrob Agents Chemother* 59: 1745–50.

Gest H (2004) The discovery of microorganisms by Robert Hooke and Antoni van Leeuwenhoek, fellows of the Royal Society. *Notes Rec R Soc Lond* 58: 187–201.

Guarner J and Brandt ME (2011) Histopathologic diagnosis of fungal infections in the 21st century. *Clin Microbiol Rev* 24: 247–80.

Hammond SP, Bialek R, Milner DA, et al. (2011) Molecular methods to improve diagnosis and identification of mucormycosis. *J Clin Microbiol* 49: 2151–3.

Hibbett DS, Binder M, Bischoff JF, et al. (2007) A higher-level phylogenetic classification of the Fungi. *Mycol Res* 111: 509–47.

Katragkou A, Walsh TJ and Roilides E (2013) Why is mucormycosis more difficult to cure than more common mycoses? *Clin Microbiol Infect* 20 (Suppl. 6): 74–81.

Marty FM, Ostrosky-Zeichner L, Cornely O, et al. (2016) Isavuconazole treatment for mucormycosis: a single-arm open-label trial and case-control analysis. *Lancet Infect Dis* 16: 828–37.

Mitchell SJ, Gray J, Morgan MEI, Hocking MD and Durbin GM (1996) Nosocomial infection with *Rhizopus microsporus* in pre-term infants: association with wooden tongue depressors. *Lancet* 348: 441–3.

Odabasi Z, Paetznick VL, Rodriguez JR, et al. (2006) Differences in beta-glucan levels in culture supernatants of a variety of fungi. *Med Mycol* 44: 267–72.

Petrikkos G, Skiada A and Drogari-Apiranthitou M (2014) Epidemiology of mucormycosis in Europe. *Clin Microbiol Infect* 20 (Suppl. 6): 67–73.

Riches ML, Trifilio S, Chen M, et al. (2016) Risk factors and impact of non-Aspergillus mold infections following allogeneic HCT: a CIBMTR infection and immune reconstitution analysis. *Bone Marrow Transplant* 51: 277–82.

Robin C, Alanio A and Cordonnier C (2014) Mucormycosis: a new concern in the transplant ward? *Curr Opin Hematol* 21: 482–90.

Roden MM, Zaoutis TE, Buchanan WL, et al. (2005) Epidemiology and outcome of zygomycosis: a review of 929 reported cases. *Clin Infect Dis* 41: 634–53.

Schaal JV, Leclerc T, Soler C, et al. (2015) Epidemiology of filamentous fungal infections in burned patients: A French retrospective study. *Burns* 41: 853–63.

Terry AR, Kahle KT, Larvie M, et al. (2016) Case 5-2016: a 43-year-old man with altered mental status and a history of alcohol use. *N Engl J Med* 374: 671–80.

Trzaska WJ, Correia JN, Villegas MT, et al. (2015) pH manipulation as a novel strategy for treating mucormycosis. *Antimicrob Agents Chemother* 59: 6968–74.

Vazquez R, Vazquez-Guillamet MC, Suarez J, et al. (2015) Invasive mould infections in lung and heart-lung transplant recipients: Stanford University experience. *Transpl Infect Dis* 17: 259–66.

Vercillo MS, Liptay MJ and Seder CW (2015) Early pneumonectomy for pulmonary mucormycosis. *Ann Thorac Surg* 99: e67–8.

Wahba H, Truong MT, Lei X, Kontoyiannis DP and Marom EM (2008) Reversed halo sign in invasive pulmonary fungal infections. *Clin Infect Dis* 46: 1733–7.

CHAPTER 19

Pneumocystis jirovecii

Stuart Flanagan

Overview of pneumocystis species and pathological associations in humans

Members of the ascomycetic genus *Pneumocystis* are microscopic yeast-like fungi that reside in mammalian lung tissue, usually without ill effect. However, in immunocompromised hosts they become pathogenic and cause respiratory infection. Originally identified by Carlos Chagas in 1909, the organism was thought to be protozoan in nature, and termed *Pneumocystis carinii*. In 1952, the Czech parasitologist Otto Jírovec identified *Pneumocystis* pneumonia (PCP) in humans, and in the late 1990s, DNA analysis showed significant difference in the *Pneumocystis* found in each mammalian species, leading to the human species being renamed as *Pneumocystis jirovecii* (Stringer et al. 2002) in honour of Jírovec.

Initially, PCP was associated with children with congenital immune defects and adults with acquired immune deficiencies, associated either with malignancy or treatments thereof. In 1981, clusters of adult PCP infection in previously healthy individuals raised the question of an acquired immunosuppressive condition, and subsequently led to the definition of the acquired immune deficiency syndrome (AIDS), a consequence of HIV (human immunodeficiency virus) infection. The introduction of highly active antiretroviral therapy (HAART) has considerably reduced the incidence of PCP infection amongst HIV-positive individuals, but it remains a health concern for patients with congenital immune defects, immunodeficiency secondary to malignancy, autoimmune disease, or treatment which may lead to immunosuppression such as chemotherapy and disease-modifying agents such as tumour necrosis factor-alpha inhibitors (Miller and Huang 2004).

Taxonomy

After identification of *Pneumocystis* species in 1909, they were erroneously considered to be part of the life cycle of the protozoan *Trypanosoma cruzi* until 1914, when they were given the genus and species designation *Pneumocystis carinii*. For most of the twentieth century, *Pneumocystis* was considered a protozoan (based on morphology, response to protozoal therapy, and absence of more usual appearances of fungi), until DNA analysis in the late 1980s identified *Pneumocystis* as an atypical fungus which characteristically lacks ergosterol in the cell membrane and is difficult to culture (Edman et al. 1988; Stringer et al. 1989).

The organism was named *Pneumocystis carinii* in 1914 to reflect its propensity for the lungs of mammals, its cystic morphology, and the Italian investigator Antonio Carini, who provided the slides for study. In the 1950s, the human specific form of *Pneumocystis* was first described by the Czech parasitologist Otto Jírovec; however, it was not until the DNA analysis of the 1980s that the *Pneumocystis* organisms in various mammals were shown to be quite different.

Significant species

The human form was renamed *Pneumocystis jirovecii*, with other species-specific forms being renamed *P. murina* (found in mice), *P. oryctolagi* (rabbits), and *P. wakefieldiae* joining the previously described *P. carinii* as being found in rats (Cushion 2010).

Pathogenesis

In common with other fungi, the cell wall of *Pneumocystis* species contains chitin and proteins, particularly β-1,3-glucan. The main cell surface antigen is major surface glycoprotein (MSG), which binds to both host macrophages via mannose receptors and also host surfactant protein D. MSG may cause a host inflammatory response and damage to alveolar epithelium, while variability of the antigen by recombination is a likely means of evading host immune defences (Stringer 2007; Keely and Stringer 2009; George et al. 2015).

Pneumocystis resides within the host mammal's lung tissue in trophic and cystic forms. Trophozoites measure 1–4 μm diameter and asexually reproduce via binary fission. After conjugation of the haploid trophic forms, a diploid zygote is produced, undergoing meiosis and mitosis to develop into a mature cyst measuring 8–10 μm diameter. The mature cysts burst and release trophic cells (Stringer et al. 2002).

Epidemiology

Pneumocystis shows strong species specificity, which may suggest that the species is an obligate parasite which has co-evolved with its host. However, this hypothesis of host acquisition is challenged by the finding of *P. jirovecii* outside the human body, in environmental samples of airborne fungus and pond water. Exposure to environmental *Pneumocystis* in childhood, the development of antibodies, and persistence of the organisms in a latent phase during adulthood were long thought to be the source for potential infection, with the organism remaining dormant until immunosuppression allowed an opportunity to cause respiratory infection. However, studies have shown a lack of *Pneumocystis* in the lungs of healthy individuals and clearing of the organisms in immunocompetent humans. This may be explained by episodes of recent (rather than reactivated) colonization, supported by the findings of genotypically different *Pneumocystis* organisms in patients with recurrent episodes of *Pneumocystis* pneumonia (Stringer et al. 2002; Miller and Huang 2004).

Clinical presentations

Almost 90% of PCP cases in humans occur in HIV-seropositive persons with CD4 T-cell counts of less than 200 cells per microlitre (or CD4 T-cell percentage of all lymphocytes <14%). Typical presentation is exertional dyspnoea, malaise, and a dry cough. Low-grade fever and poor inspiratory effort may also be present. Associated symptoms include pleuritic chest pain, haemoptysis, and presentation with spontaneous or infection-associated pneumothorax. Physical examination reveals tachypnoea and normal breath sounds or, rarely, end-inspiratory crackles. Radiological findings often reflect severity of the illness, and may include perihilar interstitial infiltrates, pneumatoceles, and pneumothoraces, although up to 39% of patients have a normal chest X-ray despite substantial hypoxaemia (see Chapters 30 and 33).

Diagnosis

Demonstration of a decrease in oxygenation levels (SpO_2) between rest and exercise is a reasonably specific test for PCP in those with normal chest X-rays with no history of the infection. However, as no clinical features are specific to PCP, microbiological investigations are required to confirm infection and to exclude alternative diagnoses and co-pathology. Sputum samples collected non-invasively from induced sputum (diagnostic sensitivity 50–90%), or alternatively via bronchoalveolar lavage (BAL; sensitivity >90%), should be examined for direct visualization of *P. jirovecii* using either histochemical silver stains (e.g. Grocott-Gomori methenamine silver stain) or immunofluorescent stains (Figure 19.1).

Nucleic acid amplification tests have increased sensitivity but reduced specificity compared with direct visualization and are not recommended as a sole diagnosis technique.

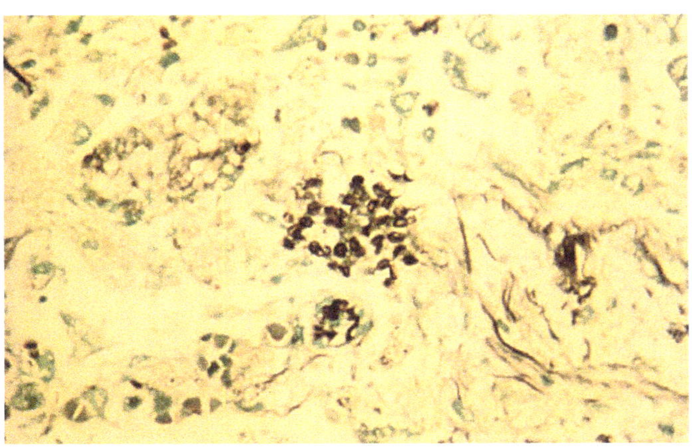

Figure 19.1 Section of lung stained with GMS (Gomori methenamine silver), showing a cluster of *Pneumocystis jirovecii* cysts within an alveolus. A nearby alveolus contains characteristic foamy macrophages.

Treatment

Treatment should not be delayed in a presumed case of PCP while awaiting adequate sputum samples. First-line treatment for moderate-to-severe PCP (PaO_2 ≤9.3 kPa) is with high-dose intravenous trimethoprim-sulphamethoxazole (TMP-SMX) for 21 days at a divided dose of 120 mg/kg/day intravenously for three days, reduced to 90 mg/kg/day intravenously for a further 18 days. Oral or intravenous corticosteroids should be commenced in all cases of suspected moderate-to-severe PCP with a PCP <9.3 kPa or SpO_2 <92%, starting at 40 mg prednisolone twice daily and slowly reduced over 21 days. First-line treatment for mild-to-moderate disease PaO_2 >9.3 kPa is with oral TMP-SMX 1920 mg/kg/day or 90 mg/kg/day in divided three-times-a-day or four-times-a-day dosages (Toma et al. 1998). Efficacy for TMP-SMX is 70–90%. Alternative therapies for those allergic or intolerant of TMP-SMX include dapsone, pentamidine, and atovaquone. Glucose-6-phosphate dehydrogenase deficiency levels should be checked prior to TMP-SMX, dapsone, or primaquine use as haemolysis can be triggered by oxidant drugs or higher dose sulphamethoxazole (Nelson et al. 2011).

A favourable treatment response can take up to seven days. All patients who are HIV-infected should be commenced on HAART, although the optimal time of introduction remains to be determined. Many clinicians introduce HAART early (i.e. within two weeks of commencing PCP therapy), which has shown a reduced mortality compared with deferred HAART (Zolopa et al. 2009).

Overall survival following an episode of PCP is up to 90%. In those individuals who deteriorate and require respiratory support, early use of continuous positive airway pressure for hypoxia in the absence of hypercapnia may avoid intubation and mechanical ventilation. Discussion with local ICU (intensive care unit) services is recommended in such cases.

PCP prophylaxis with TMP-SMX 480 mg once daily should be used in all HIV-seropositive individuals with a CD4 T-cell count persistently less than 200 cells per microlitre, or oral candidiasis or previous AIDS-defining illness. Individuals on established HAART who subsequently sustain a CD4 T-cell count of less than 200 cells per microlitre for more than three months run a very low risk of *Pneumocystis* pneumonia, and prophylaxis can be discontinued in this population.

References

Cushion MT (2010) Are members of the fungal genus *Pneumocystis* (a) commensals; (b) opportunists; (c) pathogens; or (d) all of the above? PLoS Pathog 6: e1001009. doi: 10.1371/journal.ppat.1001009 http://www.ncbi.nlm.nih.gov/pmc/articles/PMC2944789/

Edman JC, Kovacs JA, Masur H, Santi DV, Elwood HJ and Sogin ML (1988) Ribosomal RNA sequence shows *Pneumocystis carinii* to be a member of the fungi. *Nature* 334: 519–22.

George MP, Gingo KR and Morris A (2015) *Pneumocystis (carinii) jirovecii, Antimicrobe—Infectious Disease and Antimicrobial Agents*, http://www.antimicrobe.org/f11.asp, accessed 08 May 2017.

Keely SP and Stringer JR (2009) *Pneumocystis carinii*: sequence from ribosomal RNA implies a close relationship with fungi. *BMC Genomics* 10: 367. doi: 10.1186/1471-2164-10-367

Miller R and Huang L (2004) *Pneumocystis jirovecii* infection. *Thorax* 59: 731–33. doi: 0.1136/thx.2004.021436 http://www.ncbi.nlm.nih.gov/pmc/articles/PMC1747136/pdf/v059p00731.pdf

Nelson M, Dockrell DH, Edwards S, et al. (2011) British HIV Association and British Infection Association Guidelines for the Treatment of Opportunistic Infection in HIV-seropositive Individuals. *HIV Med* 12 (Suppl. 2): 1–140.

Stringer JR (2007) Antigenic variation in pneumocystis. *J Eukaryot Microbiol* 54: 8–13.

Stringer JR, Beard CB, Miller RF and Wakefield AE (2002) A new name for *Pneumocystis* from humans and new perspectives on the host-pathogen relationship. *Emerg Infect Dis* 8: 891–96. http://wwwnc.cdc.gov/eid/article/8/9/02-0096_article

Stringer SL, Stringer JR, Blaser MA, Walzer PD and Cushion MT (1989) *Pneumocystis carinii*: sequence from ribosomal RNA implies a close relationship with fungi. *Exp Parasitol* 68: 450–61.

Toma E, Thorne A, Singer J, et al., for the CTN-PCP Study Group (1998) Clindamycin with primaquine vs. Trimethoprim-sulfamethoxazole therapy for mild and moderately severe *Pneumocystis carinii* pneumonia in patients with AIDS: a multicentre, double-blind, randomized trial (CTN 004). *Clin Infect Dis* 27: 524–30.

Zolopa AR, Andersen J, Komarow L, et al., for the ACTG A5164 study team (2009) Early antiretroviral therapy reduces AIDS progression/death in individuals with acute opportunistic infections: a multicenter randomized strategy trial. PLoS One 4: e5575.

SECTION 3

Fungal diseases

CHAPTER 20

Fungal bone and joint infections

Damien Mack, Simon Warren, Shara Palanivel, and Christopher P. Conlon

Introduction to fungal bone and joint infection

Musculoskeletal infections due to fungi are relatively rare, but because of the complexity of modern medicine, are probably on the increase. Their rarity, coupled with relatively subtle clinical presentations, means that diagnosis is often delayed until the infection is well established and significant tissue damage has occurred.

Epidemiology

The clinical presentations and the types of causative fungi differ somewhat depending on the age of the patient. Problems with making an accurate diagnosis of fungal bone and joint infection probably lead to under-reporting of the prevalence of these infections. There are no robust studies of the incidence of fungal bone and joint infections. Although invasive fungal infections are increasing, there are no data to confirm that bone and joint infections are also rising. Case reports and case series suggest an increase, but this might just be reporting bias and an increased awareness of, and interest in, fungal infections.

Fungi reach bones and joints by a variety of means. Haematogenous spread from a distant focus is common and may be a particular feature in the immunocompromised host. The synovium is particularly vascular and is thus a potential site for pathogens in the bloodstream to settle. However, infection can also affect the bones and joints by spread from a contiguous focus of infection, or the fungus might be directly inoculated into the joint during surgery, for example. Mycetoma, the consequence of inoculation into the cutaneous and subcutaneous tissues, will eventually spread to deeper tissues, including bones and joints (see Chapter 23).

Children may be more at risk of direct inoculation infection with moulds through trauma from falls or road traffic accidents. In such cases the knee is often affected by direct puncture wounds.

There are certain risk factors that make bone and joint fungal infections more likely. Trauma and surgery, as outlined above, increase the risk of environmental or nosocomial fungi being directly inoculated into a joint or a bone. Immunosuppression increases the risk of fungal disease. This includes chemotherapy or bone marrow transplantation for malignancy, particularly haematological disease, HIV (human immunodeficiency virus) infection, and solid organ transplantation (Kumashi et al. 2006). In addition, there is a variety of inherited or genetic causes of immunodeficiency that can increase the risk of invasive fungal infection. Finally, the increasing complexity of modern medicine is itself a risk factor (Allan et al. 2015). The use of broad-spectrum antibiotics, admission to an intensive care unit, and multiple comorbidities are all associated with an increased probability of fungal infection (Taccone et al. 2015). Prosthetic material, particularly joint replacements, can be a nidus for fungal infection or can be infected at the time of insertion.

Causative fungi

Aspergillus and *Candida* species are the most common fungi associated with bone and joint infection, particularly in immunocompromised hosts and in nosocomial settings. However, a variety of other fungal species have been found to infect the skeleton. Dimorphic fungi are particularly likely to affect immunocompetent individuals.

Candida

Many cases of bone and joint infection with *Candida* species arise after candidaemia.

In one study, *Candida* osteomyelitis was first identified as the site of infection in nearly 50% of cases (Gamaletsou et al. 2012), whilst up to 15% had concomitant candidaemia. Approximately 50% had candidaemia as their initial presentation. Spondylodiscitis is recognized as a late complication of candidaemia, presenting as much as a year afterwards (Chia et al. 2005). Mortality in candidal osteomyelitis is approximately 6%—lower than with other forms of invasive candidal infections (Slenker et al. 2012). The most common site for osteomyelitis is vertebral, but it is also seen in long bones and the sternum (Gamaletsou et al. 2012; Pappas et al. 2016). Almost a quarter of vertebral osteomyelitis cases also have an epidural abscess (Gamaletsou et al. 2012). Although the majority of these infections are due to *C. albicans*, non-*albicans* species are on the increase (Pfaller et al. 2014) (see Chapters 11 and 25).

When considering cases of bone and joint infection due to *Candida* species, about 30% of cases affect more than one joint and most arise from candidaemia. In one study 60% of cases were caused by *C. albicans*, with *C. tropicalis* and *C. parapsilosis* making up the bulk of the rest (Gamaletsou et al. 2015). The knee joint was the most commonly affected joint, with the hip and shoulder more commonly affected than other smaller joints.

Paediatric cases are usually confined to neonates and infants. The risk in neonates most likely comes from umbilical catheters and the use of broad-spectrum antibiotics in special care baby units.

Most cases result from haematogenous spread of the *Candida* and result in either arthritis or osteomyelitis. The femur is the most common site of osteomyelitis in this group.

Although adults are also more likely to have had candidaemia before or at the time they develop bone and joint infections with *Candida*, the proportion resulting from haematogenous spread is less than that seen in children. Only about 15% have candidaemia at the time their bone or joint infection is diagnosed. Some cases result from direct inoculation at the time of surgery, or from trauma, and some relate to contiguous spread from an adjacent infection. Adults are much more likely to get discitis or vertebral osteomyelitis than children. Most adults with haematogenous spread are immunocompromised. However, intravenous drug use is a risk factor, particularly for discitis and vertebral infection (Dupont and Drouhet 1985). *Candida* infection of prosthetic joints is rare, but can arise directly from surgery or be a complication of haematogenous spread.

The clinical features of *Candida* bone and joint infections can be subtle and may only emerge some time distant from an episode of candidaemia. Fever is relatively uncommon, being present in less than 30% of adult cases, and less than 20% present with a sinus (Gamaletsou et al. 2012). Pain and local tenderness, sometimes with overlying oedema, are the most common features of joint involvement and long bone osteomyelitis. Back pain is a feature of discitis and vertebral osteomyelitis. Compared with pyogenic infections, inflammatory markers such as white cell count and C-reactive protein are only moderately elevated.

Diagnosis can be difficult, but may be suggested by the patient's risk factors. Patients with candidaemia and musculoskeletal symptoms and signs might have positive cultures from joint aspiration, but 50% of cases of *Candida* bone and joint infections in one series did not have documented candidaemia. Most cases require appropriate imaging followed by some sort of invasive investigation such as synovial or bone biopsy. Generally, MRI (magnetic resonance imaging) of the spine or bones is the preferred modality of imaging, though ultrasound might suffice for infected joints. The most common findings on imaging include: bone destruction, extension into soft tissues, increased uptake on radionuclide scan, decreased intervertebral disc space, and epidural abscess (Ganesh et al. 2015). MRI can also show decreased signal intensity on T1-weighted images and increased signal intensity on T2-weighted images (Figure 20.1). The frequently multifocal nature of *Candida* osteomyelitis suggests that radionuclide scanning, in addition to other modalities, may be appropriate for detecting all infected sites (Gamaletsou et al. 2012). In one series, 74% were diagnosed by culture alone. Some cases can be culture negative, but yeasts are found on histology of bone or synovial biopsies. The utility of available antigen detection assays and tissue PCR (polymerase chain reaction) has not been systematically investigated in bone and joint disease due to *Candida* species. Treatment usually involves a combination of surgical debridement and antifungal therapy (Nyofytos et al. 2014). There are no randomized clinical trials to guide either the choice or duration of treatment. Most cases in the literature have been treated with azoles. The most recent IDSA (Infectious Diseases Society of America) guidelines for *Candida* osteomyelitis recommend (level of evidence B-III) fluconazole 400 mg (6 mg/kg) daily for 6–12 months, or a lipid formulation of amphotericin B, 3–5 mg/kg daily for several weeks, followed by fluconazole for 6–12 months, possibly with a two-week induction phase using either an echinocandin or liposomal amphotericin B (Pappas et al. 2016). There are no data on the management of prosthetic joint infections with *Candida*, but consensus suggests that cure is unlikely if the infected prosthesis is retained. Better outcomes would be expected with a two-stage procedure so that appropriate antifungal therapy can be given before the new implant is placed.

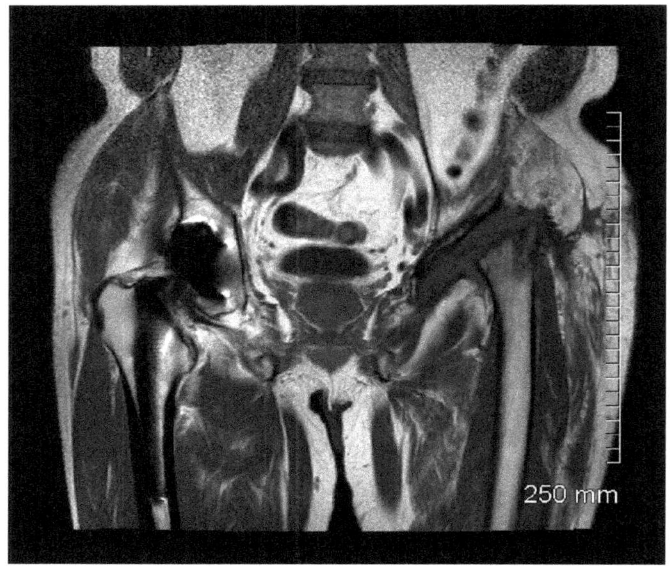

Figure 20.1 Coronal T1-weighted MR image of pelvis and femur. This patient previously had a left Girdlestone procedure (where the femoral head had been removed) and presented with pain and a discharging sinus. MRI scan shows bone marrow oedema of proximal femur suggestive of proximal femoral osteomyelitis and joint effusion. There is a right-sided total hip replacement with expected artefact.

Reproduced courtesy of Royal National Orthopaedic Hospital, Stanmore.

Aspergillus

Aspergillus species are the second most common causes of fungal bone and joint infections, but make up less than 5% of all cases of bone and joint infections (Koehler et al. 2014). *A. fumigatus* accounts for the majority of cases, with *A. flavus* the second most common. All of the other *Aspergillus* species account, in total, for less than 5% of cases. Generally, *Aspergillus* as a cause of musculoskeletal infection occurs in patients who are immunocompromised. Bone marrow transplant recipients and those with haematological malignancy are clearly at risk, but these infections are also more common in diabetics, solid organ transplant recipients, those on long-term steroid therapy, and those with HIV infection. One study found that a group of patients with skull base *Aspergillus* infection had specific defects in Th17 cytokine responses, leading to reduced production of IL-17 and IL-22 (Delsing et al. 2015). Infection of prosthetic joints or infections secondary to trauma or as a complication of surgery are uncommon. Infants and children with some primary immunodeficiencies, especially chronic granulomatous disease (CGD), are at a much increased risk of aspergillosis. Interestingly, the group with CGD are more likely to become infected with *A. nidulans* than other types of patients. Rib infections are more common in this age group than in adults. In any of the age groups, there is a mixture of bone and joint involvement via haematogenous spread of *Aspergillus* and contiguous spread from an adjacent site of primary infection. Contiguous spread appears to be more common in patients undergoing cancer therapy. Vertebral and base of skull infections are the most common sites, whereas long bone infection is relatively rare.

The clinical presentation of *Aspergillus* infection depends on the site affected. Vertebral infection often presents with back pain and tenderness, but can progress to neurological symptoms and signs. Paraparesis is associated with particularly poor clinical outcomes. Base of skull infection may arise from adjacent sinus infection and is associated with headaches and nausea. Tinnitus, deafness, proptosis, peri-orbital cellulitis, and cranial nerve palsies might also occur. Long bone and joint infections usually give rise to local pain, tenderness, and swelling. Sinus tracts sometimes form, particularly with joint infections.

Systemic symptoms are often lacking, although low-grade fever and, in chronic cases, weight loss have been reported.

Diagnosis can be difficult, and in 75% of cases the finding of bone and joint infection is the first indication of invasive aspergillosis. Unlike *Candida* bone infection, it is extremely rare to have concurrent fungaemia, so blood cultures are almost always negative. While there is increasing literature on the use of galactomannan levels in the blood, or the use of PCR in peripheral blood, to diagnose invasive pulmonary aspergillosis, there are no data to suggest that these are of use in diagnosing musculoskeletal infections. Imaging is an important adjunct to diagnosis, with MRI the preferred modality. MRI might show bone inflammation or destruction and will show adjacent soft tissue involvement in about a quarter of cases. Such imaging is important to establish the presence of spinal cord compression in vertebral disease, or cavernous sinus involvement in base of skull infection. FDG PET-CT (18F-fluorodeoxyglucose positron emission tomography/computed tomography) might also be helpful for localizing disease, but there are insufficient data at present to indicate whether this type of imaging adds to the diagnostic process. Aetiological diagnosis is usually made by either percutaneous or CT-guided biopsy, or open surgical biopsy. Proven diagnoses with positive cultures are less common than with *Candida* infection so that up to half are diagnoses based on histology. The finding of calcium oxalate crystals in tissue has been associated with *A. niger* infection in one study (Shelton et al. 2002).

Treatment with antifungal agents needs to be targeted on the culture results whenever possible. Most experience suggests that the best outcomes result from a combination of good surgical debridement in combination with systemic antifungal therapy. The use of surgery is more likely to reduce the risk of relapse. There are no clinical trials to guide the choice of antifungal agent, and case series have not shown clear differences in outcomes related to different agents. However, current guidelines favour the use of voriconazole in this setting as voriconazole has been shown to have particularly good bone penetration (Stratov et al. 2003). The increasing concern about azole-resistant *Aspergillus* should be borne in mind, and every effort to obtain material for culture should be made (Verweij et al. 2016). There are no convincing data to suggest that using a combination of antifungal agents offers better outcomes. Equally, there are no data about duration of treatment, but consensus is that at least 90 days are required. As with bacterial joint infection, there is some evidence for the use of voriconazole-impregnated cement in the treatment of prosthetic joint infections (Miller et al. 2013).

Non-*Aspergillus* filamentous fungi

Although rare, moulds other than *Aspergillus* species sometimes cause bone and joint infections (Taj-Aldeen et al. 2015). Hyalohyphomycetes are the most common group and *Scedosporium*, *Lomentospora*, and *Fusarium* the most common genera causing musculoskeletal infection. Dematiaceous fungi, particularly *Alternaria* species and some of the Mucorales (which mostly cause rhinocerebral infection—see Chapter 24), such as *Rhizopus* species, are rarer causes. Lower limbs and the axial skeleton are the most common sites of infection. With these moulds, in contrast to *Candida* and *Aspergillus* infection, direct inoculation is more common as a cause of bone and joint infection, either through road traffic accidents with fractures, or contaminated penetrating wounds, or as a complication of surgery. Direct inoculation infection appears to be more common in children than adults. Haematogenous spread to bones and joints does occur with these moulds and is more common in adults than children, usually in the setting of some form of immunocompromise. Adults are more likely to have vertebral infections.

The clinical features depend on the site of infection but include local pain, tenderness, and swelling. Vertebral and base of skull infections might be associated with neurological symptoms and signs. Fever occurs in less than half of the cases but is more common in children than adults. As with other fungal infections of the bones and joints, inflammatory markers are often raised, but not to very high levels.

Diagnosis relies on adequate imaging, usually with MRI, along with appropriate biopsy specimens obtained either percutaneously or by surgery. Obtaining a good specimen for culture and identification to species level is particularly important because of the varying susceptibility of these fungi to the available antifungal agents. Whereas *Scedosporium apiospermum* will usually respond to voriconazole (Farina et al. 2006), the susceptibility of *Fusarium* species is variable, and these two species may be difficult to distinguish on histological grounds.

Treatment requires the appropriate antifungal agent along with adequate surgical debridement. This combination results in better survival rates than the use of antifungal agents alone. There are no data to prove that combining two antifungal agents leads to better outcomes, but this is sometimes reported to be effective, particularly in *Fusarium* infections.

Prevention of musculoskeletal infection due to non-*Aspergillus* moulds can be achieved by good surgical technique along with laminar flow in the operating room. Similarly, good surgical debridement after trauma or penetrating injuries might prevent the establishment of fungal infection.

Dimorphic fungi

Although a rare occurrence, there are a variety of dimorphic fungi that have affected bones and joints (Rammaert et al. 2014). (Table 20.1) Some, such as *Sporothrix schenckii*, particularly affect joints, whereas others, such as *Blastomyces dermatitidis*, predominantly cause osteomyelitis. Vertebral bodies are the most frequently involved bones, although long bones are also infected. Generally, only one vertebra is involved with infections due to *B. dermatitidis*, *Coccidioides* spp., and *Histoplasma capsulatum*, but infections with *S. schenckii* and *Talaromyces marneffei* usually involve multiple bones. *Emmonsia* species have not yet been reported to infect bones and joints.

Table 20.1 Osteoarticular infections due to dimorphic fungi

Fungus	Bone or joints commonly involved	Comorbidities common?	Treatment
Sporothrix schenckii	Vertebrae Long bones Joints	Yes	Amphotericin B Itraconazole
Histoplasma capsulatum	Long bones Large joints	No (HIV)	Ampho B Itraconazole
Blastomyces dermatitidis	Vertebrae Long bones Large joints	No (HIV)	Ampho B + 5-fluorocytosine Itraconazole
Talaromyces marneffei	Long bones Large joints	Yes (HIV)	Ampho B Itraconazole
Coccidioides immitis	Small bones Knee	No	Ampho B Fluconazole
Paracoccidioides brasiliensis	Long bones Large joints	No	Co-trimoxazole

Patient profiles also vary in terms of risks of particular fungal infections. Males seem to be more likely to be infected, and this could be because of increased rates of trauma, alcoholism, and HIV infection. Children are rarely infected with dimorphic fungi. *Sporothrix* infections frequently follow trauma but are also seen in patients with impaired immunity—particularly alcoholics and those with diabetes mellitus, and sometimes in those with HIV infection. Alcoholics seem more prone to disseminated disease. Bone infections due to *Blastomyces* or *Coccidioides* species usually occur in people without significant comorbidities. *Histoplasma capsulatum* var. *duboisii* can lead to bone infection in immunocompetent individuals, whereas *H. capsulatum* var. *capsulatum* bone infections are usually only seen in immunocompromised individuals. However, arthralgia and erythema nodosum have been described with *H. capsulatum* var. *capsulatum* in immunocompetent patients. HIV infection accounts for most cases of disseminated *T. marneffei* infections with arthritis and a considerable number of those with *H. capsulatum*. The former are often associated with skin lesions. With good treatment for HIV infection now becoming widespread, it can be expected that many of these infections will become less common. However, the use of immunosuppressive treatment in organ transplantation, for example, means that these dimorphic fungal infections will remain a problem. There is an increasing literature of these infections becoming reactivated during therapy with anti-TNF (tumour necrosis factor) agents, such as infliximab. There are also case reports of patients with HIV having immune reconstitution inflammatory syndrome and joint involvement with histoplasmosis.

As outlined in Table 20.1, the site of infection varies with the type of fungus. Generally, however, there is local tenderness, pain, or inflammation. Systemic features are unusual except in the case of disseminated disease, when the bone and joint involvement may not be the central focus. Many of these infections are subacute or chronic and there is a considerable delay in diagnosis as a consequence. Imaging studies, particularly MRI, are important in localizing the infection and its extent. In the setting of disseminated infection, involvement of the joint or bone may be inferred indirectly if the fungal infection is proven from a non-articular source. When the primary diagnosis is made from the bone or joint, this can be done either by direct culture from biopsies or surgical specimens, or by finding compatible histological features in the face of other clinical findings, along with appropriate serological tests.

Treatment of bone and joint infections caused by dimorphic fungi will depend on the organism isolated. Case series have shown that itraconazole or amphotericin B, either alone or sequentially, has resulted in good outcomes. The IDSA guidelines for treating *Sporothrix* bone and joint infections recommend itraconazole 200 mg twice daily for 12 months, with consideration given to initial treatment with liposomal amphotericin B (3–5 mg/kg per day) for two weeks, followed by itraconazole (Kauffman et al. 2007). Similar recommendations are made for *Blastomyces* and *Histoplasma* infections (Wheat et al. 2007). It is important to measure itraconazole levels early on to ensure correct dosing. In patients with immunosuppression that cannot be reversed, lifelong suppressive therapy with itraconazole is suggested.

In one series of bone and joint infections due to dimorphic fungi, mortality was as low as 6% and was largely related to underlying conditions such as advanced HIV disease. Surgical debridement can be a useful adjunct to antifungal therapy but may not always be needed, unlike in the case of mould infections. The role of the extended-spectrum azoles, such as voriconazole and posaconazole, has not been fully evaluated for bone and joint disease with these fungi, but their good bone penetration suggests that they are useful alternatives. For *Paracoccidioides brasiliensis* infection, itraconazole is currently recommended, although co-trimoxazole has been used successfully for many years in South America. There are no trials of the duration of therapy for any of these disorders, but guidelines suggest that at least 12 months should be the goal.

Cryptococcosis

Musculoskeletal infections with *Cryptococcus neoformans* are very rare. Although they usually occur in the setting of disseminated infection in immunocompromised patients, particularly in HIV infection (Burton et al. 2009), they can also occur in immunocompetent hosts (Al-Tawfij and Ghandour 2007). The portal of entry is usually via the lungs in either case. The spine, humerus, and skull seem to be the most common sites of infection, with osteomyelitis more common than septic arthritis. Bone lesions can be mistaken for bone tumours if there is no evidence of cryptococcal infection elsewhere (Chen et al. 2005). MRI scanning is the preferred imaging modality, but a definite diagnosis can only be made by culturing the fungus from a lesion. Positive blood cultures in association with bone lesions are clearly helpful. Although many patients with immunosuppression will have circulating cryptococcal antigen (CRAG), this might be absent in up to 35% of immunocompetent patients with cryptococcal disease. The IDSA guidelines recommend amphotericin B plus flucytosine (5-fluorocytosine) as initial treatment for two to three weeks, followed by high-dose fluconazole (Perfect et al. 2010). It is probable that high-dose fluconazole alone is sufficient for immunocompetent patients. The role of surgical debridement is not clear, but it may be needed for bone abscesses or spinal involvement.

Special settings

Intravenous drug users

The majority of infective complications seen in those who inject drugs are due to bacteria, predominantly *Staphylococcus aureus*. However, fungal infections do occur and often affect bones and joints. The most common problem is *Candida* infection of vertebrae, with the lumbar spine most likely to be involved. The propensity for *Candida* infections may stem from the common practice of licking needles prior to use, but was also, in the past, associated with the use of proprietary lemon juice to dissolve heroin before injection, with the juice colonized by *Candida*.

The candidaemia that results leads to initial infection of the intervertebral disc and involvement of the adjacent vertebrae (Figure 20.2). This can be an indolent process and might be associated with psoas abscesses. A small number of cases will also have bacterial infection at the same time. Fever is rarely present and the usual presentation is with back pain. In some cases, cord compression occurs so that neurological symptoms and signs appear. MRI or CT are the imaging choices that can then guide percutaneous or open biopsy. Cases usually present some time after the original candidaemia, but it is important to take blood cultures. In addition, these patients should have echocardiography to look for *Candida* endocarditis and an ophthalmic review to exclude endophthalmitis.

The mainstay of treatment in these cases is antifungal therapy, with surgery reserved for those who need debridement or spinal stabilization. Echinocandins or high-dose fluconazole are the treatments of choice, although compliance with an oral regimen can be a problem in this patient group. Any intravenous drug user diagnosed with *Candida* bone infection should have tests for blood-borne viruses.

HIV infection

Invasive fungal infections in the setting of HIV have become less common with the advent of better and more widely available antiretroviral therapy. Invasive *Candida* and *Aspergillus* infections are more common in HIV-infected patients, but the most common fungi causing bone and joint infections in this population are the dimorphic fungi. The risk of different fungi varies geographically, but the rise in global travel means that HIV-infected patients may

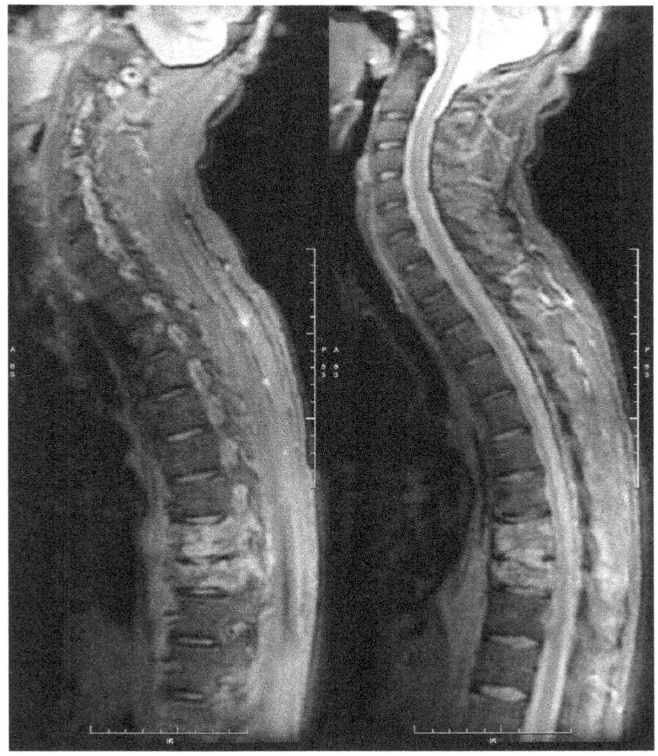

Figure 20.2 Discitis and osteomyelitis due to *Candida albicans* in an intravenous drug user.

present with a fungus that is not endemic in the area where they seek help. In essence, the clinical presentations do not differ materially from those seen in other patients with different immunodeficiencies. The management involves careful choice of antifungal agent so that drug interactions with antiretrovirals is minimized.

The other important issue to be borne in mind is the immune reconstitution inflammatory syndrome (IRIS), which is occasionally seen when patients are started on antiretroviral therapy but have subclinical infection with another organism (see Chapter 33). This is most commonly seen with tuberculosis but is well-described with fungal infections, particularly cryptococcosis and histoplasmosis. In this context, the improvement in T-cell function with antiretroviral treatment can lead to recognition of fungal antigens and a brisk inflammatory reaction. This can take the form of arthralgia or even arthritis and might be mistaken for fungal arthritis. In some settings, notably sub-Saharan Africa, patients are screened for CRAG (for cryptococcal disease) before the initiation of antiretroviral therapy in order to minimize the risk of IRIS.

Use of biological treatments

The use of biological agents, particularly anti-TNF therapies, is increasingly common. There are a large number of conditions for which these treatments are now used, but their use in rheumatological diseases is probably the most common. The risk of reactivation of tuberculosis is now well-described with these drugs, but there are also increasing numbers of reports of fungal joint infections in this setting. Diagnosis can be difficult to distinguish from a flare of joint disease, but consideration should be given to obtaining synovial fluid or synovial tissue for culture and ensuring that cultures are set up for fungi as well as mycobacteria and conventional bacteria.

Iatrogenic infection

Although a proportion of prosthetic joint infections occur as a result of haematogenous spread, some will be the result of nosocomial infection at the time of the implant. Physicians should be alert to unusual presentations of fungal infections acquired nosocomially. In 2012, a large outbreak of an unusual fungal infection was recognized in the United States associated with injections of methylprednisolone to treat back pain or inflammatory arthritis. Batches of the steroid were contaminated with a dematiaceous mould, *Exserohilum rostratum*, a rare human pathogen (Chiller et al. 2013). A large proportion of the more than 700 cases affected presented with fungal meningitis (see Chapter 22). About 20% had para-spinal abscesses, discitis, and vertebral osteomyelitis. Patients with meningitis presented earlier (average about two weeks) than those with bone involvement, and in the meningitis group the mortality was around 10%, mainly due to strokes. There were no reported deaths in those with only bone or disc involvement. Most patients were treated with either liposomal amphotericin B or voriconazole, or both. As experience grew, voriconazole became the agent of choice, largely because of better CNS penetration than with either itraconazole or posaconazole. A treatment of at least six months was recommended for those with bone involvement.

Prosthetic joint infections

Approximately 1% of prosthetic joint infections (PJIs) are of fungal aetiology, most commonly *Candida* species (Dutronc et al. 2010). As in *Candida* osteomyelitis, mixed infections are also observed—up to 15–20% (Tande and Patel 2014), commonly with Staphylococci (Kuiper et al. 2013). The risk factors for PJI are similar to those for all forms of invasive candidiasis (Box 20.1).

Diagnosis

Clinical and radiological signs are often similar to PJIs of bacterial cause, and the condition can be difficult to distinguish from aseptic loosening. Adequate sampling pre- and perioperatively is one of the most informative diagnostic tools in suspected PJI. Preoperatively, a synovial leukocyte count will help distinguish aseptic loosening from a low-grade infection, particularly in implants more than six months old. Culture of the synovial fluid may identify a causative organism if incubated for long enough in enrichment media such as blood culture bottles (Osmon et al. 2013).

Box 20.1 Risk factors for *Candida* prosthetic joint infections
Diabetes mellitus
Renal disease
Rheumatoid arthritis
Malignancy
Immunosuppression
Previous prosthetic joint infection
Malnutrition
Prolonged antimicrobial treatment
Vascular catheters

Intraoperatively, it is still advisable to collect at least five to six tissue samples to obtain optimal culture and positive histopathology results, with two to three positive cultures considered highly suggestive of infection (Atkins et al. 1998).

Like other organisms causing PJI, *Candida* (particularly *C. albicans*) can create a biofilm at the interface between implant and tissue, resulting in a different, more resilient phenotype. In the biofilm the organism is able to withstand antimicrobial therapy it would otherwise be susceptible to in its planktonic state (Kuhn et al. 2002), e.g. fluconazole. Removal of the infected implant is, therefore, almost always required for cure.

Treatment

Treatment requires a combination of antifungal agents with surgical intervention. Staged re-implantation is most associated with optimal outcome, with approximately 85% success (Dutronc et al. 2010; Kuiper et al. 2013), but more evidence is needed in this area. Conservative management has been seen as most likely to result in treatment failure (Kuiper et al. 2013).

Some studies have included implants with and without antifungal in cement. Most evidence is available for amphotericin B, particularly in older studies (Kuiper et al. 2013). However, voriconazole added to cement is also associated with good outcome (Miller et al. 2013), but doses are not consistent in these studies.

If the implant is removed, there is evidence that using a shorter duration of systemic antifungal therapy than for osteomyelitis will suffice. IDSA guidelines state that six weeks of treatment are appropriate (Pappas et al. 2016) and that oral fluconazole can be used owing to its good bioavailability. Caspofungin is also listed in the IDSA guidelines, but caution should be exercised in *C. parapsilosis* infections as the organism might be less susceptible.

Periostitis due to voriconazole

The increasing use of voriconazole has highlighted some of the adverse effects of this drug. Of particular relevance to this chapter is the increasing recognition that voriconazole usage, particularly long-term, can lead to bone pain and radiological periostitis. This could lead to confusion if patients have been prescribed this drug for musculoskeletal infections. This complication might be associated with drug-induced increases in fluoride blood levels (Moon et al. 2014).

References

Allan P, Stevens P, Chadwick P, et al. (2015) Osteomyelitis in adult patients on long-term parenteral nutrition: 2745 patient-years of experience in a national referral centre. *Clin Nutr* 35: 1135–9, http://dx.doi.org/10.1016/j.clnu.2015.09.002, accessed 1 June 2017.

Al-Tawfij JA and Ghandour J (2007) Cryptococcus neoformans abscess and osteomyelitis in an immunocompetent patient with tuberculous lymphadenitis. *Infection* 35: 377–82.

Atkins BL, Athanasou N, Deeks JJ, et al. (1998) Prospective evaluation of criteria for microbiological diagnosis of prosthetic-joint infection at revision arthroplasty. The OSIRIS Collaborative Study Group. *J Clin Microbiol* 36: 2932–9.

Burton R, Gogela N, Rebe K, McNally M and Meintjes G (2009) Cryptococcal immune reconstitution inflammatory syndrome presenting with erosive bone lesions, arthritis and subcutaneous abscesses. *AIDS* 23: 2371–3.

Chen J, Liu S, Xiong Z, et al. (2005) Cryptococcal infection of the femoral bone similar with pathological features of vascular tumors: a case report and review of literature. *Int J Clin Exp Pathol* 8: 8551–4.

Chia SL, Tan BH, Tan CT and Tan SB (2005) Candida spondylodiscitis and epidural abscess: management with shorter courses of anti-fungal therapy in combination with surgical debridement. *J Infect* 51: 17–23.

Chiller TM, Roy M, Nguyen D, et al. (2013) Clinical findings for fungal infections caused by methylprednisolone injections. *N Engl J Med* 369: 1610–19.

Delsing CE, Becker KL, Simon A, et al. (2015) Th-17 cytokine deficiency in patients with Aspergillus skull base osteomyelitis. *BMC Infect Dis* 15: 140. doi: 10.1186/s12879-015-0891-2

Dupont B and Drouhet E (1985) Cutaneous, ocular and osteoarticular candidiasis in heroin addicts: new clinical and therapeutic aspects in 38 patients. *J Infect Dis* 152: 577–91.

Dutronc H, Dauchy FA, Cazanave C, et al. (2010) Candida prosthetic infections: case series and literature review. *Scand J Infect Dis* 42: 890–5.

Farina C, Gotti E, Suter F and Goglio A (2006) *Scedosporium apiospermum* soft tissue infection: a case report and review of kidney transplant literature. *Transplant Proc* 38: 1333–5.

Gamaletsou MN, Kontoyiannis DP, Sipsas NV, et al. (2012) Candida osteomyelitis: analysis of 212 pediatric and adult cases (1970-2011). *Clin Infect Dis* 55: 1338–51.

Gamaletsou MN, Rammaert B, Bueno MA, et al. (2015) Candida arthritis: analysis of 112 pediatric and adult cases. *Open Forum Infect Dis* 3: ofv207.

Ganesh D, Gottlieb J, Chan S, Martinez O and Eismont F (2015) Fungal infections of the spine. *Spine* 40: E719–28.

Kauffman CA, Bustamante B, Chapman SW and Pappas PG (2007) Clinical practice guideline for the management of sporotrichosis: 2007 update by the Infectious Diseases Society of America. *Clin Infect Dis* 45: 1255–65.

Koehler P, Tacke D and Cornely OA (2014) Aspergillus of bones and joints—a review from 2002 until today. *Mycoses* 57: 323–35.

Kuhn DM, Chandra J, Mukherjee PK and Ghannoum MA (2002) Comparison of biofilms formed by Candida albicans and Candida parapsilosis on bioprosthetic surfaces. *Infect Immun* 70: 878–88.

Kuiper JW, van den Bekerom MP, van der Stappen J, et al. (2013) 2-stage revision recommended for treatment of fungal hip and knee prosthetic joint infections. Acta Orthop 84: 517–23.

Kumashi PR, Safdar A, Chamilos G, Chemaly RF, Raad II and Kontoyiannis DP (2006) Fungal osteoarticular infections in patients treated at a comprehensive cancer center: a 10-year retrospective review. *Eur J Clin Microbiol Infect Dis* 12: 621–6.

Miller RB, McLaren AC, Pauken C, et al. (2013) Voriconazole is delivered from antifungal-loaded bone cement. Clin Orthop Relat Res 471: 195–200.

Moon WJ, Scheller EL, Suneja A, et al. (2014) Plasma fluoride level as a predictor of voriconazole-induced periostitis in patients with skeletal pain. *Clin Infect Dis* 59: 1237–45.

Nyofytos D, Huprikar S, Reboli A, et al. (2014) Treatment and outcomes of Candida osteomyelitis: review of 53 cases from the PATH Alliance® registry. *Eur J Clin Microbiol Infect Dis* 33: 135–41.

Osmon DR, Berbari EF, Berendt AR, et al. (2013) Diagnosis and management of prosthetic joint infection: clinical practice guidelines by the Infectious Diseases Society of America. *Clin Infect Dis* 56: e1–25.

Pappas PG, Kauffman CA, Andes DR, et al. (2016) Clinical practice guideline for the management of candidiasis: 2016 update by the Infectious Diseases Society of America. *Clin Infect Dis* 62: 409–17.

Perfect JR, Dismukes WE, Dromer F, et al. (2010) Clinical practice guideline for the management of cryptococcal disease: 2010 update by the Infectious Diseases Society of America. *Clin Infect Dis* 50: 291–322.

Pfaller MA, Andes DR, Diekema DJ, et al. (2014) Epidemiology and outcomes of invasive candidiasis due to non-albicans species of Candida in 2,496 patients: data from the Prospective Antifungal Therapy (PATH) Registry 2004–2008. *PLOS One* 9: e101510.

Rammaert B, Gamaletsou MN, Zeller V, et al. (2014) Dimorphic fungal osteoarticular infections. *Eur J Clin Microbiol Infect Dis* 33: 2131–40.

Shelton JC, Antonelli PJ and Hackett R (2002) Skull base fungal osteomyelitis in an immunocompetent host. *Otolaryngol Head Neck Surg* 126: 76–8.

Slenker AK, Keith SW and Horn DL (2012) Two hundred and eleven cases of Candida osteomyelitis: 17 case reports and a review of the literature. *Diagn Microbiol Infect Dis* 73: 89–93.

Stratov I, Korman TM and Johnson PDR (2003) Management of aspergillus osteomyelitis: report of failure of liposomal amphotericin B and response to voriconazole in an immunocompetent host and literature review. *Eur J Clin Microbiol Infect Dis* 22: 227–83.

Taccone FS, Van den Abeele A-M, Bulpa P, et al. (2015) Epidemiology of invasive aspergillus in critically ill patients: clinical presentation, underlying conditions, and outcomes. *Crit Care* 19: 7.

Taj-Aldeen SJ, Rammaert B, Gamaletsou M, et al. (2015) Osteoarticular infections caused by non-Aspergillus filamentous fungi in adult and pediatric patients. A systematic review. *Medicine (Baltimore)* 94: e2078.

Tande AJ and Patel R (2014) Prosthetic joint infection. *Clin Microbiol Rev* 27: 302–45.

Verweij PE, Chowdhary A, Melchers WJG and Meis JF (2016) Azole resistance in Aspergillus fumigatus: can we retain the clinical use of mold-active antifungal azoles? *Clin Infect Dis* 62: 362–8.

Wheat LJ, Freifeld AG, Kleiman LB, et al. (2007) Clinical practice guideline for the management of patients with histoplasmosis: 2007 update by the Infectious Diseases Society of America. *Clin Infect Dis* 45: 807–25.

CHAPTER 21

Fungal cardiovascular infections

Sarah Drake and Jonathan Sandoe

Introduction to cardiovascular fungal infections

Cardiovascular fungal infections present as four main conditions.

1) Infective endocarditis

Infective endocarditis (IE) comprises a heterogeneous mixture of infections that can involve any part of the native endocardium (characteristically the heart valves), prosthetic heart valves, implantable cardiac electronic devices (ICEDs), and other implantable cardiac devices. IE is uncommon; a recent analysis in the United States (US) found an incidence of 12.7 cases per 100,000 population in 2009 (Bor et al. 2013). However, the incidence is increasing in both the US and the UK (Bor et al. 2013; Dayer et al. 2015). The pathological lesion of IE is a 'vegetation' which consists of microorganisms, fibrin, platelets, and other host/microbe-derived products. Bacteria cause the vast majority of IE cases, while fungi contribute 2–4% of cases (Gould et al. 2012).

2) Mycotic aneurysms

An aneurysm is an abnormal focal arterial dilation. Osler first coined the term 'mycotic aneurysm' in 1885 to describe a mushroom-shaped aneurysm that developed in a patient with IE (Osler 1885). Ironically the term 'mycotic' aneurysm is usually a misnomer as fungi are rarely the cause. A mycotic aneurysm refers to all extra-cardiac aneurysms of infective aetiology. They are a serious clinical condition, associated with significant morbidity and mortality. Mycotic aneurysms develop via several mechanisms: 1) haematogenous seeding during bacteraemia/fungaemia, 2) trauma to the arterial wall with direct contamination, 3) extension from a contiguous infected focus, or 4) secondary to septic microemboli.

3) Vascular graft infections

Vascular grafts are used to revascularize tissues deprived of a blood supply because of disease or trauma. They can be fashioned from native vascular material harvested from other body sites or made from man-made materials. Infection complicates graft implantation in 0.5–4% of patients (Darouiche 2004; Hobbs et al. 2010). These infections are associated with a high mortality (25–88% of cases) and amputation rate (5–25%) (Seeger 2000; Swain et al. 2004; O'Connor et al. 2006). Microbial contamination of vascular grafts can occur via several routes, including microbial seeding at the time of implantation, infection in a contiguous anatomic area, surgical site infection, or haematogenous spread. Fungal vascular graft infections are rare.

4) Intravascular catheter-related infections

Central venous catheters (CVCs) are being increasingly used to provide long-term venous access, but infection is a major, sometimes life-threatening, complication. Intravascular catheter-related bloodstream infection is the most common fungal cardiovascular infection.

Causative fungi

The fungal genera most often associated with cardiovascular infections are summarized in Table 21.1.

Candida and *Aspergillus* spp. account for the large majority of fungal IE cases (Ellis et al. 2001; Pierrotti and Baddour 2002). Although approximately 25% of fungal IE cases are caused by rare fungi (Ellis et al. 2001), publication bias may be responsible for this finding.

Epidemiology

Infective endocarditis

Fungal IE is rare. It is associated with several predisposing conditions, including: intravenous drug use (Sousa et al. 2012), indwelling medical devices, diabetes, renal disease, and malignancy (Baddley et al. 2008; Bongiorni et al. 2012). Mortality rates remain high particularly for mould-related IE (<20% survival) (Baddour et al. 2005).

Candida IE is usually a healthcare-associated infection (Falcone et al. 2009), frequently associated with short-term indwelling vascular catheters and prosthetic valves (Baddley et al. 2008). *Aspergillus* IE mostly follows cardiac surgery. It has occurred in clusters related to contaminated operating room air (Mehta 1990) and in association with high spore counts in a ward environment (Jensen et al. 2010). Fungi account for 0.4–2% of all ICED infections (Sandoe et al. 2015).

Mycotic aneurysms

Fungal mycotic aneurysms are extremely rare. Cases have occurred in patients with immune suppression (Fernandez and Morena 2005), following near drowning (Ortmann et al. 2010) and following treatment of disseminated fungal disease (Brunner et al. 2008).

Vascular graft infections

Fungal vascular graft infections are also rare, but possible predisposing factors include perianeurysmal fibrosis, multiple graft revisions,

Table 21.1 A summary of the fungal causes of cardiovascular infections

Infective endocarditis	Mycotic aneurysms	Vascular graft infections	Intravascular catheter-related infections
Candida spp.	*Candida* spp.	*Candida* spp.	*Candida* spp.
◆ *C. albicans*	*Cryptococcus* spp.	*Aspergillus* spp.	◆ *C. albicans*
◆ *C. parapsilosis*	*Aspergillus* spp.	*Penicillium* spp.	◆ *C. glabrata*
◆ *C. glabrata*	*Pseudallescheria boydii*	*Histoplasma capsulatum*	◆ *C. parapsilosis*
◆ *C. tropicalis*		*Mucorales*	◆ *C. tropicalis*
◆ *C. krusei*		Mycelia sterilia	◆ *C. krusei*
◆ *C. lusitaniae*			
◆ *C. zeylanoides*			
◆ *C. kefyr*			
◆ *C. guilliermondii*			
Aspergillus spp.			
Histoplasma capsulatum			
Talaromyces (Penicillium) spp.			
Mucorales			
Trichosporon spp.			
Paecilomyces spp.			
Lodderomyces elongisporus			
Fusarium spp.			
Exophiala dermatitidis			
Cryptococcus neoformans			
Pseudallescheria boydii			
Exophiala jeanselmei			
Curvularia lunata			
Trichophyton spp.			
Microsporum spp.			
Rhodotorula spp.			
Conidiobolus spp.			
Scedosporium spp.			
Engyodontium album			
Saccharomyces spp.			
Pichia anomala			
Phaeoacremonium parasiticum			
Acremonium spp.			
Phialemonium curvatum			
Microascus cinereus			
Bipolaris spicifera			
Scopulariopsis brevicaulis			

systemic fungal infection, and immunosuppression (Doscher et al. 1987).

Intravascular catheter-related infections

Fungi, especially *Candida* spp., account for 9% of systemic infections associated with CVCs (Wisplinghoff et al. 2004). Risk factors can be divided between host and catheter. Host factors include chronic illness, immunosuppression, total parenteral nutrition administration, and extremes of age (Tokars et al. 1999; Reunes et al. 2011). Catheter factors include location of catheter, duration, type of catheter material, conditions of insertion, and catheter site care.

Clinical features

Infective endocarditis

The clinical presentation of fungal IE is highly variable and there are no clinical features that reliably distinguish fungal and bacterial causes (Baddley et al. 2008). Patients with the former tend to be younger and have had cardiac surgery, recent broad-spectrum antibiotic treatment, and intravascular access devices (Pierrotti and Baddour 2002). The main presenting feature is fever (~90% of patients). This is often associated with systemic symptoms of chills, poor appetite, and weight loss. Heart murmurs are a common feature and new or changing murmurs occur in 77% of cases (Pierrotti and Baddour 2002). Peripheral stigmata of IE are increasingly uncommon outside the developing world, as patients tend to present at an early stage of disease (Murdoch et al. 2009).

The clinical features of ICED infections depend on which part of the device is infected. Generator pocket infections are characterized by localized inflammation (Klug et al. 2004; Uslan et al. 2007). This may progress to wound dehiscence, purulent discharge, skin erosion, or sinus formation (Sohail et al. 2008). Systemic signs of infection may also be present in generator pocket infections. ICED lead infections or ICED-IE cases often present with non-specific signs and symptoms of systemic infection such as fevers, chills, night sweats, malaise, and anorexia. Fewer than 10% of patients present with septic shock (Cacoub et al. 1998).

Mycotic aneurysms

The clinical presentation of fungal mycotic aneurysms does not appear to differ from bacterial cases and depends on the site of the aneurysm. For superficial locations (e.g. the common femoral artery), symptoms may include a painful, pulsatile, and enlarging mass, together with systemic features of infection such as fever (Johnson et al. 1983). For aneurysms located in deeper sites, such as the aorta, the aneurysm may not be palpable and may only be apparent on imaging. Patients with aortic or iliac aneurysms may present with abdominal or back pain, or alternatively, aneurysms may only present with fever of unknown origin, some of which may remain undiagnosed until rupture. Infected aneurysms of the intracranial vessels may present as a stroke or subarachnoid haemorrhage. If infected aneurysms remain undiagnosed they can lead to progressive infection, sepsis, thrombosis, or haemorrhage, with the manifestations depending on the location of the aneurysm.

Vascular graft infections

The clinical presentation of fungal vascular graft infections is highly variable, does not differ significantly from presentation with bacterial infection, and depends on when the infection develops post implantation. Symptoms of early graft infection (within three months of implantation) include surgical site infection, local abscess/sinus tract formation, haemorrhage, graft occlusion, pseudoaneurysm formation, and graft exposure. Septic emboli and distal tissue ischaemia may also be seen. Systemic signs of infection are generally present in the setting of fungaemia.

Late graft infections are more often characterized by graft healing complications than by systemic toxicity, including cutaneous sinus tracts, lack of graft incorporation by surrounding tissue, anastomotic aneurysms, and graft enteric erosions or the development of fistulae. Some patients exhibit little or no apparent inflammatory response. Other patients may develop local pain with or without a palpable mass. Aortic graft-related enteric erosions and fistulae can present with signs of systemic infection, abdominal pain, and gastrointestinal tract bleeding.

Intravascular catheter-related infections

Catheter-related bloodstream infection (CRBSI) should be suspected in patients with CVCs and symptoms or signs of systemic infection. Clinical manifestations include fever, inflammation, or purulence at the catheter insertion site, haemodynamic instability, altered mental state, catheter dysfunction and clinical signs of sepsis that start soon after catheter use. These clinical findings have poor sensitivity and specificity (Mermel et al. 2009). Clinical improvement following catheter removal suggests CRBSI, but this is insufficient for a definitive diagnosis (Mayhall 1992).

Diagnosis

Infective endocarditis

IE continues to be a diagnostic challenge because of the non-specific clinical features. Blood cultures and echocardiography are key investigations, and tools such as the Duke criteria and their modifications may assist in the diagnosis (Durack et al. 1994; Li et al. 2000).

In *Candida* IE, blood cultures are usually positive (Baddour et al. 2005). In contrast, blood cultures are rarely positive in *Aspergillus* IE, and it is usually diagnosed following culture or histology of excised heart valve tissue (Figure 21.1).

There is currently insufficient evidence to recommend the use of either *Candida* antibody or antigen testing in the diagnosis of IE (Gould et al. 2012).

Generator pocket infections are generally diagnosed based on clinical features at the site of the generator. Echocardiography is used to establish the presence of endocardial or pacing lead involvement and any complication of lead or valve infection (Figure 21.2). However, leads can be infected without lead vegetations being seen on echocardiography. Therefore, a negative scan does not rule out a diagnosis of ICED infection (Sandoe et al. 2015). Positive blood cultures are an important part of diagnosis.

Mycotic aneurysms

The diagnosis of fungal mycotic aneurysms has been based upon imaging the aneurysm and culturing a fungus from blood or aneurysm tissue (Kim 2010). Any patient with a positive blood culture and an arterial aneurysm should be considered to have a mycotic

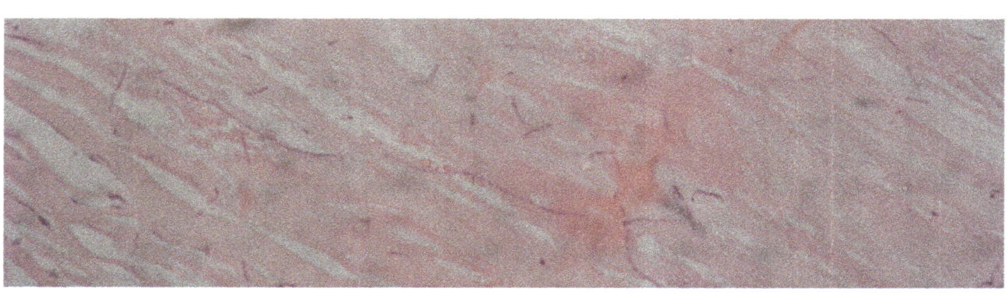

Figure 21.1 Fungal mycelia in heart valve tissue.

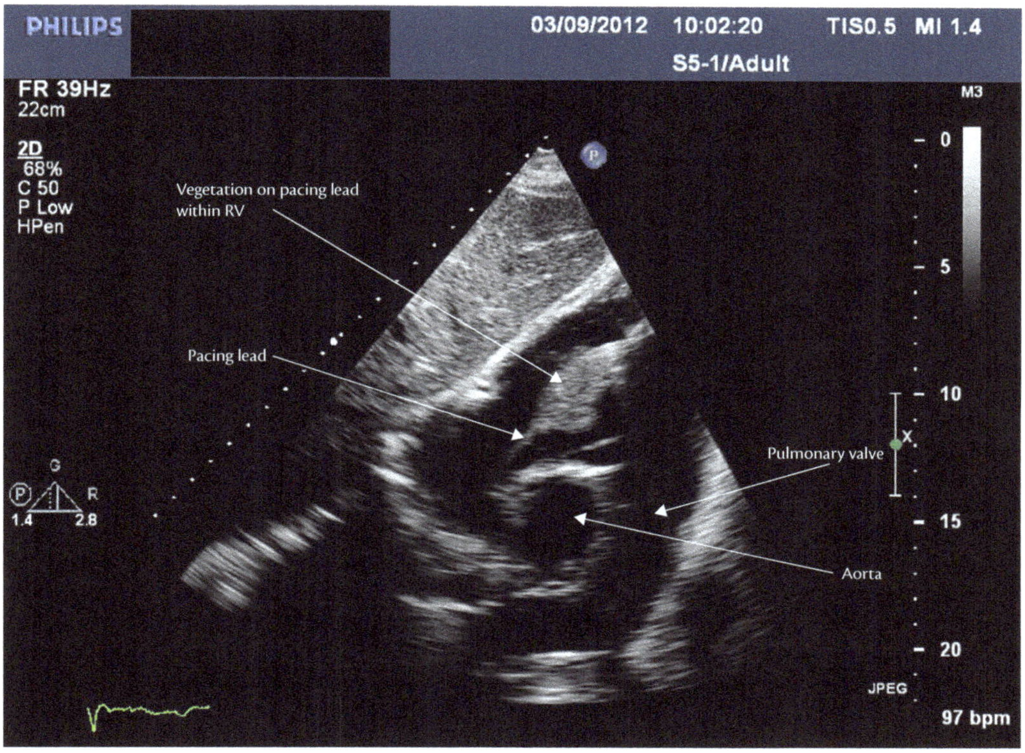

Figure 21.2 Echocardiographic image showing a vegetation attached to a pacemaker lead.
Image courtesy of Dr. Saif-El-Dean Abdel-Rahman.

aneurysm until proven otherwise, especially in the absence of any obvious source of infection.

Contrast-enhanced CT (computed tomography) scanning is a useful initial diagnostic test for investigating patients with suspected aortic aneurysms (Kim 2010). MRI (magnetic resonance imaging) can also be used, especially when contrast-enhanced CT is contraindicated (Walsh et al. 1997). More recently, 18F-fluorodeoxyglucose positron-emission tomography with CT scanning (FDG-PET/CT) has been applied to aid in the diagnosis of aneurysms (Reeps et al. 2008).

Vascular graft infections

There is no internationally accepted definition for prosthetic vascular graft infection and no agreed criteria to confirm the diagnosis. The diagnosis is usually made on the basis of clinical findings, supported by radiological and microbiological investigations. Appropriate samples for culture include explanted graft tissue and material aspirated from peri-graft collection. Blood cultures are often negative, particularly in the setting of late-onset infection (FitzGerald et al. 2005).

CT is a well-established imaging modality for the diagnosis of graft infections, with a reported sensitivity and specificity of 94% and 85%, respectively (Orton et al. 2000). CT may also permit the aspiration of infection fluid for culture in order to confirm the diagnosis and to guide appropriate antimicrobials. CT findings that support the diagnosis include ectopic gas, peri-graft fluid/inflammatory changes, anastomotic pseudoaneurysm, and thickening of adjacent bowel (Modrall and Clagett 1999). Other imaging modalities include MRI, ultrasonography, and FDG-PET/CT imaging.

Intravascular catheter-related infections

Diagnosis of fungal CRBSI requires demonstration of fungaemia and evidence that the catheter is involved. Microbiological confirmation of CRBSI can be established by meeting one of the following two criteria (Mermel et al. 2009): 1) culture of the same organism from both peripheral blood cultures and from the catheter tip, and 2) culture of the same organism from both the catheter and peripheral vein which meets the criteria for quantitative blood cultures or differential time to positivity (Raad et al. 2004; Safdar et al. 2005).

For quantitative blood cultures, a colony count from the catheter blood sample that is greater than, or equal to, three-fold higher than the colony count from the peripheral blood culture supports a diagnosis of CRBSI (Chatzinikolaou et al. 2004; Safdar et al. 2005). Differential time to positivity refers to growth detected from the catheter blood culture at least two hours before growth is detected from the peripheral sample. This method has a sensitivity of 85% and a specificity of 91% (Raad et al. 2004; Safdar et al. 2005). It should be noted that these criteria have not been specifically evaluated for fungi.

Treatment

Infective endocarditis

The management of fungal IE usually involves both medical and surgical therapy, the former being determined by the causative fungi and susceptibility testing.

For IE caused by susceptible *Candida* isolates, first-line therapy is either liposomal amphotericin B or an echinocandin (most experience is with caspofungin). Many authorities recommend the addition of flucytosine to amphotericin B (Gould et al. 2012). Surgical valve replacement is undertaken in approximately 50% of episodes (Baddley et al. 2008). Intravenous therapy is given for a minimum of four weeks, but prolonged follow-on or long-term suppressive oral therapy is advised. For example, for those with susceptible organisms and retained prosthetic material, long-term fluconazole may be appropriate (Pappas et al. 2009).

Surgical valve replacement is considered mandatory in *Aspergillus* IE, but it is challenging to establish the diagnosis pre-operation. Voriconazole is recommended as first-line therapy for IE caused by *Aspergillus* (Gould et al. 2012). In patients who cannot tolerate voriconazole, or where azole resistance has been documented, lipid-associated amphotericin B would be an appropriate alternative, possibly with flucytosine. For *Aspergillus* spp. resistant to amphotericin B (*A. terreus* and *A. nidulans*), oral posaconazole is an option (Gould et al. 2012).

Cases of endocarditis caused by other fungi form a very heterogeneous group lacking standardized treatment options.

ICED infections caused by fungi are rare and there are currently no guidelines for treatment. Antifungal therapy is based on the causative fungi identified and susceptibilities. There has been documented success in curing a *Candida* ICED infection with anidulafungin with the device *in situ* (Glockner 2011), but removal is usually required.

Mycotic aneurysms

Treatment of mycotic aneurysms usually requires antimicrobial therapy combined with surgical debridement with or without revascularization (Reddy et al. 1991). Antifungals should be tailored to culture and susceptibility results. Optimal duration of antifungal therapy is uncertain, but at least six months of intravenous and/or oral therapy is often administered, depending on surgical management (Wilson et al. 2016).

Vascular graft infections

There are no guidelines with regards to the treatment of prosthetic graft infections; fungal vascular graft infections are usually managed on a case-by-case basis. Treatment ideally involves complete graft excision and local debridement followed by extra-anatomical bypass revascularization through a non-infected field (McKinsey 1995). However, this procedure is associated with significant mortality and morbidity (Kimmel et al. 1994; Henke et al. 1998). Other treatment methods include conservative treatment (i.e. antimicrobials alone), drainage, removal of graft and drainage, removal of graft, and *in situ* reconstruction.

Antifungal therapy is a vital adjunct to surgical management where fungi are involved, usually guided by culture and susceptibility results. While there is no evidence to guide duration of therapy, six weeks of intravenous therapy followed by up to six months of oral therapy has been recommended (FitzGerald et al. 2005) as long-term suppressive therapy (Wilson et al. 2016).

Intravascular catheter-related infections

Several studies have investigated the outcomes of candidaemia and the impact of CVC removal. Most have shown that CVC retention was associated with a worse outcome (Nguyen et al. 1995; Rex et al. 1995; Hung et al. 1996; Nucci et al. 1998; Karlowicz et al. 2000; Almirante et al. 2005). While a retrospective data review showed no benefit of early catheter removal (Nucci et al. 2010), a subsequent analysis of seven randomized controlled trials of candidaemia therapy demonstrated a significant impact on mortality with CVC removal (Andes et al. 2012). Unfortunately, it is unlikely that a definitive study of this issue will ever be performed, given the difficulties of patient selection bias, randomization, and severity of illness that all impact in such a patient group. Current guidelines continue to recommend catheter removal where possible, and this seems unlikely to change (Brass and Edwards 2010).

Antifungal therapy is recommended for all cases (Nucci et al. 1998). For candidaemia caused by azole-susceptible *Candida albicans*, fluconazole 400 mg daily for 14 days from the first negative blood culture is appropriate (Mermel et al. 2009). This regimen has been shown to be equivalent to the use of amphotericin B in the treatment of candidaemia (Rex et al. 1994), but may be less effective than treatment with echinocandins (Reboli et al. 2007). For *Candida* spp. with decreased susceptibility to azoles (e.g. *C. glabrata* and *C. krusei*), echinocandins or lipid formulations of amphotericin B (Ambisome) have been shown to be highly effective (Mora-Duarte et al. 2002; Kuse et al. 2007; Reboli et al. 2007). Indeed, echinocandins are now recommended as first-line therapy in candidaemia in some international guidelines (Cornely et al. 2012).

Antifungal lock therapy is still under investigation and is not routinely recommended (Mermel et al. 2009). Where catheters cannot be removed, antifungal agents, which have an impact on biofilm formation, such as lipid formulations of amphotericin B or echinocandins, are probably appropriate (Cornely 2012).

Patients with candidaemia should undergo examination to exclude *Candida* endophthalmitis. Echocardiography is also recommended for all patients with candidaemia. Follow-up blood cultures should be obtained to ensure clearance of *Candida* from the bloodstream. It is recommended that cultures be taken every other day until they become negative (Pappas et al. 2009).

Prevention

Infective endocarditis

Specific antifungal prophylaxis for patients at increased risk of IE is not recommended. As CVCs are a risk factor for fungal IE, measures to reduce fungal CRBSI should reduce the risk of subsequent IE. Fungal ICED infections are so rare that antifungal prophylaxis is not recommended as routine prophylaxis for ICED insertion (Sandoe et al. 2015).

Mycotic aneurysms

Prevention of these rare and poorly understood events is not currently a realistic proposal.

Vascular graft infections

Measures to prevent the development of fungal prosthetic graft infections centre on meticulous aseptic surgical technique and postoperative wound care.

Intravascular catheter-related infections

Preventive measures for fungal CRBSI are derived from general infection prevention methods and include: strict aseptic technique during catheter insertion and subsequent use, avoiding groin insertion where possible, ensuring proper catheter site care, ensuring removal of catheters when no longer essential and optimal antimicrobial stewardship to reduce use of broad-spectrum antibacterial agents that predispose to fungal infection (O'Grady et al. 2002, 2003, 2011; Schiffer et al. 2013).

References

Almirante B, Rodriguez D, Park BJ, et al. (2005) Epidemiology and predictors of mortality in cases of *Candida* bloodstream infection: results from population-based surveillance, Barcelona, Spain, from 2002 to 2003. *J Clin Microbiol* 43: 1829–35.

Andes DR, Safdar N, Baddley JW, et al. (2012) Impact of treatment strategy on outcomes in patients with candidemia and other forms of invasive candidiasis: a patient-level quantitative review of randomized trials. *Clin Infect Dis* 54: 1110–22.

Baddley JW, Benjamin DK Jr, Patel M, et al. (2008) International Collaboration on Endocarditis-Prospective Cohort Study Group (ICE-PCS). *Candida* infective endocarditis. *Eur J Clin Microbiol Infect Dis* 27: 519–29.

Baddour LM, Wilson WR and Bayer AS (2005) Infective endocarditis: diagnosis, antimicrobial therapy, and management of complications: a statement for healthcare professionals from the Committee on Rheumatic Fever, Endocarditis, and Kawasaki Disease, Council on Cardiovascular Disease in the Young, and the Councils on Clinical Cardiology, Stroke, and Cardiovascular Surgery and Anesthesia, American Heart Association: endorsed by the Infectious Diseases Society of America. *Circulation* 111: e394–434.

Bongiorni MG, Tascini C, Tagliaferri E, et al. (2012) Microbiology of cardiac implantable electronic device infections. *Europace* 14: 1334–9.

Bor DH, Woolhandler S, Nardin R, Brusch J and Himmelstein DU (2013) Infective endocarditis in the U.S., 1998-2009: a nationwide study. *PLoS One* 8: e60033.

Brass EP and Edwards JE (2010) Should the guidelines for management of central venous catheters in patients with candidemia be changed now? *Clin Infect Dis* 51: 304–6.

Brunner S, Engelmann MG and Näbauer M (2008) Thoracic mycotic pseudoaneurysm from Candida albicans infection. *Eur Heart J* 29: 1515.

Cacoub P, Leprince P, Nataf P, et al. (1998) Pacemaker infective endocarditis. *Am J Cardiol* 82: 480–4.

Chatzinikolaou I, Hanna H, Hachem R, Alakech B, Tarrand J and Raad I (2004) Differential quantitative blood cultures for the diagnosis of catheter-related bloodstream infections associated with short- and long-term catheters: a prospective study. *Diagn Microbiol Infect Dis* 50: 167–72.

Cornely OA, Bassetti M, Calandra T, et al. (2012) ESCMID Fungal Infection Study Group. ESCMID guideline for the diagnosis and management of Candida diseases 2012: non-neutropenic adult patients. *Clin Microbiol Infect* 18 (Suppl. 7): 19–37.

Darouiche RO (2004) Treatment of infections associated with surgical implants. *N Engl J Med* 350: 1422–9.

Dayer MJ, Jones S, Prendergast B, Baddour LM, Lockhart PB and Thornhill MH (2015) Incidence of infective endocarditis in England, 2000-13: a secular trend, interrupted time-series analysis. *Lancet* 385: 1219–28.

Doscher W, Krishnasastry KV and Deckoff SL (1987) Fungal graft infections: case report and review of the literature. *J Vasc Surg* 6: 398–402.

Durack DT, Lukes AS and Bright DK (1994) New criteria for diagnosis of infective endocarditis: utilization of specific echocardiographic findings. Duke Endocarditis Service. *Am J Med* 96: 200–9.

Ellis ME, Al-Abdely H, Sanbridge A, Greer W and Ventura W (2001) Fungal endocarditis: evidence in the world literature, 1965-1995. *Clin Infect Dis* 32: 50–62.

Falcone M, Barzaghi N, Carosi G, et al. (2009) Italian study on endocarditis. Candida infective endocarditis: report of 15 cases from a prospective multicenter study. *Medicine (Baltimore)* 88: 160–8.

Fernandez B and Morena O (2005) Mycotic aneurism in aortic arch by Aspergillus fumigatus: contribution of a case and review of the literature. *An Med Interna* 22: 437–40.

FitzGerald SF, Kelly C and Humphreys H (2005) The diagnosis and treatment of prosthetic aortic graft infections: confusion and inconsistency in the absence of consensus. *J Antimicrob Chemother* 56: 996–9.

Glockner A (2011) Recurrent candidaemia and pacemaker wire infection with Candida albicans. *Mycoses* 54 (Suppl. 4): 20–3.

Gould FK, Denning DW, Elliott TS, et al. (2012) Guidelines for the diagnosis and antibiotic treatment of endocarditis in adults: a report of the Working Party of the British Society for Antimicrobial Chemotherapy. *J Antimicrob Chemother* 67: 269–89.

Henke PK, Bergamini TM, Rose SM, et al. (1998) Current options in prosthetic vascular graft infection. *Am Surg* 64: 39–46.

Hobbs SD, Kumar S and Gilling-Smith GL (2010) Epidemiology and diagnosis of endograft infection. *J Cardiovasc Surg (Torino)* 51: 5–14.

Hung CC, Chen YC, Chang SC, Luh KT and Hsieh WC (1996) Nosocomial candidemia in a university hospital in Taiwan. *J Formos Med Assoc* 95: 19–28.

Jensen J, Guinea J, Torres-Narbona M, et al. (2010) Post-surgical invasive aspergillosis: an uncommon and under-appreciated entity. *J Infect* 60: 162–7.

Johnson JR, Ledgerwood AM and Lucas CE (1983) Mycotic aneurysm. New concepts in therapy. *Arch Surg* 118: 577–82.

Karlowicz MG, Hashimoto LN, Kelly RE Jr and Buescher ES (2000) Should central venous catheters be removed as soon as candidemia is detected in neonates? *Pediatrics* 106: E63.

Kim YW (2010) Infected aneurysm: current management. *Ann Vasc Dis* 3: 7–15.

Kimmel RM, Murphy RX Jr and Chowdary RP (1994) Optimal management of inguinal vascular graft infections. *Ann Plast Surg* 32: 623–9.

Klug D, Wallet F, Lacroix D, et al. (2004) Local symptoms at the site of pacemaker implantation indicate latent systemic infection. *Heart* 90: 882–6.

Kuse ER, Chetchotisakd P, da Cunha CA, et al. (2007) Micafungin versus liposomal amphotericin B for candidaemia and invasive candidosis: a phase III randomised double-blind trial. *Lancet* 369: 1519–27.

Li JS, Sexton DJ, Mick N, et al. (2000) Proposed modifications to the Duke criteria for the diagnosis of infective endocarditis. *Clin Infect Dis* 30: 633–8.

McKinsey JF (1995) Extra-anatomic reconstruction. *Surg Clin North Am* 75: 731–40.

Mayhall CG (1992) Diagnosis and management of infections of implantable devices used for prolonged venous access. *Curr Clin Top Infect Dis* 12: 83–110.

Mehta G (1990) Aspergillus endocarditis after open heart surgery: an epidemiological investigation. *J Hosp Infect* 15: 245–53.

Mermel LA, Allon M, Bouza E, et al. (2009) Clinical Practice Guidelines for the Diagnosis and Management of Intravascular Catheter-Related Infection: 2009 Update by the Infectious Diseases Society of America. *Clin Infect Dis* 49: 1–45.

Modrall JG and Clagett GP (1999) The role of imaging techniques in evaluating possible graft infections. *Semin Vasc Surg* 12: 339–47.

Mora-Duarte J, Betts R, Rotstein C, et al. (2002) Comparison of caspofungin and amphotericin B for invasive candidiasis. *N Engl J Med* 347: 2020–9.

Murdoch DR, Corey GR, Hoen B, et al. (2009) Clinical presentation, etiology, and outcome of infective endocarditis in the 21st century: the International Collaboration on Endocarditis-Prospective Cohort Study. *Arch Intern Med* 169: 463–73.

Nguyen MH, Peacock JE Jr, Tanner DC, et al. (1995) Therapeutic approaches in patients with candidemia. Evaluation in a multicenter, prospective, observational study. *Arch Intern Med* 155: 2429–35.

Nucci M, Anaissie E, Betts RF, et al. (2010) Early removal of central venous catheter in patients with candidemia does not improve outcome: analysis of 842 patients from 2 randomized clinical trials. *Clin Infect Dis* 51: 295–303.

Nucci M, Colombo AL, Silveira F, et al. (1998) Risk factors for death in patients with candidemia. *Infect Control Hosp Epidemiol* 19: 846–50.

O'Connor S, Andrew P, Batt M, et al. (2006) A systematic review and meta-analysis of treatments for aortic graft infection. *J Vasc Surg* 44: 38–45.

O'Grady NP, Alexander M, Burns LA, et al. (2011) Guidelines for the prevention of intravascular catheter-related infections. *Clin Infect Dis* 52: 162–93.

O'Grady NP, Alexander M, Dellinger EP, et al. (2002) Guidelines for the prevention of intravascular catheter-related infections. *Centers for Disease Control and Prevention. MMWR Recomm Rep* 51: 1–29.

O'Grady NP, Gerberding JL, Weinstein RA and Masur H (2003) Patient safety and the science of prevention: the time for implementing the Guidelines for the prevention of intravascular catheter-related infections is now. *Crit Care Med* 31: 291–2.

Ortmann C, Wüllenweber J, Brinkmann B and Fracasso T (2010) Fatal mycotic aneurysm caused by Pseudallescheria boydii after near drowning. *Int J Legal Med* 124: 243–7.

Orton DF, LeVeen RF, Saigh JA, et al. (2000) Aortic prosthetic infections: radiologic manifestations and implications for management. *Radiographics* 20: 977–93.

Osler W (1885) The Gulstonian lectures on malignant endocarditis. *Br Med J* 1: 467–70.

Pappas PG, Kaufmann CA, Andes D, et al. (2009) Clinical Practice Guidelines for the Management of Candidiasis: 2009 Update by the Infectious Diseases Society of America. *Clin Infect Dis* 48: 503–35.

Pierrotti LC and Baddour LM (2002) Fungal endocarditis, 1995–2000. *Chest* 122: 302–10.

Raad I, Hanna HA, Alakech B, Chatzinikolaou I, Johnson MM and Tarrand J (2004) Differential time to positivity: a useful method for diagnosing catheter-related bloodstream infections. *Ann Intern Med* 140: 18–25.

Reboli AC, Rotstein C, Pappas PG, et al. (2007) Anidulafungin versus fluconazole for invasive candidiasis. *N Engl J Med* 356: 2472–82.

Reddy DJ, Shepard AD, Evans JR, Wright DJ, Smith RF and Ernst CB (1991) Management of infected aortoiliac aneurysms. *Arch Surg* 126: 878–9.

Reeps C, Essler M, Pelisek J, Seidl S, Eckstein HH and Krause BJ (2008) Increased 18F-fluorodeoxyglucose uptake in abdominal aortic aneurysms in positron emission/ computed tomography is significantly associated with inflammation, aortic wall instability, and acute symptoms. *J Vasc Surg* 48: 417–23.

Reunes S, Rombaut V, Vogelaers D, et al. (2011) Risk factors and mortality for nosocomial bloodstream infections in elderly patients. *Eur J Intern Med* 22: 39–44.

Rex JH, Bennett JE, Sugar AM, et al. (1994) A randomized trial comparing fluconazole with amphotericin B for the treatment of candidemia in patients without neutropenia. Candidemia Study Group and the National Institute. *N Engl J Med* 331: 1325–30.

Rex JH, Bennett JE, Sugar AM, et al. (1995) Intravascular catheter exchange and duration of candidemia. NIAID Mycoses Study Group and the Candidemia Study Group. *Clin Infect Dis* 21: 994–6.

Safdar N, Fine JP and Maki DG (2005) Meta-analysis: methods for diagnosing intravascular device-related bloodstream infection. *Ann Intern Med* 142: 451–66.

Sandoe JAT, Barlow G, Chambers JB, et al. (2015) Guidelines for the diagnosis, prevention and management of implantable cardiac electronic device infection. *J Antimicrob Chemother* 70: 325–59.

Schiffer CA, Mangu PB, Wade JC, et al. (2013) Central venous catheter care for the patient with cancer: American Society of Clinical Oncology clinical practice guideline. *J Clin Oncol* 31: 1357–70.

Seeger JM (2000) Management of patients with prosthetic vascular graft infection. *Am Surg* 66: 166–77.

Sohail MR, Uslan DZ, Khan AH, et al. (2008) Infective endocarditis complicating permanent pacemaker and implantable cardioverter-defibrillator infection. *Mayo Clin Proc* 83: 46–53.

Sousa C, Botelho C, Rodrigues D, et al. (2012) Infective endocarditis in intravenous drug users: an update. *Eur J Clin Microbiol Infect Dis* 31: 2905–10.

Swain TW III, Calligaro KD and Dougherty MD (2004) Management of infected aortic prosthetic grafts. *Vasc Endovascular Surg* 38: 75–82.

Tokars JI, Cookson ST, McArthur MA, Boyer CL, McGeer AJ and Jarvis WR (1999) Prospective evaluation of risk factors for bloodstream infection in patients receiving home infusion therapy. *Ann Intern Med* 131: 340–7.

Uslan DZ, Sohail MR, St Sauver JL, et al. (2007) Permanent pacemaker and implantable cardioverter defibrillator infection: a population-based study. *Arch Intern Med* 167: 669–75.

Walsh DW, Ho VB and Haggerty MF (1997) Mycotic aneurysm of the aorta: MRI and MRA features. *J Magn Reson Imaging* 7: 312–15.

Wilson WR, Bower TC, Creager MA, et al. (2016) Vascular Graft Infections, Mycotic Aneurysms, and Endovascular Infections: A Scientific Statement From the American Heart Association. *Circulation* 134: e412–e460.

Wisplinghoff H, Bischoff T, Tallent SM, Seifert H, Wenzel RP and Edmond MB (2004) Nosocomial bloodstream infections in US hospitals: analysis of 24,179 cases from a prospective nationwide surveillance study. *Clin Infect Dis* 39: 309–17.

CHAPTER 22

Fungal central nervous system infections

Tihana Bicanic and Thomas S. Harrison

Introduction to CNS fungal diseases

Infections of the central nervous system (CNS) are amongst the most devastating and difficult-to-treat of invasive fungal infections. Incidence is rising in the context of increasing at-risk populations owing to increasingly sophisticated iatrogenic immunosuppression and the global HIV (human immunodeficiency virus) epidemic. Infection can involve any part of the CNS, but distinctive clinical syndromes offer clues to specific fungal aetiologies. Clinical suspicion, early diagnosis, prompt institution of appropriate antifungal therapy, management of complications, and restoration of host immunity are key elements in mitigating the high morbidity and mortality associated with these infections.

Causative fungi

Cryptococcus neoformans is an important global cause of adult meningitis, and in high HIV prevalence countries, is much more frequent than bacterial causes (Jarvis et al. 2010). *C. gattii* is generally confined to the tropics, although it has recently emerged in the Northwest of North America (Ma et al. 2009). *Candida* spp. cause meningitis in premature babies and those with prosthetic material (shunts or drains) in the CNS. The dimorphic fungi *Histoplasma, Blastomyces, Coccidioides, Paracoccidioides,* and *Talaromyces* (*Penicillium*) spp. cause meningitis in endemic areas. Mould CNS infections usually present as intracranial mass lesions: common pathogens are *Aspergillus* spp. and the mucormycetes (*Rhizopus, Mucor, Lichtheimia*), whilst *Fusarium* spp., *Scedosporium* spp., and the dematiaceous (pigmented) moulds are less common (Table 22.1).

Epidemiology

For most fungi, the respiratory tract is the usual portal of entry. Spores or desiccated yeasts inhaled into the lung cause an initial pulmonary infection, the outcome of which, determined by pathogen virulence and the underlying immune status of the host, is either clearance of infection, control and latency with dissemination upon subsequent immunosuppression, local progression, or haematogenous dissemination to multiple organs, including the brain. Direct fungal inoculation into the CNS can also occur through trauma, surgery, or contaminated injections, as highlighted by the recent US outbreak of meningitis due to epidural methylprednisolone injections contaminated with the black-pigmented mould *Exserohilum rostratum*, causing 751 cases of meningitis and resulting in 64 deaths (Smith et al. 2013).

The vast majority of CNS fungal infections are opportunistic infections in profoundly immunocompromised hosts. In general, phagocytic dysfunction predisposes to CNS aspergillosis, mucormycosis, and candidiasis, while cell-mediated immune defects, such as in advanced HIV (CD4 count <200 cells/uL), predispose to meningitis due to *Cryptococcus neoformans* and the dimorphic fungi (Table 22.1). In haematopoietic stem cell transplant recipients, there is a bimodal peak in the risk of fungal infection during the first 100 days and during episodes of graft-versus-host disease (Kontoyiannis et al. 2010). In solid organ transplant (SOT) recipients, disease can be either secondary (reactivation) or primary infection, including from the donor organ itself, with infections presenting up to several years post transplant (Pappas et al. 2010). Other risk factors include receipt of prolonged high-dose corticosteroids and TNF-α inhibitors, diabetes, and iron overload (Table 22.1).

Immunocompetent hosts can develop CNS fungal infection: sinocranial *Aspergillus* infections in India usually occur in immunocompetent hosts, whilst cryptococcal meningitis in China occurs largely in non-HIV-infected individuals (Zhu et al. 2010). Inherited defects in innate immunity are known to predispose to invasive fungal infection (Lionakis 2012). Recent studies have highlighted Fc-ϒ receptor and mannose-binding lectin polymorphisms and anti-GM-CSF (granulocyte-macrophage colony-stimulating factor) antibodies as risk factors for cryptococcal meningitis in apparently healthy hosts (Meletiadis et al. 2007; Ou et al. 2011; Saijo et al. 2014). Clinical involvement of the CNS occurs in 5–20% of extrapulmonary infections with the dimorphic fungi (Wheat et al. 1990; Bariola et al. 2010) in residents of endemic areas, including in apparently immunocompetent hosts.

Clinical features

Two main clinical syndromes are the usual presenting feature of CNS fungal infection: subacute or chronic meningitis (Figure 22.1) or brain abscess (Figure 22.2) (Scully et al. 2008). Meningitis usually arises following haematogenous spread, whilst brain abscesses can be as a result of direct extension from adjacent sinuses, mastoid bone or the orbits into the frontal or temporal lobes, or haematogenous spread, when multiple abscesses can be seen. Rhino-orbital-cerebral involvement is more common

Table 22.1 Fungal organism, host risk factor, clinical presentation, and recommended antifungal and adjunctive treatment in CNS fungal infection

Fungal genera	Common causative organisms	Host risk factors	Clinical presentation	Recommended treatment	Adjunctive therapies
Candida	*C. albicans*	Broad-spectrum antibiotics; prematurity; presence of ventricular drain/shunt	Meningitis with microabscesses	Liposomal AmB (L-AmB) 3–5 mg/kg/day plus 5-FC followed by fluconazole	Removal of infected ventricular devices
Cryptococcus	*C. neoformans* *C gattii*	HIV, SOT (lung), glucocorticoids Anti GM-CSF antibodies	Meningoencephalitis	AmB deoxycholate 0.7–1 mg/kg/day, or L-AmB (3–6 mg/kg/day), plus 5-FC 25 mg/kg q.d.s. followed by fluconazole	Immunotherapy unproven and dependent on host status: IFN-gamma in HIV-associated CM
Histoplasma	*H. capsulatum*	HIV, SOT, anti TNF-alpha therapies	Meningitis	L-AmB 5 mg/kg followed by itraconazole	
Coccidioides	*C. immitis* *C. posadasii*	HIV, SOT, anti-TNF-alpha therapies	Meningitis	Fluconazole 400–1,200 mg/day or AmBd 0.7–1 mg/kg/day	Intrathecal AmBd 0.1–1.5 mg used by some practitioners as adjunct to fluconazole
Blastomyces	*B. dermatitidis*	DM, HIV, SOT, glucocorticoids, anti-TNF-alpha therapies	Meningitis (scans may mimic TBM) or brain abscess, extraneural skin, lung, or prostate involvement	L-AmB 5 mg/kg/day, step-down to itraconazole or voriconazole	
Talaromyces (Penicillium)	*T. marneffei*	HIV (SE Asia)	Meningitis Umbilicated skin lesions in 50%	AmB deoxycholate followed by itraconazole	
Aspergillus	*A. fumigatus*	Neutropenia, HSCT, glucocorticoids (systemic or paraspinal), SOT	Brain abscess (direct or haematogenous spread) with focal deficits and seizures Meningitis rare	Voriconazole IV 6 mg/kg b.i.d. loading, then 4mg/kg b.i.d. (use TDM)	Some authorities may consider addition of echinocandin initially
Mucorales	*Mucor circinelloides* *Rhizopus oryzae* *Lichtheimia corymbifera*	DM, iron overload, neutropenia, IVDU, glucocorticoids, HSCT, SOT	Brain abscess (direct spread): commonly aggressive sino-orbital disease, complicated by cavernous sinus thrombosis with multiple cranial nerve palsies	L-AmB 5–7.5mg/kg/day, step-down to posaconazole	Control of DM; Deferasirox not effective in RCT; Surgical resection
Fusarium	*F. solani*	Prolonged neutropenia, HSCT, SOT	Stroke-like presentation; Skin and peri-ungual lesions are a diagnostic clue; Bilateral endophthalmitis	L-AmB 5–7.5 mg/kg/day plus voriconazole until susceptibility known	Surgical resection
Scedosporium	*S. apiospermum* *S. prolificans*	HSCT, SOT *S. apiospermum*: near drowning *S. prolificans*: trauma	Similar to *Aspergillus*	*S. apiospermum*: voriconazole *S. prolificans*: voriconazole plus terbinafine	Surgical resection
Dematiaceous (melanized) moulds (phaeo-hyphomycosis)	*Cladophialophora bantiana* *Rhinocladiella mackenziei* *Exophiala dermatitidis* *Exserohilum rostratum*	One-third immunocompetent Trauma, inoculation, SOT, corticosteroids	Brain abscess (direct or haematogenous) *E. rostratum*: meningitis, arachnoiditis	L-AmB 3–5 mg/kg/ day combined with voriconazole	Surgical resection

AmBd amphotericin B deoxycholate; b.i.d. = twice a day; CM = cryptococcal meningitis; DM = diabetes mellitus; 5-FC = 5-fluorocytosine (flucytosine); GM-CSF = granulocyte-macrophage colony-stimulating factor; HIV = human immunodeficiency virus; HSCT = haematopoietic stem cell transplant; IFN = interferon; IV = intravenous; IVDU = intravenous drug use; L-AmB = liposomal amphotericin B; q.d.s. = four times a day; RCT = random controlled trial; SOT = sold organ transplant; TBM = tuberculous meningitis; TDM = therapeutic drug monitoring; TNF tumour necrosis factor

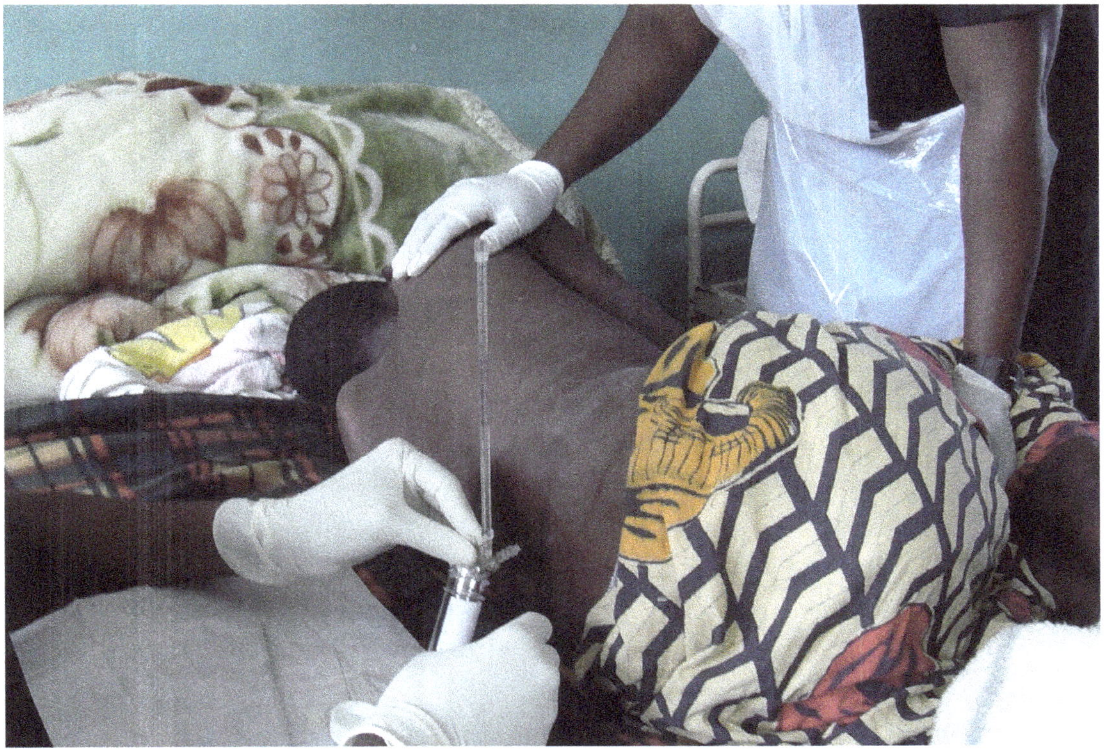

Figure 22.1 Lumbar puncture showing measurement of CSF opening pressure in a patient with cryptococcal meningitis.
Reproduced courtesy of Tihana Bicanic and Thomas S. Harrison.

in mucormycosis, whilst skull base involvement can follow sinus aspergillosis (Murthy 2007) (Table 22.2). Owing to its anatomical location, infection of the ethmoid sinus, in particular, can be complicated by cavernous sinus thrombosis and eye involvement, resulting in catastrophic visual loss.

Fungal meningitis presents with meningism (headache, neck stiffness and photophobia) of subacute onset, which may or may not be accompanied by fever. This may be associated with altered mental status (confusion or reduced conscious level, seizures, personality change)—a feature of accompanying brain involvement (encephalitis) and indicative of a poor prognosis in cryptococcal meningitis (Bicanic et al. 2009). Although usually due to the yeasts or the dimorphic fungi, *Aspergillus* spp. can also cause meningitis (Antinori et al. 2013).

Brain abscesses present with signs and symptoms of a space-occupying lesion (focal neurology, seizures). Frontal or temporal lobe abscesses should prompt a search for pre-existing fungal sinus or middle ear disease that may be amenable to biopsy and surgical debridement. Stroke-like presentations may be seen with infection with angio-invasive moulds such as

Table 22.2 CNS clinical syndromes by organism

Fungal infection	Meningitis	Brain abscess (mass lesions)	Rhino-orbital-cerebral	Skull base syndrome	Stroke syndrome	Spinal syndrome
Aspergillosis	+	++	+	+++	+	+
Mucormycosis	–	++	+++	+	+	–
Cryptococcosis	+++	+	–	–	+	+
Phaeohyphomycosis	+	+++	–	–	–	+
Candidiasis	+	+/–	–	–	+	–
Histoplasmosis	+	+	–	–	+	+
Coccidioidomycosis	+	–	–	–	+	–
Blastomycosis	+	+	–	–	–	+

Adapted with permission from Murthy J., 'Fungal infections of the central nervous system: the clinical syndromes', *Neurology India*, Volume 55, Issue 3, pp. 221–5, Copyright © 2007 Wolters Kluwer Medknow Publications. DOI: 10.4103/0028-3886.35682

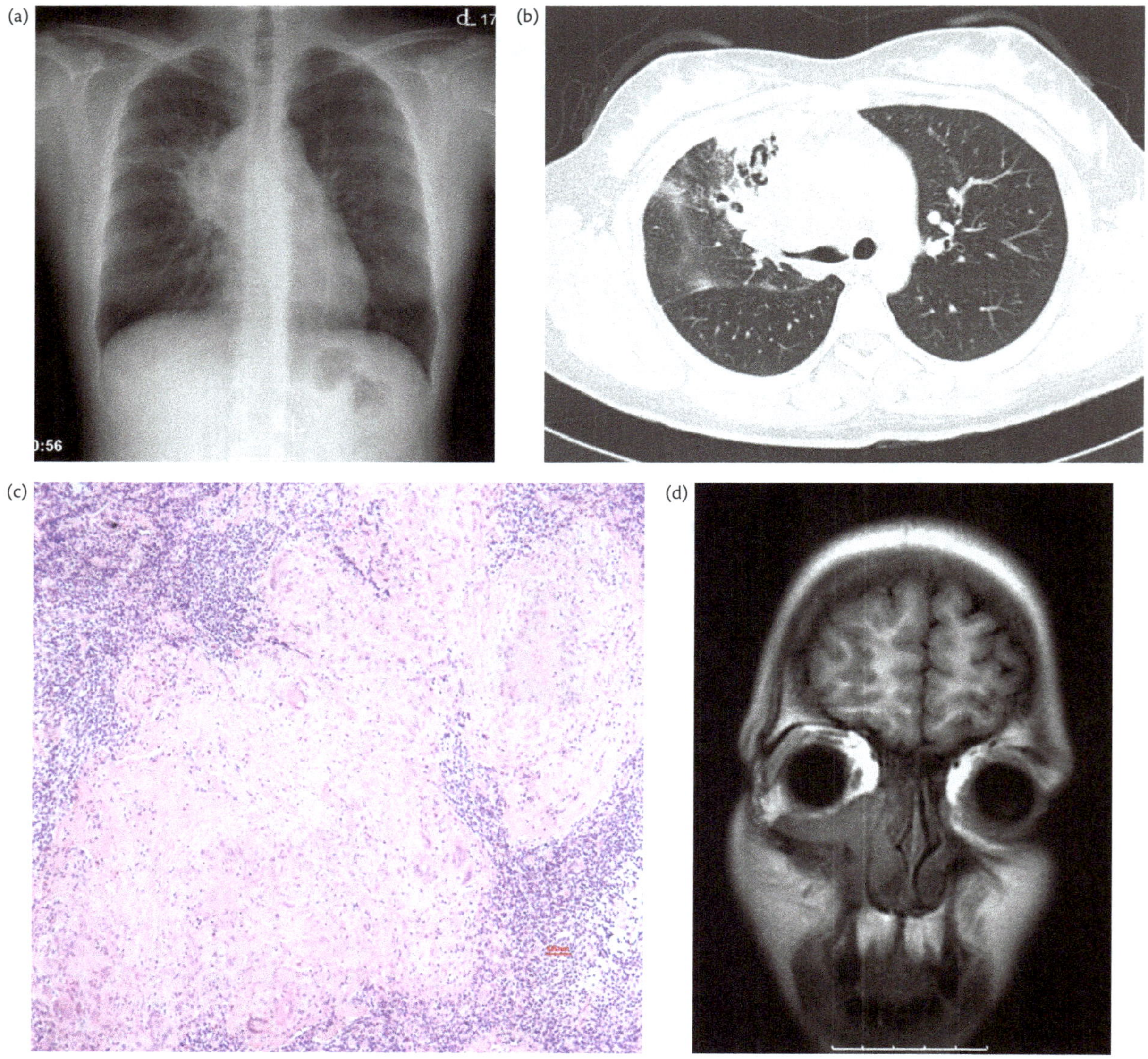

Figure 22.2 Disseminated aspergillosis involving lung, sinuses, orbit, and brain: 24-year-old immunocompetent patient from India. Initially asymptomatic with chest radiograph (**a**) and chest computed tomography image (**b**) showing right hilar lymphadenopathy with right upper lobe bronchiectasis.

c Mediastinoscopy and paratracheal lymph node biopsy showed non-necrotizing granulomata, microscopy, and cultures negative for tuberculosis; fungal stains not done. Later developed cough, treated with prednisolone for suspected sarcoidosis for three months before developing right eye swelling and left-sided hemiparesis.

d Coronal MRI demonstrates bulky abnormal soft tissue inferiorly within right nasal cavity and ethmoid air cells invading the right orbit and resulting in exophthalmos.

e T2-weighted MRIs of the brain (three slices) show multiple enhancing lesions within the right cerebral hemisphere, cerebellum, and lower medulla (one with associated mass effect and midline shift).

f Orbital biopsy ×600 magnification (haematoxylin & eosin stain, left; Grocott stain, right) shows narrow, septate hyphae with dichotomous (Y-shaped) branching. Cultures grew *Aspergillus flavus*. Patient was treated successfully with two weeks' intravenous voriconazole and anidulafungin followed by oral voriconazole for 12 months, with complete neurological recovery.

Reproduced courtesy of Tihana Bicanic and Thomas S. Harrison.

Aspergillus spp. owing to secondary thrombosis and haemorrhagic infarction, vasculitis with *Cryptococcus* and *Coccidioides* spp., and embolic events during *Candida* infective endocarditis (Table 22.2).

Less commonly, CNS fungal infections can present as myelopathy or myeloradiculopathy secondary to intramedullary or epidural abscesses, or spinal arachnoiditis. The upper thoracic spine may be affected by contiguous spread of lung aspergillosis, and blastomycosis may cause vertebral osteomyelitis. In the *Exserohilum rostratum* meningitis outbreak, when the organism was inoculated into the CNS contained within an immunosuppressive steroid carrier, spinal arachnoiditis was common, resulting in cauda equina syndrome and urinary retention, as well as posterior circulation strokes (Lyons et al. 2012).

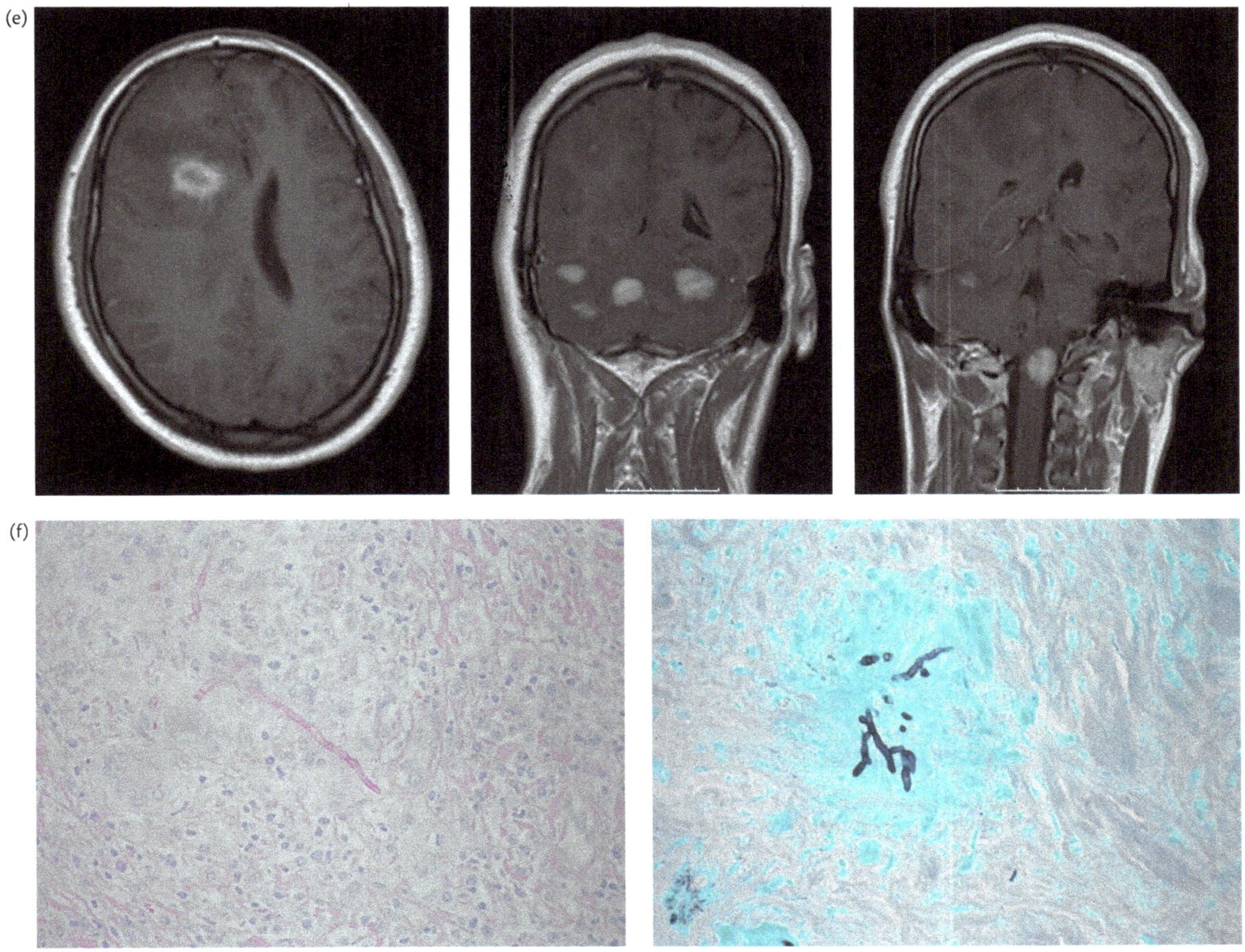

Figure 22.2 (Continued)

Diagnosis

CNS fungal infection should be considered in any at-risk host presenting with neurologic symptoms and signs. Given their poor prognosis, early consideration of fungal CNS infection in the differential diagnosis and obtaining appropriate samples for culture and histology are critical. Diagnosis requires close liaison between colleagues working in infectious diseases and microbiology, ENT (ear, nose & throat) services, neurosurgery, and histopathology.

While computed tomography (CT) of the brain may demonstrate single or multiple brain lesions and sinus or mastoid disease, MRI (magnetic resonance imaging) of the brain is the neuroimaging modality of choice. Fungal brain lesions are typically located at the grey-white matter junction (Starkey et al. 2014). Masses may show post-contrast ring enhancement and associated oedema (Figure 22.2e). Differential diagnosis includes bacterial abscesses, toxoplasmosis, tuberculosis, and primary and secondary malignancy. Infarction and/or haemorrhage may be seen with angio-invasive moulds. In HIV-associated cryptococcal meningitis, scan appearances can be unremarkable even in the context of markedly raised intracranial pressure (ICP), though dilated Virchow-Robin spaces and gelatinous pseudocysts (cryptococcomas) can occur (Figure 22.3) (Loyse et al. 2015). *Candida* CNS infection manifests as enhancing microabscesses (<3 mm) in the context of candidaemia. Coccidioidal meningitis causes contrast enhancement of the basal cisterns. Blastomycosis and histoplasmosis cause leptomeningeal enhancement and multifocal small (<2 cm) enhancing lesions (Starkey et al. 2014). Imaging may also reveal a fungal source outside the CNS, notably chest and sinuses (Figure 22.2a, b, d), allowing access to more readily and safely obtainable diagnostic specimens.

For patients with suspected fungal meningitis, unless there are contraindications, lumbar puncture should be performed with measurement of cerebrospinal fluid (CSF) opening pressure using a manometer (and therapeutic drainage in patients with cryptococcal meningitis [CM]; Figure 22.1). Typical CSF findings are a lymphocytic pleocytosis (though neutrophils, eosinophils, or a mixed picture may also be seen), moderately raised protein, and a low glucose level. In any high-risk host with meningitis, an adequate volume of CSF (at least 5–10 mL) should be cultured on fungal media (Sabouraud dextrose) at 30°C for 14–21 days.

Fungal-specific tests on CSF include the use of India ink to diagnose cryptococcal meningitis (Figure 22.4). The pan-fungal marker (1→3) β-D-glucan may be useful for diagnosing or excluding a fungal CNS infection (with the exception of mucormycoses and probably cryptococcosis) (Lyons et al. 2015).

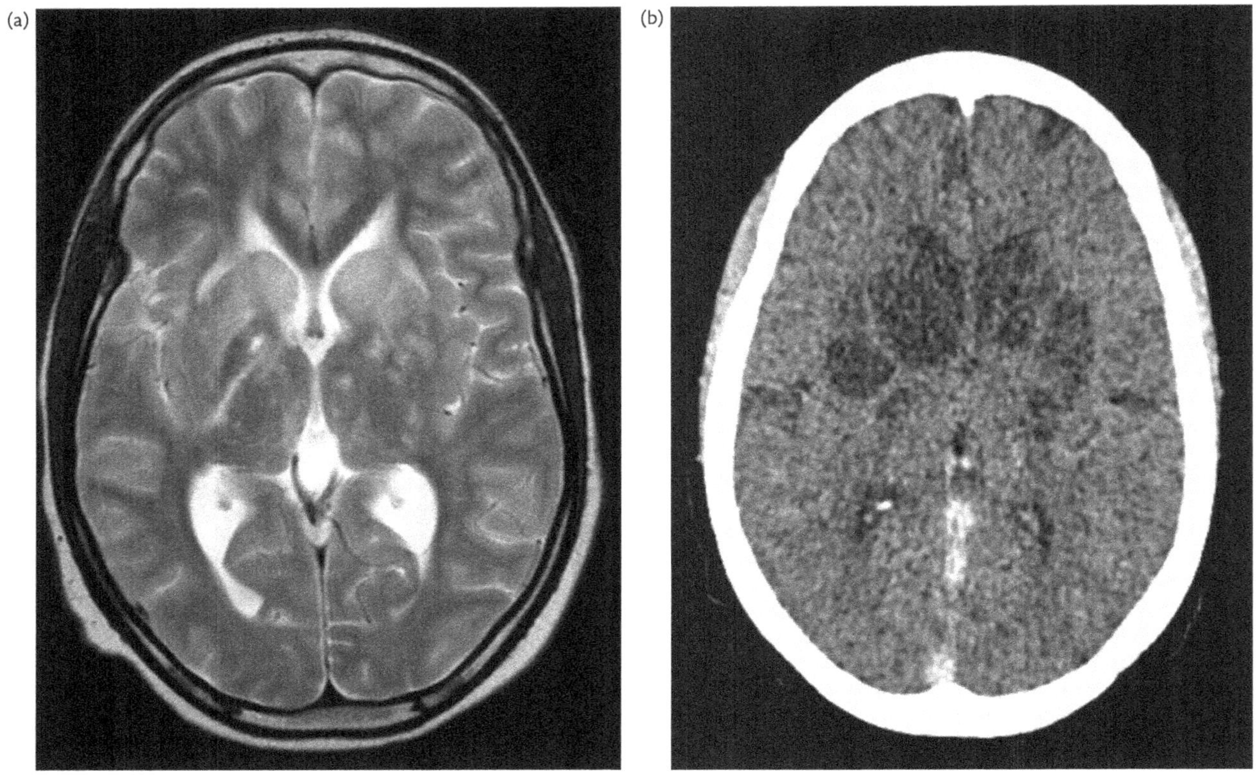

Figure 22.3 **a** Axial T2-weighted magnetic resonance image of brain of HIV-infected patient with cryptococcal meningitis showing multiple abnormally dilated perivascular (Virchow-Robin) spaces in the basal ganglia, thalamus, and internal capsules. Spaces are distended owing to collections of mucoid capsular material; larger collections can form large gelatinous pseudocysts, as seen in the computed tomography scan of the brain (**b**).
Reproduced courtesy of Tihana Bicanic and Thomas S. Harrison.

Cryptococcal and *Histoplasma* antigen assays are highly sensitive and specific for blood and CSF (Jarvis et al. 2011). These antigens are also present in urine but false positives occur when the cryptococcal antigen test is used on urine. Both have been developed as point-of-care lateral flow assays for bedside diagnosis (Immuno-Mycologics Inc, Norman OK; Figure 22.5). CSF culture is insensitive for *Blastomyces dermatitidis*: the antigen test is useful but is not widely available and has cross-reactivity with *Histoplasma capsulatum* (Bariola et al. 2010). CSF galactomannan has a higher sensitivity than *Aspergillus* culture (Klont et al. 2004; Soeffker et al. 2013). *Aspergillus* PCR is also available, but currently lacks a standardized platform. If antigen tests are unavailable, *Histoplasma* serology (immunodiffusion and complement fixation tests) on serum and CSF can be useful, but may be falsely negative in severe immunocompromise, or cross-react with other fungi. If both serology and cultures are negative in a high-risk host, application of a pan-fungal PCR—for example, of the 18S rRNA gene—to tissue or CSF samples, coupled with a genus-specific PCR, may identify the fungal pathogen (Khot and Fredricks 2009).

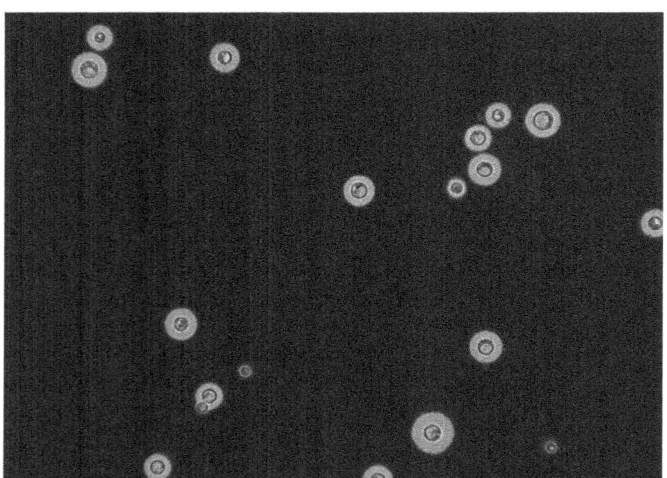

Figure 22.4 Diagnosis of cryptococcal meningitis by India ink stain (showing capsular 'halo' around yeast cells).
Reproduced courtesy of Tihana Bicanic and Thomas S. Harrison.

Blood cultures may yield the yeasts or the dimorphic fungi, though the latter can take weeks to grow and should be cultured in specialized mycobacterial/fungal blood culture bottles. In patients with focal lesions that are neurosurgically accessible, definitive diagnosis through tissue biopsy of brain or meninges is important to determine the likely aetiology and guide treatment. On histology, the H&E (haematoxylin & eosin) stain may show granulomatous inflammation and the presence of identifying features such as yeast budding, capsule, hyphae (septation and branching), and pigment (dematiaceous fungi). The fungal-specific stains Grocott silver, PAS (periodic acid-Schiff), mucicarmine (capsule), and Masson-Fontana (melanin) may further aid identification.

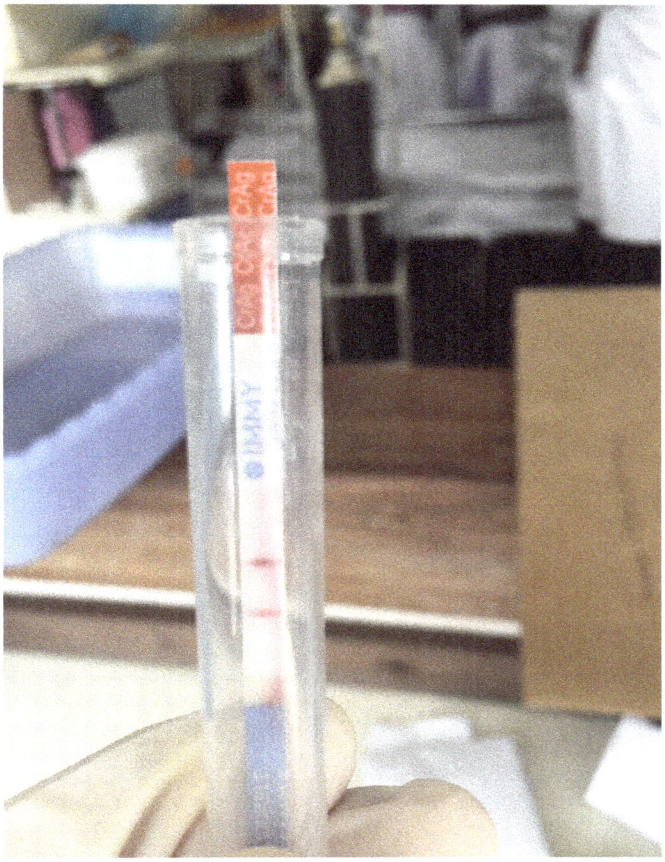

Figure 22.5 The point-of-care cryptococcal antigen lateral flow diagnostic assay can be used on blood or cerebrospinal fluid at the bedside.
Reproduced courtesy of Tihana Bicanic and Thomas S. Harrison.

Treatment

The CNS is an immune-privileged site with difficult penetration by antifungals. Despite improvements in antifungal therapy and host immune restoration therapies, outcomes of CNS fungal infections remain poor, with disease-specific mortality of up to 70%. Those that survive may be left with permanent focal neurological deficits, or visual or hearing loss. Treatment is often prolonged—for 6–12 months or longer—and initially given intravenously to achieve highest drug levels, followed by step-down to an oral azole for the continuation phase. Aside from cryptococcal meningitis, recommendations for treating CNS mycoses are usually supported by case series and expert opinion rather than data from adequately powered randomized controlled trials. For most CNS mycoses, an amphotericin B (AmB) preparation is the first-line agent, with the exception of CNS aspergillosis, where voriconazole is preferred (McCarthy et al. 2014) (Table 22.1).

Selection of an antifungal agent for CNS infections must incorporate both microbiological and pharmacokinetic parameters. Local epidemiology, including resistance patterns and prior antifungal exposure, is important to consider when selecting empiric therapy. If cultures are available, selection of drug must be tailored according to susceptibility testing.

Achieving adequate drug concentrations in the CNS is an important goal. There is marked variability in CNS penetration of antifungals (Table 22.3). Moreover, the CNS is not a single compartment: whilst CSF penetration may be poor (although this may be higher in the presence of meningitis), brain tissue concentrations generally exceed this and are a better predictor of antifungal efficacy (Kethireddy and Andes 2007). In the case of AmB (and its lipid preparations) with very low CSF penetration, levels in brain parenchyma have been shown to be above minimum inhibitory concentrations for common fungal pathogens. As penetration reflects a ratio of CSF:serum concentrations, drugs such as liposomal AmB, with much higher serum concentrations than the other formulations of AmB, may well achieve higher absolute brain tissue levels (Groll et al. 2000). Historically, clinicians have tried to overcome the low CSF penetration by administering AmB intrathecally, reported in both cryptococcal and coccidioidal meningitis, but this route is not generally recommended owing to the risk of local toxicities, including chemical arachnoiditis, seizures, and radiculopathy, and the higher parenchymal concentrations achieved using the intravenous route (Galgiani et al. 2005; Perfect et al. 2010). Flucytosine (5-fluorocytosine) has excellent CSF penetration and is synergistic with AmB against *Candida* and *Cryptococcus* spp.; thus, combination therapy is recommended for meningitis due to these organisms (Pappas et al. 2009; Perfect et al. 2010).

The azoles voriconazole and fluconazole are highly orally bioavailable, small molecular weight, moderately lipophilic molecules which both achieve CSF penetration of 50% or greater, making them useful for long-term therapy of CNS infection (Table 22.3) (Kethireddy and Andes 2007). Voriconazole is the first-line agent for CNS aspergillosis (Walsh et al. 2008), and fluconazole is used in the long-term treatment of cryptococcal and coccidioidal meningitis. Itraconazole and the newer posaconazole are larger, highly protein-bound, lipophilic molecules, with resultant poor CSF penetration (<1%) (Table 22.3). Nevertheless, brain concentrations of hydroxyl-itraconazole, an active metabolite of itraconazole, were found to be approaching those of serum in a murine *Histoplasma* meningitis model, and therapeutic efficacy was similar to that of fluconazole in cryptococcal, *Coccidioides*, and *Histoplasma* meningitis models (Kethireddy and Andes 2007). Brain penetration of posaconazole is unknown; however, again despite its negligible penetration into CSF, the efficacy of this drug has similarly been demonstrated in animal models of CNS infection and it has been successfully used to treat a range of human CNS fungal infections (Pitisuttithum et al. 2005). The echinocandins are very large molecular weight, protein-bound molecules with undetectable CSF concentrations, yet brain parenchymal penetration with this class of antifungal drugs is a little higher (Table 22.3). The drugs have shown therapeutic efficacy in animal CNS infection models, with demonstrable dose-microbiological responses in a *Candida* meningoencephalitis rabbit model (Hope and Drusano 2009). Although echinocandins are not recommended as first-line treatment in CNS infection, they have been used in combination with other antifungal classes and in salvage therapy.

With the exception of cryptococcal meningitis, where the superior effectiveness of the combination of amphotericin B and flucytosine has been demonstrated in a randomized trial (Day et al. 2013), there are no clinical trial data to support the use of combination antifungal therapy for CNS fungal infection. Combination therapy using voriconazole plus an echinocandin appeared to be more effective than voriconazole alone in a randomized trial of

Table 22.3 Antifungal drug CNS pharmacokinetics, therapeutic drug monitoring, and relevant drug interactions

Antifungal drug (class)	Route of administration	CSF penetration	Brain penetration	Therapeutic drug monitoring (TDM)*	Drug-drug interaction by class
Amphotericin B deoxycholate	IV	<1%	3–18%	–	
Liposomal AmB	IV	<5%	3%—superior to that of other lipid formulations	–	
Flucytosine (5-fluorocytosine)	IV/PO	75%		Not routinely needed when used in HIV-associated CM for 2 weeks. Recommended, if available, in renal impairment or suspected toxicity, or if 5-FC used for >2 weeks	
Fluconazole	IV/PO	40–80%	50–100%		
Voriconazole	IV/PO	60–100%	Brain biopsies show drug concentrations above/near MIC_{90} for common fungal pathogens	Aim for trough concentration of >2 mg/L and <5.5 mg/L, or a trough:MIC ratio of 2–5. Perform TDM 2–5 days after starting therapy and regularly thereafter	Levels decreased by anti-epileptics, rifamycins (rifampicin and rifabutin), some antiretrovirals Levels increased by some antiretrovirals, OCP, and proton pump inhibitors
Itraconazole	IV/PO	<1%	Concentrations of active metabolite hydroxyl-itraconazole approaching that of serum	Aim for trough >0.5 mg/L 5–7 days after starting therapy	Levels decreased by anti-epileptics, rifamycins, some antiretrovirals, H2 blockers, and proton pump inhibitors Levels increased by clarithromycin and most protease inhibitors
Posaconazole	PO	<1%	No data	Aim for trough >1 mg/L 7 days after starting therapy	Levels decreased by anti-epileptics, H2 blockers, and proton pump inhibitors Long list of drugs increasing levels; toxicity not a concern
Echinocandins	IV	0	10–20%	–	

* All ranges for therapeutic drug monitoring apply to concentrations in serum.

AmB = amphotericin B; CM = cryptococcal meningitis; 5-FC = 5-fluorocytosine; HIV = human immunodeficiency virus; IV = intravenous; MIC = minimum inhibitory concentration; OCP = oral contraceptive pill; PO = *per os* (orally); TDM = therapeutic drug monitoring

invasive aspergillosis, and some authorities would use the combination initially in patients with CNS aspergillosis (Marr et al. 2015). Combination therapy using a polyene with an azole should be used for CNS phaeohyphomycosis and fusariosis (AmB plus voriconazole) (Revankar et al. 2004; McCarthy et al. 2014) and is an option in cryptococcal meningitis (AmB plus fluconazole [Day et al. 2013]). In rhino-orbital-cerebral mucormycosis, murine data and a retrospective clinical case series lend some support to the combination of amphotericin B with an echinocandin (Spellberg et al. 2012a), whilst the iron chelator deferasirox, which showed promise as adjunctive therapy to amphotericin B in murine models, was ultimately unsuccessful in a clinical trial (Spellberg et al. 2012b). An oral combination of fluconazole and flucytosine is currently being trialled in HIV-associated cryptococcal meningitis in Africa, where amphotericin B is often not available (http://www.isrctn.com/ISRCTN45035509).

Therapeutic drug monitoring (TDM) is recommended for all azoles except fluconazole. Voriconazole in particular has large inter- and intra-patient pharmacokinetic variability, and higher trough levels are recommended in CNS infection (>2 mg/L, as compared with >1 mg/L for non-CNS invasive fungal infections) (Ashbee et al. 2014). TDM may also have a role in preventing toxicity of azoles and flucytosine (Table 22.3). Voriconazole liver toxicity may be associated with the higher doses used in CNS infection, so regular monitoring is required. Neurological symptoms and signs, serial imaging in the case of brain abscesses, and serial lumbar punctures to track biomarkers in the fungal meningitides can be used to monitor treatment response. In HIV-associated cryptococcal meningitis, microbiological clearance of the organism from CSF using serial quantitative cultures has been shown to correlate with survival and risk of relapse, whereas serial cryptococcal antigen (CRAG) testing is less useful as raised titres may persist for months (Jarvis et al. 2014). Other potentially useful treatment response CSF fungal biomarkers include *Histoplasma* antigen (Wheat et al. 2007), CSF galactomannan indices (Soeffker et al. 2013), and *Coccidioides* complement-fixing antibody titres (Galgiani et al. 2005). Serial β-D-glucan levels showed utility in monitoring clinical response in the *Exserohilum* meningitis outbreak (Litvintseva et al. 2014).

In terms of complications, raised intracranial pressure secondary to communicating hydrocephalus is common in patients with cryptococcal meningitis and is associated with potentially reversible visual and hearing loss. This must be managed with daily high-volume therapeutic lumbar punctures (Perfect et al. 2010). In CNS fungal infections involving the skull base, the development of obstructive hydrocephalus may require a temporary external drain or placement of a ventriculo-peritoneal shunt. Provided that a patient has received appropriate antifungal treatment, there is usually little risk of seeding of the CNS fungal infection into the abdomen. Bulk excision of intracranial abscesses, particularly within functional areas, should not be performed. In the spinal cord, intervention may be needed for focal lesions causing spinal cord compression.

Addressing host immunity can be an overlooked aspect of treatment of CNS fungal infections. In immunocompromised hosts, reversal of immunosuppression by immune restoration through antiretroviral therapy (ART), use of adjunctive cytokines such as G-CSF (granulocyte-CSF) and GM-CSF, or lowering doses of immunosuppressive agents in SOT recipients is as important as antifungal treatment in ensuring a successful outcome. In HIV-associated cryptococcal meningitis, augmentation of pro-inflammatory immune responses, using as few as two doses of adjunctive interferon gamma, was associated with improved fungal clearance (Jarvis et al. 2012).

Paradoxically, excess inflammation can also be harmful, especially in the closed compartment of the CNS: dysregulated, over-exuberant immune responses to residual fungal antigens can be associated with the immune reconstitution inflammatory syndrome (IRIS), which can result in oedema, raised intracranial pressure, and additional mortality. There is no established biomarker of IRIS and no clinical trials of management: provided that CSF cultures are negative, a reducing course of steroids is used empirically alongside antifungals (Longley et al. 2013; Williamson et al. 2017). Steroids however are not recommended for treatment of first episode (culture-positive) HIV-associated cryptococcal meningitis: a large randomised trial of adjunctive steroids showed no difference in 10-week mortality; and increased disability and slower fungal clearance in the group that received steroids in addition to amphotericin-B based treatment (Beardsley et al. 2016).

Prevention

As fungi are ubiquitous, preventing exposure is challenging. HSCT (haematopoietic stem cell transplantation) patients are usually nursed in positive-pressure rooms with high-efficiency particulate air (HEPA) filters. No fungal vaccines are currently available for the at-risk population. Antifungal prophylaxis with mould-active drugs is routinely used before engraftment, and during episodes of graft-versus-host disease in HSCT recipients, and during episodes of chemotherapy-induced neutropenia in high-risk patients. Universal, or targeted, prophylaxis based on pre-transplant serological status, is used in some centres for SOT recipients in regions of endemic mycoses (Galgiani et al. 2005). In HIV-infected patients, early institution of ART, before the onset of severe immunocompromise, is the best primary prevention. Secondary prevention using an azole following meningitis due to *Cryptococcus neoformans* and the dimorphic fungi is recommended until CD4 counts stabilize above 100–200 cells per μL and HIV viral load is undetectable. Detectable cryptococcal antigen in the blood (antigenaemia), which precedes meningitis symptoms by weeks, offers an opportunity for intervention to prevent HIV-associated cryptococcal meningitis. CRAG prevalence in global cohorts with CD4 counts of less than 100 cells per μL ranges from 2% to 21% (Rajasingham et al. 2012). Both reflex CRAG screening using the point-of-care test prior to start of ART and the treatment of antigenaemic patients with fluconazole are being implemented in high-burden countries in Africa and have been shown to be both cost-effective (Jarvis et al. 2013) and associated with improved survival in ART implementation programmes (Mfinanga et al. 2015).

References

Antinori S, Corbellino M, Meroni L, et al. (2013) Aspergillus meningitis: a rare clinical manifestation of central nervous system aspergillosis. Case report and review of 92 cases. *J Infect* 66: 218–38.

Ashbee HR, Barnes RA, Johnson EM, et al. (2014) Therapeutic drug monitoring (TDM) of antifungal agents: guidelines from the British Society for Medical Mycology. *J Antimicrob Chemother* 69: 1162–76.

Bariola JR, Perry P, Pappas PG, et al. (2010) Blastomycosis of the central nervous system: a multicenter review of diagnosis and treatment in the modern era. *Clin Infect Dis* 50: 797–804.

Beardsley J, Wolbers M, Kibengo FM, et al. 2016 CryptoDex Investigators. Adjunctive Dexamethasone in HIV-Associated Cryptococcal Meningitis. *N Engl J Med* 374(6): 542–54.

Bicanic T, Muzoora C, Brouwer AE, et al. (2009) Independent association between rate of clearance of infection and clinical outcome of HIV-associated cryptococcal meningitis: analysis of a combined cohort of 262 patients. *Clin Infect Dis* 49: 702–9.

Day JN, Chau TT, Wolbers M, et al. (2013) Combination antifungal therapy for cryptococcal meningitis. *N Engl J Med* 368: 1291–302.

Galgiani JN, Ampel NM, Blair JE, et al. (2005) Coccidioidomycosis. *Clin Infect Dis* 41: 1217–23.

Groll AH, Giri N, Petraitis V, et al. (2000) Comparative efficacy and distribution of lipid formulations of amphotericin B in experimental Candida albicans infection of the central nervous system. *J Infect Dis* 182: 274–82.

Hope W and Drusano G (2009) Antifungal pharmacokinetics and pharmacodynamics: bridging from the bench to bedside. *Clin Microbiol Infect* 15: 602–12.

Jarvis J, Bicanic T, Loyse A, et al. (2014) Determinants of mortality in a combined cohort of 501 patients with HIV-associated Cryptococcal meningitis: implications for improving outcomes. *Clin Infect Dis* 58: 736–45.

Jarvis JN, Harrison TS, Lawn SD, et al. (2013) Cost effectiveness of cryptococcal antigen screening as a strategy to prevent HIV-associated cryptococcal meningitis in South Africa. *PloS One* 8: e69288.

Jarvis JN, Meintjes G, Rebe K, et al. (2012) Adjunctive interferon-γ immunotherapy for the treatment of HIV-associated cryptococcal meningitis: a randomized controlled trial. *AIDS* 26: 1105–13.

Jarvis JN, Meintjes G, Williams A, et al. (2010) Adult meningitis in a setting of high HIV and TB prevalence: findings from 4961 suspected cases. *BMC Infect Dis* 10: 67.

Jarvis JN, Percival A, Bauman S, et al. (2011) Evaluation of a novel point-of-care cryptococcal antigen test on serum, plasma, and urine from patients with HIV-associated cryptococcal meningitis. *Clin Infect Dis* 53: 1019–23.

Kethireddy S and Andes D (2007) CNS pharmacokinetics of antifungal agents. Expert Opin Drug Metab Toxicol vol. 3, no. 4, pp. 573–81

Khot, P.D. & Fredricks, D.N. 2009, 'PCR-based diagnosis of human fungal infections', *Expert Rev Anti Infect Ther* 7: 1201–21.

Klont RR, Mennink-Kersten MA and Verweij PE (2004) Utility of Aspergillus antigen detection in specimens other than serum specimens. *Clin Infect Dis* 39: 1467–74.

Kontoyiannis DP, Marr KA, Park BJ, et al. (2010) Prospective surveillance for invasive fungal infections in hematopoietic stem cell transplant recipients, 2001-2006: overview of the Transplant-Associated Infection

Surveillance Network (TRANSNET) Database. *Clin Infect Dis* 50: 1091–100.

Lionakis MS (2012) Genetic susceptibility to fungal infections in humans. *Curr Fungal Infect Rep* 6: 11–22.

Litvintseva AP, Lindsley MD, Gade L, et al. (2014) Utility of (1-3)-beta-D-glucan testing for diagnostics and monitoring response to treatment during the multistate outbreak of fungal meningitis and other infections. *Clin Infect Dis* 58: 622–30.

Longley N, Harrison TS and Jarvis JN (2013) Cryptococcal immune reconstitution inflammatory syndrome. *Curr Opin Infect Dis* 26: 26–34.

Loyse A, Moodley A, Rich P, et al. (2015) Neurological, visual, and MRI brain scan findings in 87 South African patients with HIV-associated cryptococcal meningoencephalitis. *J Infect* 70: 668–75.

Lyons JL, Gireesh ED, Trivedi JB, et al. (2012) Fatal Exserohilum meningitis and central nervous system vasculitis after cervical epidural methylprednisolone injection. *Ann Intern Med* 157: 835–6.

Lyons JL, Thakur KT, Lee R, et al. (2015) Utility of measuring (1,3)-beta-d-glucan in cerebrospinal fluid for diagnosis of fungal central nervous system infection. *J Clin Microbiol* 53: 319–22.

Ma H, Hagen F, Stekel DJ, et al. (2009) The fatal fungal outbreak on Vancouver Island is characterized by enhanced intracellular parasitism driven by mitochondrial regulation. *Proc Natl Acad Sci U S A* 106: 12980–5.

McCarthy M, Rosengart A, Schuetz AN, et al. (2014) Mold infections of the central nervous system. *N Engl J Med* 371: 150–60.

Marr KA, Schlamm HT, Herbrecht R, et al. (2015) Combination antifungal therapy for invasive aspergillosis: a randomized trial. *Ann Intern Med* 162: 81–9.

Meletiadis J, Walsh TJ, Hwa Choi E, et al. (2007) Study of common functional genetic polymorphisms of FCGR2A, 3A and 3B genes and the risk for cryptococcosis in HIV-uninfected patients. *Med Mycol* 45: 513–18.

Mfinanga S, Chanda D, Kivuyo SL, et al. (2015) Cryptococcal meningitis screening and community-based early adherence support in people with advanced HIV infection starting antiretroviral therapy in Tanzania and Zambia: an open-label, randomised controlled trial. *Lancet* 385: 2173–82.

Murthy JM (2007) Fungal infections of the central nervous system: the clinical syndromes. *Neurol India* 55: 221–5.

Ou X, Wu J, Zhu L, et al. (2011) Genotypes coding for mannose-binding lectin deficiency correlated with cryptococcal meningitis in HIV-uninfected Chinese patients. *J Infect Dis* 203: 1686–91.

Pappas PG, Alexander BD, Andes DR, et al. (2010) Invasive fungal infections among organ transplant recipients: results of the Transplant-Associated Infection Surveillance Network (TRANSNET). *Clin Infect Dis* 50: 1101–11.

Pappas PG, Kauffman CA, Andes D, et al. (2009) Clinical practice guidelines for the management of candidiasis: 2009 update by the Infectious Diseases Society of America. *Clin Infect Dis* 48: 503–35.

Perfect JR, Dismukes WE, Dromer F, et al. (2010) Clinical practice guidelines for the management of cryptococcal disease: 2010 update by the Infectious Diseases Society of America. *Clin Infect Dis* 50: 291–322.

Pitisuttithum P, Negroni R, Graybill JR, et al. (2005) Activity of posaconazole in the treatment of central nervous system fungal infections. *J Antimicrob Chemother* 56: 745–55.

Rajasingham R, Meya DB and Boulware DR (2012) Integrating cryptococcal antigen screening and pre-emptive treatment into routine HIV care. *J Acquir Immune Defic Syndr* 59: e85–91.

Revankar S, Sutton D and Rinaldi M (2004) Primary central nervous system phaeohyphomycosis: a review of 101 cases. *Clin Infect Dis* 38: 206–16.

Saijo T, Chen J, Chen SC, et al. (2014) Anti-granulocyte-macrophage colony-stimulating factor autoantibodies are a risk factor for central nervous system infection by Cryptococcus gattii in otherwise immunocompetent patients. *MBio* 5: e00912–14.

Scully EP, Baden LR and Katz JT (2008) Fungal brain infections. *Curr Opin Neurol* 21: 347–52.

Smith RM, Schaefer MK, Kainer MA, et al. (2013) Fungal infections associated with contaminated methylprednisolone injections. *N Engl J Med* 369: 1598–609.

Soeffker G, Wichmann D, Loderstaedt U, et al. (2013) Aspergillus galactomannan antigen for diagnosis and treatment monitoring in cerebral aspergillosis. *Prog Transplant* 23: 71–4.

Spellberg B, Ibrahim A, Roilides E, et al. (2012a) Combination therapy for mucormycosis: why, what, and how? *Clin Infect Dis* 54 (Suppl. 1): S73–8.

Spellberg B, Ibrahim AS, Chin-Hong PV, et al. (2012b) The Deferasirox-AmBisome Therapy for Mucormycosis (DEFEAT Mucor) study: a randomized, double-blinded, placebo-controlled trial. *J Antimicrob Chemother* 67: 715–22.

Starkey J, Moritani T and Kirby P (2014) MRI of CNS fungal infections: review of aspergillosis to histoplasmosis and everything in between. *Clin Neuroradiol* 24: 217–30.

Walsh TJ, Anaissie EJ, Denning DW, et al. (2008) Treatment of aspergillosis: clinical practice guidelines of the Infectious Diseases Society of America. *Clin Infect Dis* 46: 327–60.

Wheat LJ, Connolly-Stringfield PA, Baker RL, et al. (1990) Disseminated histoplasmosis in the acquired immune deficiency syndrome: clinical findings, diagnosis and treatment, and review of the literature. *Medicine* 69: 361–74.

Wheat LJ, Freifeld AG, Kleiman MB, et al. (2007) Clinical practice guidelines for the management of patients with histoplasmosis: 2007 update by the Infectious Diseases Society of America. *Clin Infect Dis* 45: 807–25.

Williamson PR, Jarvis JN, Panackal AA, et al. (2017) Cryptococcal meningitis: epidemiology, immunology, diagnosis and therapy. *Nat Rev Neurol* 13(1): 13–24.

Zhu L, Wu J, Xu B, Ou X, Zhang Q and Weng X (2010) Cryptococcal meningitis in non-HIV-infected patients in a Chinese tertiary care hospital, 1997-2007. *Med Mycol* 48: 570–9.

CHAPTER 23

Fungal infections of the skin and subcutaneous tissue

Roderick J. Hay

Introduction to fungal infections affecting the skin

Fungal infections that affect the skin include some of the more common human diseases, such as tinea pedis (or 'athlete's foot'), which present no threat to life. Fungal skin infections may also be cutaneous manifestations of deep mycoses—sometimes rare, and occasionally life threatening. The latter category includes diseases, such as cryptococcosis, in which bloodstream dissemination to the skin may occur. Imported (or endemic) infections may be seen in all of these categories, although clinical presentation may occur years after the individual has left their country of origin. So, in taking a history, it is important to include sufficient information on travel and potential for exposure.

Further details of these infections are described in Section 2 and in the literature (Anaissie et al. 2009; Hay and Ashbee 2016); this section will describe the presentation of different mycoses in the skin.

Epidemiology

The superficial infections are world-wide in distribution, although there are regional variations, particularly where infections affect children, e.g. tinea capitis. They include the dermatophyte or ringworm infections, superficial candidiasis or thrush, and *Malassezia* infections of which the common skin disease, pityriasis versicolor, is an example. These are the fourth most common cause of non-fatal human disabilities, affecting just under 1 billion people at any given time (Hay et al. 2014). These figures do not include *Candida* infections of the oral mucosa or vulvovaginal tract. They also conceal local peaks of infection. For instance, there are areas of tinea capitis in sub-Saharan Africa where prevalence rates can exceed 25% of the community in schools (Hogewoning et al. 2011). Likewise, areas endemic for *Trichophyton concentricum*, causing tinea imbricata in the West Pacific, can affect over 20% of the community. In many industrialized countries the prevalence of tinea pedis, or dermatophytosis of the feet, is approximately 15% (Ameen 2010).

Figures for the prevalence of onychomycosis are variable, depending on the ascertainment method. However, the Achilles study in Europe showed prevalence rates of fungal nail infection of at least 22%, and higher in the over-60 age group (Burzykowski et al. 2003). The prevalence was higher in northern Europe than southern Europe. Similar changes in distribution are seen in Asia, where northern areas of China and Japan have higher onychomycosis prevalence rates than are seen in Malaysia and other southern countries.

The subcutaneous mycoses are seldom common although there are some epicentres of higher prevalence, such as Mexico and Sudan (Fahal et al. 2015). Mycetoma, chromoblastomycosis and other deep mycoses have recently been designated Neglected Tropical Diseases by the World Health Organisation.

By definition, the systemic infections involve internal organs. But in all systemic mycoses the skin may be affected either through bloodstream spread or, less frequently, if the infection is introduced directly into the skin. However, some infections affecting patients with AIDS are more likely to show cutaneous involvement, e.g. infections due to *Talaromyces (Penicillium) marneffei,* histoplasmosis, or cryptococcosis. In *Talaromyces* infection, approximately 70% of patients with HIV/AIDS show skin involvement (Kawila et al. 2013). Cryptococcosis skin involvement is particularly associated with AIDS (10–15%; Garman and Tyring 2002). In addition, strains of *C. neoformans* serotype D (var. *neoformans*) are more likely to be found in skin lesions.

Examples of direct inoculation of the skin by organisms that cause systemic infections include following a laboratory accident, after a natural disaster such as an earthquake or flooding (Lee et al. 2006), or with the insertion of medical devices such as cannulae.

Finally, with the endemic systemic mycoses, some skin signs, such as erythema nodosum and erythema multiforme, are not the direct result of cutaneous invasion but rather the host's immune response, although they are usually accompanied by other signs of immune complex mediated reactions such as arthritis or iritis (Braverman 1999).

Immunosuppression

In immunosuppressed patients both the prevalence and the clinical presentation of fungal infections affecting the skin may be altered. This depends on both the nature of the immune defect as well as the normal route of infection. In dermatophytosis, for instance, the clinical presentation may alter in patients with HIV/AIDS and in recipients of solid organ transplants, although the prevalence of infection is usually not increased (Torssander et al. 1988; Güleç et al. 2003). Examples include a higher risk of tinea faciei (facial dermatophytosis) or proximal subungual onychomycosis, an aggressive invasion of the nail plate (Garman and Tyring 2002). *Malassezia* infection (tinea versicolor) is not more prevalent in HIV-positive individuals, whereas the inflammatory reaction to

Malassezia yeasts, seborrhoeic dermatitis, is commoner in early HIV, reflecting defective regulation of the normal human immune response. In patients with defects of the immune system affecting neutrophils, again there is no evidence to suggest a greater prevalence of superficial mycoses.

This pattern is different with deep mycoses. In sporotrichosis, for instance, there is a higher risk of cutaneous dissemination of skin infections in patients with underlying HIV/AIDS (Kauffman et al. 2000). With the endemic mycoses there appears to be a higher risk of cutaneous dissemination in patients with HIV/AIDS (Wheat 1995). However, it is not known whether this simply reflects a higher underlying disease prevalence rate or a higher predilection for dermatotropism in the presence of HIV.

Main clinical syndromes

Superficial mycoses

Dermatophyte infections

The dermatophyte infections are common in all environments. However, their clinical presentation is variable, depending on the part of the body affected. Certain common clinical patterns of infection are seen regularly (Hay and Ashbee 2016):

1) Scaling annular patches on the skin with a raised edge. This is the essential sign of ringworm or dermatophyte infection affecting the body or limbs. There are variants, particularly when an anthropophilic fungus is involved, when the border of the lesion is often not clearly defined and may be difficult to discern, particularly on areas such as the back or face. By contrast, zoophilic infections, or those caused by *Microsporum gypseum*, are often more inflamed and the rim of the lesions more easily discernible. On the soles of the feet there is seldom a visible lesion edge and the infection causes scaling sometimes in small circles less than 1 cm in diameter. However, the scaling is often most obvious at the side of the foot—moccasin-type tinea pedis.

   An unusual variant on the annular patch is the presence of multiple concentric rings of scales, typical of the infection caused by *T. concentricum*, tinea imbricata. Sometimes these patients have sheets of large scales (Hay et al. 1984).

2) Vesicles or blisters (bullae). These may be caused by dermatophyte infection on the feet. Typically these are due to *T. interdigitale*. These lesions can occur either between the toe webs, usually the lateral web spaces, or on the soles. It is important to recognize that, in some patients, inflammatory forms of tinea pedis may trigger an immunological reaction—an acute form of eczema, or pompholyx—which also presents with vesicles on the feet. This is known as an 'id' (interface dermatitis) reaction and can occur on the contralateral foot as well as the hands.

3) Patchy hair loss with or without scaling and itching is the most important feature of tinea capitis or scalp ringworm (Fuller et al. 1997; Ghannoum et al. 2003). This is variable, and some patients present with an infection which mainly consists of scales resembling severe dandruff. In infections where there is a heightened immune response, the skin may become very inflamed and boggy with, in some cases, pus. This very inflammatory lesion of the scalp is a kerion; it is commoner with zoophilic infection but can occur with anthropophilic organisms such as *T. tonsurans*. Usually, a patient can be reassured that they will recover hair growth once treated.

   The clinical pattern of favus is very distinctive as the hair shafts are usually surrounded by greyish scales or crusts which are confluent between individual hair shafts. As the infection develops, the hair follicles are usually destroyed—'scarring alopecia'. Scarring is not common with other forms of tinea capitis.

4) Other patterns of skin infection occur in dermatophytosis, although they are less common. They include the formation of tender dermal nodules. These typically occur on the legs and follow hair follicle invasion by the fungus—'nodular perifolliculitis' (Das et al. 2007).

5) Immunosuppression, particularly due to HIV or topical or systemic steroid therapy, may modify these appearances (Pernicario and Peters 1986). Generally, the outer rim of the infection is very indistinct. However, there is often accentuation of the hair follicle infection, suggesting a form of folliculitis.

One common clinical diagnostic dilemma is the patient with interdigital infection where there is intense maceration of the skin and erosion of the surface (Howell et al. 1988). Often, such patients present with pain rather than itching (Figures 23.1 and 23.2) and may show greenish skin discolouration in the affected area. Such cases often represent secondary bacterial infection, usually due to gram-negative bacteria such as *Pseudomonas aeruginosa*. Other secondary invaders are *Candida albicans* and *Corynebacterium minutissimum* (Al-Sogair et al. 1991). If initial fungal investigations are negative, it is helpful to swab for bacterial growth and treat as appropriate. However, the original dermatophyte infection may resurface and will also require treatment.

Onychomycosis

Fungal nail disease is usually described according to the presumed route of invasion of the nail plate and whether or not it involves the proximal nail fold, which, as a result, becomes inflamed and swollen—a paronychium (Midgley and Moore 1996; Hay and Baran 2011). Most dermatophytes do not cause paronychia, whereas nail infection due to *Candida*, *Neoscytalidium*, and *Fusarium* spp. are all often accompanied by nail fold swelling. In the case of *Candida* infection, subsequent invasion of the nail plate itself is not invariable.

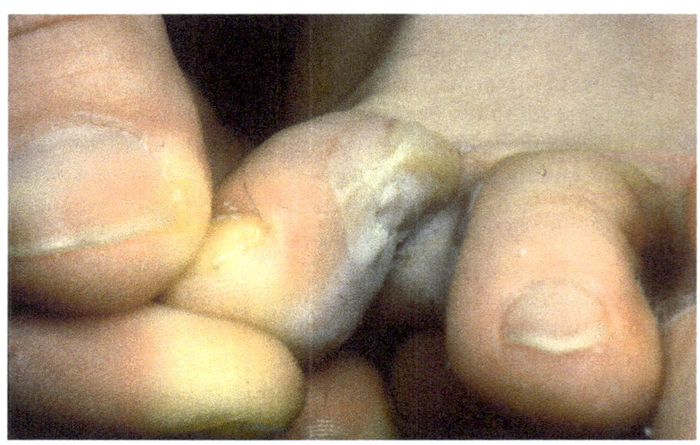

Figure 23.1 Interdigital tinea pedis (athlete's foot) due to *Trichophyton interdigitale*.

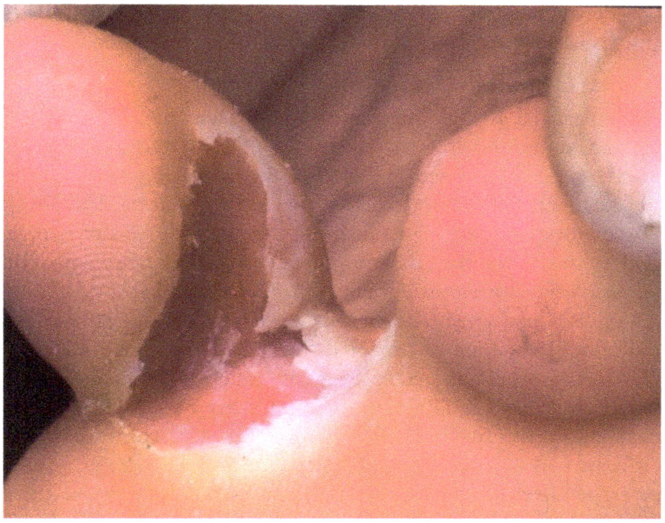

Figure 23.2 Interdigital Gram-negative infection.

The current clinical classification of onychomycosis is shown in Box 23.1. Key clinical aspects are a consequence of the route of infection.

1) The commonest form, in over 85% of cases, is distal and lateral subungual onychomycosis, as the infection develops under the nail plate and proceeds from the distal tip proximally. The nail plate is usually discoloured and may be thickened, although less so in certain infections, such as those caused by *Neoscytalidium*. Onycholysis is an accompanying feature.
2) Superficial infection of the top surface of the nail plate can be caused by certain dermatophytes such as *T. interdigitale* or *Fusarium* and *Acremonium* spp. The infection appears as a cloudy patch which can be scraped away using a scalpel blade.
3) Infection of the proximal nail plate is much less common and the infection may present as cloudy patches on the nail plate or as linear bands (striate pattern) which develop with nail growth into superficial onychomycosis. Rarely, in immunosuppressed patients, the fungi penetrate through the nail plate to cause a deep infection of the hard keratin.
4) A rarer pattern of infection—endonyx onychomycosis—is seen in patients infected with some dermatophytes that cause tinea capitis, such as *T. soudanense*. Here, the fungus penetrates from the top surface but grows within the nail plate, often leaving scales on the surface which can come away to leave pits along with discolouration.
5) If the nail plate is destroyed completely (totally dystrophic onychomycosis), it is difficult to define the origin of the infection, but this occurs as an end stage of untreated dermatophyte infections. It can also occur very rapidly in patients with the rare syndrome of chronic mucocutaneous candidiasis (Perheentupa 2006).

In all these forms of nail plate infection the nail is often discoloured, and usually white or yellowish. But in *Scopulariopsis brevicaulis* infection, for instance, there is often an orange-brown colour due to the presence of pigmented arthroconidia in the nail. *T. rubrum* and *Neoscytalidium* spp. can cause black pigmentation of the nail—melanonychia.

Box 23.1 Onychomycosis clinical classification (after Hay and Baran 2011)

Distal and lateral subungual onychomycosis—DLSO

Superficial onychomycosis (white or black)—SO

a) *patchy* or *transverse*
b) *originating from beneath the proximal nail fold*
   - patchy
   - transverse (striate)
c) *with deep penetration*—the fungi invade from superficial to deep aspects of the nail plate

Endonyx onychomycosis—EO

Proximal subungual onychomycosis—PSO

a) *patchy*
b) *transverse (striate, longitudinal)*

Mixed onychomycosis—MO, e.g. DLSO plus SO, SO plus PSO

Totally dystrophic onychomycosis—TDO

The infection may also be described by organism and colour, e.g. black DLSO due to *T. rubrum*.

Adapted from *Journal of the American Academy of Dermatology*, Volume 65, Issue 6, Hay R. J. & Baran R., 'Onychomycosis: A proposed revision of the clinical classification', pp. 1219–27, Copyright © 2010 American Academy of Dermatology, Inc., Published by Mosby Inc., with permission from Elsevier, http://www.sciencedirect.com/science/article/pii/S0190962210018244

Some patients may produce a mixed pattern, with some nails showing distal and lateral onychomycosis, for instance, and others superficial onychomycosis.

Clues to the correct diagnosis are often subtle. However, with dermatophyte nail infection it is unusual for the nail to be invaded without clinical signs of either tinea pedis or tinea manuum. Likewise, *Candida* infection of the nail plate is rare in the absence of paronychia, but it can occur particularly in patients with Raynaud's disease. However, it usually presents only with finger nail involvement. Patients with *Neoscytalidium* infections may show scaling of the skin or toe webs, and on the fingers the nail fold is often swollen.

Candidiasis of the skin

Candida infections of the skin surface, other than the nail fold or nail plate, are usually found on areas which are occluded, such as the groin, the toe or finger web spaces, and under the breasts (Edwards 2015). In all sites there is usually a variable degree of itching and the skin surface is generally red, although between the fingers and in the toe web spaces the skin is white, soggy, and macerated, with erosion of the surface. An important clue to candidiasis in the flexures is the presence of small pustules outside the border of the erythematous rash—satellite pustules. These may also be solid without pus, but their location is similar.

Other superficial mycoses

Tinea nigra, caused by *Hortaea* (*Phaeoannellomyces*) *werneckii*, presents as a black or brown macule, usually on the palms (Rossetto and Cruz 2012). There is scaling, but generally this is not easy to define. It may be mistaken for an acral lentigo, but skin scraping with demonstration of the presence of pigmented hyphae in direct microscopy is the best way of establishing the diagnosis. In white piedra—caused by *Trichosporon asahii, ovoides*, or *inkin*—the hairs, usually in the axillae or groins, are coated with small but firm white plaques adhering to the hair shafts (Kalter et al. 1986); these must be distinguished from the soft and more extensive plaques on hair associated with trichomycosis axillaris caused by overgrowth of commensal bacteria associated with hyperhidrosis.

Neoscytalidium infections due to *N. hyalinum* and *N. dimidiatum* (formerly *Scytalidium dimidiatum*) normally present as a scaly rash affecting the palms, soles, and toe webs, or onychomycosis (Hay and Moore 1984). Most patients originate from a tropical region. Clinically, these infections mimic the dry-type infections caused by *Trichophyton rubrum* such as tinea pedis, but seldom respond well to conventional antifungals.

Malassezia infections. Pityriasis versicolor is a common dermatosis in warmer climates but is also seen regularly in northern countries, often after the patient has returned from a holiday in the sun (Crespo Erchiga and Delgado Florencio 2002). Patients have a mildly symptomatic rash with either an increase in pigment or loss of pigment associated with well-defined, slightly scaly patches which may become confluent, covering a wide area on the trunk or neck. Rare variants affect other areas such as the groins. Other dermatoses that present similarly, such as vitiligo, do not show scaling, which may be best elicited by gently scratching the affected area. The main cause is *M. globosa*. This organism can also produce a form of folliculitis, often presenting after a holiday in a sunny climate. Unlike other causes of folliculitis or acne, the rash is concentrated on the upper trunk and consists of itchy pustules without comedones.

Malassezia is also associated with seborrhoeic dermatitis due to an aberrant inflammatory response to the presence of commensal *Malassezia* yeasts (Naldi 2010). It is not clear whether this is restricted to certain species or even variants within several species. The rash also consists of scaling and erythema. The key sites affected are on the face around the nasolabial folds, the eyebrows, behind the ears, the scalp, and the centre of the chest. The scalp lesions are similar to common dandruff. Indeed, there is strong evidence that dandruff is a milder version of seborrhoeic dermatitis. Seborrhoeic dermatitis is also associated with untreated HIV infections (Mathes and Douglas 1985)

Key features of laboratory diagnosis

Failure to confirm the diagnosis of superficial mycoses is often due to the poor quality and amount of material submitted. Skin samples should be taken by scraping the skin surface firmly with the blunt side of a scalpel or a solid blade. Nail clippings should be taken from as far proximally on the nail as can be reached with comfort (Midgley and Moore 1996). Scalp brushings are taken using a disposable toothbrush or hairbrush. If scrapings are taken, the sample needs to contain hairs rather than skin scale alone.

In onychomycosis, the samples, even with careful sampling and processing, are often negative. An aid to diagnosis is to take skin samples from the soles, as the chances of a positive fungal identification are higher. If the laboratory uses molecular diagnostic techniques, the samples have a higher yield (Gräser et al. 2012).

Interpreting the laboratory results is also important. With nail infections, fungi with variable pathogenicity such as aspergilli may cause invasive infection, but equally they may be commensal and repeated samples may be needed. Likewise, *Candida* spp. can colonize onycholytic nails without causing disease, and the presence of yeasts and hyphae in direct microscopy is critical (Midgley and Moore 1996)

Treatment strategies

All superficial fungal infections require treatment, as few will resolve spontaneously. Generally the approach to treatment is pragmatic, with well-defined infection of the skin being treated with topical therapy (e.g. tinea pedis and tinea cruris) (Rotta et al. 2013). More widespread infections or those affecting the nails or hair, as well as those that have not responded to topical treatments, are treated with systemic antifungal drugs (Bell-Syer et al. 2012).

In fungal nail infections there is evidence favouring using both topical and systemic treatment in those where the nail matrix—that is, the proximal sixth of the nail plate—is infected (Gupta/Onychomycosis Combination Therapy Study Group 2005; Baran et al. 2007). This involves use of nail lacquer such as amorolfine or ciclopirox, as well as either oral terbinafine or itraconazole. In some cases, removal of infected nail sections, particularly where there are longitudinal streaks in the nail plate, with topically applied 40% urea may be necessary to successfully complete therapy (Joseph and Mozena 2007).

With kerions, it may be necessary to remove any crusted material from the scalp. This can be painful, so gentle soaking of the infected area with saline-soaked gauze may facilitate the process.

In dermatophyte infection, treatment failure is seldom associated with antifungal resistance, and other issues affecting outcome such as compliance and drug absorption have to be considered.

Preventive strategies are rarely employed in superficial mycoses with the exception of tinea capitis, where it is usual practice to screen the family of patients with anthropophilic infection (Health Protection Agency 2008). Current strategy is to treat all those without clinical signs and symptoms, but with positive scalp cultures for fungus, with topical therapy such as ketoconazole shampoo. Generally, if the organism is *T. tonsurans*, any child with fungal growth on culture should be treated with oral therapy.

Subcutaneous infection and the skin

Sporotrichosis

Subcutaneous sporotrichosis includes two main forms: lymphangitic and fixed infections. The lymphangitic form usually develops on exposed skin sites such as hands or feet. The first sign of infection is the appearance of a dermal nodule that breaks down into a small ulcer. Draining lymphatics become inflamed and swollen, and a chain of secondary nodules develops along the course of the lymphatic; these may also break down and ulcerate (Barros et al. 2011) The diagnosis has to be confirmed by culture and histology of a biopsy sample as there are other infections which present in a very similar pattern (Figures 23.3 and 23.4). The commonest of these are *Mycobacterium marinum* infection, leishmaniasis, and primary cutaneous *Nocardia* infection. However, rarely, other organisms behave in the same way in immunosuppressed individuals. It is important to recognize the various infectious causes of sporotrichoid spread; using a careful travel history or a history of exposure to a potential source, such as an aquarium or fish for *M. marinum*, may help to direct investigation.

In the fixed variety, which accounts for about 15% of cases, the infection remains localized to a single site, such as the face, and an inflamed granulomatous lesion develops that may subsequently ulcerate. Fixed lesions can closely mimic cutaneous leishmaniasis.

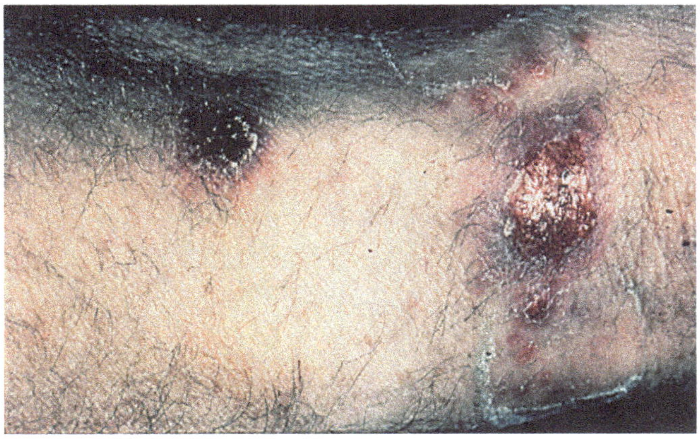

Figure 23.3 Lymphangitic (sporotrichoid spread) of sporotrichosis.

All patients with cutaneous sporotrichosis need antifungal therapy (Table 23.1).

Mycetoma (maduromycosis, Madura foot)

Mycetoma is characterized by the formation of visible aggregates of the causative organisms, grains, which are surrounded by abscesses. The key to patient management is to identify whether the infection is due to a fungus (eumycetoma) or an actinomycete (actinomycetoma) as this will determine the best course of treatment (van de Sande et al. 2014).

The clinical features of both eu- and actino-mycetomas are very similar. They are most common on the foot, lower leg, or hand, although head or back involvement may also occur. Infection of the chest wall can occur with *Nocardia* infections. In actinomycetomas, the openings of the sinus tract often protrude above the skin surface—a subtle but not invariable clinical pointer to the diagnosis. Patients may describe the appearance of black or white granular material from sinuses. An increase in skin surface sweating may occur over mycetomas and is an important diagnostic clue.

All patients need imaging studies (X-ray or magnetic resonance scans) to determine the true extent of infection, which tends to involve bone in the later stages.

Mycetoma grains may be obtained by opening a pustule or sinus tract with a sterile needle and gently squeezing the edges. If simple removal, by incising an unruptured sinus with a small collection of pus below the surface, fails to produce grains, a deep surgical biopsy will be necessary. Ideally, as many grains should be obtained as possible and part-placed in sterile saline for culture, and part in formal saline for histopathology.

All mycetomas require treatment (Table 23.1).

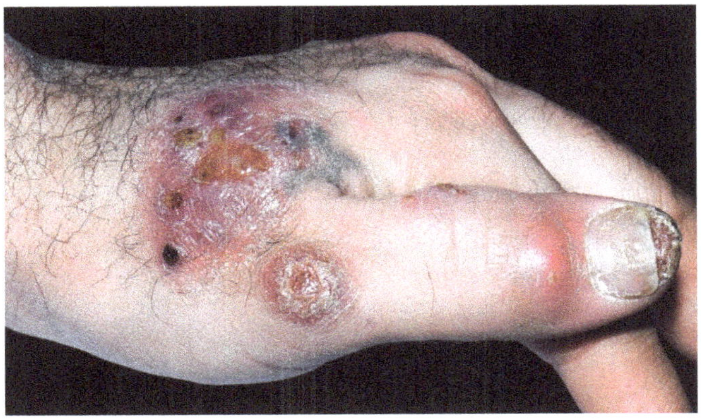

Figure 23.4 Lymphangitic (sporotrichoid spread) of *Mycobacterium marinum* infection.

Chromoblastomycosis (chromomycosis)

Chromoblastomycosis is a chronic fungal infection of the skin and subcutaneous tissues caused by pigmented or dematiaceous fungi that are implanted into the dermis from the environment.

The initial site of the infection is usually the feet, legs, or arms (Lu et al. 2013). These early lesions are small, painless and firm nodules that slowly expand over months or years. Established lesions are usually large verrucose nodules or flat atrophic plaques, but sometimes a combination of both patterns. Individual lesions may be thick and often develop secondary bacterial infection which causes the lesions to smell. The warty changes may have developed from other conditions such as verrucous tuberculosis, and more extensive lesions have to be distinguished from mossy foot secondary to chronic lymphoedema caused by lymphatic filariasis or podoconiosis, although the latter is usually bilateral.

The typical brown sclerotic or muriform fungal cells can be seen in skin scrapings using potassium hydroxide (KOH) mounts taken from the skin surface of lesions. Their location can sometimes be detected in areas on the lesion's surface where there is a small dark spot. Histology of biopsied material is also useful as the pathological changes and presence of muriform cells are both typical.

All cases require treatment (Table 23.1).

Phaeohyphomycosis (phaeomycotic cyst, cystic chromomycosis)

Phaeohyphomycosis is a rare infection characterized by the formation of subcutaneous inflammatory cysts (Isa-Isa et al. 2012). The lesions present as large subcutaneous cysts (e.g. around the knee) which may be surgically removed, the diagnosis becoming apparent after excision. They may mimic other conditions such as Baker's cysts. The treatment is surgical excision without chemotherapy, although relapse can occur, particularly in immunocompromised patients.

Other subcutaneous infections

Subcutaneous mucormycosis occasionally presents as a subcutaneous infection. There are two forms, caused respectively by *Basidiobolus ranarum* (*B. haptosporus*) and *Conidiobolus coronatus* (Prabhu and Patel 2004). They present as localized firm swellings in the skin located around the limb girdles in the case of the former, and the central facial tissues of the nose and mouth in the latter.

The main skin features are shown in Table 23.1.

Systemic mycoses and the skin

The systemic mycoses, by definition, invade deep structures such as the lungs, liver, and spleen, but they may also affect the skin as well as mucosal surfaces. Skin involvement usually follows spread via the bloodstream to produce generalized or localized infections affecting the skin (Ramos-e-Silva et al. 2012) (Table 23.1). There are two main varieties: the opportunistic and the endemic respiratory mycoses. Of the two, the endemic mycoses are more usually associated with skin lesions. The endemic (respiratory) mycoses are histoplasmosis (classic and African types), blastomycosis,

Table 23.1 Skin manifestations of subcutaneous mycoses

Disease	Endemic areas	Presenting skin features	Diagnosis (most useful)	Treatment
Mycetoma	Tropics - mainly dry tropics of Africa, Middle East, Latin America and Asia	Hard subcutaneous swelling. Sinus openings showing papules with pus. In actinomycetomas these are often protuberant	Direct microscopy of grains, Culture, Histology	Actinomycetomas – Cotrimoxazole/ Rifampiciin, Dapsone/Streptomycin Alternatives – amikacin, moxifloxacin Eumycetomas – Trial of antifungals eg itraconazole. Surgery
Sporotrichosis	Tropics and subtropics. Southern USA, Latin America, South Africa, Far East, Australia, Japan	Solitary granulomas with ulceration Ascending nodules/ulcers on lymphatic drainage channels (sporotrichoid) Multiple cutaneous ulcers in immunosuppressed	Culture Direct microscopy Histology	Itraconazole Terbinafine Potassium iodide (saturated solution)
Chromoblastomycosis	Tropics and subtropics (high rainfall). Latin America, sub-Saharan Africa, India, Far East, West Pacific	Warty nodules and/or large plaques. May have scarring in centre. Black dots on surface – good sampling points for histology/ microscopy	Direct microscopy Culture Histology	Itraconazole Terbinafine Heat
Subcutaneous mucoromycete infections		Hard subcutaneous swellings Due to *Basidiobolus* – limbs and trunk Due to *Conidiobolus* - face	Culture Histology	Itraconazole and/or Potassium iodide
Phaeomycotic cyst	Tropics and subtropics	Defined subcutaneous lump (cyst)	Culture Histology	Surgical excision

Source: data from Barros, de Almeida Paes, & Schubach, 2011; van de Sande et al., 2014; Lu et al., 2013; Isa-Isa, García, Isa, & Arenas, 2012; Prabhu & Patel, 2004.

coccidioidomycosis, paracoccidioidomycosis, infections due to *Talaromyces marneffei*, and the recently described emmonsiosis (Kenyon et al. 2014). In all endemic mycoses, direct implantation of the organism into the skin, for example as a result of a laboratory accident, will result in a local nodule or ulcer with enlargement of the draining lymph nodes. These are known as primary cutaneous infections and are rare (Smith et al. 2013).

Histoplasmosis

There are a number of different clinical syndromes due to *Histoplasma capsulatum* that may involve the skin in addition to primary cutaneous infection:

1. In acute pulmonary histoplasmosis, patients are thought to have been exposed to large quantities of conidia. The main symptoms are cough, chest pain, and fever, but this is often with accompanying joint pains and rash—toxic erythema, erythema multiforme, or erythema nodosum (Friedman et al. 1984). These skin rashes are not common, occurring in fewer than 10% of patients, but they may be precipitated by antifungal treatment of the acute infection.
2. In acute forms of disseminated histoplasmosis there is spread to other organs such as the liver and spleen, lymphoreticular system, and bone marrow (Sun et al 2014; Moreno-Coutiño et al. 2015). This is most likely to occur in untreated AIDS patients, some of whom develop skin lesions as a manifestation of disseminated bloodstream infection. These are papules, small nodules, or molluscum contagiosum-like lesions that may subsequently develop into shallow ulcers.
3. In African histoplasmosis caused by *H capsulatum* var. *duboisii*, isolated or multiple skin lesions, papules, nodules, or abscesses may be the presenting signs of infection.

The diagnosis and treatment of histoplasmosis is discussed elsewhere. The symptoms and rash of patients who have erythema multiforme associated with acute histoplasmosis can be worsened or triggered by antifungal therapy.

Table 23.2 summarizes the clinical skin lesions that may occur with the other systemic mycoses.

Coccidioidomycosis may present with erythema nodosum or erythema multiforme or with disseminated skin ulcers or granulomas (Crum-Cianflone et al. 2006). Erythema nodosum and erythema multiforme occur after acute exposure and are thought to be an immunological response to the infection; the former presents with tender subcutaneous nodules, usually on the lower limbs, and is more common than erythema multiforme (Braverman 1999). Patients with erythema nodosum rarely develop progressive disease and it is regarded as a good prognostic sign.

Paracoccidioidomycosis may also present with disseminated skin granulomas (Ramos-E-Silva and Saraiva Ldo 2008), although these are often located around the mucocutaneous junctions, e.g. mouth or conjunctivae. The granulomas are irregular and erode the skin and mucosal surfaces.

Talaromyces marneffei infection of the skin is also seen in patients who are HIV positive. It often presents with disseminated umbilicated skin papules on the face and trunk (Kawila et al. 2013). These closely resemble the viral infection molluscum contagiosum, although the lesion sizes are variable, with some reaching 2 cm in

Table 23.2 Skin manifestations of endemic systemic mycoses other than histoplasmosis

Disease Disease	*Endemic area*	*Presenting skin features*	Diagnosis – use of the skin lesions
Blastomycosis *Blastomyces dermatitidis*	North America, Central Africa	Granulomatous and crusted skin lesions. May be solitary and over 4-5 cm in size	Culture and histology of skin biopsy
Coccididioido- mycosis *Coccidioides immitis, posadasii*	Dry west coast USA, Mexico, Colombia, Venezuela Argentina	Occasional erythema nodosum in primary infection. Ulcers, abscesses and granulomas rare	Culture and histology of skin biopsy
Paracoccidioi-domycosis *Paracoccidioides brasiliensis*	Mexico, central and south America	Ulcers and granulomas around orifices eg mouth, anus.	Culture and histology of skin biopsy
Infection due to *Talaromyces marneffei*	SE Asia, Thailand, S China, Hong Kong	Multiple papules, often with central umbilication, ulcers.	Culture and histology of skin biopsy or smear taken from skin lesion
Emmonsiosis	South Africa	Multiple papules, purulent, crusted hyperkeratotic, infiltrated, scaly or verrucous plaques, nodules, ulcers or hyperpigmented patches	Culture and histology of skin biopsy

diameter. These lesions are also often very extensive, particularly on the face.

The majority of patients with emmonsiosis (almost all of those described are HIV positive) have skin lesions. These may be papules, purulent, crusted hyperkeratotic, infiltrated, scaly, or verrucous plaques, nodules, ulcers, or hyperpigmented patches (Schwartz et al. 2015).

In cryptococcosis, systemic symptoms such as headache and fever dominate. In disseminated disease, cutaneous lesions may precede or follow the signs of involvement of the central nervous system and lungs. The most frequent types of lesions are firm, papular, or cystic, slow-growing, subcutaneous or dermal swellings (Thomas and Schwartz 2001; Khuraijam et al. 2015), Molluscum contagiosum-like papules or pustules are also characteristic of widespread systemic infection. They often occur around the nose and mouth. Any of these lesions may ulcerate, or ulcers may develop in primarily unaffected skin.

Often, the term primary cutaneous cryptococcosis is used to describe solitary, or occasional multiple, lesions on the skin (Du et al. 2015). But in many such cases there is evidence of systemic spread, implying that the skin lesion has developed after bloodstream spread from a primary lung focus. There are, however, some documented cases of primary cutaneous infection by inoculation, although all patients need to be investigated thoroughly for evidence of more extensive disease even if the presenting lesion is in the skin. These lesions are, however, very similar in appearance to those seen in other systemic mycoses, such as histoplasmosis and infections caused by *Talaromyces marneffei*.

All of these infections should be treated with antifungal drugs after thorough investigation for systemic spread. The optimum therapy is discussed elsewhere.

Skin lesions are seen less commonly with the opportunistic systemic mycoses.

In systemic (disseminated) candidiasis, typical skin lesions start as macules, become papular or nodular, and may show a pale centre (Mays et al. 2006). These are occasionally haemorrhagic and may break down to form ulcers. Hair follicle invasion by *Candida*, leading to pustules and nodules in the hair-bearing areas of the scalp, beard, axilla, and pubis, may occur in a very specific and characteristic infection following candidaemia in intravenous heroin abusers (Bisbe et al. 1992).

Apart from the invasion of necrotic skin or burns, or after severe trauma involving contact with soil—for example, after a landslide or tsunami—mucormycosis of the skin is rare (Petrikkos et al. 2012), but it can occur particularly in infections due to *Saksenaea vasiformis*. Necrotizing infections of the skin associated with the application of dressings contaminated with *Rhizopus rhizopodiformis* and with *R. microsporus* from wooden spatulas have been described (Antoniadou 2009). Cutaneous mucormycosis requires prompt systemic antifungal treatment. Even so, extensive debridement or removal of necrotic skin and underlying subcutis and fascia is usually necessary.

Unusual causes of skin lesions among opportunistic systemic mycoses

Other organisms that can cause skin disease include *Aspergillus*, *Trichosporon*, and *Fusarium*; all of these may affect the neutropenic patient (Mays et al. 2006).

Aspergillus and *Trichosporon* can produce large, scattered necrotic lesions, although with the latter, smaller papules and pustules have been seen. *Fusarium* and, more rarely, *Acremonium* infection may produce target-like lesions, which can show central necrosis. In some cases of *Fusarium* infection, scattered skin lesions have been accompanied by digital cellulitis and superficial white onychomycosis caused by the same organism.

References

Al-Sogair SM, Moawad MK and Al-Humaidan YM (1991) Fungal infection as a cause of skin disease in the Eastern Province of Saudi Arabia: tinea pedis and tinea manuum. *Mycoses* 1991 34: 339–44.

Ameen M (2010) Epidemiology of superficial fungal infections. *Clin Dermatol* 28: 197–201.

Anaissie EJ, McGinnis MR and Pfaller MA (2009) *Clinical Mycology* (2nd edn, London: Churchill Livingstone, Elsevier).

Antoniadou A (2009) Outbreaks of zygomycosis in hospitals. *Clin Microbiol Infect* 15 (Suppl. 5): 55–9.

Baran R, Sigurgeirsson B, de Berker D, et al. (2007) A multicentre, randomized, controlled study of the efficacy, safety and cost-effectiveness of a combination therapy with amorolfine nail lacquer and oral terbinafine compared with oral terbinafine alone for the treatment of onychomycosis with matrix involvement. *Br J Dermatol* 157: 149–57.

Barros MB, de Almeida Paes R and Schubach AO (2011) Sporothrix schenckii and Sporotrichosis. *Clin Microbiol Rev* 24: 633–54.

Bell-Syer SE, Khan SM and Torgerson DJ (2012) Oral treatments for fungal infections of the skin of the foot. *Cochrane Database Syst Rev* 10: CD003584. doi: 10.1002/14651858.CD003584.pub

Bisbe J, Miro JM, Latorre X, et al. (1992) Disseminated candidiasis in addicts who use brown heroin: report of 83 cases and review. *Clin Infect Dis* 15: 910–23.

Braverman IM (1999) Protective effects of erythema nodosum in coccidioidomycosis. *Lancet* 353: 168.

Burzykowski T, Molenberghs G, Abeck D, et al. (2003) High prevalence of foot diseases in Europe: results of the Achilles Project. *Mycoses* 46: 496–505.

Crespo Erchiga V and Delgado Florencio V (2002) *Malassezia* species in skin diseases. *Curr Opin Infect Dis* 15: 133–42.

Crum-Cianflone NF, Truett AA, Teneza-Mora N, et al. (2006) Unusual presentations of coccidioidomycosis: a case series and review of the literature. *Medicine (Baltimore)* 85: 263–77.

Das S, Saha R and Bhattacharya SN (2007) Disseminated nodular granulomatous perifolliculitis. *Indian J Med Microbiol* 25: 288–90.

Du L, Yang Y, Gu J, Chen J, Liao W and Zhu Y (2015) Systemic Review of Published Reports on Primary Cutaneous Cryptococcosi in Immunocompetent Patients. *Mycopathologia* 180: 19–25.

Edwards JE. (2015) *Candida* species., *in*: GL Mandell, JE Bennett and R Dolin, eds, *Mandell, Douglas, and Bennett's Principles and Practice of Infectious Diseases*, (8th edn, Philadelphia: Churchill Livingstone), 2879–94.

Fahal A, Mahgoub el S, El Hassan AM and Abdel-Rahman ME (2015) Mycetoma in the Sudan: an update from the Mycetoma Research Centre, University of Khartoum, Sudan. *PLoS Negl Trop Dis* 9: e0003679.

Friedman SJ, Black JL and Duffy J (1984) Histoplasmosis presenting as erythema multiforme and polyarthritis. *Cutis* 34: 396–8.

Fuller LC, Child FC and Higgins EM (1997) Tinea capitis in southeast London: an outbreak of Trichophyton tonsurans infection. *Br J Dermatol* 136: 139–45.

Garman ME and Tyring SK (2002) The cutaneous manifestations of HIV infection. *Dermatol Clin* 20: 193–214.

Ghannoum M, Isham N, Hajjeh R, et al. (2003) Tinea capitis in Cleveland: survey of elementary school students. *J Am Acad Dermatol* 48: 189–93.

Gräser Y, Czaika V and Ohst T (2012) Diagnostic PCR of dermatophytes—an overview. *J Dtsch Dermatol Ges* 10: 721–6.

Güleç AT, Demirbilek M, Seçkin D, et al. (2003) Superficial fungal infections in 102 renal transplant recipients: a case-control study. *J Am Acad Dermatol* 49: 187–92.

Gupta AK and the Onychomycosis Combination Therapy Study Group (2005) Ciclopirox topical solution, 8% combined with oral terbinafine to treat onychomycosis: a randomized, evaluator-blinded study. *J Drugs Dermatol* 4: 481–5.

Hay RJ and Ashbee R (2016) Fungal infections, *in*: C Griffiths, J Barker, T Bleiker, et al., eds, *Rook's Textbook of Dermatology*, Part 3, Chapter 32 (9th edn, Oxford: Wiley-Blackwell), 32.1–32.96.

Hay RJ and Baran R (2011) Onychomycosis: a proposed revision of the clinical classification. *J Am Acad Dermatol* 65: 1219–27.

Hay RJ and Moore MK (1984) Clinical features of superficial fungal infections caused by Hendersonula toruloidea and Scytalidium hyalinum. *Br J Dermatol* 110: 677–83.

Hay RJ, Nicols R, Williams HE, et al. (2014) The global burden of skin disease in 2010: an analysis of the prevalence and impact of skin conditions. *J Invest Dermatol* 134: 1527–34.

Hay RJ, Reid S, Talwat E, et al. (1984) Endemic tinea imbricata: a study on Goodenough Island, Papua New Guinea. *Trans R Soc Trop Med Hyg* 78: 246–51.

Health Protection Agency (2008) Tinea capitis in the United Kingdom: A report on its diagnosis, management and prevention. HPA Publications 2008, http://webarchive.nationalarchives.gov.uk/20140714084352/http://www.hpa.org.uk/webc/hpawebfile/hpaweb_c/1194947321499, accessed 15 May 2017.

Hogewoning AA, Adegnika AA, Bouwes Bavinck JN, et al. (2011) Prevalence and causative fungal species of tinea capitis among schoolchildren in Gabon. *Mycoses* 54: 354–9.

Howell SA, Clayton YM, Phan QC, et al. (1988) Tinea pedis: the relationship between symptoms and host characteristics. *Microbiol Ecol Health Dis* 1: 131–8.

Isa-Isa R, García C, Isa M and Arenas R (2012) Subcutaneous phaeohyphomycosis (mycotic cyst). *Clin Dermatol* 30: 425–31.

Joseph WS and Mozena JD (2007) Podiatric approach to the management of onychomycosis, *in*: RK Scher and CR Daniel, eds, *Nails: Diagnosis, Therapy, Surgery* (3rd edn, Philadelphia: Saunders), 133–40.

Kalter DCA, Tschen JA, Cernoch PL, et al. (1986) Genital white piedra: epidemiology, microbiology and therapy. *J Am Acad Dermatol* 14: 982–93.

Kauffman CA, Hajjeh R and Chapman SW (2000) Practice guidelines for the management of patients with sporotrichosis. For the Mycoses Study Group. Infectious Diseases Society of America. *Clin Infect Dis* 30: 684.

Kawila R, Chaiwarith R and Supparatpinyo K (2013) Clinical and laboratory characteristics of penicilliosis marneffei among patients with and without HIV infection in Northern Thailand: a retrospective study. *BMC Infect Dis* 2013 13: 464. doi: 10.1186/1471-2334-13-464

Kenyon C, Corcoran C and Govender NP (2014) An emmonsia species causing disseminated infection in South Africa. *N Engl J Med* 370: 284.

Khuraijam R, Lungran P, Yoihenba K, Laishram RS and Pukhrambam P (2015) Pancytopenia and cutaneous cryptococcosis as an indicator disease of acquired immune deficiency syndrome. *Indian J Med Microbiol* 33: 439–4.

Lee SH, Choi CP, Eun HC and Kwon OS (2006) Skin problems after a tsunami. *J Eur Acad Dermatol Venereol* 20: 860–3.

Lu S, Lu C, Zhang J, Hu Y, Li X and Xi L (2013) Chromoblastomycosis in mainland China: a systematic review on clinical characteristics. *Mycopathologia* 175: 489–95.

Mathes BM and Douglas MC (1985) Seborrheic dermatitis in patients with acquired immunodeficiency syndrome. *J Am Acad Dermatol* 13: 947–51.

Mays SR, Bogle MA and Bodey GP (2006) Cutaneous fungal infections in the oncology patient: recognition and management. *Am J Clin Dermatol* 7: 31–43.

Midgley G and Moore MK (1996) Nail infections. *Dermatol Clin* 14: 41–9.

Moreno-Coutiño G, Hernández-Castro R, Toussaint-Caire S, Montiel-Robles M, Sánchez-Pérez FS and Xicohtencatl-Cortés J (2015) Histoplasmosis and skin lesions in HIV: a safe and accurate diagnosis. *Mycoses* 58: 413–15.

Naldi L (2010) Seborrhoeic dermatitis. *BMJ Clin Evid* (online). Dec 7. pii: 1713.

Perheentupa J (2006) Autoimmune polyendocrinopathy-candidiasis-ectodermal dystrophy. *J Clin Endocrinol Metabol* 91: 2843–50.

Pernicario C and Peters MS (1986) Tinea faciale mimicking seborrheic dermatitis in a patient with AIDS. *N Engl J Med* 314: 315–16.

Petrikkos G, Skiada A, Lortholary O, Roilides E, Walsh TJ and Kontoyiannis DP. (2012) Epidemiology and clinical manifestations of mucormycosis. *Clin Infect Dis* 54 (Suppl. 1): S23–34.

Prabhu RM and Patel R (2004) Mucormycosis and entomophthoramycosis: a review of the clinical manifestations, diagnosis and treatment. *Clin Microbiol Infect* 10 (Suppl. 1): 31–47.

Ramos-e-Silva M, Lima CM, Schechtman RC, Trope BM and Carneiro S. (2012) Systemic mycoses in immunodepressed patients (AIDS). *Clin Dermatol* 30: 616–27.

Ramos-E-Silva M and Saraiva Ldo E (2008) Paracoccidioidomycosis. *Dermatol Clin* 26: 257–69.

Rossetto AL and Cruz RC (2012) Tinea nigra: successful treatment with topical butenafine. *An Bras Dermatol* 87: 939–41.

Rotta I, Ziegelmann PK, Otuki MF, et al. (2013) Efficacy of topical antifungals in the treatment of dermatophytosis: a mixed-treatment comparison meta-analysis involving 14 treatments. *JAMA Dermatol* 149: 341–9.

Schwartz IS, Govender NP, Corcoran C, et al. (2015) Clinical characteristics, diagnosis, management, and outcomes of disseminated emmonsiosis: a retrospective case series. *Clin Infect Dis* 61: 1004–12.

Smith JA, Riddell J 4th and Kauffman CA (2013) Cutaneous manifestations of endemic mycoses. *Curr Infect Dis Rep* 15: 440–9.

Sun NZ, Augustine JJ and Gerstenblith MR (2014) Cutaneous histoplasmosis in renal transplant recipients. *Clin Transplant* 28: 1069–74.

Thomas I and Schwartz RA (2001) Cutaneous manifestations of systemic cryptococcosis in immunosuppressed patients. *J Med* 32: 259–66.

Torssander J, Karlsson A, Morfeldt-Månson L, Putkonen PO and Wasserman J (1988) Dermatophytosis and HIV infection. A study in homosexual men. *Acta Derm Venereol* 68: 53–6.

van de Sande WW, Maghoub el S, Fahal AH, Goodfellow M, Welsh O and Zijlstra E. (2014) The mycetoma knowledge gap: identification of research priorities. *PLoS Negl Trop Dis* 8: e2667. doi: 10.1371/journal.pntd.0002667

Wheat J (1995) Endemic mycoses in AIDS: a clinical review. *Clin Microbiol Rev* 8: 149–58.

CHAPTER 24

Fungal diseases of the ear, nose, and throat

Arunaloke Chakrabarti

Introduction to fungal diseases of the ear, nose, and throat

Fungal diseases of the ear (otomycosis), nose (fungal rhinosinusitis), and throat (oropharyngeal candidiasis) are increasingly recognized problems and are common diseases. Less commonly, fungal laryngeal diseases and invasive otomycosis are reported, especially in immunosuppressed hosts. The first two common fungal diseases are described here in detail. Fungal infections of the pharynx and larynx are dealt with together at the end of this chapter.

Fungal diseases affecting the ear

Otomycosis

Acute or chronic superficial fungal infection of the external auditory canal with rare involvement of the middle ear is called otomycosis or fungal otitis externa.

Epidemiology

The disease has worldwide distribution, affecting young people (aged 20–40 years) and commonly occurring in the summer months with an estimated prevalence of 4 per 1,000 population (Saki et al. 2013). Fungal aetiology accounts for 9% of otitis externa and 30% of symptomatic cases of otitis (Munguia and Daniel 2008). The infection rate is higher in tropical and subtropical climates. Several predisposing factors have been described for the disease, such as swimming, foreign body in the ear canal, traumatic inoculation (while cleaning the external ear canal with an ear bud or wooden stick), reduced or excessive cerumen, poor hygiene, use of hearing aids, working in dusty environments, diabetes mellitus, ear surgery, open mastoid cavity, tympanic membrane perforation, instilling oil in the ear canal, and ear wax. A considerable number of patients give a history of topical application of broad-spectrum antibiotics and steroids (Prasad et al. 2014; Gharaghani et al. 2015).

Nearly 60 species of mould or yeast are incriminated in the aetiology of otomycosis. However, *Aspergillus* spp. are the predominant isolates across the globe (80% of cases) and *Aspergillus niger* is the commonest species. Different species of *Candida* have been isolated in 20% of cases, especially from immunosuppressed hosts, and *C. parapsilosis* is the commonest yeast. Dermatophytes, *Scedosporium apiospermum* and *Malassezia* spp. are rarely isolated. In some reports, two fungal species or mixed fungal–bacterial infections are noted (Gharaghani et al. 2015).

Clinical features

The patients usually present with subacute or chronic symptoms such as otalgia, pruritis, aural fullness, tinnitus, and hearing loss. Occasionally the presentation may be acute. Physical examination with an otoscope reveals white, grey, black, or creamy coloured masses in the external auditory canal (Figure 24.1). *Aspergillus fumigatus* and yeasts produce fluffy white debris, while *A. niger* forms a black mass. *Aspergillus* otomycosis presents as mild inflammation of the deep ear canal with large shed sheets of keratin looking like wet tissue paper within the lumen. *Candida* spp. produce gross oedema of the ear canal with curd-like material in the lumen (Prasad et al. 2014). Dermatophytes are usually associated with tinea barbae in adults and tinea capitis in children (Kazemi and Ghiaei 2005). Patients on long-term topical steroid therapy for atopic dermatitis or psoriasis may develop fungal otitis externa on the auricle and within the auditory canal (Vennewald and Klemm 2010). In immunosuppressed patients, there is a possibility of involvement of the middle ear following perforation of tympanic membrane with consequent invasion of contiguous bone and brain. The disease may occasionally lead to the fatal acute invasive form following mastoid bone destruction and meningitis; otherwise, otitis media in otomycosis is rare. Mastoid surgery for otitis media may lead to fungal infection of the mastoid ear cells. Pain in the mastoid area with discharge is suggestive of such cases.

Diagnosis

This depends on clinical history, physical examination, microscopy, and culture of samples collected on otoscopic examination. Imaging is unhelpful unless there is invasion of bones or brain. Nuclear imaging including technetium (Tc99)-labelled scintigraphy and gallium scan, may help in the early diagnosis of osteomyelitis. Histopathology of skin biopsy specimens or surgical material and direct microscopy of debris from the auditory canal can easily identify the morphology of the causative fungus—yeast or mycelium (coloured or hyaline). Occasionally, the fruiting head of the fungus may be visible on direct microscopy and helps in presumptive identification of the fungus. The isolation and identification of the fungus help with appropriate therapy (Vennewald and Klemm 2010).

Treatment strategies

Though the disease is rarely fatal, treatment is challenging and sometimes frustrating for the otolaryngologists and patients, as long-term therapy is required and recurrence is not uncommon.

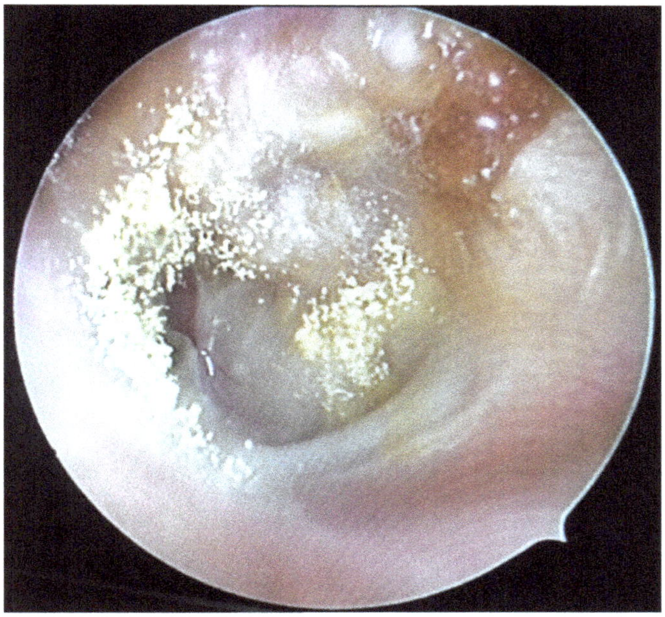

Figure 24.1 Clinical appearance of otomycosis includes thick accumulation of creamy coloured debris in the external auditory canal.

The treatment includes elimination of predisposing factors, otoscopic debridement of all debris, and topical antifungal treatment. Syringing should be avoided; gentle suctioning is sufficient to clear the debris. Clotrimazole (1%), miconazole (0.25%), bifonazole (1%), econazole (1%), fluconazole, tolnaftate, ciclopirox olamine (1%), naftifine, nystatin, and amphotericin B (3%)—as solution, cream, gel, powder, or ointment—are used as topical therapy (Stern et al. 1988). In cases of perforation of the tympanic membrane, cream, ointment, and gel should be avoided, as the small particles of these substances may cause inflammation and the formation of granulation tissue in the middle ear. In such cases, antifungal agents in solution are recommended. Self-medication with clotrimazole solution on Q-tips may be allowed, as it increases patient satisfaction levels (Abou-Halawa et al. 2012). Ear drops containing a 7.5% povidone-iodine solution have been found to be equally as effective as a 1% clotrimazole and lignocaine solution (Philip et al. 2013). Fluconazole may be used when yeast is isolated. Ear drops containing alcohol, acids, and antiseptics may lead to ototoxicity. Acetic acid, cresyl acetate, gentian violet, 50% propylene glycol, and 70% isopropyl alcohol, used for treatment, may penetrate and damage the inner ear. Therefore, patients on treatment should be monitored carefully on follow up. Mercurochrome along with thiomersal (Merthiolate) is used in some countries to minimize cost of therapy, though the preparation is not approved by the FDA (Food and Drug Administration) as it contains mercury. In rare refractory or immunosuppressed patients, systemic antifungal therapy with amphotericin B or a triazole may be required (Munguia and Daniel 2008; Vennewald and Klemm 2010; Prasad et al. 2014).

Prevention

As swimming is an important predisposing factor in these patients, it is advisable to avoid swimming during the treatment period; otherwise, frequent cleaning and drying of the ear canal with a hair dryer after each swim are recommended. Patients' nails and other body sites should be inspected and treated if necessary when dermatophytic otomycosis is suspected, to prevent reinfection. Use of ear-buds or wooden sticks to clean the auditory canal should be avoided (Vennewald and Klemm 2010).

Fungal diseases affecting the nose and paranasal sinuses

Fungal rhinosinusitis

Rhinosinusitis is an inflammatory disease affecting the nose and paranasal sinuses. The inflammation may be due to microorganisms, allergens, drugs, irritants, or trauma. During the disease process, inflammatory material and the swollen epithelium of the nose and paranasal sinuses obstruct the sinus opening and normal mucosal drainage, leading to pain, swelling, nasal blockage, and fetid discharge. The disease can be acute or chronic depending on the aetiology and host immunity. Chronic rhinosinusitis affects up to 20% of the population in some areas (Meltzer et al. 2004). Fungus as a cause of rhinosinusitis has gained importance over the last two decades. Simultaneously, there has been much controversy and confusion regarding the role of fungi, as well as in the classification, pathogenesis, and management of fungal rhinosinusitis (FRS).

Acute FRS occurs in immunosuppressed hosts, especially in patients with haematological malignancies who are undergoing chemotherapy, and transplant recipients. This entity is well characterized. *Mucorales* and *Aspergillus* spp. are common aetiological agents (Chakrabarti et al. 2009a,b). However, there is a great deal of controversy regarding the classification of chronic FRS as a consequence of the perceived role of fungi, which ranges from 'bystander' to the cause of all cases of chronic rhinosinusitis (Chakrabarti et al. 2009a). Depending on the histopathological findings, host immunity, and fungal invasion across the mucosa, chronic FRS is classified as either invasive or non-invasive. The invasive disease is further classified into granulomatous and chronic invasive types, whereas non-invasive FRS may present as localized colonization, fungal ball formation, or eosinophil-related FRS including allergic fungal rhinosinusitis (AFRS). FRS is prevalent worldwide with a high prevalence rate in tropical areas of Asia and Africa, including Sudan, Saudi Arabia, Pakistan, and India (Chakrabarti et al. 2009a,b; Telmesani 2009). The magnitude of the disease has been assessed in the villages of North India. The prevalence of chronic FRS was found to be 0.11% of the village population and 8.1% of all chronic rhinosinusitis cases (Chakrabarti et al. 2015). The epidemiology, pathology, diagnosis, and management of FRS are summarized in Table 24.1.

Acute invasive FRS including rhinocerebral mucormycosis

This disease is considered a fungal emergency owing to its dramatic course and high mortality (approximately 50%).

Epidemiology

Acute invasive FRS is seen worldwide, with an increasing incidence in recent years, and the number of cases in India is phenomenal compared with that in other countries. In India, acute FRS is largely due to *Mucorales* (rhinocerebral mucormycosis), whereas *Aspergillus fumigatus* and *Mucorales* spp. are isolated nearly in equal proportion in other countries. The disease is observed in immunosuppressed hosts such as in patients with haematological malignancy

Table 24.1 Epidemiology, pathology, clinical features, diagnosis and management of FRS

	Acute invasive FRS	Chronic invasive FRS	Granulomatous FRS	Fungal ball	Allergic FRS	Eosinophil-related FRS
Geographic distribution	Worldwide	Worldwide	Tropical regions of Africa and Asia	Worldwide common in southern France	Worldwide, high rate in tropical region	Worldwide
Host	Immunocompromised mainly. ◆ Haematological malignancy on chemotherapy ◆ Haematopoietic stem cell transplant recipients and other transplant recipients ◆ Uncontrolled diabetes and ketoacidosis	Mildly immunocompromised ◆ Diabetes ◆ On long-term steroid therapy at low dose	Immunocompetent	Immunocompetent	Atopic host	Immunocompetent
Fungi	*Mucorales Aspergillus* spp.	*Aspergillus* spp.	*Aspergillus flavus* commonly	*Aspergillus* spp., hyaline & dematiaceous moulds	Dematiaceous fungi in the USA, *A. flavus* in Asia	Dematiaceous fungi in the USA, *A. flavus* in Asia
Role of fungus in disease	Pathogen	Pathogen	Pathogen	Colonizer	Allergen	Not clear
Pathology	Necrosis, acute inflammation, invasion of blood vessels, thrombosis	Mixed inflammation with plenty of hyphae	Granulomatous reaction with few hyphae	Dense conglomeration of hyphae without invasion, non-specific mucosal inflammation	Allergic mucin with few hyphae, allergic inflammation	Eosinophilic mucin with few hyphae
Duration of disease	Acute: <4 weeks	Chronic: >12 weeks	Chronic: >12 weeks	Chronic: >12 weeks	Chronic: >12 weeks	Chronic: >12 weeks
Clinical feature	Fever, swelling of nose, protrusion of orbit after orbital involvement; eschar formation is common; fungal emergency as the disease occasionally progresses in hours	Swelling, nasal discharge, and blockade; orbital involvement common	Swelling, nasal discharge, and blockade; extension to orbit and brain common	Swelling, nasal obstruction, and discharge	Swelling, nasal obstruction, loss of smell, pressure sensation on face, and orbital protrusion following eye involvement	Swelling, nasal obstruction, facial pain or fullness, and rhinorrhoea
Diagnosis	Endoscopic biopsy of necrosed tissue (direct microscopy and culture); CT scan to evaluate extent of lesion	Endoscopic biopsy; histopathology to differentiate from granulomatous type; CT scan – sphenoid and ethmoid sinus commonly involved	Endoscopic biopsy; histopathology to differentiate from chronic invasive disease; CT scan – similar to chronic invasive type	Endoscopic biopsy; direct microscopy and culture; radiology – commonly one sinus involved	◆ Type-I hypersensitivity ◆ Nasal polyposis ◆ Eosinophilic mucin without mucosal invasion ◆ Positive fungal stain ◆ CT scan –heterogeneous opacity	◆ Eosinophilic mucin without mucosal invasion ◆ Nasal polyposis ◆ Positive fungal stain
Treatment	1. Aggressive debridement 2. Amphotericin B, posaconazole/isavuconazole salvage therapy 3. Reversal/control of predisposing factors 4. Immuno-potentiation	1. Surgical removal of mass 2. Systemic antifungal (voriconazole/ itraconazole/ amphotericin B)	1. Surgical removal of mass 2. Systemic antifungal (itraconazole/ voriconazole/ amphotericin B)	Surgery	1. Surgery 2. Oral and/or local steroid 3. Immunotherapy	1. Surgery 2. ? Steroid/? Antifungal therapy
Prognosis	High mortality ~50%	Good prognosis, occasional recurrence	Good prognosis, occasional recurrence	Good prognosis	Recurrence common	Not clear

undergoing chemotherapy, or with uncontrolled diabetes and diabetic ketoacidosis, in haematopoietic stem cell recipients, and in solid organ transplant recipients (Chakrabarti and Singh 2011). The risk factors for mucormycosis differ significantly between India and other western countries (USA and Europe). While haematological malignancy and transplants are common predisposing factors for mucormycosis in Europe and the USA, the overwhelming numbers of cases of mucormycosis with uncontrolled diabetes in India overshadow all other risk factors. In a computational model, the overall mucormycosis rate in India is calculated as 0.14 cases per 1,000 population (Chakrabarti et al. 2013).

Clinical features

The presentation starts with non-specific symptoms such as facial pain, headache, fever, and lethargy, making early diagnosis difficult. Progression of the disease results in proptosis, visual loss, palatal ulcer, and cranial nerve defects. Both *A. fumigatus* and *Mucorales* spp. are angio-invasive fungi, and the step-wise progression of clinical features indicates infarction at different sites. The infarction also leads to dusky/black coloration of skin and tissue (eschar formation). Untreated disease is universally fatal. Mortality is also high in patients with delayed therapy. The progress is rapid and death may occur within a few days. Peri-nasal cellulitis and paraesthesia are early signs of the disease. Facial symptoms include weakness, numbness, and pain; nasal symptoms include purulent discharge, hypoaesthesia, stuffiness, and rhinorrhoea; ocular symptoms include peri-orbital or retro-orbital pain, diplopia, and blurred vision leading to blindness; neurological symptoms include convulsions, altered mental status, dizziness, and unsteady gait (Nithyanandam et al. 2003; Chakrabarti et al. 2009b).

Diagnosis

The diagnosis of the disease is not difficult, once the condition is established. Computed tomography scans demonstrate the extent of the disease, opacification and bony destruction of the sinuses (especially the ethmoid and sphenoid sinuses), and orbital and cranial involvement. Magnetic resonance imaging may help to detect vascular invasion and extension of the disease process along peripheral nerves. Direct microscopy or histopathology of endoscopic biopsy/scraping material may rapidly detect the fungus. *Aspergillus* hyphae are hyaline and septate and branch at an acute angle. *Mucorales* spp. have broad, aseptate, and ribbon-like hyphae with branching at right angles. On histopathology, bland tissue necrosis in the infarcted area should increase the suspicion of fungal aetiology (Figure 24.2a). For culture, the biopsy tissue should not be crushed or vortexed as this will damage the hyphae and reduce the chances of isolating the fungus. The sample may be minced with fine scissors before culture.

Treatment

The management of acute invasive FRS should use a three-pronged strategy: extensive surgical debridement, reversal or removal of immunosuppression, and antifungal therapy. Liposomal amphotericin B (3–5 mg/kg/day) or amphotericin B lipid complex (up to 5 mg/kg/day) is the treatment of choice for rhinocerebral mucormycosis; and voriconazole (6 mg/kg) intravenous twice daily for the first 48 hours, and then 400 mg orally daily, when acute invasive FRS is due to *Aspergillus* spp. The patient should be monitored closely. If the patient responds well to amphotericin B therapy, oral posaconazole or isavuconazole may replace intravenous amphotericin B. If the response is poor, escalation of the lipid-associated amphotericin B dose (up to 10 mg/kg/day) or the addition of posaconazole/isavuconazole and immunopotentiation (granulocyte-monocyte cell stimulating factor, interferon gamma) therapy are the choices. Hyperbaric oxygen therapy may be useful in rhinocerebral mucormycosis and extensive cutaneous disease. In neutropenic patients neutrophil transfusion may also help. The therapy should be continued until the symptoms are relieved (Kontoyiannis and Lewis 2011, 2014; Ananda-Rajah and Kontoyiannis 2015).

Chronic FRS and granulomatous FRS

Both chronic FRS and granulomatous FRS are categorized as invasive forms of fungal rhinosinusitis (invasion of fungi across the nasal mucous membrane), with a time course of more than 12 weeks.

Epidemiology

Chronic invasive FRS due to *A. fumigatus* is seen worldwide in patients with diabetes or in those receiving long-term steroid therapy. In contrast, the granulomatous invasive type due to *A. flavus* occurs in immunocompetent hosts in Sudan, India, Pakistan, and Saudi Arabia, and rarely in Europe and the United States. Occasionally, other *Aspergillus* spp., and rarely *Bipolaris* spp., *Curvularia* spp., and *Schizophyllum communae* spp., have been isolated from both clinical types.

Clinical features

These diseases progress slowly as enlarging masses in the cheek, orbit, nose, maxillae, and paranasal sinuses. Ethmoid and sphenoid sinuses are commonly affected, but there may be involvement of any paranasal sinus. Patients often seek medical attention late when proptosis or cranial nerve palsies develop.

Diagnosis

The lesions are often mistaken for malignancy owing to their mass-like appearance. Histopathological examination of biopsy specimens is needed for diagnosis and can differentiate other forms of FRS. Granulomatous invasive FRS is characterized by a non-caseating granulomatous reaction with considerable fibrosis, occasional vasculitis, vascular proliferation, and perivascular fibrosis. Hyphae are scanty and present inside giant cells (Figure 24.2b). In contrast, dense accumulation of hyphae in mixed inflammatory cells with occasional vascular proliferation and vascular invasion by fungi are noted in chronic invasive FRS. The isolation of fungi is not difficult. Occasionally, molecular techniques can be used to identify the fungus. Precipitating antibody against *Aspergillus* spp. may also help in diagnosis and prognosis.

Treatment

Surgical removal of the inflammatory mass combined with systemic antifungal therapy are the mainstay of therapy for both varieties. Amphotericin B, voriconazole and itraconazole have been used in these patients until the symptoms are relieved. Recurrence is rare.

Paranasal sinus fungal ball

This disease has been given several names in the literature, such as mycetoma, aspergilloma, and chronic non-invasive granuloma.

Epidemiology

Though the cases are reported worldwide, the incidence is high in southern France, where it is common in middle-aged and elderly

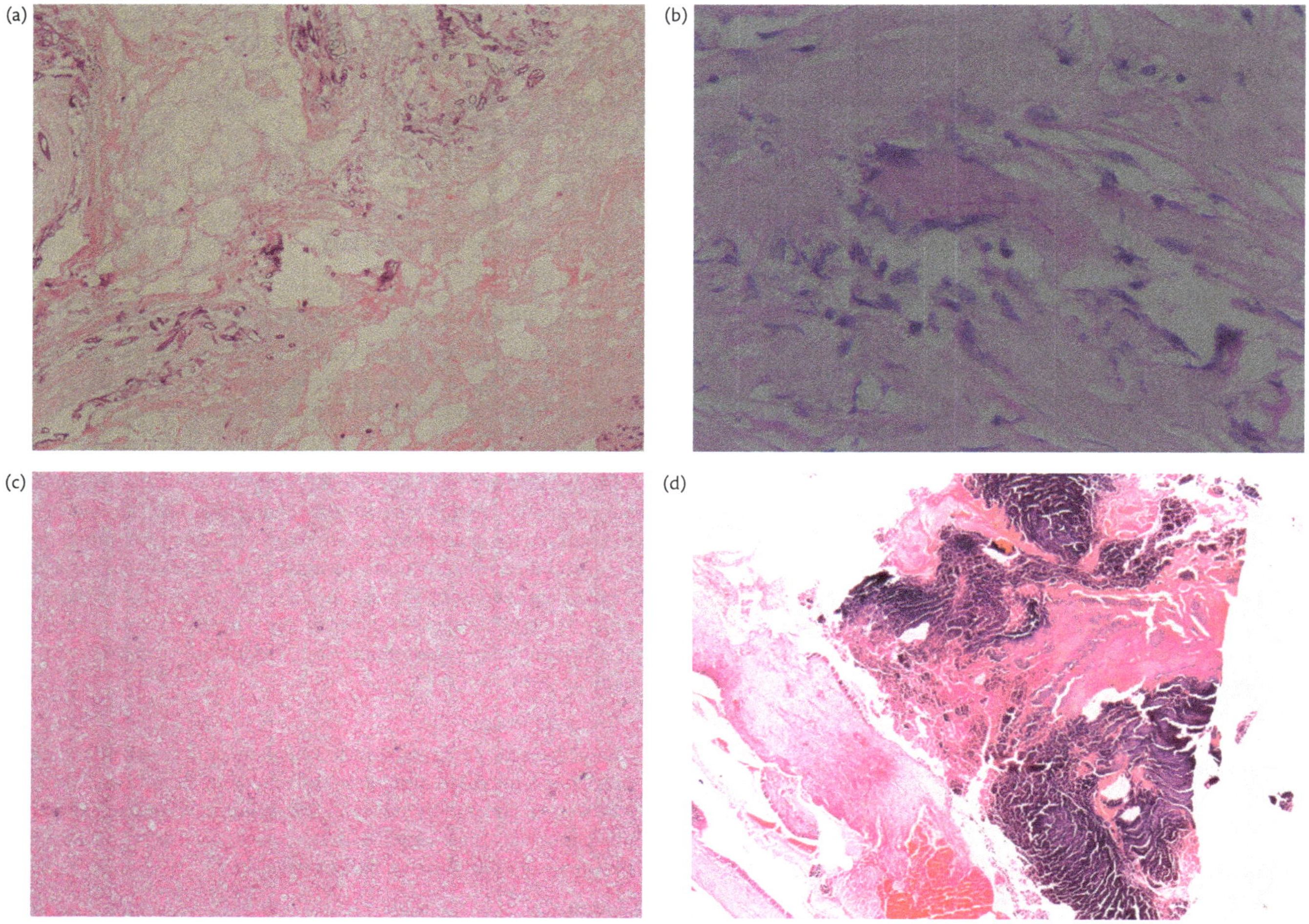

Figure 24.2 **a** Acute invasive fungal rhinosinusitis with bland necrosis and plenty of hyphae.
b Chronic granulomatous fungal rhinosinusitis with fungal hyphae inside giant cell.
c Paranasal sinus fungal ball due to dense accumulation of fungal hyphae.
d Allergic fungal rhinosinusitis with allergic (eosinophilic) mucin.

women (Dufour et al. 2006). In Brazil, this condition is also prevalent, as the disease was diagnosed in 3.7% of 890 endoscopic sinus surgeries (Dall'Igna et al. 2005). Root filling has been implicated as a risk factor.

Clinical features

Patients present with chronic non-specific sinus symptoms, including nasal obstruction, fullness, nasal discharge, and facial discomfort. Nearly 10% of patients may remain asymptomatic for a long time. Unilateral single sinus (maxillary) involvement is common.

Diagnosis

Computed tomography scans typically show opacification of a unilateral maxillary sinus without discrete calcification. Occasionally, bony erosion may be seen. The sinus mass, when removed by endoscopic surgery, appears as mucopurulent cheesy and clay-like material. On histopathology, hyphal concretion with occasional flocculent calcium and without any mucosal invasion is seen (Figure 24.2c). A non-granulomatous inflammatory response in the mucosa may take place on account of a pressure effect. *A. fumigatus* is the commonest isolate, though culturing fails in multiple cases (Chakrabarti et al. 2009a,b). Other *Aspergillus* spp. and *Scedosporium apiospermum* are occasionally isolated.

Treatment

Endoscopic sinus surgery is required to remove the entire mass. No antifungal therapy is required.

Eosinophilic fungal rhinosinusitis, including allergic fungal rhinosinusitis

Major confusion remains regarding the classification and diagnosis of this condition. The role of fungus in the pathogenesis of the disease is also questioned and the therapy is not standardized. Safirstein (1976), Millar et al. (1981), and Katzenstein et al. (1983) independently described a few cases of chronic rhinosinusitis as having mucosal plugs in their sinuses resembling allergic bronchopulmonary aspergillosis. Bent and Khun (1994) finally defined allergic fungal rhinosinusitis (AFRS) with five major criteria and a few minor criteria (Box 24.1). This definition was seriously challenged by Ponikau et al. (1999) and subsequently by other workers (Braun et al. 2003). They demonstrated the presence of fungus in mucinous material of

Box 24.1 Diagnosis of AFRS

Major criteria

1 Type I hypersensitivity described by skin test or *in vitro* testing

2 Nasal polyposis

3 Characteristic CT findings: unilateral or asymmetric involvement of the sinuses presenting as heterogeneous signal intensity; central areas of hyper-attenuation on CT scan corresponding with hypo-intensity on T1-weighted MR images, and signal void on T2-weighted MR images

4 Allergic mucin without tissue invasion

5 Positive fungal stain

Minor criteria

1 Asthma

2 Unilateral disease

3 Bone erosion

4 Fungal culture

5 Presence of Charcot-Leyden crystals

6 Peripheral blood eosinophilia

Adapted with permission from Bent J. P., Kuhn F. A., 'Diagnosis of Allergic Fungal Sinusitis', *Otolaryngology—head and neck surgery*, Volume 111, Issue 5, pp. 580–8, Copyright © 1994 SAGE Publications. DOI: 10.1177/019459989411100508.

the sinuses in chronic rhinosinusitis patients independently of type I hypersensitivity and coined a new term—eosinophilic fungal rhinosinusitis (EFRS). They claimed that the majority of cases of chronic rhinosinusitis are due to fungus, as fungi could be detected in sinus material from nearly all patients. However, fungi could be detected as colonizers in many healthy individuals as well. They believed that in this patient group, colonizing fungi attract eosinophils into the sinuses, and that the high level of eosinophil-granule major basic protein damages the mucosal epithelium, leading to secondary bacterial infection and rhinosinusitis (Ponikau et al. 2005). This view was challenged by several workers (Ferguson 2000a; Orlandi et al. 2007). Ferguson stated that 'Eosinophilia or eosinophilic mucin is not synonymous with allergic mucin. Allergies may be associated with eosinophilic mucin, but eosinophilic mucin can be present without evidence of allergies'. She later described a few patients as having eosinophilic mucin in their sinuses without the presence of fungi, and coined a new term for these patients—eosinophilic mucin rhinosinusitis (EMRS) (Ferguson 2000b). These patients had asthma, increased aspirin hypersensitivity, and IgG1 deficiency. However, considerable overlap exists between AFRS, EFRS, and EMRS without a clear-cut definition of each entity (Saravanan et al. 2006), though many consider AFRS as a distinct entity.

Allergic fungal rhinosinusitis (AFRS)

Epidemiology

AFRS is the form most commonly seen in tropical countries (Das et al. 2009; Chakrabarti and Singh 2011, 2015), where the patients are young agricultural workers. In temperate climates, such a rural link is not described. The aetiological agents differ in the two regions. In the USA, melanized fungi—including *Alternaria* spp., *Bipolaris* spp. and *Curvularia* spp.—are common isolates (Cody et al. 1994; Schubert 2009), whereas *A. flavus* is common across South Asia, the Middle East, and Sudan (Saravanan et al. 2006; Al-Dousary 2008).

Clinical features

The patients present with non-specific symptoms of chronic rhinosinusitis such as nasal obstruction, loss of smell, fullness and nasal discharge. However, the history of unilateral or asymmetric involvement of paranasal sinuses, atopy (asthma) and polyposis without significant pain may help in suspecting the disease. Recurrence is common. Occasionally the patient may have an acute presentation with double vision or visual loss, distortion of facial features due to pressure effect and complete nasal obstruction. Nasal crust of green, brown or black mucin with the consistency of clay are usually observed in endoscopic examination. Occasionally the disease is named as Sino-bronchial Allergic Mycosis (SAM Syndrome) when simultaneous allergic bronchopulmonary aspergillosis is noted in the same patient (Venarske and deShazo 2002).

Diagnosis

CT or MRI shows complete opacification of more than one sinus with heterogeneity and bony erosion (Figure 24.3). Occasionally, displacement of adjacent anatomical structures is seen. On microscopy of nasal crusts, tight clusters of eosinophil and eosinophilic degraded product (allergic/eosinophilic mucin) with Charcot-Leyden crystals are observed (Figure 24.2d). Fungal hyphae may be scanty in the mucinous material. On histopathology the fungus may be missed if mucus is not processed with tissue.

Treatment

General principles of management include avoidance of allergen and control of allergy with the use of local or systemic corticosteroids and antihistamines, together with surgical clearing of nasal passages. The role of immunotherapy is still debatable. Surgical clearing of mucinous materials with permanent drainage and aeration is the cornerstone of management. Oral corticosteroids in place of nasal corticosteroids therapy may be more effective in preventing recurrence (Rupa et al. 2010). There is no role for antifungal therapy in the present treatment protocol.

Diseases of the nose other than fungal rhinosinusitis

Besides fungal rhinosinusitis, two fungal diseases of the nose have been found in tropical regions across the globe—Conidiobolomycosis and Rhinosporidiosis. The aetiological agents of conidiobolomycosis are the *Conidiobolus* spp. Rhinosporidiosis is caused by *Rhinosporidium seeberi*, which is now classified as a fish parasite (DRIP clade).

Conidiobolomycosis

Epidemiology

The disease is found in tropical regions, such as northeastern Brazil, Central America, Caribbean Islands, Africa, India and a few other Southeast Asian countries. The disease is rarely seen in the USA and Australia. Immunocompetent adults engaged in farming and outdoor activities in rural villages acquire this infection, possibly

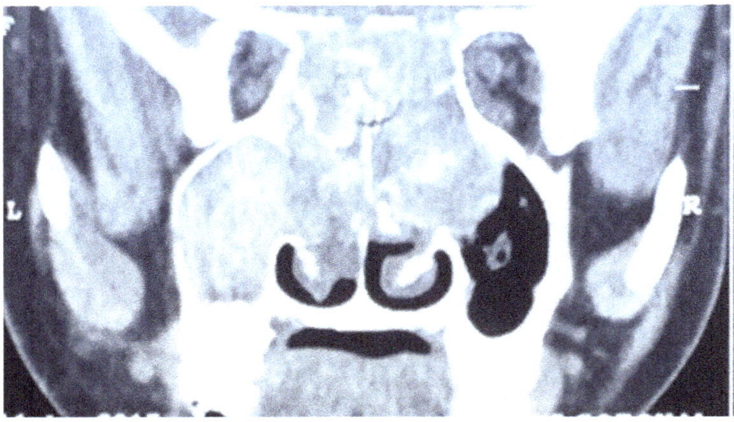

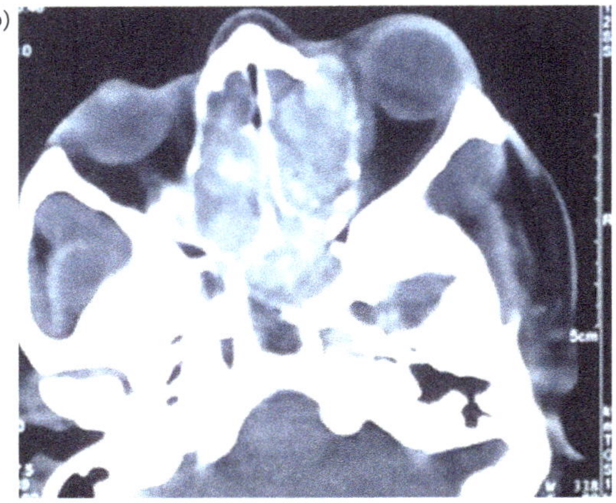

Figure 24.3 Computed tomography scan of a patient with allergic fungal rhinosinusitis affecting multiple sinuses bilaterally and bony erosion.
a Coronal plane; **b** Axial plane.

by inoculation or inhalation. The aetiological agents—*Conidiobolus coronatus* and *C. incongruous* live in soil and rotting plant material and can infect humans, insects and domestic animals. (Hoogendijk et al. 2006; Fischer et al. 2008; Isa-Isa et al. 2012).

Clinical features

The disease often mimics malignancy or granulomatous lesions. It progresses slowly from subcutaneous nodular lesions and mucosal inflammation, leading to nasal obstruction, discharge and facial deformity in central structures (cheeks, forehead and lips). No ulceration is seen. In later stages the pharynx, paranasal sinuses, muscular layers of face, mediastinum or lungs are involved. Rarely the brain may be involved (Hoogendijk et al. 2006). However, no vascular involvement or thrombosis is seen on tissue biopsy. As the lesion is superficial, a finger can be passed between the nodular swelling and deep tissue.

Diagnosis

As exudate from lesions is rarely seen, biopsy samples are needed. Short, broad (4-10μ), aseptate hyphae with suppurative granulomatous inflammation are seen on direct microscopy. The granulomas contains lymphocytes, histiocytes, multi-nucleated giant cells, plasma cells and eosinophils. The hyphae may be surrounded by an eosinophilic halo (Splendore-Hoeppli phenomenon). When isolation of fungus fails, real time polymerase chain reaction helps in diagnosis (Hoogendijk et al. 2006).

Treatment

The optimal therapy of conidiobolomycosis is not known. Conventional treatment includes surgical debridement, correction of deformities and antifungal therapy. Monotherapy or combination therapy with amphotericin B, itraconazole, fluconazole, voriconazole, terbinafine, potassium iodide, dapsone, 5-fluorocytosine, and trimethoprim/sulfamethoxazole have been used in these patients. Though dosage and duration of therapy are not well defined, long term antifungal therapy is required. Best results are achieved with the use of itraconazole (300 mg/day) for at least six months (Isa-Isa et al. 2012).

Rhinosporidiosis

This is a chronic granulomatous disorder involving the mucous membranes caused by *Rhinosporidium seeberi*. The disease is characterized by unilateral vascular pedunculated polyps, most commonly in the nasal cavity (70-80%). It is common in the coastal regions of India and Sri Lanka and the frequency may be high as 1.4% of the pediatric population in hyper-endemic zones (Moses and Shanmugham 1987). Occasional cases have been reported from the United States, South America, Italy, Iran and Turkey (Das et al. 2011; Kaushal et al. 2011). It is not clear how humans acquire the infection. Possibly the organism enters through a traumatized nasal epithelium from an aquatic source as the disease is found in rural areas among people who are in contact with stagnant water. The disease takes a chronic course leading to nasal obstruction and epistaxis and can spread to the pharynx and paranasal sinuses. Rarely, the skin is involved. Diagnosis can easily be achieved by direct microscopy of aspirated material or a biopsy of the pedunculated polyp. The organism presents as sporangia at various stages of maturation (20-300 μm in size) with endospores inside the sac along with chronic inflammatory cells. As the organism cannot be cultured, histopathology or direct microscopy remains the gold standard. The treatment is challenging as no medication is known to act against the agent. Surgical removal of the mass/polyp is the treatment of choice, though recurrence is frequent. Dapsone has been used with limited success to prevent recurrence (Das et al. 2011).

Nasal histoplasmosis

Histoplasmosis caused by *Histoplasma capsulatum* presents with pulmonary manifestations and dissemination in immunosuppressed hosts. Histoplasmosis with mucocutaneous lesions has been reported in immunocompetent hosts. Some of these cases have nasal involvement and they present with nasal swelling, obstruction and congestion. Histopathology of the biopsy samples demonstrates intra-histiocytic small (2-4μ) yeast cells with budding. The patients respond well to oral itraconazole therapy (Sood et al. 2007).

Fungal infections of the pharynx and larynx

Fungal infection of the pharynx and larynx is uncommon except as the consequence of progression of oral candidiasis in HIV positive or seriously immunosuppressed patients. These sites may be involved as part of disseminated disease especially in histoplasmosis (Rajah and Essa 1993; Gerber et al. 1995), paracoccidioidomycosis

(Tristano and Diaz 2007), and coccidioidomycosis (Drutz and Catanzaro 1978). The patients present with hoarseness of voice, cough and pharyngeal pain. On laryngoscopy the ulcerative and granulomatous lesion becomes visible. Histopathology of biopsy sample helps in diagnosis, as each fungus has a different morphological form in tissue. Isolation on culture finally helps in identification of the fungus. Itraconazole therapy is usually successful as the patients are commonly immunocompetent.

Oropharyngeal candidiasis

The disease is common in HIV/AIDS and other immunosuppressed patients such as those with haematological malignancy and transplant recipients. The disease is also seen in premature newborns and patients receiving head and neck radiotherapy. Asthmatics who are taking inhaled steroids for a long period may also develop the disease. The patients may remain asymptomatic until the *Candida* pseudomembrane obstructs the digestive or respiratory tract leading to difficulty in ingestion or respiration. A few patients may present with a painful mouth and loss of taste. Associated denture related candidiasis or angular chelitis may be seen. Direct microscopy and culture of the pseudomembrane helps with the diagnosis. Even observation of the typical white patches at the infected site may make the diagnosis with great certainty. Topical nystatin, amphotericin B, or clotrimazole, or oral fluconazole, itraconazole, or voriconazole can easily clear the white patches. However, only improvement of the immunocompromised status will prevent recurrence of the disease (Li et al. 2013; Pankhurst 2013).

References

Abou-Halawa AS, Khan MA, Alrobaee AA, Alzolibani AA and Alshobaili HA (2012) Otomycosis with perforated tympanic membrane: self-medication with topical antifungal solution versus medicated ear wick. *Int J Health Sci (Qassim)* 6: 73–7.

Al-Dousary SH (2008) Allergic fungal sinusitis: radiological and microbiological features of 59 cases. *Ann Saudi Med* 28: 17–21.

Ananda-Rajah MR and Kontoyiannis D (2015) Isavuconazole: a new extended spectrum triazole for invasive mold diseases. *Future Microbiol* 10: 693–708.

Bent JP and Kuhn FA (1994) Diagnosis of allergic fungal sinusitis. *Otolaryngol Head Neck Surg* 111: 580–8.

Braun H, Buzina W, Freudenschuss K, Beham A and Stammberger H (2003) 'Eosinophilic fungal rhinosinusitis': a common disorder in Europe? *Laryngoscope* 113: 264–9.

Chakrabarti A, Das A and Panda NK (2009a) Controversies surrounding the categorization of fungal sinusitis. *Med Mycol* 57 (Suppl. 1): S299–308.

Chakrabarti A, Denning DW, Ferguson BJ, et al. (2009b) Fungal rhinosinusitis: a categorization and definitional schema addressing current controversies. *Laryngoscope* 119: 1809–18.

Chakrabarti A, Rudramurthy SM, Panda N, Das A and Singh A (2015) Epidemiology of chronic fungal rhinosinusitis in rural India. *Mycoses* 58: 294–302.

Chakrabarti A and Singh R (2011) The emerging epidemiology of mould infections in developing countries. *Curr Opin Infect Dis* 24: 521–6.

Chakrabarti A, Sood P and Denning D (2013) Estimating fungal infection burden in India using computational models: mucormycosis burden as a case study (Poster No. 1044). Presented at 23rd ECCMID Conference: Berlin, Germany, April 27–30.

Cody DT 2nd, Neel HB 3rd, Ferreiro JA and Roberts GD (1994) Allergic fungal sinusitis: the Mayo Clinic experience. *Laryngoscope* 104: 1074–9.

Dall'Igna C, Palombini BC, Anselmi F, Araújo E and Dall'Igna DP (2005) Fungal rhinosinusitis in patients with chronic sinusal disease. *Braz J Otorhinolaryngol* 71: 712–20.

Das A, Bal A, Chakrabarti A, Panda N and Joshi K (2009) Spectrum of fungal rhinosinusitis; histopathologist's perspective. *Histopathology* 54: 854–9.

Das S, Kashyap B, Barna M, et al. (2011) Nasal rhinosporidiosis in humans: new interpretations and a review of the literature of this enigmatic disease. *Med Mycol* 49: 311–15.

Drutz DJ and Catanzaro A (1978) Coccidioidomycosis. Part I. *Am Rev Respir Dis* 117: 559–85.

Dufour X, Kauffmann-Lacroix C, Ferrie JC, Goujon JM, Rodier MH and Klossek JM (2006) Paranasal sinus fungus ball: epidemiology, clinical features and diagnosis. A retrospective analysis of 173 cases from a single medical center in France, 1989–2002. *Med Mycol* 44: 61–7.

Ferguson BJ (2000a). Eosinophilic mucin rhinosinusitis: a distinct clinicopathological entity. *Laryngoscope* 110: 799–813.

Ferguson BJ (2000b) Definition of fungal rhinosinusitis. *Otolaryngol Clin North Am* 33: 227–35.

Fischer N, Ruef Ch, Ebnöther C and Bächli EB (2008) Rhinofacial Conidiobolus coronatus infection presenting with nasal enlargement. *Infection* 36: 594–6.

Gerber ME, Rosdeutscher JD, Seiden AM and Tami TA (1995) Histoplasmosis: the otolaryngologist's perspective. *Laryngoscope* 105: 919–23.

Gharaghani M, Seifi Z and Zarei Mahmoudabadi A (2015) Otomycosis in Iran: a review. *Mycopathologia* 179: 415–24.

Hoogendijk CF, van Heerden WF, Pretorius E, Vismer HF and Jacobs JF (2006) Rhino-orbitocerebral entomophthoramycosis. *Int J Oral Maxillofac Surg* 35: 277–80.

Isa-Isa R, Arenas R, Fernández RF and Isa M (2012) Rhinofacial conidiobolomycosis (entomophthoramycosis). *Clin Dermatol* 30: 409–12.

Katzenstein AL, Sale SR and Greenberger PA (1983) Allergic Aspergillus sinusitis: a newly recognized form of sinusitis. *J Allergy Clin Immunol* 72: 89–93.

Kaushal S, Mathur SR, Mallick SR and Ramam M (2011) Disseminated cutaneous, laryngeal, nasopharyngeal, and recurrent obstructive nasal rhinosporidiosis in an immunocompetent adult: a case report and review of literature. *Int J Dermatol* 50: 340–2.

Kazemi AH and Ghiaei S (2005) Survey of otomycosis in north-western area of Iran 1997-2004. *J Mazand Univ Med Sci* 48: 112–19.

Kontoyiannis DP and Lewis RE (2011) How I treat mucormycosis. *Blood* 118: 1216–24.

Kontoyiannis DP and Lewis RF (2014) Treatment principles for the management of mold infections. *Cold Spring Harb Perspect Med* 5: pii: a019737.

Li X, Lei L, Tan D, et al. (2013) Oropharyngeal Candida colonization in human immunodeficiency virus infected patients. *APMIS* 121: 375–402.

Meltzer EO, Hamilos DL, Hadley JA, et al. (2004) Rhinosinusitis: establishing definition for clinical research and patient care. *J Allergy Clin Immunol* 114 (6 Suppl.): S155–212.

Millar JW, Johnston A and Lamb D (1981) Allergic aspergillosis of the maxillary sinuses [abstract]. *Thorax* 36: 710.

Moses JS and Shanmugham A (1987) Epidemiological survey of rhinosporidiosis in man—a sample survey in a high school located in a hyperendemic area. *Indian Vet J* 64: 34–8.

Munguia R and Daniel SJ (2008) Ototopical antifungals and otomycosis: a review. *Int J Pediatr Otorhinolaryngol* 72: 453–9.

Nithyanandam S, Jacob MS, Battu RR, Thomas RK, Correa MA and D'Souza O (2003) Rhino-orbito-cerebral mucormycosis. A retrospective analysis of clinical features and treatment outcomes. *Indian J Ophthalmol* 51: 231–6.

Orlandi RR, Thibeault SL and Ferguson BJ (2007) Microarray analysis of allergic fungal sinusitis and eosinophilic mucin rhinosinusitis. *Otolaryngol Head Neck Surg* 136: 707–13.

Pankhurst CL (2013) Candidiasis (oropharyngeal). *BMJ Clin Evid* 2013: 1304.

Philip A, Thomas R, Job A, Sundaresan VR, Anandan S and Albert RR (2013) Effectiveness of 7.5% providone iodine in comparison to 1%

clotrimazole with lignocaine in the treatment of otomycosis. *ISRN Otolaryngol* 2013: Article ID 239730.

Ponikau JU, Sherris DA, Kephart GM, et al. (2005) Striking deposition of toxic eosinophil major basic protein in mucus: implication for chronic rhinosinusitis. *J Allergy Clin Immunol* 116: 362–9.

Ponikau JU, Sherris DA, Kern EB, et al. (1999) The diagnosis and incidence of allergic fungal sinusitis. *Mayo Clin Proc* 74: 877–84.

Prasad SC, Kotigadde S, Shekhar M, et al. (2014) Primary otomycosis in the Indian subcontinent: predisposing factors, microbiology and classification. *Int J Microbiol* 2014: 636493.

Rajah V and Essa A (1993) Histoplasmosis of the oral cavity, oropharynx and larynx. *J Laryngol Otol* 107: 58–61.

Rupa V, Jacob M, Mathews MS and Seshadri MS (2010) A prospective, randomised, placebo-controlled trial of postoperative oral steroid in allergic fungal sinusitis. *Eur Arch Otorhinolaryngol* 267: 233–8.

Safirstein BH (1976). Allergic broncho-pulmonary aspergillosis with obstruction of the upper respiratory tract. *Chest* 70: 788–90.

Saki N, Rafiei A, Nikakhlagh S, Amirrajab N and Saki S (2013) Prevalence of otomycosis in Khouzestan Province, south-west Iran. *J Laryngol Otol* 127: 25–7.

Saravanan K, Panda NK, Chakrabarti A, Das A and Bapuraj RJ (2006) Allergic fungal rhinosinusitis: an attempt to resolve the diagnosis dilemma. *Otolaryngol Head Neck Surg* 132: 173–8.

Schubert MS (2009) Allergic fungal sinusitis: pathophysiology, diagnosis and management. *Med Mycol* 47 (Suppl. 1): S324–30.

Sood N, Gugnani HE, Batra R, Ramesh V and Padhye AA (2007) Mucocutaneous nasal histoplasmosis in an immunocompetent young adult. *Indian J Dermatol Venereol Leprol* 73: 182–4.

Stern JC, Shah MK and Lucente FE (1988) In vitro effectiveness of 13 agents in otomycosis and review of the literature. *Laryngoscope* 98: 1173–7.

Telmesani LM (2009) Prevalence of allergic fungal sinusitis among patients with nasal polyps. *Ann Saudi Med* 29: 212–14.

Tristano AG and Diaz L (2007) A case of laryngeal paracoccidioidomycosis masquerading as chronic obstructive lung disease. *South Med J* 100: 709–11.

Venarske DL and deShazo RD (2002) Sinobronchial allergic mycosis: the SAM syndrome. *Chest* 121: 1670–6.

Vennewald I and Klemm E (2010) Otomycosis: diagnosis and treatment. *Clin Dermatol* 28: 202–11.

CHAPTER 25

Fungaemia and disseminated infection

Rebecca Lester and John H. Rex

Introduction to the clinical aspects of invasive fungal disease

Invasive fungal disease (IFD) can present without localization or obvious target organ involvement. Such disseminated mycoses occur more commonly in patients who are immunocompromised, particularly from haematological malignancy. Fever is the most common manifestation of disseminated fungal infection and may occur with or without localizing clinical features. As mortality from IFD is high, early recognition and treatment are essential. This chapter reviews the common and emerging pathogens implicated in disseminated fungal infection, together with key aspects of epidemiology, clinical presentation, diagnosis, and management.

Causative fungi

Whilst almost any fungus has the potential to cause invasive disease (Table 25.1), *Candida, Cryptococcus*, and *Aspergillus* are the most commonly isolated in clinical practice (Lamagni et al. 2001). Mycoses due to non-*Aspergillus* moulds such as *Fusarium, Mucor*, and *Scedosporium* have, however, become increasingly common, and infections with the thermally dimorphic endemic fungi remain important in limited geographic regions (Nucci and Marr 2005).

Candida spp.

Candida spp. are ubiquitous in the environment and normal human commensals, particularly of the skin, gastrointestinal tract, and female genital tract. More than 150 *Candida* spp. exist, but only a small number are pathogenic to humans. Although decreasing in overall incidence, *C. albicans* is still the most frequently isolated in invasive infection, and *C. albicans, C. glabrata, C. parapsilosis, C. tropicalis*, and *C. krusei* account for 95–97% of invasive disease (Pappas et al. 2003; Wisplinghoff et al. 2004; Horn et al. 2009). Widespread use of azole antifungal agents in treatment and prophylaxis has led to a rise in non-*albicans* spp., in particular *C. glabrata* (Tortorano et al. 2002, 2006; Guinea 2014). Recently, *C. auris*, another species commonly resistant to fluconazole, has emerged as a cause of hospital-acquired outbreaks of candidaemia in a number of countries (Satoh et al. 2009; Lee et al. 2011; Chowdhary et al. 2013; Magobo et al. 2014; Emara et al. 2015).

Other invasive yeasts

Cryptococcus spp. are saprophytic encapsulated yeasts, and *C. neoformans and C. gattii* are the two major pathogenic species implicated in invasive infection. *C. neoformans* is ubiquitous, causing invasive disease worldwide predominantly in patients with impaired T-cell-mediated immunity. *C. gattii* has caused smaller outbreaks in tropical, subtropical, and more recently, temperate climates (Stephen et al. 2002), usually in the non-immunosuppressed host.

Malassezia furfur is a lipophilic yeast which may cause invasive fungaemia in premature neonates receiving lipid-containing parenteral nutrition (Dankner et al. 1987) as well as intravenous catheter-related fungaemia in both immunosuppressed and healthy adult hosts (Myers et al. 1992; Barber et al. 1993). *Trichosporon* spp. (*T. asahii* and *T. mucoides*) and *Blastoschizomyces capitatus* occasionally cause fungaemia, predominantly in patients with haematological malignancy (Martino et al. 2004; Girmenia et al. 2005).

A number of less common yeasts have been reported as causes of fever and fungaemia, occasionally with widespread organ involvement and usually in severe immunosuppression. *Rhodotorula* spp. (most often, *R. rubra*) and *Saccharomyces cerevisiae* have caused intravascular catheter-related fungaemia (Kiehn et al. 1992). *Pichia anomala* and *Saccharomyces cerevisiae* have been associated with intravenous catheter-related fungaemia, and *Pichia* with endovascular infections (Nohinek et al. 1987; Haron et al. 1988).

Aspergillus spp.

Only a few species of the hyaline mould *Aspergillus* are pathogenic to humans. The majority of invasive infections are caused by *A. fumigatus, A. flavus, A. niger*, and *A. terreus* (Baddley et al. 2001; Perfect et al. 2001; Marr et al. 2002). *A. fumigatus* is the most commonly isolated species in invasive infection, but in recent years the relative incidence of other species, in particular *A. terreus*, has increased (Marr et al. 2002).

Non-*Aspergillus* moulds

Non-*Aspergillus* moulds usually present with localized infection, but a number are capable of causing disseminated disease, particularly in immunosuppression. Mucormycosis is the second most common invasive mould infection, with *Rhizopus, Mucor*, and *Rhizomucor* spp. the most frequently isolated causative fungi (Kontoyiannis et al. 2010). *Fusarium* (most often *F. solani*) and *Scedosporium* (most often *S. apiospermum/boydii* and *Lomentospora prolificans [formerly S. prolificans]*) are important causes of invasive disease in the transplant population (Perfect and Schell 1996; Pfaller and Diekema 2004). Note that *Scedosporium* spp. and their

Table 25.1 Fungi that may present with disseminated infection

Fungus	Usual patient and clinical setting	Principal manifestations other than fever
Candida spp.	ICU patients	Endophthalmitis, endocarditis
	Neonates	Meningitis
	Severely neutropenic or transplant patients	Papular, macronodular or purpuric skin lesions, hepatosplenic involvement, endocarditis
Aspergillus spp.	Severely neutropenic or transplant patients	Pulmonary syndrome, ulcerated necrotic skin lesions, focal neurological deficit
H. capsulatum	Acute DH: infants, immunosuppressed adults (e.g. lymphoma)	Hepatosplenomegaly, marrow involvement (pancytopenia), lymphadenopathy, interstitial pneumonia
	Acute DH in HIV	Maculopapular rash, interstitial pneumonia, marrow involvement (pancytopenia), septic shock
	Subacute DH: healthy and immunosuppressed adults	Hepatosplenomegaly, marrow involvement, oral ulcerations, adrenal deficiency
	Chronic DH: apparently healthy adults	Oropharyngeal ulcers or nodules, weight loss, hepatosplenomegaly
B. dermatitidis/gilchristii	Healthy or severe immunosuppression	Persistent mild pneumonia, chronic ulcerative skin lesions
C. immitis/posadasii	Healthy or severe immunosuppression	Variable: skin, bone, meningitis, and lung involvement
C. neoformans	Severe immunosuppression	CNS involvement and nodular rash
S. schenckii	Severe immunosuppression	Nodular skin lesions plus multifocal bone and joint involvement
P. brasiliensis/lutzii	Male patients residing in Central or South America	Destructive lesions of the oropharynx or nares, bone involvement, lung involvement
Fusarium spp.	Severely neutropenic or transplant patients	Paronychia and nodular skin lesions that often become necrotic
Trichosporon spp.	Severely neutropenic or transplant patients	Nodular skin lesions
Malassezia spp.	Associated with use of lipid-rich TPN solutions	Undifferentiated fever
B. capitatus	Severely neutropenic or transplant patients	Hepatosplenic involvement
T. marneffei	Travel to Southeast Asia/China	Disease is similar to acute disseminated histoplasmosis
Emmonsia spp.	Severe immunosuppression	Disease is similar to disseminated histoplasmosis or blastomycosis
Other agents*	Severely neutropenic or transplant patients	Fever and fungaemia

* *Paecilomyces* spp., *Pichia* spp., *Saccharomyces* spp., *Rhodotorula* spp.

CNS = central nervous system; DH = disseminated histoplasmosis; ICU = intensive care unit; TPN = total parenteral nutrition

Adapted from *Clinical Mycology*, Second Edition, Baer S. L., Pappas P. G., 'Haematogenously Disseminated Fungal Infections', pp. 609–22, Copyright © 2009 Elsevier Inc. with permission from Elsevier, http://www.sciencedirect.com/science/book/9781416056805

related teleomorphs in the genus *Pseudallescheria* have a complex and evolving nomenclature and are herein referred to collectively as *Scedosporium* spp.

Endemic fungi

The thermally dimorphic fungi *Histoplasma capsulatum*, *Blastomyces dermatitidis* (and *B. gilchristii*), *Paracoccidioides brasiliensis* (and *P. lutzii*), *Coccidioides immitis* (and *C. posadasii*), *Sporothrix schenckii*, and *Talaromyces* (formerly *Penicillium*) *marneffei* may cause invasive disease within a relatively restricted geographic range (Figure 25.1).

Epidemiology

Disseminated fungal infection occurs primarily in immunosuppressed patients, and advances in organ and stem cell transplantation, chemotherapy, and intensive care management have greatly increased the population at risk in recent years.

Candida spp. are the most common cause of invasive fungaemia amongst hospitalized patients and the fourth most common cause of all nosocomial bloodstream infections in some settings (Edmond et al. 1999). Patients in intensive care account for the majority of cases of invasive candidiasis, with candidaemia the most common presentation (Wisplinghoff et al. 2004; Playford et al. 2008, 2010). Risk factors for invasive disease include central venous catheters, parenteral nutrition, antibiotic use, mechanical ventilation, and haemodialysis. Abdominal and cardiac surgery put patients at increased risk of invasive disease, as do diabetes, renal failure, transplant, and steroid use (Eggimann et al. 2003; Pappas et al. 2010; Harrison et al. 2013). Mortality from invasive candidiasis is high—often in excess of 25% (Kibbler et al. 2003; Berdal et al. 2014; Klingspor et al. 2015)—and candidaemia has been independently associated with adverse outcomes in bloodstream infection (Pittet et al. 1997).

Invasive aspergillosis (IA) occurs predominantly in patients with prolonged neutropenia in the context of haematological malignancy

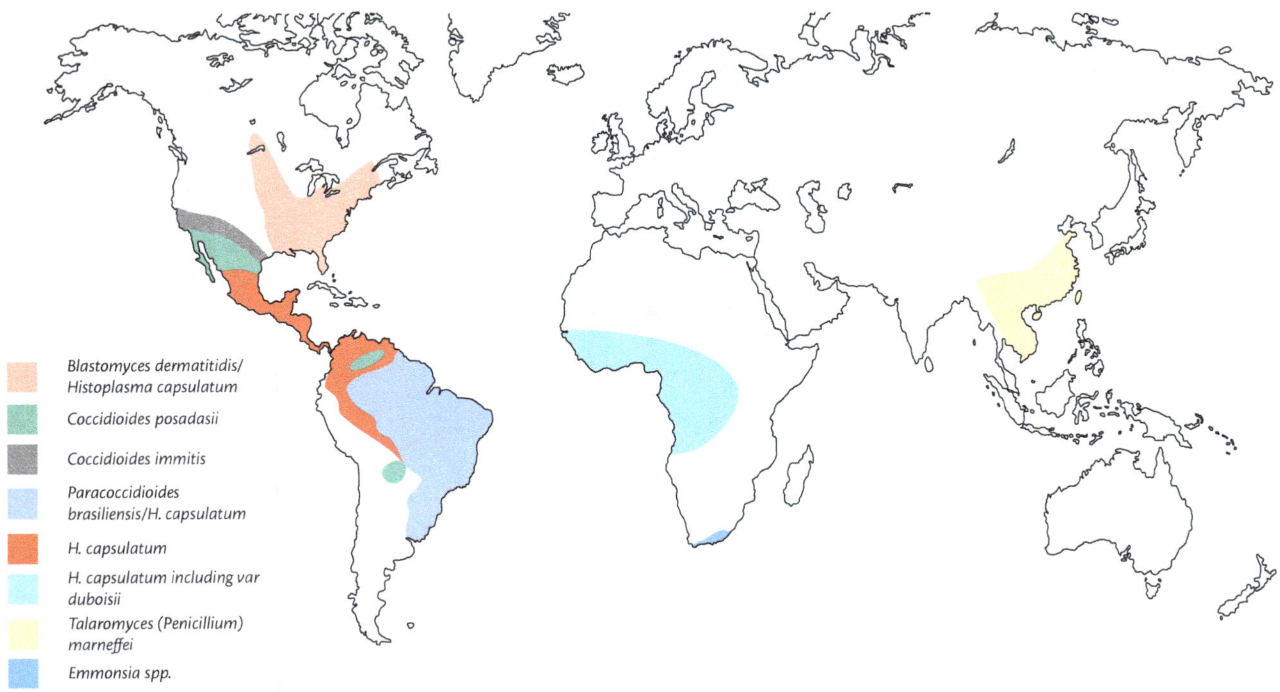

Figure 25.1 Major geographic distribution of the endemic mycoses.

Adapted from *Clinical Mycology*, Second Edition, Baer S. L., Pappas P. G., 'Haematogenously Disseminated Fungal Infections', pp. 609–22, Copyright © 2009 Elsevier Inc. with permission from Elsevier, http://www.sciencedirect.com/science/book/9781416056805.

and in haematopoietic stem cell transplantation (HSCT) or solid-organ transplant recipients (Kontoyiannis et al. 2010; Pappas et al. 2010). Other risk factors include advanced HIV (human immunodeficiency virus) infection (Barnes and Marr 2006), chronic granulomatous disease, and iatrogenic immunosuppression from steroids or anti-TNF agents (Tsiodras et al. 2008). Mortality from IA is high, often exceeding 50% in neutropenic patients and 85% in allogeneic HSCT recipients (Yeghen et al. 2000; Lin et al. 2001).

An increase in the use of voriconazole prophylaxis is thought, in part, to account for the rising incidence of disseminated infection from non-*Aspergillus* moulds (Marty et al. 2004). Most infections occur in the context of profound immunosuppression, particularly in HSCT (Nucci and Anaissie 2002) and solid-organ transplant recipients (Husain et al. 2003), but poorly controlled diabetes and renal failure are well-defined risk factors for invasive mucormycosis (Ribes et al. 2000).

Endemic fungi

Invasive disease from these organisms usually occurs in immunocompromised patients, in particular those with impaired T-cell immunity, but infection in healthy hosts is also well described. Histoplasmosis has a worldwide distribution; however, the Mississippi-Ohio River Valley region in the USA is considered to be the major endemic region. The other agents of endemic mycoses have a more limited geographic range (Figure 25.1).

Clinical features

The clinical features of disseminated fungal infection are frequently non-specific, and fever with or without a sepsis syndrome may be the sole manifestation (Denning et al. 2003). Patterns of signs and symptoms—when considered in the context of the patient—and risk factors can often narrow the diagnosis, but there are no pathognomonic clinical features.

Candidaemia in critical care patients frequently manifests as undifferentiated septic shock, and blood cultures may not become positive until late in the course of the infection (Kibbler et al. 2003). A persistent fever in a critical care patient who has risk factors and no other established source of fever should therefore raise suspicion of candidiasis and may prompt empirical treatment. Disseminated disease may be complicated by visceral involvement, most commonly affecting brain, myocardium, heart valves, and eyes. Candida retinitis occurs in up to 15% of cases (Donahue et al. 1994), whereas endophthalmitis (with vitreous involvement) (Figure 25.2) is classical but rarely seen. All patients with documented candidaemia should have a detailed ophthalmic assessment and echocardiogram (Ullmann et al. 2012a).

An invasive pulmonary syndrome with cough, pleuritic chest pain, fever, and occasionally haemoptysis is the most common form of invasive aspergillosis. Although these symptoms are non-specific, the clinical syndrome—combined with radiographic features of pulmonary parenchymal invasion in at-risk patients—should raise suspicion. Sinusitis and skin lesions are the other most frequently reported features of invasive disease, and progressive haematogenous dissemination—which may involve any organ, but most commonly the central nervous system (CNS)—carries a poor prognosis (Patterson et al. 2000).

Disseminated fusariosis can mimic IA, but skin lesions and positive blood cultures are more common. Up to 60–90% of patients will have a maculopapular or nodular rash, typically with ulceration and central necrosis of lesions (Nucci et al. 2004).

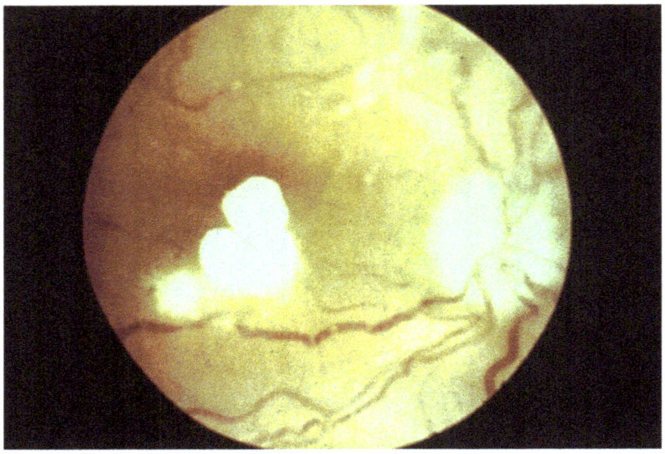

Figure 25.2 *Candida* endophthalmitis; multiple creamy white retinal lesions.

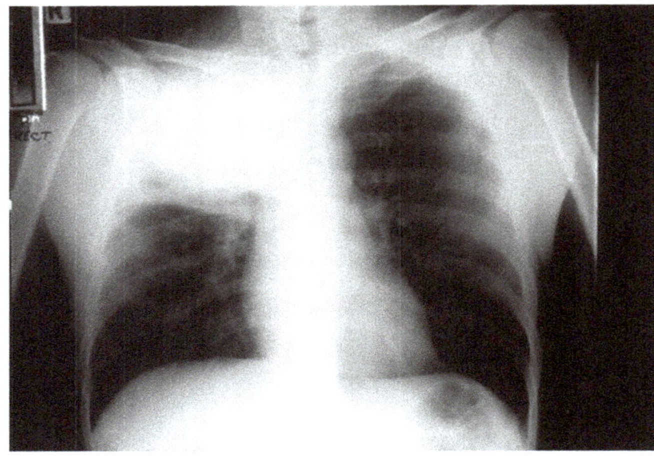

Figure 25.4 Radiograph showing pulmonary cryptococcal infection (right upper lobe disease)

The hallmark of mucormycosis is tissue necrosis and infarction, usually manifesting as rhino-orbital cerebral disease (Figure 25.3) or rapidly progressive pneumonia. Contiguous infection from the lungs or haematogenously disseminated disease is rare but carries high mortality (Roden et al. 2005).

Cryptococcal infection classically presents with CNS or pulmonary disease (Figure 25.4), and subacute meningitis in a patient with HIV is the most common scenario. However, cryptococcosis can occur in patients who are mildly immunosuppressed or in normal hosts, and presentation with only mild headaches, subtle cognitive impairment, or fever alone is well described. A low threshold for CSF (cerebrospinal fluid) sampling is required.

Acute disseminated histoplasmosis in infants and immunosuppressed adults is associated with massive reticuloendothelial involvement, causing a syndrome of fever, weight loss, lymphadenopathy, hepatosplenomegaly, and pancytopenia. Patients with HIV are at risk for severe disease with septic shock and multi-organ involvement (Goodwin et al. 1980; Wheat et al. 1990). Subacute dissemination is more common in older patients with chronic immunosuppression, for example those taking steroids, and may cause fever, hepatosplenomegaly, and gastrointestinal ulceration. Chronic disseminated histoplasmosis may be the hardest to diagnose, causing low-grade fevers and mild constitutional symptoms, sometimes in a normal host. A single painful oropharyngeal ulcer is a common manifestation, but almost any organ can be involved. Adrenal involvement with insufficiency can occur in any form of the disease.

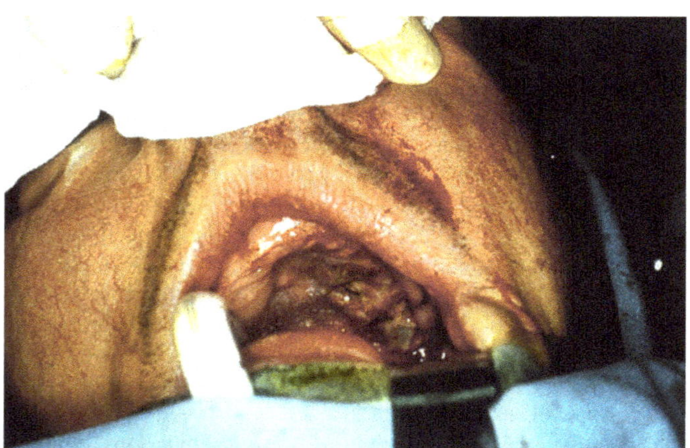

Figure 25.3 Rhinocerebral zygomycosis with palatal involvement.

The other endemic mycoses more commonly present with focal organ involvement, particularly respiratory infection. Rapidly fatal disseminated blastomycosis with respiratory failure, skin lesions, and multi-organ failure can occur, most commonly in cases of advanced HIV (Pappas et al. 1992). *Coccidioides* spp. are more likely to disseminate in certain patient groups, particularly pregnant women, Filipinos, African-Americans, and immunosuppressed hosts. Progression from primary pulmonary infection causes fever, skin lesions, meningitis, and bony involvement. Reticuloendothelial dissemination in paracoccidioidomycosis is the norm, causing hepatosplenomegaly, lymphadenopathy, and pancytopenia. Chronic dissemination with fever, weight loss, and cough may also occur. *Talaromyces* (formerly *Penicillium) marneffei*) typically causes disseminated infection in HIV, but can occur in other forms of immunosuppression and in healthy hosts. The clinical syndrome mimics chronic disseminated histoplasmosis, with fever, malaise, lymphadenopathy, hepatosplenomegaly, and pancytopenia. Umbilicated nodular or pustular skin lesions are classical.

The recently described endemic disease emmonsiosis may also mimic histoplasmosis or blastomycosis and almost always occurs in immunocompromised individuals (see Chapter 16).

Diagnosis

Early diagnosis and prompt initiation of antifungal therapy reduce mortality in disseminated fungal infection (Morrell et al. 2005; Garey et al. 2006), and the absence of pathognomonic clinical features means that a low threshold for tissue sampling and culture is required. Available guidelines recommend a unified approach to diagnosis involving microbiology, histopathology, and imaging (Pappas et al. 2009; Ullmann et al. 2012a; Schelenz et al. 2015).

Positive culture from blood or other sterile body fluids, or the presence of fungal elements in tissue or sterile body fluids, is the only way to be certain of invasive or disseminated infection, and biopsy of affected areas is essential where possible. However, tissue sampling is often logistically difficult in patients who are critically unwell, and sampling error can lead to low sensitivity.

Blood cultures should be taken in all cases of suspected IFD, but yield a diagnosis only for some fungi. The sensitivity of blood cultures approaches 50% for detecting disseminated *Candida* infection (Berenguer et al. 1993; Kibbler et al. 2003) and 40% for *Fusarium* infection, but other fungi are rarely isolated. Isolation of *Candida* from non-sterile sites can present diagnostic difficulty and does not always indicate infection. The presence of *Candida* in respiratory samples usually implies airway colonization or contamination rather than invasive pulmonary disease, and candiduria almost invariably represents colonization. However, in intensive care, candiduria may correlate with invasive disease and predict subsequent infection (Pittet et al. 1994). In general, guidelines suggest empirical therapy in septic patients who are not responding to appropriate antibacterial therapy rather than pre-emptive treatment of colonized patients in these settings (Pappas et al. 2009).

In immunocompromised patients the isolation of *Aspergillus* from respiratory samples has correlated well with invasive disease, but is far more likely to represent colonization in the normal host (Horvath and Dummer 1996). Tissue sampling and histopathological confirmation is the gold-standard for diagnosing IA, but host factors such as pancytopenia and respiratory failure frequently prohibit sampling in the most unwell patients.

Serological testing is a useful adjunct to diagnosis in some infections. The *Aspergillus* galactomannan ELISA (enzyme-linked immunosorbent assay) is more sensitive than culture in IA (Leeflang et al. 2008); twice-weekly screening is recommended in high-risk patient groups (Schelenz et al. 2015). A lateral flow device is now available for the rapid detection of a different antigen and appears of value in the diagnosis of IA, particularly when using bronchoalveolar lavage fluid (Hoenigl et al. 2014).

(1→3) β-D-glucan is a component of many fungal cell walls, and commercially available assays are sensitive with high negative predictive value. These assays may be useful in the diagnosis of IFD (although they are negative in cryptococcosis and mucormycosis), but positive tests require further investigation (Schelenz et al. 2015). Antigen testing using latex agglutination or lateral flow technology is well established in detecting cryptococcal antigen in CSF and serum, with high sensitivity and specificity. Antigen testing of body fluids is useful in the diagnosis of disseminated histoplasmosis, and urine antigen testing has the highest sensitivity of up to 90% in progressive disseminated disease (Kauffman 2006). Complement fixation serology is available for the diagnosis of *Coccidioides immitis and Paracoccidioides brasiliensis* infection, but may give false-negative results in patients with depressed immune systems. A number of *Blastomyces dermatitidis* antigen tests are available, and urinary assays in particular are sensitive but cross-react with other antigens, including those of *Histoplasma, Penicillium, and Paracoccidioides* (Kauffman 2006).

A number of rapid techniques have been developed to aid timely diagnosis of IFD. The *C. albicans* peptide nucleic acid (PNA) fluorescence *in situ* hybridization (FISH) test identifies *Candida* directly from blood cultures and can differentiate *albicans* from non-*albicans* spp. in a matter of hours with high sensitivity (Rigby et al. 2002; Wilson et al. 2005; Shepard et al. 2008; Stone et al. 2013). Matrix-assisted laser desorption/ionization–time-of-flight mass spectrometry (MALDI-TOF MS) can detect fungi directly from blood cultures, but currently with less sensitivity and specificity than PNA-FISH (Gorton et al. 2014)). Nucleic acid amplification tests have the potential to improve IFD diagnosis, but fully standardized data on most species-specific and 'pan-fungal' PCRs are not yet available, with their use currently limited to reference laboratories (Alanio and Bretagne 2014).

Treatment

Diagnostic difficulty and the need for prompt treatment frequently necessitate empiric or pre-emptive antifungal therapy in suspected IFD (Walsh et al. 2008). Empirical therapy involves use of antifungals in patients with undifferentiated fever and risk factors for IFD, whilst pre-emptive strategies involve treatment in the presence of suggestive laboratory tests or radiology but in the absence of confirmed microbiology or histopathology (Vazquez et al. 2013). There are many possible clinical settings, and good evidence for the value of one strategy over another is lacking. Pre-emptive strategies do seem to lead to an increase in confirmed diagnosis, but a difference in all-cause mortality has not yet been shown (Cordonnier et al. 2009).

Guidelines for the treatment of candidaemia in neutropenic and non-neutropenic patients are available (Cornely et al. 2012; Lortholary et al. 2012; Ullmann et al. 2012b). All candidaemic patients should be treated, and empirical therapy with fluconazole in intensive-care patients who have fever in the absence of usual causes has been shown to reduce mortality in uncontrolled studies (Garey et al. 2006). Removal of intravascular catheters improves outcomes in candidaemic patients and should form part of routine management where possible (Andes et al. 2012). In general, an echinocandin is recommended for empirical treatment in neutropenic patients owing to the risk of resistant non-*albicans* species, but fluconazole can be used first-line in non-neutropenic hosts. Treatment should be continued for two weeks after the last positive blood culture.

The specifics of other antifungal therapies are reviewed in Sections 2 and 4. Table 25.2 summarizes the treatment of selected disseminated fungal infections.

Prevention

Antifungal prophylaxis has been shown to reduce mortality from IFD amongst high-risk haematology and oncology patients, and a number of azole agents are effective (Morgenstern et al. 1999; Robenshtok et al. 2007; Marks et al. 2011). Antifungal prophylaxis in the intensive-care setting has been studied extensively but is currently only recommended in certain patient groups—in units with high rates of invasive candidiasis despite standard infection-control procedures (Pappas et al. 2009). In neutropenic patients, hand-washing, use of positive pressure and high-efficiency particulate air (HEPA)-filtered airflow, and care-bundles for intravenous catheter-insertion are all effective in lowering the incidence of fungal infections (Manuel and Kibbler 1998). Careful infection-control policies are therefore essential alongside any use of antifungal prophylaxis.

Table 25.2 Treatment of selected invasive fungal diseases

Disease	Primary therapy	Alternatives	Duration	Comments
Aspergillosis	Voriconazole	Amphotericin B/ L-AMB Isavuconazole Itraconazole Posaconazole (refractory disease) Echinocandin*	Minimum 2 weeks	Poor response unless neutrophil recovery Reduction in iatrogenic immunosuppression where possible
Candidiasis	Echinocandin	Fluconazole Amphotericin B/L-AMB	Minimum 2 weeks from first negative blood culture	Fluconazole may be used as primary therapy in stable non-neutropenic patients with no recent azole exposure
Blastomycosis				
Severe	Amphotericin B		6–12 months	In severe disease, step-down to itraconazole once patient stabilizes
Mild/moderate	Itraconazole			
Coccidioidomycosis				
Severe	Amphotericin B/L-AMB	Itraconazole	At least 6 months	Step-down to azole once patient stabilizes
Stable/slowly progressive	Fluconazole			
Histoplasmosis				
Non-immunosuppressed/ mild/moderate disease	Itraconazole	Amphotericin B	At least 12 months	
Severe disease	Amphotericin B/L-AMB			AmB for 1–2 weeks, then itraconazole for at least 12 months
Mucormycosis	L-AMB	Posaconazole Isavuconazole	Variable	Surgical debridement Control of predisposing condition Posaconazole as step-down once patient is improving
Paracoccidioidomycosis	Itraconazole		6 months	Relapses common

* As salvage combination therapy with voriconazole or mphotericin B.

AmB = amphotericin B; L-AMB = liposomal amphotericin B.

References

Alanio A and Bretagne S (2014) Difficulties with molecular diagnostic tests for mould and yeast infections: where do we stand? *Clin Microbiol Infect* 20 (Suppl. 6): 36–41.

Andes DR, Safdar N, Baddley JW, et al. (2012) Impact of treatment strategy on outcomes in patients with candidemia and other forms of invasive candidiasis: a patient-level quantitative review of randomized trials. *Clin Infect Dis* 54: 1110–22.

Baddley JW, Stroud TP, Salzman D and Pappas PG (2001) Invasive mold infections in allogeneic bone marrow transplant recipients. *Clin Infect Dis* 32: 1319–24.

Barber GR, Brown AE, Kiehn TE, Edwards FF and Armstrong D (1993) Catheter-related Malassezia furfur fungemia in immunocompromised patients. *Am J Med* 95: 365–70.

Barnes PD and Marr KA (2006) Aspergillosis: spectrum of disease, diagnosis, and treatment. *Infect Dis Clin North Am* 20: 545–61.

Berdal JE, Haagensen R, Ranheim T and Bjornholt JV (2014) Nosocomial candidemia; risk factors and prognosis revisited; 11 years experience from a Norwegian secondary hospital. *PLoS One* 9: e103916.

Berenguer J, Buck M, Witebsky F, et al. (1993) Lysis-centrifugation blood cultures in the detection of tissue-proven invasive candidiasis. Disseminated versus single-organ infection. *Diagn Microbiol Infect Dis* 17: 103–9.

Chowdhary A, Sharma C, Duggal S, et al. (2013) New clonal strain of Candida auris, Delhi, India. *Emerg Infect Dis* 19: 1670–3.

Cordonnier C, Pautas C, Maury S, et al. (2009) Empirical versus preemptive antifungal therapy for high-risk, febrile, neutropenic patients: a randomized, controlled trial. *Clin Infect Dis* 48: 1042–51.

Cornely OA, Bassetti M, Calandra T, et al. (2012) ESCMID* guideline for the diagnosis and management of Candida diseases 2012: non-neutropenic adult patients. *Clin Microbiol Infect* 18 (Suppl. 7): 19–37.

Dankner WM, Spector SA, Fierer J and Davis CE (1987) Malassezia fungemia in neonates and adults: complication of hyperalimentation. *Rev Infect Dis* 9: 743–53.

Denning DW, Kibbler CC, Barnes RA and British Society for Medical Mycology (2003) British Society for Medical Mycology proposed standards of care for patients with invasive fungal infections. *Lancet Infect Dis* 3: 230–40.

Donahue SP, Greven CM, Zuravleff JJ, et al. (1994) Intraocular candidiasis in patients with candidemia. Clinical implications derived from a prospective multicenter study. *Ophthalmology* 101: 1302–9.

Edmond MB, Wallace SE, Mcclish DK, et al. (1999) Nosocomial bloodstream infections in United States hospitals: a three-year analysis. *Clin Infect Dis* 29: 239–44.

Eggimann P, Garbino J and Pittet D (2003) Epidemiology of Candida species infections in critically ill non-immunosuppressed patients. *Lancet Infect Dis* 3: 685–702.

Emara M, Ahmad S, Khan Z, et al. (2015) Candida auris candidemia in Kuwait, 2014. *Emerg Infect Dis* 21: 1091–2.

Garey KW, Rege M, Pai MP, et al. (2006) Time to initiation of fluconazole therapy impacts mortality in patients with candidemia: a multi-institutional study. *Clin Infect Dis* 43: 25–31.

Girmenia C, Pagano L, Martino B, et al. (2005) Invasive infections caused by Trichosporon species and Geotrichum capitatum in patients with hematological malignancies: a retrospective multicenter study from Italy and review of the literature. *J Clin Microbiol* 43: 1818–28.
Goodwin RA Jr, Shapiro JL, Thurman GH, Thurman SS and Des Prez RM (1980) Disseminated histoplasmosis: clinical and pathologic correlations. *Medicine (Baltimore)* 59: 1–33.
Gorton RL, Seaton S, Ramnarain P, Mchugh TD and Kibbler CC (2014) Evaluation of a short, on-plate formic acid extraction method for matrix-assisted laser desorption ionization-time of flight mass spectrometry-based identification of clinically relevant yeast isolates. *J Clin Microbiol* 52: 1253–5.
Guinea J (2014) Global trends in the distribution of Candida species causing candidemia. *Clin Microbiol Infect* 20 (Suppl. 6): 5–10.
Haron E, Anaissie E, Dumphy F, Mccredie K and Fainstein V (1988) Hansenula anomala fungemia. *Rev Infect Dis* 10: 1182–6.
Harrison D, Muskett H, Harvey S, et al. (2013) Development and validation of a risk model for identification of non-neutropenic, critically ill adult patients at high risk of invasive Candida infection: the Fungal Infection Risk Evaluation (FIRE) Study. *Health Technol Assess* 17: 1–156.
Hoenigl M, Prattes J, Spiess B, et al. (2014) Performance of galactomannan, beta-d-glucan, Aspergillus lateral-flow device, conventional culture, and PCR tests with bronchoalveolar lavage fluid for diagnosis of invasive pulmonary aspergillosis. *J Clin Microbiol* 52: 2039–45.
Horn DL, Neofytos D, Anaissie EJ, et al. (2009) Epidemiology and outcomes of candidemia in 2019 patients: data from the prospective antifungal therapy alliance registry. *Clin Infect Dis* 48: 1695–703.
Horvath JA and Dummer S (1996) The use of respiratory-tract cultures in the diagnosis of invasive pulmonary aspergillosis. *Am J Med* 100: 171–8.
Husain S, Alexander BD, Munoz P, et al. (2003) Opportunistic mycelial fungal infections in organ transplant recipients: emerging importance of non-Aspergillus mycelial fungi. *Clin Infect Dis* 37: 221–9.
Kauffman CA (2006) Endemic mycoses: blastomycosis, histoplasmosis, and sporotrichosis. *Infect Dis Clin North Am* 20: 645–62.
Kibbler CC, Seaton S, Barnes RA, et al. (2003) Management and outcome of bloodstream infections due to Candida species in England and Wales. *J Hosp Infect* 54: 18–24.
Kiehn TE, Gorey E, Brown AE, Edwards FF and Armstrong D (1992) Sepsis due to Rhodotorula related to use of indwelling central venous catheters. *Clin Infect Dis* 14: 841–6.
Klingspor L, Tortorano AM, Peman J, et al. (2015) Invasive Candida infections in surgical patients in intensive care units: a prospective, multicentre survey initiated by the European Confederation of Medical Mycology (ECMM) (2006-2008). *Clin Microbiol Infect* 21: 87. e1–87.e10.
Kontoyiannis DP, Marr KA, Park BJ, et al. (2010) Prospective surveillance for invasive fungal infections in hematopoietic stem cell transplant recipients, 2001-2006: overview of the Transplant-Associated Infection Surveillance Network (TRANSNET) Database. *Clin Infect Dis* 50: 1091–100.
Lamagni TL, Evans BG, Shigematsu M and Johnson EM (2001) Emerging trends in the epidemiology of invasive mycoses in England and Wales (1990-9). *Epidemiol Infect* 126: 397–414.
Lee WG, Shin JH, Uh Y, et al. (2011) First three reported cases of nosocomial fungemia caused by Candida auris. *J Clin Microbiol* 49: 3139–42.
Leeflang MM, Debets-Ossenkopp YJ, Visser CE, et al. (2008) Galactomannan detection for invasive aspergillosis in immunocompromized patients. *Cochrane Database Syst Rev*: CD007394.
Lin SJ, Schranz J and Teutsch SM (2001) Aspergillosis case-fatality rate: systematic review of the literature. *Clin Infect Dis* 32: 358–66.
Lortholary O, Petrikkos G, Akova M, et al. (2012) ESCMID* guideline for the diagnosis and management of Candida diseases 2012: patients with HIV infection or AIDS. *Clin Microbiol Infect* 18 (Suppl. 7): 68–77.
Magobo RE, Corcoran C, Seetharam S and Govender NP (2014) Candida auris-associated candidemia, South Africa. *Emerg Infect Dis* 20: 1250–1.
Manuel RJ and Kibbler CC (1998) The epidemiology and prevention of invasive aspergillosis. *J Hosp Infect* 39: 95–109.
Marks DI, Pagliuca A, Kibbler CC, et al. (2011) Voriconazole versus itraconazole for antifungal prophylaxis following allogeneic haematopoietic stem-cell transplantation. *Br J Haematol* 155: 318–27.
Marr KA, Carter RA, Crippa F, Wald A and Corey L (2002) Epidemiology and outcome of mould infections in hematopoietic stem cell transplant recipients. *Clin Infect Dis* 34: 909–17.
Martino R, Salavert M, Parody R, et al. (2004) Blastoschizomyces capitatus infection in patients with leukemia: report of 26 cases. *Clin Infect Dis* 38: 335–41.
Marty FM, Cosimi LA and Baden LR (2004) Breakthrough zygomycosis after voriconazole treatment in recipients of hematopoietic stem-cell transplants. *N Engl J Med* 350: 950–2.
Morgenstern GR, Prentice AG, Prentice HG, et al. (1999) A randomized controlled trial of itraconazole versus fluconazole for the prevention of fungal infections in patients with haematological malignancies. U.K. Multicentre Antifungal Prophylaxis Study Group. *Br J Haematol* 105: 901–11.
Morrell M, Fraser VJ and Kollef MH (2005) Delaying the empiric treatment of candida bloodstream infection until positive blood culture results are obtained: a potential risk factor for hospital mortality. *Antimicrob Agents Chemother* 49: 3640–5.
Myers JW, Smith RJ, Youngberg G, Gutierrez C and Berk SL (1992) Fungemia due to Malassezia furfur in patients without the usual risk factors. *Clin Infect Dis* 14: 620–1.
Nohinek B, Zee-Cheng CS, Barnes WG, Dall L and Gibbs HR (1987) Infective endocarditis of a bicuspid aortic valve caused by Hansenula anomala. *Am J Med* 82: 165–8.
Nucci M and Anaissie E (2002) Cutaneous infection by Fusarium species in healthy and immunocompromised hosts: implications for diagnosis and management. *Clin Infect Dis* 35: 909–20.
Nucci M and Marr KA (2005) Emerging fungal diseases. *Clin Infect Dis* 41: 521–6.
Nucci M, Marr KA, Queiroz-Telles F, et al. (2004) Fusarium infection in hematopoietic stem cell transplant recipients. *Clin Infect Dis* 38: 1237–42.
Pappas PG, Alexander BD, Andes DR, et al. (2010) Invasive fungal infections among organ transplant recipients: results of the Transplant-Associated Infection Surveillance Network (TRANSNET). *Clin Infect Dis* 50: 1101–11.
Pappas PG, Kauffman CA, Andes D, et al. (2009) Clinical practice guidelines for the management of candidiasis: 2009 update by the Infectious Diseases Society of America. *Clin Infect Dis* 48: 503–35.
Pappas PG, Pottage JC, Powderly WG, et al. (1992) Blastomycosis in patients with the acquired immunodeficiency syndrome. *Ann Intern Med* 116: 847–53.
Pappas PG, Rex JH, Lee J, et al. (2003) A prospective observational study of candidemia: epidemiology, therapy, and influences on mortality in hospitalized adult and pediatric patients. *Clin Infect Dis* 37: 634–43.
Patterson TF, Kirkpatrick WR, White M, et al. (2000) Invasive aspergillosis. Disease spectrum, treatment practices, and outcomes. I3 Aspergillus Study Group. *Medicine (Baltimore)* 79: 250–60.
Perfect JR, Cox GM, Lee JY, et al. (2001) The impact of culture isolation of Aspergillus species: a hospital-based survey of aspergillosis. *Clin Infect Dis* 33: 1824–33.
Perfect JR and Schell WA (1996) The new fungal opportunists are coming. *Clin Infect Dis* 22 (Suppl. 2): S112–18.
Pfaller MA and Diekema DJ (2004) Rare and emerging opportunistic fungal pathogens: concern for resistance beyond Candida albicans and Aspergillus fumigatus. *J Clin Microbiol* 42: 4419–31.

Pittet D, Li N, Woolson RF and Wenzel RP (1997) Microbiological factors influencing the outcome of nosocomial bloodstream infections: a 6-year validated, population-based model. *Clin Infect Dis* 24: 1068–78.

Pittet D, Monod M, Suter PM, Frenk E and Auckenthaler R (1994) Candida colonization and subsequent infections in critically ill surgical patients. *Ann Surg* 220: 751–8.

Playford EG, Marriott D, Nguyen Q, et al. (2008) Candidemia in nonneutropenic critically ill patients: risk factors for non-albicans Candida spp. *Crit Care Med* 36: 2034–9.

Playford EG, Nimmo GR, Tilse M and Sorrell TC (2010) Increasing incidence of candidaemia: long-term epidemiological trends, Queensland, Australia, 1999–2008. *J Hosp Infect* 76: 46–51.

Ribes JA, Vanover-Sams CL and Baker DJ (2000) Zygomycetes in human disease. *Clin Microbiol Rev* 13: 236–301.

Rigby S, Procop GW, Haase G, et al. (2002) Fluorescence *in situ* hybridization with peptide nucleic acid probes for rapid identification of Candida albicans directly from blood culture bottles. *J Clin Microbiol* 40: 2182–6.

Robenshtok E, Gafter-Gvili A, Goldberg E, et al. (2007) Antifungal prophylaxis in cancer patients after chemotherapy or hematopoietic stem-cell transplantation: systematic review and meta-analysis. *J Clin Oncol* 25: 5471–89.

Roden MM, Zaoutis TE, Buchanan WL, et al. (2005) Epidemiology and outcome of zygomycosis: a review of 929 reported cases. *Clin Infect Dis* 41: 634–53.

Satoh K, Makimura K, Hasumi Y, et al. (2009) Candida auris sp. nov., a novel ascomycetous yeast isolated from the external ear canal of an inpatient in a Japanese hospital. *Microbiol Immunol* 53: 41–4.

Schelenz S, Barnes RA, Barton RC, et al. (2015) British Society for Medical Mycology best practice recommendations for the diagnosis of serious fungal diseases. *Lancet Infect Dis* 15: 461–74.

Shepard JR, Addison RM, Alexander BD, et al. (2008) Multicenter evaluation of the Candida albicans/Candida glabrata peptide nucleic acid fluorescent *in situ* hybridization method for simultaneous dual-color identification of C. albicans and C. glabrata directly from blood culture bottles. *J Clin Microbiol* 46: 50–5.

Stephen C, Lester S, Black W, Fyfe M and Raverty S (2002) Multispecies outbreak of cryptococcosis on southern Vancouver Island, British Columbia. *Can Vet J* 43: 792–4.

Stone NR, Gorton RL, Barker K, Ramnarain P and Kibbler CC (2013) Evaluation of PNA-FISH yeast traffic light for rapid identification of yeast directly from positive blood cultures and assessment of clinical impact. *J Clin Microbiol* 51: 1301–2.

Tortorano AM, Biraghi E, Astolfi A, et al. (2002) European Confederation of Medical Mycology (ECMM) prospective survey of candidaemia: report from one Italian region. *J Hosp Infect* 51: 297–304.

Tortorano AM, Kibbler C, Peman J, et al. (2006) Candidaemia in Europe: epidemiology and resistance. *Int J Antimicrob Agents* 27: 359–66.

Tsiodras S, Samonis G, Boumpas DT and Kontoyiannis DP (2008) Fungal infections complicating tumor necrosis factor alpha blockade therapy. *Mayo Clin Proc* 83: 181–94.

Ullmann AJ, Cornely OA, Donnelly JP, et al. (2012a) ESCMID* guideline for the diagnosis and management of Candida diseases 2012: developing European guidelines in clinical microbiology and infectious diseases. *Clin Microbiol Infect,* 18 (Suppl. 7): 1–8.

Ullmann AJ, Akova M, Herbrecht R, et al. (2012b) ESCMID* guideline for the diagnosis and management of Candida diseases 2012: adults with haematological malignancies and after haematopoietic stem cell transplantation (HCT). *Clin Microbiol Infect* 18 (Suppl. 7): 53–67.

Vazquez JA, Miceli MH and Alangaden G (2013) Invasive fungal infections in transplant recipients. *Ther Adv Infect Dis* 1: 85–105.

Walsh TJ, Anaissie EJ, Denning DW, et al. (2008) Treatment of aspergillosis: clinical practice guidelines of the Infectious Diseases Society of America. *Clin Infect Dis* 46: 327–60.

Wheat LJ, Connolly-Stringfield PA, Baker RL, et al. (1990) Disseminated histoplasmosis in the acquired immune deficiency syndrome: clinical findings, diagnosis and treatment, and review of the literature. *Medicine (Baltimore)* 69: 361–74.

Wilson DA, Joyce MJ, Hall LS, et al. (2005) Multicenter evaluation of a Candida albicans peptide nucleic acid fluorescent *in situ* hybridization probe for characterization of yeast isolates from blood cultures. *J Clin Microbiol* 43: 2909–12.

Wisplinghoff H, Bischoff T, Tallent SM, et al. (2004) Nosocomial bloodstream infections in US hospitals: analysis of 24,179 cases from a prospective nationwide surveillance study. *Clin Infect Dis* 39: 309–17.

Yeghen T, Kibbler CC, Prentice HG, et al. (2000) Management of invasive pulmonary aspergillosis in hematology patients: a review of 87 consecutive cases at a single institution. *Clin Infect Dis* 31: 859–68.

CHAPTER 26

Fungal diseases of the gastrointestinal tract

Silke Schelenz

Introduction to fungal gastrointestinal tract infections

A number of fungi are able to cause a variety of diseases which manifest themselves in the gastrointestinal (GI) tract, affecting the oropharynx, oesophagus, stomach, or intestine. Certain fungi can be acquired through contaminated food and drink products, while others, such as *Candida* spp., form part of the normal healthy gut microflora. The commonest clinical setting is the overgrowth of *Candida* in the GI tract following disruption of microflora by agents such as broad-spectrum antibiotics, leading to colonization and infection of the mucosal lining. If unmanaged, patients often develop oral and oesophageal candidiasis, or in severe cases *Candida* bloodstream infection and dissemination to other organs. Other yeasts, including *Saccharomyces* spp., acquired via the oral route are also able to cause mucosal and systemic infections, although this is less common and more prevalent in cancer patients.

The majority of tissue-invasive GI fungal diseases are due to environmental moulds that are ingested via either contaminated food or water products. These serious infections with primary focus in the gut are rare but often life-threatening in patients who are immunocompromised. In some cases invasive fungal infections with a primary focus elsewhere, including the lung, can disseminate to the GI tract, but this is a less common event. The main problem is the non-specific nature of clinical presentation and relative difficulty in confirming the diagnosis of the invasive fungal infection. As a consequence, diagnosis and appropriate treatment are delayed, contributing to significant morbidity and high mortality. Other non-infective GI fungal diseases related to fungal toxins or immune dysregulation are discussed in Chapters 9 and 31.

Causative fungi and brief discussion of fungi involved

Amongst fungi causing disease in humans, *Candida* is the commonest cause of GI fungal infections, whereas moulds are rare but emerging pathogens. Most cases of oropharyngeal and oesophageal candidiasis are due to *C. albicans*. Other non-*C. albicans* spp., including *C. glabrata, C. tropicalis*, and *C. krusei,* have been reported and are more prevalent in immunocompromised patients (Phillips et al. 1996). Identifying the particular *Candida* species is relevant for the appropriate choice of empirical treatment as some species are intrinsically resistant to certain antifungal agents; one example is *C. krusei*, which expresses natural resistance to fluconazole.

Saccharomyces is another yeast reported to cause GI tract infections, particularly in immunocompromised patients, including those with neutropenia and malignancies. The two main pathogens are *Saccharomyces cerevisiae* and *subtype S. boulardii*—found in food products and probiotics. *S. cerevisiae*, also known as 'brewer's yeast' or 'baker's yeast', is used in wine-, beer-, and bread-making.

Cryptococcosis may also involve the GI tract. Although this is rare, it should be considered in AIDS or severely immunocompromised patients (Colebunders et al. 1988; Washington et al. 1991). The basidiospores of *C. neoformans* are commonly found in soil and bird droppings worldwide, and *C. gattii* has been isolated from many different tree species around the world. Infections of the gut may occur as a result of dissemination of infection from the lungs.

Mould infections have emerged over recent years and are increasingly recognized as a cause of life-threatening GI tract infections. The two most common filamentous groups of fungi involved are *Aspergillus* and Mucorales spp. (*Mucor, Rhizopus, Absidia*, and *Cunninghamella*). They are able to cause life-threatening infections, particularly in immunocompromised patients.

Aspergillus spores are ubiquitous in the environment, in particular present in decaying organic matter such as compost. Infection normally occurs in the respiratory tract following inhalation of spores, but infections of the GI tract have also been found to be a consequence of ingesting contaminated food products such as nuts and spices. *A. fumigatus, A. flavus*, and *A. niger* are the most common species causing infection in humans.

Fungi of the order Mucorales are also typically found in soil, plants, and rotting organic matter. These fungi are classically known to cause life-threatening sinusitis in diabetic and immunocompromised patients, and cases of gut mucormycosis have been reported after presumed ingestion of contaminated food products.

Cases of GI tract infections with endemic dimorphic fungi such as *Paracoccidioides, Histoplasma*, and *Talaromyces marneffei* (formerly *Penicillium marneffei*) occur mainly in countries with a high endemicity. *Paracoccidioides brasiliensis* is endemic to Latin America (Brazil, Columbia, Venezuela). Its natural habitat remains unknown, although the fungus has been found in soil and areas of coffee cultivation.

Histoplasma capsulatum is endemic to the USA (Ohio River valley, Mississippi River), Canada, parts of Africa, and some areas of India (West Bengal). It is commonly found in soil but is also associated with bird and bat droppings, particularly in caves. *Histoplasma capsulatum* var. *duboisii*, which is mainly prevalent in Uganda, Nigeria, Zaire, the Ivory Coast, and Senegal, is the cause of African histoplasmosis and usually affects the skin and bones, though rare cases of GI disease have been reported in HIV (human immunodeficiency virus) patients (Ehui et al. 2011).

Talaromyces marneffei is endemic to Southeast Asian countries such as Thailand, Vietnam, Hong Kong, Taiwan, southern China, and India, particularly Manipur. The pathogen is associated with rats, but the natural habitat is uncertain.

For further information about these fungi, please refer to Section 2.

Epidemiology

The prevalence of serious fungal GI infections depends largely on the fungal species and their geographic endemicity as well as on the underlying risk factors among patients.

Candida is the commonest cause of GI tract infections. The yeast is a commensal of the human healthy gut and co-exists within the bowel microbial flora. Colonization occurs in infants as early as day five after birth and is more prevalent in preterm babies. *Candida* is present in the gut in up to 70% of healthy adults, but certain factors, including broad-spectrum antibiotics or steroid inhalers, promote an over-growth of *Candida*, resulting in mucosal infection. This process is augmented if there is impaired cellular immunity (diabetes, pregnancy, HIV/AIDS, or malignancies), mucosal damage such as mucositis following cytotoxic cancer chemotherapy, or low gastric pH.

Candida infections range from oral thrush to oesophagitis, gastritis, and in severe cases to translocation of yeasts into the bloodstream, causing candidaemia and dissemination to other organs. *Candida* can lead to gastric perforation in otherwise healthy patients with low gastric pH due to the use of antacids (Gupta 2012).

The overall prevalence of GI candidiasis has been reported in previous studies to be around 4–6%, and the most commonly affected sites are the oral cavity and the oesophagus, followed by the stomach, the small intestine, and the large intestine (Ears et al. 1972; Tsukamoto 1986).

Saccharomyces is another yeast found in food sources that colonizes the gut and is able to cause oesophagitis or systemic infection. Cases of *S. cerevisiae var boulardii* fungaemia have been reported following the use of *S. cerevisiae var boulardii* containing probiotics for the treatment of diarrhoea in critically ill patients (Lolis et al. 2008). Yeasts can easily translocate from the intestine into the bloodstream as a consequence of septic shock and intestinal ischaemia.

Cryptococcus infections are normally associated with meningoencephalitis following transient pneumonia. A review of an autopsy series showed GI tract involvement in 8 out of 24 (33%) *Cryptococcus* cases, suggesting that this pathogen is causing GI tract infections more often than was previously suspected (Washington et al. 1991). Most case reports are of infections in AIDS patients, but other predisposing factors are haematological malignancy and corticosteroid therapy. Infections are reported to involve the caecum, oesophagus, stomach, terminal ileum, colon, gallbladder, and small bowel. *Cryptococcus neoformans* has also been found in a small proportion of AIDS patients presenting with persistent diarrhoea, suggesting that this yeast may be causing gastroenteritis (Colebunders et al. 1988).

Mould infections of the GI tract are much rarer than yeast infections but are considered an emerging group of fungal infections associated with a high mortality. Moulds such as *Aspergillus* and Mucorales are able to enter the GI tract via the food chain. Secondary dissemination of invasive aspergillosis also occurs in the gut from other primary sites (mainly the lung) with an incidence of 4–23% in case series (Hori et al. 2002; Eggiman et al. 2006). Aspergillosis involving the GI tract has a high mortality rate of 47–60%, which may relate to late diagnosis and treatment, as well as the severity of the underlying pathological process in mainly immunocompromised patients (Eggiman et al. 2006).

The incidence of primary gut aspergillosis related to ingestion of spores is rare, with a reported frequency of around 1% amongst invasive aspergillosis cases (Eggiman et al. 2006). Particular risk factors for both *Aspergillus* and Mucorales infections are prolonged immunosuppression and neutropenia.

Mucormycosis of the GI tract is a rare but emerging invasive fungal infection. A review of 929 mucormycosis cases showed that 7% (66 cases) of patients had GI involvement (Roden et al. 2005). The infection is usually acquired through ingestion of contaminated foods such as fermented milk, dried bread products, and fermented porridge. The stomach is the most common site of GI infection, followed by the colon, small intestine, and oesophagus (Agha et al. 1985). Underlying predisposing factors include diabetes, haematological malignancy, immunosuppressive treatment, malnutrition, burns, metabolic acidosis, and iron chelation therapy (Lehrer et al. 1980; Roden et al. 2005; Spellberg 2012). The mortality is 85–98% (Cherney et al. 1999; Martinello et al. 2012).

Dimorphic fungi are also able to cause GI pathology, particularly as part of secondary infection, but in many cases the infection is not clinically recognized until post-mortem examination owing to non-specific symptoms and lack of awareness. GI tract involvement in histoplasmosis can affect both immunocompetent and immunocompromised patients. It is particularly common (70–90%) in patients with disseminated infection (Goodwin et al. 1980; Spivak et al. 1996). Based on autopsy studies of *P. brasiliensis* cases, involvement of the lower intestine occurs in 10–30% of cases, whereas upper GI tract infection is less common (3–10% duodenal infection) (Goldani 2011).

The majority of *T. marneffei* infections are seen in immunocompromised individuals such as HIV or solid organ transplant patients. In some endemic regions infections have been reported in 7.7% of AIDS patients, but the exact incidence of GI involvement is unclear (Low and Lee 2002). GI infections are mainly a result of disseminated disease and affect the oropharynx and intestine.

Clinical features

The clinical presentation of invasive gut mycosis depends on the location of the affected area and underlying risk factors such as immunosuppression (Table 26.1). Signs and symptoms are not pathognomonic for any specific fungus, although speed of progression may point to certain more acute and rapidly occurring infections such as mucormycosis rather than more chronic infections such as oesophageal candidiasis.

Oropharyngeal candidiasis presents classically as 'oral thrush' with pseudomembranous white lesions in the mouth, but

Table 26.1 Presentations of gut mycosis, underlying risk factors, and symptoms in selective case reports

Pathogen	Disease range	Risk factors	Symptoms	References
Aspergillus spp.	Small bowel infarction	AML, immunosuppression, transplant	Persistent fever, weight loss	Catalano et al. 1997
	Toxic megacolon	Sarcoma	Fever, abdominal pain, extensive abdominal distention	Mohite et al. 2007
	Gut aspergilloma	No risk factors	Mechanical bowel obstruction	Li et al. 2014
Candida spp.	Oesophagitis	Diabetes, neutropenia, AIDS, T-cell immunodeficiency	Oesophagitis: retrosternal pain, dysphagia; rarely haemorrhages Gastric perforation	Pappas et al. 2009
	Gastritis and gastric-perforation	Antacids—otherwise healthy, not immunosuppressed	Peritonitis, fever, abdominal pain Candidaemia	Gupta 2012
Saccharomyces cerevisiae var boulardii	Bloodstream infection	Probiotics	Signs of sepsis	Lolis et al. 2008
Histoplasma capsulatum	Predominantly the small bowel, but the large bowel, duodenum, stomach, and oesophagus can be affected	Immunosuppressed as well as non-immunocompromised patients	Intestinal ulcerations and inflammation	Lamps et al. 2000
Mucorales	Upper GI bleeding	Diabetes, phagocyte defects, corticosteroids, organ or stem cell transplantation, use of desferrioxamine	Acute abdomen, peritonitis	Nandu et al. 2009 Spellberg 2012 Martinello et al. 2012
Paracoccidioides brasiliensis	Colitis of the large intestine	Severe malnutrition in a child	Diarrhoea with fresh blood and mucus, severe malnutrition	Penna 1979
Talaromyces marneffei	Perforated sigmoid colon	Renal transplant	Abdominal pain and diarrhoea, septic shock	Hart et al. 2011

AML = acute myeloid leukaemia; GI = gastrointestinal

atrophic erythematous lesions are also common as well as glossitis and angular cheilitis. *Candida* oesophagitis may present with chest pain, difficulty swallowing, or—in infants—poor feeding. In a recent study 58% of patients were asymptomatic, and the symptomatic population presented with acid regurgitation (21.7%), epigastric pain (18.9%), dyspepsia (13.5%), or nausea (10.3%), but only 11.7% had typical oesophageal symptoms (dysphagia, odynophagia, or chest discomfort) (Choi et al. 2013). It is important to note that the majority (90%) of patients may not have concomitant oral candidiasis.

Patients with acute leukaemia or other haematological malignancies may also have ulceration of the stomach, and less commonly of the duodenum or intestine. Perforation can lead to peritonitis and haematogenous spread to the liver, spleen, and other organs. GI tract infections with *Saccharomyces* spp. are able to mimic signs and symptoms of candidiasis and cannot clinically be distinguished.

A number of case reports have shown that *Cryptococcus* infections can cause secondary infection of the GI tract, affecting caecum, oesophagus, stomach, terminal ileum, colon, gallbladder, and small bowel (Washington et al. 1991). Clinical presentation will depend upon the part of the GI tract that is infected. Prolonged and chronic diarrhoea in AIDS patients may be associated with cryptococcal gastroenteritis (Colebunders et al. 1988). Symptoms of oesophagitis have been reported as gastroesophageal reflux, including odynophagia, and are similar to those caused by *Candida* (Washington et al. 1991). Clinical symptoms of GI cryptococcal infection may be the first indication of disseminated disease.

Invasive aspergillosis of the gut can be primary, or secondary due to dissemination from other sites. Primary infections of the gut are rare but have been described in high-risk immunocompromised patients such as those with acute myeloid leukaemia undergoing chemotherapy (Li et al. 2014). Presenting symptoms depend on the location, but abdominal pain, severe abdominal distention, and persistent fever despite broad-spectrum antibiotics are common features (Mohite et al. 2007). In an autopsy review of 107 cases of invasive aspergillosis, 25 (23%) demonstrated secondary GI involvement (Hori et al. 2002). The majority (16/25 cases) had upper GI tract infections, including oesophagitis, gastric, and duodenal disease. Clinical symptoms included upper abdominal pain and severe melaena, but some cases were asymptomatic. Nine cases had lower GI tract involvement of the large or small intestine with signs and symptoms of bloody diarrhoea, intestinal or colon mass, pan-peritonitis, or ileus.

GI mucormycosis is a rapidly developing angio-invasive aggressive infection, although the diagnosis is often delayed because of the non-specific presentation. Infection may present with an abdominal mass (appendix, caecum, or ileum) or this can be mistaken for an intra-abdominal abscess. Abdominal pain, distention, and vomiting are the most common presenting symptoms. Gut mucormycosis should be considered in patients with typical risk factors, such as diabetes, neutropenia and iron-chelating therapy, or presenting with pain or bleeding, in combination with abnormal endoscopic findings.

In patients who are, or have been, in countries where dimorphic fungi are endemic, clinicians should also consider these as causes of GI tract infections. Paracoccidioidomycosis has two main clinical presentations: juvenile acute/subacute infection and the more common chronic infection in adults. The infection should therefore be considered in patients with a past medical history of having visited endemic areas of South America. GI tract involvement is more common in the chronic adult disease and involves mainly the small and large intestine presenting with abdominal lymphadenopathy, dilated loops, mucosal nodules, and ulceration. Infection of the oesophagus or stomach is uncommon (Goldani 2011).

Histoplasmosis can be subacute or severe, depending on the cellular host immune response. A review of GI histoplasmosis showed, in the majority of cases, an involvement of the ileum, but other sites—including jejunum, colon, oesophagus, and stomach—can also be affected (Lamps et al. 2000). The infected lesions mainly present as ulcers and mucosal inflammation. Clinical symptoms are again non-specific and clinical suspicion should be high in immunocompromised patients from endemic areas (Goldani 2011).

Another mycosis causing GI tract infection in immunocompromised hosts is infection with *Talaromyces marneffei*. Again, signs and symptoms are non-specific and may include fever, abdominal pain, and diarrhoea (Hart et al. 2011). These are often in association with the molluscum contagiosum-like skin lesions of the disseminated infection. Clinical suspicion is essential in particular in patients who have had contact with endemic areas such as Southeast Asia.

Diagnosis

The clinical diagnosis of GI fungal diseases, other than oral candidiasis, is often not easy, as there are no pathognomonic signs or symptoms. There are, however, three main approaches to diagnosing severe disease, which are: imaging (endoscopy, ultrasound, computed tomography [CT]/magnetic resonance imaging), serology (fungal biomarkers, fungal specific antibody, and antigen detection), and microscopy of tissue using special fungal stains (Grocott methenamine silver stain, Calcofluor, PAS [periodic acid-Schiff]) and cultures. Molecular diagnostic assays such as PCR (polymerase chain reaction) remain less commonly used although they can be applied to tissue samples if available.

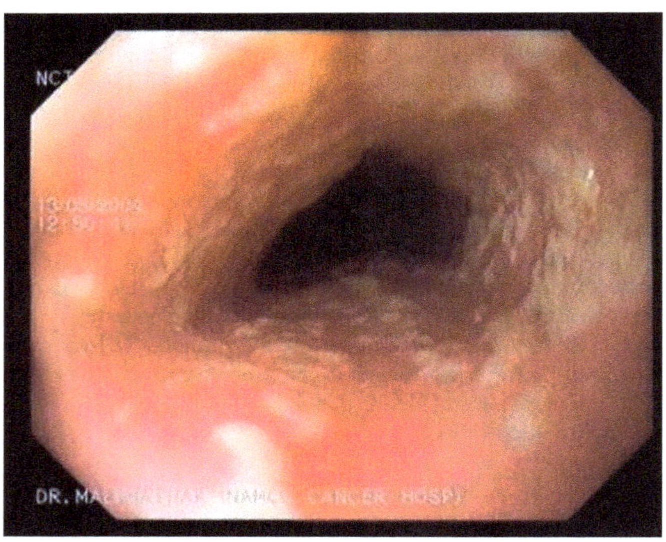

Figure 26.1 *Candida* oesophagitis showing typical white and yellow plaques adherent to the mucosa.
Reproduced courtesy of Vijay Malpathak and Wiley Blackwell.

The diagnosis of oropharyngeal candidiasis is relatively easy to establish. Oral candidiasis is characterized by white patchy lesions, ulcerations, or red painful patches that can be swabbed and cultured to confirm the causative organism, but other yeasts such as *Saccharomyces* or *Cryptococcus* can also cause this presentation. Fungal oesophagitis is diagnosed by endoscopy, showing white or yellow plaques (Figure 26.1). Biopsy or mucosal brushings provide direct evidence of invasive infection, and fungal elements may be seen as magenta-stained structures using PAS stain or black with Grocott silver stain. Microabscesses are usually visible with polymorphonuclear infiltrates, although less so in neutropenia.

In suspected cryptococcal disease a serum cryptococcal antigen test should be performed. Upper GI endoscopy has been useful in diagnosing cryptococcal oesophagitis and has also demonstrated gastric nodules in AIDS patients (Washington et al. 1991). Some cases are only diagnosed at post mortem because of lack of clinical suspicion.

Diagnosis of invasive mould infection of the GI tract is more difficult to confirm owing to the more obscure presentation and less accessible location, which means that a diagnosis is often only achieved on tissue histology after surgery or post mortem. All cases benefit from a CT of the abdomen and endoscopy to identify the location of any potentially affected tissues.

In some cases, such as invasive GI tract aspergillosis, the detection of fungal biomarkers, particularly serum galactomannan, may be useful in supporting a diagnosis, but ultimate confirmation is by histology of the affected GI tract tissue. Tissues stained by PAS or Grocott demonstrate typically acute-angled branching, septate hyphae of *Aspergillus* spp. The mucosa may show ulcers and debris containing inflammatory cells and necrosis on H&E (haematoxylin & eosin) stain.

In cases of GI mucormycosis, endoscopy has demonstrated lesions with a grey plaque-like base and necrotic slough over it resembling a tumour. Biopsies from the centre and edge of the lesion may show non-septate, right angular branched fungal hyphae indicative of Mucorales moulds on PAS and Grocott stains. While diagnosis relies extensively on the identification of the fungus in tissue histology, confirmation of the species is challenging given the frequent absence of growth on culture. Some studies have used PCR and sequencing of the internal transcribed spacer (ITS)1 of the RNA gene on formalin fixed wax-embedded blocks to establish the diagnosis (Martinello et al. 2012).

The confirmation of GI histoplasmosis is also strongly based on histology. As *Histoplasma capsulatum* particularly affects the reticuloendothelial system, fungal lesions can be found in Peyer patches and mucosal lymphoid tissue in ulcer and nodule biopsies. Unfortunately, in many patients with gut histoplasmosis, the fungal cultures, serology, and skin tests for *Histoplasma* have been reported negative (Lamps et al. 2000), but the *Histoplasma* antigen may be positive in disseminated disease.

Histopathology is also useful for the diagnosis of paracoccidioidomycosis, as Grocott-stained biopsies may demonstrate the typical 'pilot's wheel' appearance of a mother cell surrounded by multiple peripheral daughter cells. Mucosal biopsies can also be cultured, but the fungus may take some time to grow. Another useful test is serology (agar gel immunodiffusion) for the detection of anti-*P. brasiliensis* antibodies, which are highly specific for the confirmation of active infection and in monitoring clinical response to antifungal therapy. In immunocompromised patients such as those with AIDS, antibody titres may be unreliable and antigen tests should be performed (Goldani 2011).

Histology and cultures of tissue biopsies of infected mucosa in suspected infection with *T. marneffei* are useful. Blood cultures should also be taken as they are positive in some cases (Hart et al. 2011). In addition, serological tests have been described, including an indirect immunofluorescent antibody test, although antibody-based assays have limited value in severely immunocompromised patients (Yuen et al. 1994). One should be aware that monoclonal antibodies used in the Platelia *Aspergillus* galactomannan antigen test may cross-react with the galactomannan of *Talaromyces* spp.

Treatment

The specific treatment for fungal GI tract infections depends on the confirmation of fungal species and susceptibility. As symptoms are often non-specific, leading to late diagnosis, it is advisable for at-risk patients with persistent fever and GI symptoms to start empirical therapy with a broad-spectrum antifungal agent. As GI mycosis can cause gut perforation and peritonitis, positive blood cultures with bacterial gut organisms should not distract clinicians from the possibility of invasive fungal infection. Part of the general management of confirmed invasive gut mycosis should also be the minimization of underlying risk factors such as control of diabetes. There are a number of national and international guidelines available to aid antifungal treatment which are beyond the scope of this chapter and are described in Chapter 49.

The first-line treatment of oropharyngeal candidiasis is based on an azole (fluconazole, or other triazole), depending on the susceptibility. International guidelines suggest that *Candida* oesophagitis should be treated with fluconazole, or in more severe cases, or if the isolate is azole resistant, with an echinocandin or amphotericin B (Pappas et al. 2009). Cryptococcal infections will also usually respond to fluconazole or amphotericin B and should be treated in the same way as other cases of disseminated cryptococcosis.

For most invasive mould infections, surgical intervention and reduction of immunotherapy are essential in order to remove infarcted bowel and tissue and to improve the host response to infection. In one case of *Aspergillus* toxic megacolon, total colectomy and ileostomy, followed by two weeks of antifungal therapy, led to cure of the infection (Mohite et al. 2007).

Surgical debridement of necrotic tissue also seems to be critical in gut mucormycosis, combined with early antifungal therapy (high-dose liposomal amphotericin B). Other options include posaconazole or isavuconazole, adjunctive treatment (recombinant cytokines [G-CSF, GM-CSF, IFN-gamma], granulocyte transfusion) or combination therapy. In the context of GI mucormycosis, posaconazole administration and absorption may be problematic, specifically in the perioperative period, where therapeutic drug monitoring is crucial.

Specific treatment for GI paracoccidioidomycosis includes prolonged (up to 6 months) antifungal therapy with drugs such as itraconazole, which has a reported effectiveness of 95%, or voriconazole (Queiroz-Telles et al. 2007). Fluconazole has a lower response rate and higher relapse rate.

GI infection with *T. marneffei* also usually responds to antifungal therapy with agents such as liposomal amphotericin B, itraconazole, and voriconazole, but untreated disseminated infection is almost always fatal. Long-term suppressive maintenance therapy may be necessary depending on the CD4 count.

Prevention

Immunocompromised patients should receive advice on the risk associated with certain food and water to avoid or reduce the risk of potentially contaminated food sources. Public health monitoring and good food standards should assure a high quality and safe food/environment.

Primary and secondary prophylaxis with antifungal agents in some HIV positive or severely immunocompromised patients may be needed for some mycoses including candidiasis, *cryptoccocosis* and *T. marneffei* infections.

References

Agha FP, Lee HH, Boland CR, et al. (1985) Mucormycoma of the colon: early diagnosis and successful management. *AJR Am J Roentgenol* 145: 739.

Catalano J, Picardi M, Anzivino D, Insabato L, Notaro R and Rotoli B (1997) Small bowel infarction by Aspergillus. *Haematologica* 82: 182–3.

Cherney CL, Chutuape A and Fikrig MK (1999) Fatal invasive gastric mucormycosis occurring with emphysematous gastritis: case report and literature review. *Am J Gastroenterol* 94: 252.

Choi JH, Chang Geun Lee CG, Lim YJ, Kang HW, Lim CY and Choi J-S (2013) Prevalence and risk factors of esophageal candidiasis in healthy individuals: a single center experience in Korea. *Yonsei Med J* 54: 160–5.

Colebunders R, Lusakumuni K, Nelson AM, et al. (1988) Persistent diarrhoea in Zairian AIDS patients: an endoscopic and histological study. *Gut* 29: 1687–91.

Ears P, Goldstein M and Sherlock P (1972) *Candida* infections of the gastrointestinal tract. *Medicine* 51: 367–79.

Eggiman P, Chevrolet M, Starobinski M, et al. (2006) Primary invasive aspergillosis of the digestive tract: report of two cases and review of the literature. *Infection* 34: 333–8.

Ehui E, Doukouré B, Kolia-Diafouka P, et al. (2011) Intestinal histoplasmosis with *Histoplasma duboisii* in a patient infected by HIV-1 in Abidjan (Ivory Coast). *J AIDS Clin Res* 2: 125.

Goldani LZ (2011) Gastrointestinal paracoccidioidomycosis. *J Clin Gastroenterol* 45: 87–9.

Goodwin RA, Shapiro JL, Thurman GH, et al. (1980) Disseminated histoplasmosis: clinical and pathologic correlations. *Medicine* 59: 1–33.

Gupta N (2012) A rare cause of gastric perforation-candida infection: a case report and review of the literature. *J Clin Diagn Res* 6: 1564–5.

Hart J, Dyer JR, Clark BM, McLellan DG, Perera S and Ferrari P (2011) Travel-related disseminated *Penicillium marneffei* infection in a renal transplant. *Transpl Infect Dis* 14: 434–9.

Hori A, Kami M, Kishi Y, et al. (2002) Clinical significance of extra-pulmonary involvement of invasive aspergillosis: a retrospective autopsy-based study of 107 patients. *J Hosp Infect* 50: 175–82.

Lamps LW, Molina CP, West AB, Haggitt RC and Scott MA (2000) The pathologic spectrum of gastrointestinal and hepatic histoplasmosis. *Am J Clin Pathol* 113: 64–72.

Lehrer RI, Howard DH and Sypherd PS, et al. (1980) Mucormycosis. *Ann Intern Med* 93: 93–108.

Li E, Hussein H, Todiwala A and Kirby R (2014) Primary gut aspergillosis in a patient with acute myeloid leukaemia: the importance of early suspicion and definitive treatment. *BMJ Case Rep* Mar 18, 2014. pii: bcr2013202316. doi: 10.1136/bcr-2013-2316

Lolis N, Veldekis D, Moraitou H, et al. (2008) Saccharomyces boulardii fungaemia in an intensive care unit patient treated with caspofungin. *Crit Care* 12: 414.

Low K and Lee SS (2002) The pattern of aids reporting and the implications on HIV surveillance. *Public Health Epidemiol Bull* 11: 41–9.

Martinello M, Nelson A, Bignold L and Shaw D (2012) "We are what we eat!" Invasive intestinal mucormycosis: a case report and review of the literature. *Med Mycol Case Rep* 1: 52–5.

Mohite U, Kell J, Haj MA, et al. (2007) Invasive aspergillosis localised to the colon presenting as toxic megacolon. *Eur J Haematol* 78: 270–3.

Nandu V, Nagral A, Khubchandani S and Agrawal C (2009) A rare cause of upper GI bleeding. *Gut* 58: 1039–48.

Pappas PG, Kauffman CA, Andes D, et al. (2009) Clinical Practice Guidelines for the Management of Candidiasis: 2009 update by the Infectious Diseases Society of America. *Clin Infect Dis* 48: 503–35.

Penna FJ (1979) Blastomycosis of the colon resembling clinically ulcerative colitis. *Gut* 20: 896–9.

Phillips P, Zemcov J, Mahmood W, Montaner JS, Craib K and Clarke AM (1996) Itraconazole cyclodextrin solution for fluconazole-refractory oropharyngeal candidiasis in AIDS: correlation of clinical response with in vitro susceptibility. *AIDS* 10: 1369–76.

Queiroz-Telles F, Goldani LZ, Schlamm HT, et al. (2007) An open label comparative pilot study of oral voriconazole and itraconazole for long-term treatment of paracoccidioidomycosis. *Clin Infect Dis* 45: 1462–9.

Roden MM, Zaoutis TE, Buchanan WL, et al. (2005) Epidemiology and outcome of zygomycoses: a review of 929 reported cases. *Clin Infect Dis* 41: 634–53.

Spellberg B (2012) Gastrointestinal mucormycosis. *Gastroenterol Hepatol (N Y)* 8: 140–2.

Spivak H, Schlasinger MH, Tabanda-Lichauco R, et al. (1996) Small bowel obstruction from gastrointestinal histoplasmosis in acquired immune deficiency syndrome. *Am Surg* 62: 369–72.

Tsukamoto H (1986) Clinicopathological studies on fungal infections of the digestive tract. *Jpn J Gastroenterol* 83: 2341–50.

Washington K, Gottfried MR and Wilson ML (1991) Gastrointestinal cryptococcosis. *Mod Pathol* 4: 707–11.

Yuen KY, Wong SS, Tsang DN and Chau PY (1994) Serodiagnosis of *Penicillium marneffei* infection. *Lancet* 344: 444–5.

CHAPTER 27

Genito-urinary fungal infections

Jack D. Sobel

Introduction to genito-urinary fungal infections

Given the vast array of fungal genera that can cause invasive disease in multiple organ systems, it is striking that *Candida* spp. alone are responsible for the overwhelming majority of mycotic infections involving the lower genital tract and urinary tract in both sexes. The pathogenesis of *Candida* infections in the lower genital tract in both men and women reflects common asymptomatic colonization which can transform into symptomatic syndromes, while the infection remains remarkably superficial or mucosal only, without tissue invasion. In contrast, kidney and prostate infection due to any mycotic genus represents either ascending disease or is secondary to systemic bloodstream infection, but is an invasive fungal infection. Given the predominance of *Candida* spp. as genitourinary pathogens, most of the text of this chapter will be directed at candidiasis.

Female lower genital tract fungal infection

Candidal vaginitis is the second most common vaginal infection after bacterial vaginosis. During the childbearing years, 75% of women experience at least one episode of vulvovaginal candidiasis, and 40–50% of these women experience a second episode (Hurley 1981). A small subpopulation of women (6–9%) experience repeated recurrent episodes of candidal vaginitis (Foxman et al. 2013).

Asymptomatic vaginal candidiasis

Asymptomatic candidiasis is common; *Candida* organisms may be isolated from the genital tract of about 20% of asymptomatic healthy women of childbearing age. *Candida* gains access to the vaginal lumen and secretions predominantly from the adjacent perianal area, and then adheres to vaginal epithelial cells (Sobel et al. 1998; Sobel 2007).

The hormonal dependence of the infection is illustrated by the fact that *Candida* is seldom isolated from premenarchal girls, and that the prevalence of candidal vaginitis is lower after the menopause, except in women taking hormone replacement therapy (HRT).

Pathogenesis

Germination of *Candida* enhances colonization and tissue invasion. Factors that facilitate germination (e.g. oestrogen therapy, pregnancy) tend to precipitate symptomatic vaginitis; measures that inhibit germination may prevent acute vaginitis in women who are asymptomatic carriers of yeast. Other virulence factors include proteolytic enzymes, toxins, and phospholipase elaboration (see Chapter 8). In individual patients it is uncommon to find a precipitating factor that explains the transformation from asymptomatic carriage to symptomatic vaginitis, except for use of antibacterial agents (Sobel 2007).

Oestrogens: During pregnancy, the incidence of clinical episodes reaches a maximum in the third trimester, but symptomatic recurrences are common throughout pregnancy. It is generally thought that the high level of reproductive hormones increases the glycogen content of the vaginal environment and provides a carbon source for *Candida* growth and germination. Oestrogens increase vaginal epithelial cell avidity for *Candida* adherence, and a yeast cytosol receptor or binding system for female reproductive hormones has been documented. In addition, oestrogens increase the formation of yeast mycelia. Low-oestrogen oral contraceptives and HRT, especially topical therapy, may contribute to vaginitis in post-menopausal women.

Diabetes mellitus: Vaginal colonization with *Candida* is more common in diabetes mellitus; uncontrolled diabetes predisposes to symptomatic vaginitis. Type 2 diabetes selects for *C. glabrata*. Diets high in, or binges of, refined sugar may precipitate symptomatic vaginitis.

Antibiotics: Symptomatic vulvovaginal candidiasis often occurs during or after use of systemic or intravaginal antibiotics, possibly as a result of eliminating the normal protective vaginal bacterial flora. Although no antimicrobial agent is free from this complication, it is especially common following the use of broad-spectrum antibiotics (Pirotta and Garland 2005). It is hypothesized that *Lactobacillus* spp. in the natural flora provide a colonization resistance mechanism and prevent germination of *Candida*. However, most women taking antibiotics do not develop candidal vaginitis, and women deficient in lactobacilli are not at risk of developing candidal vaginitis.

Environmental factors: Factors that predispose to candidal vaginitis may include tight, poorly ventilated clothing and nylon underclothing, which increase perineal moisture levels and temperature. Chemical contact, local allergy, and hypersensitivity reactions may also predispose to symptomatic vaginitis (Sobel 2007).

Immunosuppression: In patients who are debilitated or immunosuppressed, oral and vaginal candidiasis correlate well with reduced cell-mediated immunity. This is evident in chronic mucocutaneous candidiasis and AIDS. Cell-mediated immunity (Th17) contributes to normal vaginal defence mechanisms by preventing mucosal invasion and vaginitis.

Genetic factors: These have an important role in determining the risk of both vaginal yeast colonization and symptomatic episodes. Recent studies suggest a role for mannose-binding lectin, toll-like receptors, and cytokine gene polymorphisms (Rosentul et al. 2014).

Recurrent and chronic candidal vaginitis: Various theories have been proposed to explain recurrent vaginitis (Sobel 2007).

Intestinal reservoir: The intestinal reservoir theory is based on the recovery of *Candida* on rectal culture in almost 100% of women with vulvovaginal candidiasis. DNA typing of vaginal and rectal cultures obtained simultaneously usually reveals identical strains. However, other studies have shown a lower concordance between rectal and vaginal cultures in patients with recurrent vulvovaginal candidiasis (RVVC); also, oral nystatin, which reduces intestinal yeast carriage, fails to prevent recurrence of vulvovaginal candidiasis. Repeated re-introduction of yeast into the vagina from the gut is therefore no longer considered a likely cause of recurrent candidal vaginitis.

Sexual transmission: Penile colonization with *Candida* is present in about 20% of male partners of women with RVVC; infected partners usually carry identical strains. Oral colonization of partners with an identical strain of *Candida* also occurs and may be a source of orogenital transmission. However, in most studies involving treatment of partners, there was no reduction in the frequency of episodes of vaginitis, undermining this hypothesis.

Vaginal relapse: Although antimycotic therapy may reduce the number of *Candida* organisms in the lumen and alleviate the signs and symptoms of inflammation, eradication or clearance of *Candida* from the vagina is incomplete, in part because all of the antimycotic agents are fungistatic. The small number of organisms that persist in the vagina results in continued carriage of the organism, so that when host environmental conditions permit, the colonizing organisms increase in number and undergo mycelial transformation, resulting in a new clinical episode. Host factors that determine persistence and regrowth of *Candida* organisms may include the vaginal microbiome and genetically determined host inflammatory responses.

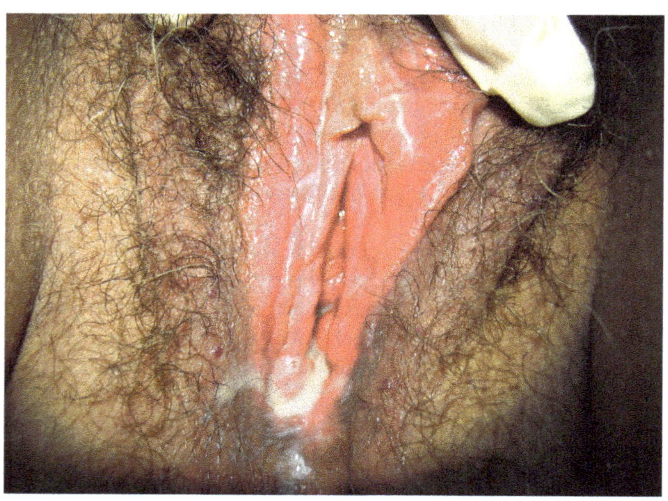

Figure 27.1 Diffuse erythema and oedema of the vulval vestibule and labia in acute *Candida* vaginitis.
Reproduced courtesy of Jack D. Sobel.

Antifungal drug resistance: This is seldom responsible for recurrent vulvovaginal candidiasis in women infected with *C. albicans*, but has been reported to be on the increase (Marchaim et al. 2012).

Clinical features

Vulval pruritus is the most common symptom of candidal vulvovaginitis and is present in most symptomatic patients (Eckert et al. 1998). Vaginal discharge is often minimal and sometimes absent. Although described as being typically 'cottage cheese-like' in character, this discharge may vary from watery to homogeneously thick. Vaginal soreness, irritation, vulval burning, dyspareunia, and external dysuria are common.

Characteristically, symptoms are exacerbated during the week before the onset of menses. The onset of menstrual flow brings some relief. Examination reveals erythema (Figure 27.1) and swelling of the labia and vulva, often with discrete, pustulopapular peripheral lesions including fissures. The cervix is normal. Vaginal mucosal erythema with adherent whitish discharge is present.

Diagnosis

In most symptomatic patients, vulvovaginal candidiasis (VVC) is readily diagnosed on the basis of microscopic examination of vaginal secretions. A wet mount or saline preparation has a sensitivity of 40–60%, and 10% potassium hydroxide preparation is more sensitive in diagnosing the presence of germinated yeast, but around half of patients with VVC are microscopy negative.

Patients with candidal vaginitis have a normal vaginal pH (4.0–4.5). A pH of more than 4.5 suggests the possibility of bacterial vaginosis, trichomoniasis, atrophic vaginitis, or a mixed infection.

Routine cultures are unnecessary, but vaginal culture should be performed in suspicious cases with negative microscopy. Although vaginal culture is the most sensitive method available for detecting *Candida*, a positive culture does not necessarily indicate that *Candida* is responsible for the vaginal symptoms.

There is no reliable serological technique for the diagnosis of symptomatic VVC. Newer tests involving DNA probes and polymerase chain reaction analysis are now available and are more sensitive (although less specific for clinical disease), but are expensive and the results are not quickly available.

Treatment of acute candidal vaginitis

Topical antimycotic agents for acute *Candida* vaginitis are available as creams, lotions, vaginal tablets, suppositories and coated tampons (Reef et al. 1995). There is little evidence that the formulation of the topical antimycotic influences its clinical efficacy. Nystatin creams and vaginal suppositories achieve a mycological cure rate of about 75–80%. The clinical and mycological cure rates achieved by azole derivatives (about 85–90%) in acute, uncomplicated candidal vaginitis appear to be slightly higher than those achieved by the polyenes (e.g. nystatin) (Reef et al. 1995; Sood et al. 2000). There is little evidence that any one azole is superior. Topical azoles are generally free from local and systemic adverse effects (Table 27.1).

There has been a significant move towards using shorter courses of treatment with progressively higher doses of antifungal drugs, culminating in single-dose regimens. Short courses and single-dose regimens are effective with most of the azole and polyene antifungals. Although anecdotal evidence suggests that individual failures are not uncommon, it seems reasonable to use single-dose and short-course therapy in pregnant and non-pregnant women with infrequent episodes of mild-to-moderate severity (uncomplicated

Table 27.1 Therapy of acute candidal vaginitis

Drug	Formulation	Dosage
Butoconazole	2% cream	5 g × 3 days
	2% cream	Single dose
Clotrimazole	1% cream	5 g × 7–14 days
	10% cream	5 g single application
	100 mg vaginal tab	1 tab × 7 days
	100 mg vaginal tab	2 tabs × 3 days
	500 mg vaginal tab	1 tab once
Miconazole	2% cream	5 g × 7 days
	100 mg vaginal supp.	1 supp. × 7 days
	200 mg vaginal supp.	1 supp. × 3 days
	1,200 mg vaginal supp.	1 supp. once
Econazole	150 mg vaginal tab	1 tab × 3 days
	150 mg vaginal supp.	Single dose
Fenticonazole	2% cream	5 g × 7 days
Sertaconazole	300 mg supp.	Single dose
Ticonazole	2% cream	5 g × 7 days
	6.5% cream	5 g single application
Terconazole	0.4% cream	5 g × 7 days
	0.8% cream	5 g × 3 days
	80 mg vaginal supp.	1 supp. × 3 days
Fluconazole	150 mg tab	Single dose
Itraconazole	100 mg tab	2 tab × 3 days
Nystatin	100,000 units vaginal supp.	Daily × 14 days

supp. = suppository.

Reproduced courtesy of Jack D. Sobel.

vaginitis). Moderate-to-severe vaginitis requires more prolonged therapy (Reef et al. 1995; Sobel et al. 1998).

Itraconazole, 200 mg/day for three days or 400 mg for one day, and fluconazole, 150 mg single daily dose, achieve clinical and mycological cure in around 90% of cases of acute, uncomplicated candidal vaginitis (Sobel et al. 1995; Watson et al. 2002). Clinical results with oral therapy are as good as, if not superior to, those with conventional topical antimycotic therapy, and several studies indicate that, given a choice, most women prefer oral therapy (Watson et al. 2002).

Any therapeutic advantage of oral therapy must be weighed against the potential adverse effects and toxicity. Oral therapy is still not recommended in pregnant women, although several studies indicate that limited fluconazole exposure may not be harmful (Mølgaard-Nielsen et al. 2013). Management of VVC during pregnancy is more difficult, because the clinical response tends to be slower and recurrences are more frequent. Most topical antifungal agents are effective, particularly when prescribed for one to two weeks; however, single-dose therapy with clotrimazole has also been shown to be effective during pregnancy.

Treatment of recurrent vulvovaginal candidiasis

Treatment of RVVC aims to control rather than cure the infection. Vulvovaginal candidiasis is considered to be recurrent if the patient has three or more attacks per year (Sobel et al. 1998). The diagnosis of RVVC must be confirmed by culture, and reversible causes eliminated when possible. However, in most women with RVVC, no underlying or predisposing factor is identified. RVVC requires long-term maintenance with a suppressive prophylactic regimen (Sobel et al. 1998; Donders et al. 2008; Rosa et al. 2013). The most widely used regimen consists of an induction regimen of fluconazole 150 mg for three doses over one week, followed by once-weekly single-dose fluconazole 150 mg given for six months (Sobel et al. 1998). During this period, symptoms remain almost entirely absent. Following cessation of therapy, approximately half the women with RVVC remain in long-term remission and half return to the identical syndrome of frequent episodes of vaginitis justifying reinstitution of effective weekly fluconazole control therapy (Sobel et al. 1998). Topical clotrimazole 500 mg, once weekly, can also be used. Oral nystatin has little proven value in long-term prophylaxis.

Resistant vaginal yeast is seldom the cause of RVVC; however, in women who do not respond to conventional therapy, unusual organisms may be involved (e.g. *Saccharomyces cerevisiae, C. glabrata, C. krusei, C. tropicalis*) that are known to have relatively higher minimum inhibitory concentrations to azoles. Patients with these infections may respond to oral imidazoles, topical 17% flucytosine, or topical boric acid 600 mg/day in a gelatin capsule given vaginally (White et al. 2001; Sobel et al. 2003; Iavazzo et al. 2011). Because non-*albicans* spp. of *Candida* are less virulent than *C. albicans*, it is essential to ensure that the isolated strain of non-*albicans Candida* is the cause of symptoms and not an innocent bystander.

RVVC is not a useful marker of HIV (human immunodeficiency virus) infection. HIV testing should be based on high-risk behaviour. There is little justification for treating the male partner, because treatment is unhelpful. There exists preliminary evidence that asymptomatic vaginal colonization and symptomatic vaginitis may be associated with increased HIV transmission.

Balanitis in males

Two forms of balanoposthitis (balanitis) are associated with *Candida* spp. Both may be acquired sexually. A true superficial but invasive infection occurs particularly in uncircumcised males and those with diabetes. It is characterized by intense pruritus, discomfort, erythema, and swelling which are localized primarily to the glans, but may extend to involve the penile shaft and scrotum. Cultures are invariably positive for *Candida* spp. Treatment comprises topical antimycotics or systemic azoles.

A milder but more common and particularly recurrent form of balanitis is also described in which penile cultures may be negative for *Candida*. Symptoms of local erythema or rash and pruritus typically appear soon after unprotected intercourse. Clinical manifestations are transient and often relieved by washing or topical corticosteroids. They represent a proposed penile, cutaneous immediate hypersensitivity reaction to the presence of *Candida* antigen in vaginal secretions, often of asymptomatic women. Cure requires eradication of *Candida* from the female vaginal source.

Fungal infections of the urinary tract

There has been a marked increase in opportunistic fungal pathogens involving the urinary tract, of which *Candida* spp. are the most prevalent (Kauffman et al. 2000; Sobel et al. 2011). The kidney and urinary tract becomes infected as a result of haematogenous spread or from an ascending infection, usually in the presence of urinary obstruction. *Candida* spp. are common causes of ascending infection in catheterized and obstructed urinary tracts, particularly in diabetic individuals. Patients receiving immunosuppression therapy for renal transplantation are at risk for invasive fungal urinary tract infections (UTIs) caused by *Candida*, *Aspergillus*, and *Cryptococcus* spp. The acquired immunodeficiency syndrome (AIDS) is associated with mucosal *Candida* infections, but not candiduria; however, disseminated histoplasmosis and cryptococcosis—both common complications of AIDS—frequently involve the urinary tract.

Candida spp. are the main fungal species commonly associated with urethritis, cystitis, and pyelonephritis. Nevertheless, many species of fungi can cause prostatitis, epididymitis, chronic bladder inflammation or ulceration, and ureteric obstruction. In the absence of obstruction, fungal infections rarely cause renal insufficiency. Fungal infection should always be considered in the differential diagnosis of filling defects in the collecting system.

Epidemiology

Candida frequently exists as a saprophyte on the external genitalia or urethra; however, yeasts in measurable quantities are found in less than 1% of clean voided urine specimens. *Candida* infections currently account for 5% of urine isolates in the general hospital and 10% of positive urinary cultures in tertiary-care centres (Kobayashi et al. 2004). Candiduria is especially common in the intensive care unit (ICU) and may represent the most common urinary infection in surgical ICUs (Alvarez-Lerma et al. 2003). Presently, 10–15% of nosocomial UTIs are caused by *Candida* spp. Most positive urine cultures are isolated or transient and represent colonization rather than true infection; however, candiduria may lead to symptomatic UTI and/or fungaemia.

Patients at most risk for candiduria are those who are elderly, female, diabetic, or taking antibiotics, or have indwelling urinary devices, and have had prior surgical procedures (Kauffman et al. 2000; Fraisse et al. 2011; Sobel et al. 2011). In the asymptomatic patient, candiduria almost always represents colonization, and the elimination of underlying risk factors, such as indwelling catheters, is often adequate to eradicate candiduria (Kauffman et al. 2000).

Multiple studies have noted that candiduria does not commonly lead to candidaemia (Ang et al. 1993; Kauffman et al. 2000; Binelli et al. 2006; Paul et al. 2007; Bougnoux et al. 2008). Several of these studies have shown that candiduria is a marker for greater mortality, but death is not related to *Candida* infection and treatment for *Candida* infection does not change mortality rates (Simpson et al. 2004; Paul et al. 2007; Viale 2009).

Microbiology

C. albicans is the most common fungal species isolated from the urine, and in one large study was found in 446 (52%) of 861 patients with funguria (Kauffman et al. 2000; Sobel et al. 2011). *C. glabrata* accounts for 25–35% of infections, whereas 8–28% of infections are due to *C. tropicalis*, *C. krusei*, and *C. parapsilosis*. Recent epidemiological studies have reported a marked increase in infections caused by *C. glabrata* and *C. tropicalis* (Fisher et al. 2011; Sobel et al. 2011). Mixed infections caused by more than one *Candida* species are not infrequent, as is concomitant bacteriuria.

Clinical features

Most patients with candiduria are asymptomatic. Patients with an indwelling bladder catheter most often are colonized rather than infected with a *Candida* species. However, patients with *Candida* cystitis may present with frequency, dysuria, urgency, haematuria, and pyuria. Cystoscopy reveals soft, pearly white, slightly elevated patches that resemble oral thrush, as well as hyperaemia and inflammation of the bladder mucosa.

Ascending infection, although rare, may result in *Candida* pyelonephritis characterized by fever, leucocytosis, rigors, and costovertebral angle tenderness. Ultrasonography and computed tomography (CT) scanning are useful in diagnosing an intrarenal and perinephric abscess. Excretory urography may reveal ureteropelvic fungus balls with or without accompanying papillary necrosis. Ascending infection with *Candida* spp. uncommonly causes candidaemia, with 3–10% of episodes of candidaemia being secondary to candiduria (Ang et al. 1993). When candidaemia occurs it invariably complicates anatomical obstruction, manipulation, or a urological procedure.

Fungal bezoars may develop anywhere in the urinary drainage system but most commonly are found in the pelvis or upper ureters in the presence of ureteral obstruction (see Chapter 29). Fungal balls in the urinary tract have also been described with *Aspergillus*, *Penicillium* spp., and zygomycetes.

Renal candidiasis secondary to haematogenous spread represents a systemic infection usually accompanied by fever and other constitutional manifestations of sepsis (see Chapter 29). Candiduria may be the only clue to the diagnosis of invasive and disseminated candidiasis (Kauffman et al. 2011). Rarely, *Candida* spp. cause localized infections in prostate, epididymis, or testicles (Sobel 2002; Wise and Shteynshlyuger 2006).

Diagnosis

Diagnostic tests on urine are often not helpful in differentiating colonization from infection or in pinpointing the involved site within the urinary tract (Sobel 2002; Kauffman et al. 2011). Pyuria in a patient with an indwelling bladder catheter does not differentiate *Candida* infection from colonization. Similarly, the colony count in the urine, especially when a catheter is present, cannot be used to define infection (Sobel 2002; Kauffman et al. 2011). Imaging of the urinary tract by ultrasound or CT scanning is helpful in defining structural abnormalities, hydronephrosis, abscesses, emphysematous pyelonephritis, and fungus ball formation (Erden et al. 2000; Sadegi et al. 2009).

Treatment of asymptomatic candiduria

Given the frequency of asymptomatic candiduria and the infrequency of clinical complications, treatment with antifungal agents is not recommended unless the patients are at high risk for dissemination, such as very low birth weight infants or patients who are to undergo urologic manipulation (Robinson et al. 2009). More controversial are neutropenic patients. Patients undergoing urological procedures, however, should be treated with oral fluconazole 400 mg daily or amphotericin B (AmB) 0.3–0.6 mg/kg daily for several days before and after the procedure.

Treatment of symptomatic *Candida* urinary tract infections

Several basic principles are important in the approach to treating *Candida* UTIs. The ability of the antifungal agent to achieve adequate concentrations in the urine is as important as the antifungal susceptibilities of the infecting species. *C. albicans*, the most common cause of fungal UTI, is relatively easy to treat because it is susceptible to fluconazole, which achieves high concentrations in the urine. Oral fluconazole, 200 mg daily for two weeks, is recommended and has been shown to be effective in a randomized, double-blind trial of patients with candiduria (Sobel et al. 2000). Removal of an indwelling bladder catheter, if feasible, is also strongly recommended.

In contrast, candiduria due to fluconazole-resistant *C. glabrata* and *C. krusei* can be extremely difficult to treat. For fluconazole-resistant *C. glabrata*, AmB deoxycholate 0.3-0.6 mg/kg daily for 1-7 days (Fisher et al. 2003) or oral flucytosine 2.5 mg/kg 4 times daily for 7-10 days is recommended (Pappas et al. 2016). For *C. krusei* an identical regimen of AmB is used. AmB deoxycholate bladder irrigation 50 mg/L daily for 5-7 days is useful for treatment of cystitis due to fluconazole-resistant species of *Candida* (Jacobs et al. 1994). In all patients with symptomatic candiduria every effort should be made to eliminate urinary tract obstruction. Similarly, nephrostomy tubes or catheters should be removed or replaced.

Flucytosine demonstrates good activity against a broad spectrum of *Candida* species with the exception of *C. krusei*. However, its use is limited by toxicity and lack of availability and it should not be used as monotherapy because of the high likelihood of the development of resistance. AmB deoxycholate has broad-spectrum activity, achieving high urinary concentrations in the absence of renal insufficiency, but needs to be given intravenously and has substantial toxicity, often contributing to the pre-existing renal dysfunction. The lipid formulations of AmB appear not to achieve adequate urine concentrations, and their use to treat candiduria is not advised (Agustin et al. 1999).

The echinocandins have minimal excretion of active drug into the urine and generally are not effective in treating *Candida* UTI, although rare successes are reported (Agustin et al. 1999; Sobel et al. 2007; Malani 2010). Echinocandins, as with all antifungal drug classes, are effective in treating renal parenchymal infections—that is, acute pyelonephritis—because renal tissue concentrations are adequate, as for any systemic fungal infection. Fungal balls (bezoars) due to *Candida* and *Aspergillus* spp. are best treated surgically in concert with the aforementioned antifungal drugs. Irrigation through nephrostomy tubes with AmB is also recommended in the presence of obstruction. Fungus balls in bladder and lower ureter can generally be removed endoscopically (see Chapter 29).

Fungal prostatitis

Fungal prostatitis may result from local inoculation (*Candida* and *Trichosporon* spp.) by contaminated or infected urine, or from haematogenous spread (blastomycosis, histoplasmosis, coccidioidomycosis, aspergillosis, cryptococcosis, candidiasis, and mucormycosis). Frequently, prostatic involvement by fungi is chronic and asymptomatic, and is discovered at the time of prostatectomy or autopsy (Wen et al. 2012).

Candida spp. are the commonest cause of prostatitis, followed by *Blastomyces* and *Cryptococcus* spp. Risk factors for candidal prostatitis are similar to those for UTI, especially diabetes mellitus, antibiotic administration, indwelling catheters, and anatomical abnormalities. Considering the high prevalence of candiduria, especially in catheterized patients, *Candida* abscesses of the prostate gland are rare.

Acute prostatitis caused by *Candida* spp. presents with fever, constitutional findings, perineal pain, discomfort, irritative bladder symptoms, and, occasionally, urinary obstruction, especially in the presence of a *Candida* prostatic abscess. In most patients, urine cultures for *Candida* are positive. The presence of an abscess is confirmed by transrectal ultrasonography, magnetic resonance imaging, or CT scans. In addition to systemic antifungal therapy, focal suppuration requires drainage, either by the percutaneous route or, occasionally, by performing a transurethral prostatectomy.

Most prostatic fungal infections other than those due to *Candida* result from haematogenous dissemination, especially dissemination of *Blastomyces dermatitidis*. Clinical features are identical for all the invasive mycoses. The diagnosis of chronic fungal prostatitis should be considered when symptomatic patients have laboratory signs of urinary inflammation (pyuria) but negative bacterial cultures. A negative fungal culture of urine or secretions should not, however, exclude a diagnosis of chronic fungal prostatitis, given the pathology of granulomatous fungal prostatitis.

Cryptococcal infection of the prostate occurs secondary to haematogenous seeding in immunocompromised patients (especially those with AIDS) and may accompany pulmonary infection or meningitis. Most cases of prostatic infection are asymptomatic and only diagnosed at autopsy. Patients with AIDS are more likely to develop prostatic abscess, which may be symptomatic and present with dysuria, frequency, nausea, and fever. Physical examination may only reveal variable prostatic enlargement. Although the mainstay of treatment remains intravenous AmB—often in combination with flucytosine—fluconazole, by virtue of its oral convenience, relative lack of toxicity, penetration, and efficacy in UTI has become the long-term treatment of choice. Nevertheless, treatment failures with fluconazole have been reported. Importantly, prostatic infection is an important site of relapse of cryptococcosis after seemingly successful treatment in patients with AIDS.

References

Agustin J, Lacson S, Raffalli J, Aguero-Rosenfeld ME and Wormser GP (1999) Failure of a lipid amphotericin B preparation to eradicate candiduria: preliminary findings based on three cases. *Clin Infect Dis* 29: 686–7.

Alvarez-Lerma F, Nolla-Salas J, León C, et al. (2003) Candiduria in critically ill patients admitted to intensive care medical units. *Intensive Care Med* 29: 1069–76.

Ang BS, Telenti A, King B, Steckelberg JM and Wilson WR (1993) Candidemia from a urinary tract source: microbiological aspects and clinical significance. *Clin Infect Dis* 17: 662–6.

Binelli CA, Moretti ML, Assis RS, et al. (2006) Investigation of the possible association between nosocomial candiduria and candidaemia. *Clin Microbiol Infect* 12: 538–43.

Bougnoux ME, Kac G, Aegerter P, d'Enfert C, Fagon JY and CandiRea Study Group. (2008) Candidemia and candiduria in critically ill patients admitted to intensive care units in France: incidence, molecular diversity, management and outcome. *Intensive Care Med* 34: 292–9.

Donders G, Bellen G, Byttebier G, et al. (2008) Individualized decreasing-dose maintenance fluconazole regimen for recurrent vulvovaginal candidiasis (ReCiDiF trial). *Am J Obstet Gynecol* 199: 613.e1–9.

Eckert LO, Hawes SE, Stevens CE, Koutsky LA, Eschenbach DA and Holmes KK (1998) Vulvovaginal candidiasis: clinical manifestations, risk factors, management algorithm. *Obstet Gynecol* 92: 757–65.

Erden A, Fitoz S, Karagülle T, Tükel S and Akyar S (2000) Radiological findings in the diagnosis of genitourinary candidiasis. *Pediatr Radiol* 30: 875–7.

Fisher JF, Woeltje K, Espinel-Ingroff A, Stanfield J and DiPiro JT (2003) Efficacy of a single intravenous dose of amphotericin B for Candida urinary tract infections: further favorable experience. *Clin Microbiol Infect* 9: 1024–7.

Fisher JF, Kavanagh K, Sobel JD, Kauffman CA and Newman CA (2011) Candida urinary tract infection: pathogenesis. *Clin Infect Dis* 52 (Suppl. 6): S437–51.

Foxman B, Muraglia R, Dietz JP, Sobel JD and Wagner J (2013) Prevalence of recurrent vulvovaginal candidiasis in 5 European countries and the United States: results from an internet panel survey. *J Low Genit Tract Dis* 17: 340.

Fraisse T, Crouzet J, Lachaud L, et al. (2011) Candiduria in those over 85 years old: a retrospective study of 73 patients. *Intern Med* 50: 1935–40.

Hurley R (1981) Recurrent Candida infection. *Clin Obstet Gynaecol* 8: 209–14. PubMed PMID: 7261523.

Iavazzo C, Gkegkes ID, Zarkada IM and Falagas ME (2011) Boric acid for recurrent vulvovaginal candidiasis: the clinical evidence. *J Womens Health (Larchmt)* 20: 1245–55.

Jacobs LG, Skidmore EA, Cardoso LA and Ziv F (1994) Bladder irrigation with amphotericin B for treatment of fungal urinary tract infections. *Clin Infect Dis* 18: 313–18.

Kauffman CA, Vazquez JA, Sobel JD, et al. (2000) Prospective multicenter surveillance study of funguria in hospitalized patients. The National Institute for Allergy and Infectious Diseases (NIAID) Mycoses Study Group. *Clin Infect Dis* 30: 14–18.

Kauffman CA, Fisher JF, Sobel JD and Newman CA (2011) Candida urinary tract infections—diagnosis. *Clin Infect Dis* 52 (Suppl. 6): S452–6.

Kobayashi CC, de Fernandes OF, Miranda KC, de Sousa ED and Silva Mdo R (2004) Candiduria in hospital patients: a study prospective. *Mycopathologia* 158: 49–52.

Malani A (2010) Failure of caspofungin for treatment of Candida glabrata candiduria: case report and review of the literature. *Infect Dis Clin Pract (Baltim Md)* 18: 271–2.

Marchaim D, Lemanek L, Bheemreddy S, Kaye KS and Sobel JD (2012) Fluconazole-resistant Candida albicans vulvovaginitis. *Obstet Gynecol* 120: 1407–14.

Mølgaard-Nielsen D, Pasternak B and Hviid A (2013) Use of oral fluconazole during pregnancy and the risk of birth defects. *N Engl J Med* 369: 830–9.

Pappas PG, Kauffman CA, Andes DR, et al. (2016) Clinical Practice Guideline for the Management of Candidiasis: 2016 update by the Infectious Diseases Society of America. *Clin Infect Dis* 62: e1–50.

Paul N, Mathai E, Abraham OC, Michael JS and Mathai D (2007) Factors associated with candiduria and related mortality. *J Infect* 55: 450–5.

Pirotta MV and Garland SM (2005) Her choice: dealing with lactobacilli, vaginitis, and antibiotics. *Curr Infect Dis Rep* 7: 445–52.

Reef SE, Levine WC, McNeil MM, et al. (1995) Treatment options for vulvovaginal candidiasis, 1993. *Clin Infect Dis* 20 (Suppl. 1): S80–90.

Robinson JL, Davies HD, Barton M, et al. (2009) Characteristics and outcome of infants with candiduria in neonatal intensive care—a Paediatric Investigators Collaborative Network on Infections in Canada (PICNIC) study. *BMC Infect Dis* 9: 183.

Rosa MI, Silva BR, Pires PS, et al. (2013) Weekly fluconazole therapy for recurrent vulvovaginal candidiasis: a systematic review and meta-analysis. *Eur J Obstet Gynecol Reprod Biol* 167: 132–6.

Rosentul DC, Delsing CE, Jaeger M, et al. (2014) Gene polymorphisms in pattern recognition receptors and susceptibility to idiopathic recurrent vulvovaginal candidiasis. *Front Microbiol* 5: 483.

Sadegi BJ, Patel BK, Wilbur AC, Khosla A and Shamim E (2009) Primary renal candidiasis: importance of imaging and clinical history in diagnosis and management. *J Ultrasound Med* 28: 507–14.

Simpson C, Blitz S and Shafran SD (2004) The effect of current management on morbidity and mortality in hospitalised adults with funguria. *J Infect* 49: 248–52.

Sobel JD, Brooker D, Stein GE, et al. (1995) Single oral dose fluconazole compared with conventional clotrimazole topical therapy of Candida vaginitis. Fluconazole Vaginitis Study Group. *Am J Obstet Gynecol* 172: 1263–8.

Sobel JD, Faro S, Force RW, et al. (1998) Vulvovaginal candidiasis: epidemiologic, diagnostic, and therapeutic considerations. *Am J Obstet Gynecol* 178: 203–11.

Sobel JD, Kauffman CA, McKinsey D, et al. (2000) Candiduria: a randomized, double-blind study of treatment with fluconazole and placebo. The National Institute of Allergy and Infectious Diseases (NIAID) Mycoses Study Group. *Clin Infect Dis* 30: 19–24.

Sobel J (2002) Controversies in the diagnosis of candiduria: what is the critical colony count? *Curr Treat Options Infect Dis* 4: 81–3.

Sobel JD, Chaim W, Nagappan V and Leaman D (2003) Treatment of vaginitis caused by Candida glabrata: use of topical boric acid and flucytosine. *Am J Obstet Gynecol* 189: 1297–300.

Sobel JD (2007) Vulvovaginal candidosis. *Lancet* 369: 1961–71.

Sobel JD, Bradshaw SK, Lipka CJ and Kartsonis NA (2007) Caspofungin in the treatment of symptomatic candiduria. *Clin Infect Dis* 44: e46–9.

Sobel JD, Fisher JF, Kauffman CA and Newman CA (2011) Candida urinary tract infections—epidemiology. *Clin Infect Dis* 52 (Suppl. 6): S433–6.

Sood G, Nyirjesy P, Weitz MV and Chatwani A (2000) Terconazole cream for non-Candida albicans fungal vaginitis: results of a retrospective analysis. *Infect Dis Obstet Gynecol* 8: 240–3.

Viale P (2009) Candida colonization and candiduria in critically ill patients in the intensive care unit. *Drugs* 69 (Suppl. 1): 51–7.

Watson MC, Grimshaw JM, Bond CM, Mollison J and Ludbrook A (2002) Oral versus intra-vaginal imidazole and triazole anti-fungal agents for the treatment of uncomplicated vulvovaginal candidiasis (thrush): a systematic review. *BJOG* 109: 85–95.

Wen SC, Juan YS, Wang CJ, et al. (2012) Emphysematous prostatic abscess: case series study and review. *Int J Infect Dis* 16: e344–9.

White DJ, Habib AR, Vanthuyne A, Langford S and Symonds M (2001) Combined topical flucytosine and amphotericin B for refractory vaginal Candida glabrata infections. *Sex Transm Infect* 77: 212–13.

Wise GJ and Shteynshlyuger A (2006) How to diagnose and treat fungal infections in chronic prostatitis. *Curr Urol Rep* 7: 320–8.

CHAPTER 28

Fungal eye infections

Heather L. Clark and Eric Pearlman

Introduction to fungal eye infections

In 2005, contact lens wearers presented to eye clinics throughout the United States, Europe, and Asia with severe corneal infections (keratitis) (Bernal et al. 2006). Most patients were treated for viral or bacterial infections, but their condition worsened, and in many cases required corneal transplants or enucleation. Eventually the causative organism was diagnosed as *Fusarium*, a genus of filamentous moulds common in the environment, and patients were then treated with antifungal agents. More than 250 cases of *Fusarium* keratitis were reported worldwide, all associated with soft contact lens use (Epstein 2007). Diagnosis was based on cultures from corneas and from the environment, and *Fusarium* was identified by morphological characteristics and by genotyping using multilocus DNA sequence typing. Of the confirmed cases, 34% did not respond to topical antifungal agents or had corneal scarring and required a corneal transplant (Chang et al. 2006). In addition to cases in the USA, multiple cases were reported in Britain, France, Singapore, and Hong Kong (Saw et al. 2007; Gaujoux et al. 2008; Ma et al. 2009; Tuft and Tullo 2009). The outbreak was linked to a lens care solution that did not effectively inhibit fungal growth, resulting in contamination from the environment. Individuals with suboptimal lens care hygiene were at increased risk which ended after the product was removed from the market (Centers for Disease Control and Prevention 2006; Chang et al. 2006).

In contrast to the cause of the keratitis outbreak, the 2012 US outbreak of fungal endophthalmitis was associated with patients who had undergone retinal surgery (Centers for Disease Control and Prevention 2012). In that outbreak, 47 cases across nine states were ultimately attributed to two contaminated compounds—Brilliant Blue G dye and triamcinolone acetonide, which came from a single compounding pharmacy, and were later recalled. The fungi identified were *Fusarium* and *Bipolaris* mould species. The majority of patients lost vision in the affected eye and several required enucleation (Mikosz et al. 2014).

In this chapter we will review the epidemiology, clinical characteristics, pathogenesis, and treatment of keratitis and endophthalmitis caused by yeasts and filamentous fungi.

Epidemiology of fungal keratitis

Corneal infection with yeasts, primarily *Candida* spp., is more commonly seen in industrialized countries and has no apparent connection to environmental or employment factors (Galarreta et al. 2007). *Candida* keratitis is generally associated with contact lens wear, prior ocular surface disease, or ocular surgery (Ritterband et al. 2006; Sengupta et al. 2012; Nielsen et al. 2015). In marked contrast, infection with filamentous moulds, including *Fusarium*, *Aspergillus*, and *Curvularia* spp., is associated with hot, humid climates mainly in the developing world, and exposure occurs mainly through trauma, although *Fusarium* is also an important cause of contact-lens-associated keratitis.

Contact-lens-associated fungal keratitis

Keratitis caused by *Fusarium* spp. came to prominence in 2005–2006 with the outbreak already described, comprising 164 confirmed cases in the USA. All of these were associated with contact lens wear and with a specific lens care product that was unable to control the growth of fungi introduced from the environment. The ability of the organisms to form biofilm on contact lenses and lens cases was also a major factor. *Fusarium* forms biofilm on silicone hydrogel lenses, and studies showed that the lens care solution was less effective on biofilm-forming clinical isolates than on the ATCC 36031 reference isolate used to evaluate the antimicrobial effects of lens disinfectants, which did not form a biofilm on soft contact lenses (Imamura et al. 2008). The US Federal Drug Administration (FDA) has since moved to utilize clinical isolates to test lens care solutions. Since that outbreak, contact lens wear has continued to be a major risk factor for fungal keratitis. *Candida albicans* can also form biofilms on contact lenses, and some cases of *Candida* keratitis are also associated with contact lens wear (Imamura et al. 2008).

Fungal infections associated with corneal injury

Filamentous fungal pathogens account for more than 50% of all corneal ulcers in tropical climates (Srinivasan et al. 1997). *Fusarium* and *Aspergillus* spp. are the most commonly identified agents (Kredics et al. 2015). Larger population studies conducted at the Aravind Eye Hospitals in southern India from 2006 to 2009 found that 63% of culture-positive microbial keratitis cases were of fungal aetiology (Lin et al. 2012). *Fusarium* spp. were the predominant cause of fungal keratitis (42.3%), and the number of cases of fungal keratitis peaked in July and January, which corresponds to the windy and harvest seasons, respectively. No significant seasonal trend was observed for bacterial keratitis. A recent study from the same region, including 25,097 presumed infectious keratitis patients seen between 2002 and 2012, also found *Fusarium* spp. to be the major cause of corneal ulcers, and the number of cases of fungal keratitis increased over this time (Figure 28.1a) (Lalitha et al. 2015). Similar findings were reported in northern and central China, where *Fusarium* spp. were the major cause of

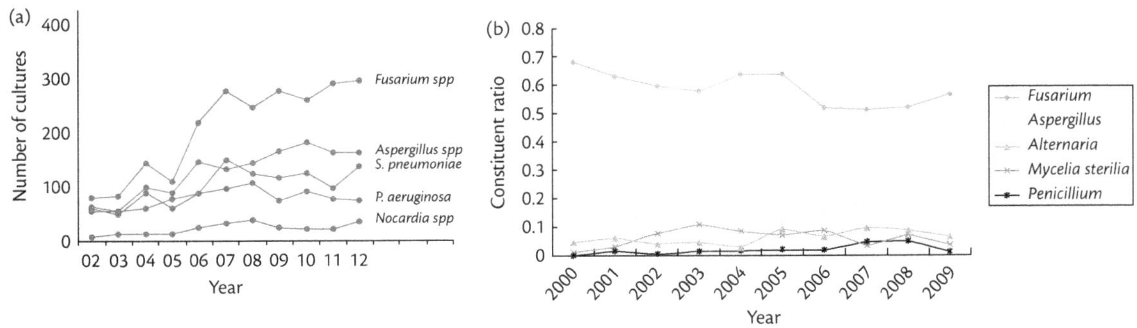

Figure 28.1 Incidence of *Fusarium* and *Aspergillus* keratitis associated with ocular injury in developing countries.

a The major bacteria and fungi isolated from corneal ulcers from 2002 to 2012 at the Aravind Eye Hospital, Madurai, India. Annual number of cultures positive for each organism.

b Percentage total cases of fungal keratitis in central China from 2000 to 2009, and represented as cumulative ratio.

a Reproduced with permission from Lalitha, P. et al, 'Trends In Bacterial and Fungal Keratitis In South India, 2002–2012', *British Journal of Ophthalmology*, Volume 99, pp. 192–4, Copyright © 2015 British Medical Journal. DOI: 10.1136/bjophthalmol-2014-305000. **b** Reproduced with permission from Wang, L., Sun, S., Jing, Y., Han, L., Zhang, H., & Yue, J., 'Spectrum of fungal keratitis in central China', *Clinical and Experimental Ophthalmology*, Volume 37, Number 8, pp. 763–71, 2009, Copyright © 2009 Royal Australian and New Zealand College of Ophthalmologists. DOI: 10.1111/j.1442-9071.2009.02155.x

corneal ulcers reported by the Shandong Eye Institute between 1999 and 2004 and the Henan Eye Institute between 2000 and 2009 (Figure 28.1b) (Xie et al. 2006; Wang et al. 2009). Both studies noted that corneal injury was the predominant underlying cause, and was associated with males in agricultural regions, where the incidence increased during the harvest season. Similar findings regarding prevalence and risk factors using smaller cohorts were reported for Africa, South America, and regions of southern and East Asia, and have been reviewed by Kredics et al. (2015). Overall, the major risk factor is agricultural work, where ocular injury and exposure to *Fusarium*, *Aspergillus*, and other filamentous fungi in soil and plant matter is common.

Ocular surgery is another major risk factor for mycotic keratitis; however, these cases are primarily due to yeasts such as *Candida albicans*. There are numerous reports of keratitis following corneal and cataract surgery, most of which involve yeast infections (Garg et al. 2003; Kanavi et al. 2007; Chen et al. 2009).

Fungal endophthalmitis

Candida spp. are also the most common aetiologic agent in endophthalmitis, either as a result of haematogenous spreading of systemic infection (endogenous), or following ocular infection (exogenous). It is estimated that up to 30% of patients with systemic candidaemia, a common nosocomial infection, develop endophthalmitis (Brooks 1989). The major risk factors associated with endogenous endophthalmitis include intravenous (IV) catheters or other medical devices, IV drug use, broad-spectrum antibiotic use, and immune suppression. In contrast, exogenous endophthalmitis is mainly caused by contamination during ocular surgery, primarily cataract removal and corneal transplant. Trauma or progression of keratitis to posterior structures may also result in exogenous endophthalmitis, where common agents include *Aspergillus*, *Fusarium*, and *Penicillium* spp. (Wykoff et al. 2008). Filamentous moulds introduced systemically by IV drug use, or in immunocompromised patients, also cause endogenous endophthalmitis (Klotz et al. 2000).

Clinical characteristics and diagnosis of fungal infections in the cornea

The mammalian cornea comprises external epithelial cells, which form tight junctions, a stromal layer (~90% of the cornea) which comprises collagen fibrils and houses resident keratocytes and macrophages, and a single endothelial cell layer (Figure 28.2a, b). These cells function independently to ensure the 80% hydration level required for corneal transparency. During infection, hyphae penetrate throughout the corneal stroma (Figure 28.2c), and can ultimately penetrate through to the anterior chamber and into the posterior eye.

Infectious keratitis patients typically present with redness, pain, photophobia, and decreased vision in the affected eye (Garg et al. 2000; Bourcier et al. 2003). Mycotic ulcers frequently appear as a dense white or yellow inflammatory infiltrate in the corneal stroma, with variable size, depth, and location. Anterior chamber inflammation and leukocyte infiltration (hypopyon) are also a common finding of such ulcers (Figure 28.2d) (Shukla et al. 2008), and consist primarily of neutrophils (Figure 28.2e, f) (Karthikeyan et al. 2011). A key distinguishing characteristic of fungal keratitis, compared with bacterial keratitis, is the presence of an irregular, feathery border around the lesion (Dalmon et al. 2012).

Delayed treatment can result in perforation of the cornea and increased risk of endophthalmitis, in which the hyphae invade the vitreous humour, resulting in loss of retinal function. Methods of diagnosing mycotic keratitis include direct examination and *in vivo* confocal microscopy of the cornea (which shows hyphae in the stroma), or corneal ulcer scrapings, culture, and morphological and DNA identification of the pathogen (Slowik et al. 2015; van Diepeningen et al. 2015). Diagnosis at the species level requires PCR (polymerase chain reaction) amplification and sequencing of multiple, specific loci within the genome. Species identification is important because of the highly variable susceptibility to antimicrobial agents (Kredics et al. 2015). DNA can be obtained from cultures or directly from corneal ulcers (Ferrer et al. 2001).

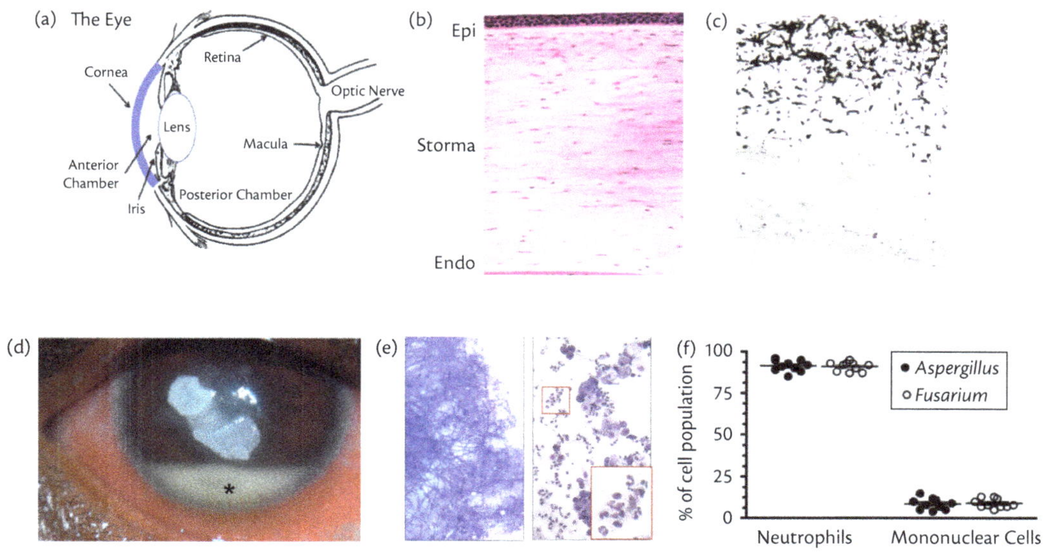

Figure 28.2 Clinical and histological features of *Fusarium* and *Aspergillus* keratitis.

a The human eye.

b Haematoxylin & eosin (H&E)-stained section of normal human cornea showing epithelium, stroma, and endothelium.

c Gomori methenamine silver (GMS)-stained cornea from a patient infected with *A. flavus* keratitis following corneal transplantation.

d *Fusarium* keratitis patient showing accumulation of neutrophils in the anterior chamber*, termed a 'hypopyon'.

e Scraping from a corneal ulcer from a short-term infection showing *A. flavus* hyphae (left panel) and cells stained with Giemsa (right panel).

f Percentage of neutrophils and mononuclear cells in corneal ulcers caused by *Fusarium* and *Aspergillus* (data points represent individual patients).

a–c Reprinted from *Cytokine*, Volume 58, Issue 1, Leal, S. M., Jr., & Pearlman, E., 'The role of cytokines and pathogen recognition molecules in fungal keratitis - Insights from human disease and animal models', pp. 107–11, Copyright © 2012 Elsevier Inc. with permission from Elsevier, http://www.sciencedirect.com/science/article/pii/S1043466611008854. All rights reserved. **d** Reprinted from '*Mycoses*, Volume 51, Issue 3, Shukla, P. K., Kumar, M., & Keshava, G. B. S., 'Mycotic keratitis: an overview of diagnosis and therapy', pp. 183–99, Copyright © The Authors, with permission from John Wiley & Sons. DOI: 10.1111/j.1439-0507.2007.01480.x. **e** and **f** Reproduced with permission from Karthikeyan, R. S., Leal, S. M., Jr., Prajna, N. V., Dharmalingam, K., Geiser, D. M., Pearlman, E., & Lalitha, P., 'Expression of innate and adaptive immune mediators in human corneal tissue infected with Aspergillus or fusarium', *Journal of Infectious Diseases*, Volume 204, Issue 6, pp. 942–50, Copyright © 2011 Oxford University Press. DOI: 10.1093/infdis/jir426

Endophthalmitis patients also present with pain and vision loss. The lesions appear as white plaques on the choroid and retina with accompanying inflammatory infiltrates in the vitreous humour and anterior chamber. Patients with mould infections present earlier and these infections result in worse visual outcomes and more frequent enucleation surgery than yeast infections (Sridhar et al. 2013). Diagnosis is based on examination of the posterior eye following pupil dilation. Biopsy and analysis of the vitreous humour, or blood in the case of systemic infection, by the methods described are necessary to identify the causative organism (Klotz et al. 2000).

Current therapies and intervention

The standard treatment for microbial keratitis is topical antimicrobial agents followed by topical steroids to control the inflammatory response and prevent corneal scarring. The effectiveness of antimycotics has been recently reviewed (Kredics et al. 2015). The first line of treatment is with topical polyenes, most commonly natamycin (5%) or amphotericin B (0.15%), which are effective against *Aspergillus* and *Fusarium*; however, hyphae invade the deeper stromal lamellae, and these polyenes have a relatively poor ability to penetrate the stroma. Azoles including ketoconazole (no longer available in most countries—see Chapter 46), imidazole, and voriconazole are also used against these organisms, although they are still considered a second-line treatment. A third line of treatment is oral, subconjunctival, or intravitreal injection of azoles or amphotericin B; however, if these are ineffective, corneal transplantation (keratoplasty) is required. Similarly, *Candida* infections are treated with amphotericin B or azoles (Slowik et al. 2015). A study comparing clinical isolates from the contact-lens-associated *Fusarium* keratitis outbreak showed differences in susceptibility to voriconazole, with *Fusarium oxysporum* isolates growing as biofilm being more resistant (minimum inhibitory concentration [MIC] 256 μg/mL) than *Fusarium solani* isolates (MIC <10 μg/mL) (Mukherjee et al. 2012).

Following antimycotic treatment, the inflammatory response is managed using topical corticosteroids; however, if the hyphae are not completely killed, any remaining live fungi can grow rapidly, resulting in uncontrolled fungal growth in the absence of an immune response, along with severe corneal damage. Therefore, there is a pressing need for more targeted antifungal and anti-inflammatory therapeutics.

Endogenous endophthalmitis requires treatment of the systemic infection, which for endogenous and exogenous endophthalmitis includes intravenous amphotericin B or oral azoles. Concurrent injections of amphotericin B or azoles, and often a combination of agents, into the vitreous humour and/or vitrectomy are also beneficial in more severe cases (Klotz et al. 2000; Wykoff et al. 2008; Mithal et al. 2015). Amphotericin B has potential for retinal toxicity; therefore azoles are favoured for intraocular use (Kernt and Kampik 2010).

Host–pathogen interactions in mycotic infections

Disease outcomes in fungal infection depend on both the virulence of the invading fungus, and the veracity of the host immune response. Corneal resident macrophages are essential for initial recognition of hyphae and chemokine secretion to recruit neutrophils, which are the major host cells that mediate fungal killing in the cornea, but also contribute to tissue damage (Leal et al. 2010, 2012; Clark et al. 2016).

Experimental models in rabbits and mice have been used to examine the interactions between the immune system and pathogenic fungi in keratitis. In a mouse model of contact-lens-associated keratitis, lenses are incubated with *Fusarium* conidia, which adhere to the lens and form a biofilm. The lens with the adherent biofilm is then placed on the cornea following abrasion of the corneal epithelium, and the hyphae then penetrate into the corneal stroma, causing severe disease associated with a pronounced neutrophil infiltration (Sun et al. 2009). A second model mimics ocular injury by injecting *Aspergillus* or *Fusarium* conidia directly into the corneal stroma, and within hours the conidia germinate, and hyphae spread throughout the cornea (Tarabishy et al. 2008; Leal et al. 2010).

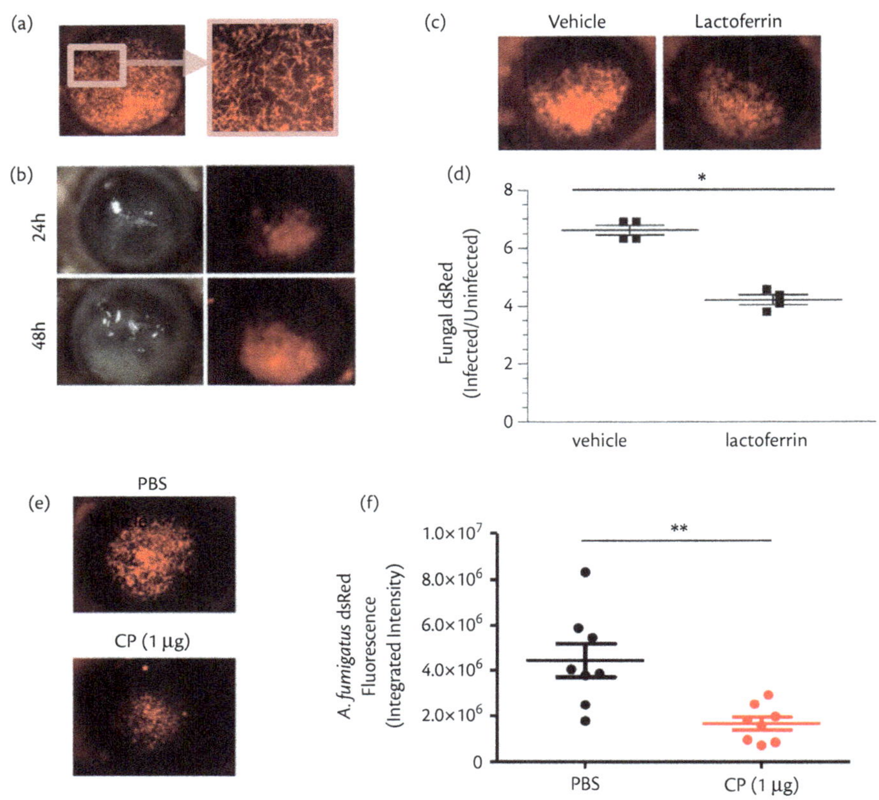

Figure 28.3 Murine model of *Aspergillus* keratitis.

a *A. fumigatus* conidia expressing red fluorescence protein (Af293.1RFP) were injected into the corneal stroma of immunosuppressed C57BL/6 mice. After 24 hours, conidia have germinated and hyphae have spread throughout the cornea.

b Corneal opacification and Af293.1RFP hyphae in immunocompetent mice 24 hours and 48 hours post infection. Note area of opacification corresponds to an RFP area expressing hyphae.

c,d Topical application of lactoferrin inhibits hyphal growth in the cornea. Total red fluorescent protein is quantified by image analysis.

e,f Subconjunctival administration of recombinant calprotectin (CP) inhibits hyphal growth in the cornea. Original magnification is ×20 (**a,b,c,e**). Data points in **d** and **f** depict individual mice.

Experimental studies of fungal endophthalmitis have examined antifungal agents rather than host–pathogen interactions. Using a neutropenic rabbit model of endogenous *Candida* endophthalmitis, intravenous injection of *C. albicans* resulted in endophthalmitic lesions significantly less frequently than in immunocompetent rabbits, suggesting that the immune response is primarily responsible for tissue damage (Henderson et al. 1980). It is likely that the host response to pathogenic fungi is similar in keratitis and endophthalmitis; therefore, we will discuss recent advances in host–pathogen interactions revealed by keratitis studies, which point to new therapeutic strategies for fungal infections.

Innate immunity in *Aspergillus* and *Fusarium* keratitis

Corneal scrapings from fungal keratitis patients reveal elevated expression of pathogen recognition molecules, C-type lectins, and toll-like receptors, as well as pro-inflammatory and chemotactic cytokines, compared with healthy donor corneas (Karthikeyan et al. 2011). Further, studies using cytokine and pathogen receptor gene knockout mice support the following sequence of events (Tarabishy et al. 2008; Leal et al. 2010; Leal and Pearlman 2012). Firstly, cell wall β-glucan is exposed on the cell wall during germination, which can activate the C-type lectin Dectin-1 on resident corneal macrophages. Dectin-1 signalling drives production of chemotactic and pro-inflammatory cytokines which recruit neutrophils to the corneal stroma (Sun et al. 2009; Leal et al. 2010). Dormant *Aspergillus* and *Fusarium* conidia have an outer hydrophobic layer incorporating the RodA protein, which blocks host recognition of the underlying cell wall carbohydrates β-1,3 glucan and α-mannan (Linder et al. 2005). The absence of RodA either genetically or following removal with hydrofluoric acid resulted in recognition of β-1,3 glucan by macrophages and dendritic cells, resulting in increased production of cytokines through Dectin-1 and Dectin-2 (Carrion Sde et al. 2013). In vivo, the Δ*RodA A. fumigatus* mutant induced a more rapid and robust host response in infected corneas than the parent strain, resulting in neutrophil infiltration and more rapid fungal killing (Aimanianda et al. 2009; Carrion Sde et al. 2013).

Individuals with mutations in genes that affect production of, or responsiveness to, IL-17, a pro-inflammatory cytokine produced by T helper 17 (Th17) cells and other immune cells, exhibit increased susceptibility to fungal infections, including mucocutaneous candidiasis (Underhill and Pearlman 2015). IL-17 levels are also elevated in fungal infected human corneas (post-transplant corneas) and in corneal ulcers from patients presenting early in infection (Figure 28.4a), where neutrophils comprised >90% of the cell population (Karthikeyan et al. 2011). Consistent with these findings, peripheral blood neutrophils from patients and from resident cohorts produced IL-17A (Karthikeyan et al. 2015).

Similarly, in murine models of keratitis caused by *Candida*, *Aspergillus*, and *Fusarium*, neutrophils were the predominant source of IL-17A at early time points, with CD4+ T cells recruited later (Zhang et al. 2013; Taylor et al. 2014a). These neutrophils also express the IL-17RC receptor subunit, and are then further activated by IL-17 to produce higher levels of reactive oxygen species (ROS). ROS enhance the capacity of neutrophils to kill *Aspergillus* in vitro, and the adoptive transfer of IL-17-producing neutrophils resulted in increased fungal killing in the cornea compared with unstimulated neutrophils or stimulated neutrophils from mice that do not produce IL-17 (IL-17$^{-/-}$ mice) (Figure 28.4b, c) (Taylor et al. 2014b). Therefore, IL-17-expressing and -responding neutrophils have an important role in the pathogenesis of fungal infections in the cornea and in other tissues.

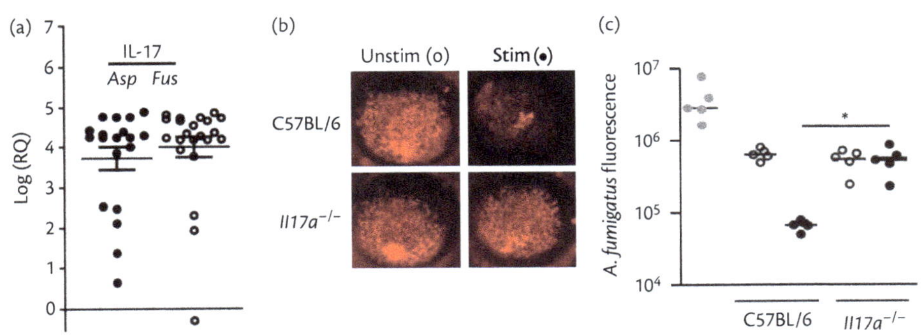

Figure 28.4 The role of IL-17-producing neutrophils in fungal keratitis.

a Quantitative polymerase chain reaction of corneal scrapings from patients infected with *Fusarium* (***Fus***) or *Aspergillus* (***Asp***) and compared with normal corneas (ΔΔCt) on a log scale. Data points depict individual patients.

b,c Af293.RFP hyphal growth in infected mouse corneas following adoptive transfer of neutrophils from C57BL/6 and IL-17$^{-/-}$ mice that were either unstimulated (no IL-17) or which had been stimulated to induce IL-17 production. There was significantly less hyphal growth in the presence of IL-17*: $P<0.05$.

b Original magnification is ×20.

c Data points represent individual mice.

a Reproduced with permission from Karthikeyan, R. S., Leal, S. M., Jr., Prajna, N. V., Dharmalingam, K., Geiser, D. M., Pearlman, E., & Lalitha, P., 'Expression of innate and adaptive immune mediators in human corneal tissue infected with Aspergillus or fusarium', *Journal of Infectious Diseases*, Volume 204, Issue 6, pp. 942–50, Copyright © 2011 Oxford University Press, DOI: 10.1093/infdis/jir426.

b Reproduced with permission from Taylor, P. R. et al., 'Activation of neutrophils by autocrine IL-17A-IL-17RC interactions during fungal infection is regulated by IL-6, IL-23, RORgammat and dectin-2', *Nature Immunology*, Volume 15, Issue 2, pp. 143–51, Copyright © 2013, Rights Managed by Nature Publishing Group, DOI: 10.1038/ni.2797.

Neutrophil anti-fungal defences in *Aspergillus* and *Fusarium* keratitis

Aspergillus and *Fusarium* hyphae are rapidly killed by ROS produced by NADPH (nicotinamide adenine dinucleotide phosphate) oxidase (NOX) activation in host cells, and individuals with mutations in NOX complex genes are highly susceptible to fungal infections (Henriet et al. 2013). Mice lacking a functional NOX complex cannot generate ROS and are unable to kill hyphae in infected corneas, despite neutrophil infiltration (Leal et al. 2012). Furthermore, *A. fumigatus* anti-oxidant activity regulated by the transcription factor Yap1 and the gene for phosphatase Z is required to combat oxidative stress and cause corneal disease (Muszkieta et al. 2014).

Fungal pathogens require nutrient metals for growth; however, the immune system effectively sequesters these nutrients during infection as a means of control (termed 'nutritional immunity') (Hood and Skaar 2012). *Aspergillus* iron acquisition requires iron-binding siderophores, synthesis of which is controlled by *Sid* genes (Schrettl et al. 2004). During corneal infection, *A. fumigatus Sid* mutants exhibited impaired growth and virulence (Leal et al. 2013), indicating a requirement for siderophores in fungal keratitis.

Trauma-induced fungal keratitis is mimicked in mice by injecting conidia directly into the corneal stroma; conidia then germinate and spread throughout the cornea, especially in immunocompromised animals (Figure 28.3a, b). Neutrophils recruited to infected corneas chelate iron through lactoferrin and lipocalin proteins; further, topical application of agents that either chelate iron (Figure 28.3c, d) (Leal et al. 2013) or block siderophore biosynthesis were found to limit hyphal growth in the cornea.

In addition to iron, *Aspergillus* hyphae require zinc for growth, which is acquired by the zinc transporters ZrfA-C, which in turn are regulated by transcription factor ZafA (Moreno et al. 2007; Amich et al. 2010). *A. fumigatus* ZafA mutants exhibit an impaired ability to grow in the cornea (Clark et al. 2016). Calprotectin is an abundant neutrophil protein comprising 40% of total cytoplasmic proteins which chelates zinc and manganese (Zackular et al. 2015). Calprotectin-deficient mice are impaired in their ability to clear *Aspergillus* hyphae from infected corneas, although this phenotype can be reversed by injection of recombinant calprotectin (Figure 28.3e, f) (Clark et al. 2016). Although not shown in a keratitis model, calprotectin also has an important role in killing *C. albicans*; therefore it is likely that nutrient acquisition is also important in yeast virulence (Urban et al. 2009).

Conclusion

Fungal keratitis and endophthalmitis represent major public health problems worldwide, causing severe pain, vision loss, and blindness. This also results in loss of income for families and communities, and continued expense of treatment and surgery. Current antifungal treatments are limited and plagued with problems of efficacy and toxicity, while anti-inflammatory treatments are non-specific. A thorough understanding of host and pathogen factors mediating defence and damage during keratitis will direct us to novel therapeutic approaches with targeted activity to fungal virulence factors or specific inflammatory pathways.

References

Aimanianda V, Bayry J, Bozza S, et al. (2009) Surface hydrophobin prevents immune recognition of airborne fungal spores. *Nature* 460: 1117–21.

Amich J, Vicentefranqueira R, Leal F and Calera JA (2010) Aspergillus fumigatus survival in alkaline and extreme zinc-limiting environments relies on the induction of a zinc homeostasis system encoded by the zrfC and aspf2 genes. *Eukaryot Cell* 9: 424–37.

Bernal MD, Acharya NR, Lietman TM, Strauss EC, Mcleod SD and Hwang DG (2006) Outbreak of Fusarium keratitis in soft contact lens wearers in San Francisco. *Arch Ophthalmol* 124: 1051–3.

Bourcier T, Touzeau O, Thomas F, et al. (2003) Candida parapsilosis keratitis. *Cornea* 22: 51–5.

Brooks RG (1989) Prospective study of Candida endophthalmitis in hospitalized patients with candidemia. *Arch Intern Med* 149: 2226–8.

Carrion Sde J, Leal SM Jr, Ghannoum MA, Aimanianda V, Latge JP and Pearlman E (2013) The RodA hydrophobin on Aspergillus fumigatus spores masks Dectin-1- and Dectin-2-dependent responses and enhances fungal survival in vivo. *J Immunol* 191: 2581–8.

Centers for Disease Control and Prevention (2006) Update: Fusarium keratitis--United States, 2005-2006. *MMWR Morb Mortal Wkly Rep* 55: 563–4.

Centers for Disease Control and Prevention (2012) Notes from the field: multistate outbreak of postprocedural fungal endophthalmitis associated with a single compounding pharmacy—United States, March-April 2012. *MMWR Morb Mortal Wkly Rep* 61: 310–11.

Chang DC, Grant GB, O'donnell K, et al. (2006) Multistate outbreak of Fusarium keratitis associated with use of a contact lens solution. *JAMA* 296: 953–63.

Chen WL, Tsai YY, Lin JM and Chiang CC (2009) Unilateral Candida parapsilosis interface keratitis after laser *in situ* keratomileusis: case report and review of the literature. *Cornea* 28: 105–7.

Clark HL, Jhingran A, Sun Y, et al. (2016) Zinc and manganese chelation by neutrophil S100A8/A9 (calprotectin) limits extracellular Aspergillus fumigatus hyphal growth and corneal infection. *J Immunol* 196: 336–44.

Dalmon C, Porco TC, Lietman TM, et al. (2012) The clinical differentiation of bacterial and fungal keratitis: a photographic survey. *Invest Ophthalmol Vis Sci* 53: 1787–91.

Epstein AB (2007) In the aftermath of the Fusarium keratitis outbreak: what have we learned? *Clin Ophthalmol* 1: 355–66.

Ferrer C, Colom F, Frases S, Mulet E, Abad JL and Alio JL (2001) Detection and identification of fungal pathogens by PCR and by ITS2 and 5.8S ribosomal DNA typing in ocular infections. *J Clin Microbiol* 39: 2873–9.

Galarreta DJ, Tuft SJ, Ramsay A and Dart JK (2007) Fungal keratitis in London: microbiological and clinical evaluation. *Cornea* 26: 1082–6.

Garg P, Gopinathan U, Choudhary K and Rao GN (2000) Keratomycosis: clinical and microbiologic experience with dematiaceous fungi. *Ophthalmology* 107: 574–80.

Garg P, Mahesh S, Bansal AK, Gopinathan U and Rao GN (2003) Fungal infection of sutureless self-sealing incision for cataract surgery. *Ophthalmology* 110: 2173–7.

Gaujoux T, Chatel MA, Chaumeil C, Laroche L and Borderie VM (2008) Outbreak of contact lens-related Fusarium keratitis in France. *Cornea* 27: 1018–21.

Henderson DK, Hockey LJ, Vukalcic LJ and Edwards JE Jr (1980) Effect of immunosuppression on the development of experimental hematogenous Candida endophthalmitis. *Infect Immun* 27: 628–31.

Henriet S, Verweij PE, Holland SM and Warris A (2013) Invasive fungal infections in patients with chronic granulomatous disease. *Adv Exp Med Biol* 764: 27–55.

Hood MI and Skaar EP (2012) Nutritional immunity: transition metals at the pathogen-host interface. *Nat Rev Microbiol* 10: 525–37.

Imamura Y, Chandra J, Mukherjee PK, et al. (2008) Fusarium and Candida albicans biofilms on soft contact lenses: model development, influence of lens type, and susceptibility to lens care solutions. *Antimicrob Agents Chemother* 52: 171–82.

Kanavi MR, Foroutan AR, Kamel MR, Afsar N and Javadi MA (2007) Candida interface keratitis after deep anterior lamellar keratoplasty: clinical, microbiologic, histopathologic, and confocal microscopic reports. *Cornea* 26: 913–16.

Karthikeyan RS, Leal SM Jr, Prajna NV, et al. (2011) Expression of innate and adaptive immune mediators in human corneal tissue infected with Aspergillus or fusarium. *J Infect Dis* 204: 942–50.

Karthikeyan RS, Vareechon C, Prajna NV, Dharmalingam K, Pearlman E and Lalitha P (2015) Interleukin 17 expression in peripheral blood neutrophils from fungal keratitis patients and healthy cohorts in southern India. *J Infect Dis* 211: 130–4.

Kernt M and Kampik A (2010) Endophthalmitis: pathogenesis, clinical presentation, management, and perspectives. *Clin Ophthalmol* 4: 121–35.

Klotz SA, Penn CC, Negvesky GJ and Butrus SI (2000) Fungal and parasitic infections of the eye. *Clin Microbiol Rev* 13: 662–85.

Kredics L, Narendran V, Shobana CS, Vagvolgyi C, Manikandan P and the Indo-Hungarian Fungal Keratitis Working Group (2015) Filamentous fungal infections of the cornea: a global overview of epidemiology and drug sensitivity. *Mycoses* 58: 243–60.

Lalitha P, Prajna NV, Manoharan G, et al. (2015) Trends in bacterial and fungal keratitis in South India, 2002-2012. *Br J Ophthalmol* 99: 192–4.

Leal SM Jr, Cowden S, Hsia YC, Ghannoum MA, Momany M and Pearlman E (2010) Distinct roles for Dectin-1 and TLR4 in the pathogenesis of Aspergillus fumigatus keratitis. *PLoS Pathog* 6: e1000976.

Leal SM Jr and Pearlman E (2012) The role of cytokines and pathogen recognition molecules in fungal keratitis—insights from human disease and animal models. *Cytokine* 58: 107–11.

Leal SM Jr, Roy S, Vareechon C, et al. (2013) Targeting iron acquisition blocks infection with the fungal pathogens Aspergillus fumigatus and Fusarium oxysporum. *PLoS Pathog* 9: e1003436.

Leal SM Jr, Vareechon C, Cowden S, et al. (2012) Fungal antioxidant pathways promote survival against neutrophils during infection. *J Clin Invest* 122: 2482–98.

Lin CC, Lalitha P, Srinivasan M, et al. (2012) Seasonal trends of microbial keratitis in South India. *Cornea* 31: 1123–7.

Linder MB, Szilvay GR, Nakari-Setala T and Penttila ME (2005) Hydrophobins: the protein-amphiphiles of filamentous fungi. *FEMS Microbiol Rev* 29: 877–96.

Ma SK, So K, Chung PH, Tsang HF and Chuang SK (2009) A multi-country outbreak of fungal keratitis associated with a brand of contact lens solution: the Hong Kong experience. *Int J Infect Dis* 13: 443–8.

Mikosz CA, Smith RM, Kim M, et al. (2014) Fungal endophthalmitis associated with compounded products. *Emerg Infect Dis* 20: 248–56.

Mithal K, Pathengay A, Bawdekar A, et al. (2015) Filamentous fungal endophthalmitis: results of combination therapy with intravitreal amphotericin B and voriconazole. *Clin Ophthalmol* 9: 649–55.

Moreno MA, Ibrahim-Granet O, Vicentefranqueira R, et al. (2007) The regulation of zinc homeostasis by the ZafA transcriptional activator is essential for Aspergillus fumigatus virulence. *Mol Microbiol* 64: 1182–97.

Mukherjee PK, Chandra J, Yu C, Sun Y, Pearlman E and Ghannoum MA (2012) Characterization of fusarium keratitis outbreak isolates: contribution of biofilms to antimicrobial resistance and pathogenesis. *Invest Ophthalmol Vis Sci* 53: 4450–7.

Muszkieta L, Carrion Sde J, Robinet P, et al. (2014) The protein phosphatase PhzA of A. fumigatus is involved in oxidative stress tolerance and fungal virulence. *Fungal Genet Biol* 66: 79–85.

Nielsen SE, Nielsen E, Julian HO, et al. (2015) Incidence and clinical characteristics of fungal keratitis in a Danish population from 2000 to 2013. *Acta Ophthalmol* 93: 54–8.

Ritterband DC, Seedor JA, Shah MK, Koplin RS and Mccormick SA (2006) Fungal keratitis at the new york eye and ear infirmary. *Cornea* 25: 264–7.

Saw SM, Ooi PL, Tan DT, et al. (2007) Risk factors for contact lens-related fusarium keratitis: a case-control study in Singapore. *Arch Ophthalmol* 125: 611–17.

Schrettl M, Bignell E, Kragl C, et al. (2004) Siderophore biosynthesis but not reductive iron assimilation is essential for Aspergillus fumigatus virulence. *J Exp Med* 200: 1213–19.

Sengupta J, Khetan A, Saha S, Banerjee D, Gangopadhyay N and Pal D (2012) Candida keratitis: emerging problem in India. *Cornea* 31: 371–5.

Shukla PK, Kumar M and Keshava GB (2008) Mycotic keratitis: an overview of diagnosis and therapy. *Mycoses* 51: 183–99.

Slowik M, Biernat MM, Urbaniak-Kujda D, Kapelko-Slowik K and Misiuk-Hojlo M (2015) Mycotic infections of the eye. *Adv Clin Exp Med* 24: 1113–17.

Sridhar J, Flynn HW Jr, Kuriyan AE, Miller D and Albini T (2013) Endogenous fungal endophthalmitis: risk factors, clinical features, and treatment outcomes in mold and yeast infections. *J Ophthalmic Inflamm Infect* 3: 60.

Srinivasan M, Gonzales CA, George C, et al. (1997) Epidemiology and aetiological diagnosis of corneal ulceration in Madurai, south India. *Br J Ophthalmol* 81: 965–71.

Sun Y, Chandra J, Mukherjee P, Szczotka-Flynn L, Ghannoum MA and Pearlman E (2009) A murine model of contact lens-associated fusarium keratitis. *Invest Ophthalmol Vis Sci* 51: 1511–16.

Tarabishy AB, Aldabagh B, Sun Y, et al. (2008) MyD88 regulation of Fusarium keratitis is dependent on TLR4 and IL-1R1 but not TLR2. *J Immunol* 181: 593–600.

Taylor PR, Leal SM Jr, Sun Y and Pearlman E (2014a) Aspergillus and Fusarium corneal infections are regulated by Th17 cells and IL-17-producing neutrophils. *J Immunol* 192: 3319–27.

Taylor PR, Roy S, Leal SM Jr, et al. (2014b) Activation of neutrophils by autocrine IL-17A-IL-17RC interactions during fungal infection is regulated by IL-6, IL-23, RORγt and dectin-2. *Nat Immunol* 15: 143–51.

Tuft SJ and Tullo AB (2009) Fungal keratitis in the United Kingdom 2003-2005. *Eye (Lond)* 23: 1308–13.

Underhill DM and Pearlman E (2015) Immune interactions with pathogenic and commensal fungi: a two-way street. *Immunity* 43: 845–58.

Urban CF, Ermert D, Schmid M, et al. (2009) Neutrophil extracellular traps contain calprotectin, a cytosolic protein complex involved in host defense against Candida albicans. *PLoS Pathog* 5: e1000639.

van Diepeningen AD, Brankovics B, Iltes J, Van Der Lee TA and Waalwijk C (2015) Diagnosis of infections: approaches to identification by the Clinical Mycology Laboratory. *Curr Fungal Infect Rep* 9: 135–143.

Wang L, Sun S, Jing Y, Han L, Zhang H and Yue J (2009) Spectrum of fungal keratitis in central China. *Clin Experiment Ophthalmol* 37: 763–71.

Wykoff CC, Flynn HW Jr, Miller D, Scott IU and Alfonso EC (2008) Exogenous fungal endophthalmitis: microbiology and clinical outcomes. *Ophthalmology* 115: 1501–7, 1507.e1–2.

Xie L, Zhong W, Shi W and Sun S (2006) Spectrum of fungal keratitis in north China. *Ophthalmology* 113: 1943–8.

Zackular JP, Chazin WJ and Skaar EP (2015) Nutritional immunity: S100 proteins at the host-pathogen interface. *J Biol Chem* 290: 18991–8.

Zhang H, Li H, Li Y, et al. (2013) IL-17 plays a central role in initiating experimental Candida albicans infection in mouse corneas. *Eur J Immunol* 43: 2671–82.

CHAPTER 29

Fungal infections of the kidney and those associated with renal failure, dialysis, and renal transplantation

Eileen K. Maziarz and John R. Perfect

Introduction

Fungal infections of the kidneys require a high index of suspicion for early diagnosis, and expertise in anticipating complications to manage them successfully. These infections may reflect disseminated fungal infection or occur in the absence of systemic disease. This chapter will review fungal infections of the kidney as well as those associated with chronic renal failure, peritoneal dialysis, and renal transplantation.

Fungal infections of the kidney

Causative fungi

As discussed in Chapter 27, funguria is a relatively common finding among hospitalized patients, with up to 10–15% of all nosocomial urinary tract infections (UTIs) caused by *Candida* spp. (Sobel et al. 2011). *Candida albicans* is the most common organism isolated from urinary specimens, though non-*albicans* species (particularly fluconazole-resistant organisms such as *C. glabrata* and *C. krusei*) have been observed in a significant minority of urinary culture specimens in patients with candiduria (Kobayashi et al. 2004). Risk factors for funguria are well established and have included: recent antimicrobial exposure (90%), concurrent (non-fungal) infection (85%), indwelling urinary devices (83%), and comorbid illnesses including diabetes mellitus (39%), urinary tract abnormalities (38%), and malignancy (22%) (Kauffman et al. 2000). Hence, funguria represents a considerable challenge to the clinician as it can reflect anything from contamination of the specimen, to colonization of a bladder catheter, to life-threatening disseminated fungal infection with renal involvement. It is therefore incumbent upon the clinician to neither dismiss these findings nor immediately treat all patients with antifungal agents; a high index of suspicion for systemic fungal infection is required when these organisms are cultured from a high-risk patient. *Candida* spp. are the most commonly isolated organisms from urinary specimens and will be the focus of this chapter. Many other fungi can involve the kidney, including *Aspergillus* spp., members of the Mucorales, *Cryptococcus* spp., the endemic mycoses, and a variety of dematiaceous moulds. These fungi infrequently cause localized kidney infections and will be discussed in Chapters 10, 12, 14, 16, and 18.

Pathophysiology and epidemiology

Fungal infections of the kidney are most commonly due to haematogenous dissemination (antegrade infection). The kidney is the organ most commonly involved in disseminated candidiasis (Louria et al. 1962; Lehner 1964) and the primary risk factors are those related to invasive candidiasis (see Chapters 11 and 25). The high frequency of renal involvement in disseminated mycoses, especially in the case of *Candida*, suggests that 'tropism' for the kidneys or local immune factors are responsible.

Animal models of infection demonstrate that when mice or rabbits undergo intravenous challenge with *Candida*, the bloodstream is cleared very quickly (Hurtrel et al. 1980). In contrast to other parenchymal sites and the bloodstream, where fungal clearance occurs rapidly, infection is not controlled in the kidney, where yeast can multiply, facilitating the persistence of infection (Hurtrel et al. 1980; Spellberg et al. 2003). Yeasts disseminate to the kidneys via the bloodstream and elicit an inflammatory response via neutrophils and macrophages. To be successful, these yeasts must penetrate capillary walls to invade the interstitium. This invasion is facilitated by attachment to capillary walls via various adherence mechanisms, which differ among *Candida* spp. (Schmid et al. 1995; Cotter and Kavanagh 2000), and penetrance, which is facilitated by hyphal and pseudohyphal forms. The correlation between an organism's ability to produce hyphal forms and virulence is highlighted by the differences seen in animal models of infection with *C. albicans*, which can form pseudohyphae and hyphae, and with other organisms including *C. glabrata*, which are monomorphic *in vivo* (incapable of producing hyphal and pseudohyphal forms) (Ryley and Ryley 1990; Brieland et al. 2001). It should be noted that while dimorphism is not an essential virulence factor for renal infection in *Candida* spp., the ability to form hyphae and pseudohyphae allows for enhanced virulence compared with hyphal-deficient mutants, which clinically present as chronic, non-fatal infections (Kauffman and Tan 1974). Furthermore, the ability to perform molecular studies on *Candida* has allowed a more precise understanding of morphology changes in the yeast (Whiteway and Oberholzer 2004) and its biofilm mechanisms (Nobile and Johnson 2015). Underlying differences in immune response have been characterized, including a shift from a Th2 to a Th1 response in models of infection with hyphal-deficient mutants (Brieland et al. 2001; Spellberg et al. 2003), so it is clear that the host interacts directly with the yeast.

Within the renal interstitium, fungi elicit a highly inflammatory response mediated primarily by neutrophils which can result in the formation of microabscesses and abscesses in the renal cortex. Further penetration into the renal tubules is again facilitated by hyphal and pseudohyphal forms. Fungal proliferation can occur within the *relatively* protected site of proximal renal tubules, and this is the proposed site of the renal acute phase responses, including upregulation of cytokines and chemokines and activation of the complement and the coagulation cascades (MacCallum and Odds 2005; Luyckx et al. 2009; MacCallum 2009; Fisher et al. 2011). From the proximal tubules, yeasts can re-penetrate the interstitium and lead to further abscess formation; extension beyond the renal cortex can lead to perinephric abscesses. Alternatively, papillitis and papillary necrosis occur, and the yeasts can aggregate with necrotic debris in the renal pelvis and other parts of the collecting system to form fungus balls, or 'bezoars' (Hurley and Winner 1963). In addition to a variety of virulence factors for particular fungi, there appears to be an inoculum effect, with high inocula resulting in rapidly fatal sepsis and multi-organ disease (Spellberg et al. 2005) and lower inocula resulting in chronic renal infection (Hurley and Winner 1963). In animal models of infection, death is directly correlated with fungal burden in the renal tissue after infection (Hurtrel et al. 1980; Spellberg et al. 2003).

Ascending fungal UTIs can also occur, although this situation is less common than haematogenous seeding. Most cases of retrograde yeast infections occur in the setting of urinary obstruction, indwelling bladder catheters, bacteriuria, and immunosuppression including diabetes mellitus. The pathogenesis of retrograde infection is less well understood, although multiple studies have demonstrated an association between concurrent gram-negative bacterial infections and risk of ascending fungal infections (Parkash et al. 1970; Levinson and Pitsakis 1987; Fisher et al. 2011) The presence of commensal bacteria and their ability to facilitate adhesion of *Candida* spp. to mucosal surfaces may indeed play a significant role in these rare infections (Nair and Samaranayake 1996). The clinical consequences of these interactions are potentially of great magnitude in the setting of indwelling urinary catheters, given the frequent occurrence of concomitant funguria and bacteriuria in hospitalized patients (Kauffman et al. 2000).

Clinical features, diagnosis, and management

As discussed, the spectrum of renal candidiasis includes both acute infections as part of disseminated *Candida* infection, and chronic, more indolent presentations from a lower urinary tract source. The latter presentation is usually localized to the kidney and genitourinary system and carries a very low risk of secondary fungaemia (Kauffman et al. 2000; Sobel et al. 2000) in the absence of urinary tract obstruction (Ang et al. 1993). These distinct entities present quite differently; the clinical presentations and management will be discussed separately (Table 29.1).

Table 29.1 Features of acute and chronic renal candidiasis

	Acute renal candidiasis	Chronic renal candidiasis
Pathogenesis	Haematogenous seeding of kidneys in disseminated candidiasis	Ascending infection from lower urinary tract source
Clinical setting	Neonates (especially preterm and low-birthweight) ICU setting Vascular catheters and parenteral nutrition Broad-spectrum antibiotics Immunosuppression*	Urinary tract obstruction Congenital abnormalities of urinary tract Indwelling bladder catheters Diabetes mellitus Urological instrumentation or surgery Concurrent bacteriuria
Findings	Bilateral kidney involvement (parenchyma +/− collecting system) Microabscesses and abscesses in renal cortex Papillary necrosis** Fungal bezoars** Perinephric abscess** Assume bloodstream infection	Unilateral kidney involvement (collecting system) Fungal bezoars*** Papillary necrosis*** Perinephric abscess Bloodstream infection rare in the absence of instrumentation or manipulation
Treatment	Systemic antifungals Monitor for and manage sequelae/complications	Systemic antifungals Invasive procedures often required

* Includes haematological malignancy, solid organ transplantation, use of chronic immunosuppressive agents, and malignancy

** Sequelae/complications of primary infection

*** Usually occur/s in the absence of renal parenchymal involvement

Acute Candida infection of the kidney: diagnosis and management

There are no specific signs or symptoms of acute renal candidiasis, and a high level of suspicion for invasive candidiasis is required whenever a critically ill patient is found to have candiduria. In these patients, signs and symptoms parallel those of invasive candidiasis (See Chapter 25), although occasionally referable urinary symptoms are reported, including abdominal or flank pain, dysuria, costovertebral angle tenderness, or the findings of a palpable mass on examination (Song et al. 2012). Obstructive renal bezoars should be suspected if oliguria/anuria, pneumaturia, or urinary debris is reported (Tennant et al. 1968; Sultana et al. 1998). Many patients will be critically ill and unable to report referable symptoms, or have attenuated host response due to underlying conditions. The diagnosis is particularly challenging in high-risk neonates, in whom thrombocytopenia (defined as a sustained decline in platelet count of 10% or more per day) may be the earliest indicator of disseminated candidiasis (Benjamin et al. 1999). This fragile group of patients appears to be at increased risk of developing obstructive bezoars and abscesses, which have been observed in up to 42% of neonates with candiduria (Bryant et al. 1999). Isolation of yeasts from urinary specimens in neonates has a high predictive value for disseminated candidiasis. A high index of suspicion for renal candidiasis cannot be overemphasized; often, these patients have shared risk factors for multiple infections and many reasons for renal dysfunction. Most experts recommend that renal ultrasonography should be requested on any high-risk preterm infant with candiduria (Benjamin et al. 1999), although it should be noted that nearly 50% of neonates with renal bezoars will have normal imaging at the time of initial candiduria (Berman et al. 1989; Bryant et al. 1999). Ultrasonography may demonstrate diffuse focal hypoechoic cortical abscesses or dilation of the renal calyces and pelvis as well as echogenic material in the collecting system without acoustic shadowing (Sadegi et al. 2009).

Although there is little argument to treat symptomatic fungal cystitis or candiduria when present in the setting of disseminated disease in high-risk patients—including neonates, neutropenic hosts, or patients with abnormal urinary structure—asymptomatic candiduria with or without indwelling bladder catheter is a more difficult (and far more common) scenario. Present data suggest that approximately 40% of candiduria cases will be eliminated with catheter removal alone. Furthermore, although treatment with fluconazole will more commonly clear the candiduria and is more effective in those with normal renal function, this does not prevent persistence, and at two-week follow up, no impact of antifungal therapy is demonstrated (Sobel et al 2000). Therefore, at present, consideration of treatment for asymptomatic candiduria must be made in the appropriate clinical context; frequently, treatment is not required.

Once identified, the evaluation and management of acute urinary tract disease should follow established management guidelines for candidaemia (see Chapter 25), including evaluation for other metastatic sites of infection, and in neonates—with their immature blood–brain barrier—lumbar puncture is indicated. Vascular and bladder catheter removal is recommended as part of management (Pappas et al. 2009). Systemic treatment should be tailored to the offending organism and a review of susceptibility data. Fluconazole is the agent of choice for susceptible *Candida* isolates; this agent achieves high tissue and urine concentrations and is less nephrotoxic than the polyenes. The available lipophilic extended-spectrum azoles, such as itraconazole, voriconazole, posaconazole, and isavuconazole, may be active against fungal pyelonephritis but they have poor pharmacokinetics for reaching the bladder, and thus are limited in their ability to treat lower urinary tract infections. Rates of infections due to azole-resistant *Candida* spp. are increasing (Kauffman et al. 2000), and in these cases intravenous amphotericin B or the echinocandins can be used. While echinocandins do not concentrate in the urine and are not recommended for treating simple candiduria, concentrations in the renal parenchyma appear to be adequate in pyelonephritis or where high urinary drug concentrations are not required (as in the case of fungus balls and cystitis) (Sobel et al. 2007). Liposomal amphotericin B should probably be used infrequently owing to poor tissue penetration in the renal tubules (Agustin et al. 1999). Patients with renal involvement and known disseminated candidiasis should be closely monitored for complications, including obstructive lesions, perinephric abscesses, and emphysematous pyelonephritis, which can develop despite appropriate systemic antifungal therapy (Bryant et al. 1999) and often require procedural intervention for a successful outcome (discussed in the section below). The length of treatment is not precisely defined, but in complicated cases, at least two weeks of therapy is often required.

Chronic Candida infection of the kidney

Another, albeit less frequent, presentation of renal candidiasis follows a more subacute and indolent course. These infections are thought to primarily develop via retrograde infection in patients with established risk factors including: anatomical or functional urinary tract obstruction, indwelling bladder catheters, recent antibacterial exposure, concomitant bacteriuria, diabetes mellitus, and other immunosuppressive conditions (Scerpella and Alhalel 1994). Glycosuria and neurogenic bladder are predisposing factors found in diabetic patients. These yeast infections can occur in both children and adults; in infancy, however, the risk factors are distinct from those associated with acute *Candida* infection in adults and often occur in term infants with congenital anomalies of the genitourinary tract with or without recent instrumentation (Bisht and VanDer Voort 2011).

In contrast to acute infections associated with systemic candidiasis, in which bilateral renal involvement is usually seen, these ascending infections are generally confined to a single kidney, and the risk of secondary candidaemia is low in the absence of urinary tract manipulation (Ang et al. 1993). Involvement is limited to the collecting system and includes the presence of fungal bezoars and papillary necrosis, and occasionally, further tissue invasion can lead to perinephric abscesses. Renal cortical involvement is not seen in these chronic infections; the finding of microabscesses in addition to these obstructive lesions should raise concern for disseminated infection.

Clinical features of chronic renal candidiasis differ from those of the acute infections described in 'Acute *Candida* infection of the kidney: diagnosis and management'. Fever and systemic signs of infection are less common. However, flank pain and costovertebral angle tenderness may be reported. There are no specific findings from urinalysis (aside from urinary leucocytes) or urine culture (including any concentration of yeasts) that discriminate infection/disease from contamination/colonization; therefore, a high index of suspicion for these infections is warranted, particularly when a clinically high risk patient is found to have persistent candiduria. Ultrasonography and computed tomography (CT) urography are useful diagnostic imaging modalities. The latter may demonstrate renal scarring, blunting of the calyces, papillary necrosis, or filling defects in the collecting system (Quaia et al. 2014) and is superior to ultrasonography in visualizing pyelonephritis and perinephric abscesses (Kauffman et al. 2011).

Management of chronic renal candidiasis, including urinary fungus balls, will often require both medical and surgical interventions (Irby et al. 1990). Goals include the prevention or elimination of systemic infection, relief of obstruction (when present), eradication of infectious pathogen, and prevention of further long-term sequelae. All patients should be treated with a systemic antifungal agent directed at the offending fungal pathogen prior to manipulation of the urinary tract to prevent secondary candidaemia. Fluconazole and amphotericin B (with or without flucytosine) are the most commonly used agents and are recommended in the present guidelines (Pappas et al. 2009). In the absence of obstruction, some authors have reported success with systemic therapy alone (Benjamin and Fisher 1999; Robinson et al. 2009); however, access to the upper urinary tract is often required to facilitate disruption of the dense fungal elements. This can be achieved via percutaneous nephrostomy (PCN) tube placement (when hydronephrosis is present) or retrograde transurethral catheters (if PCN placement is precluded). Large-bore tubes are often required to effectively drain the obstructing material and allow access for local irrigation of antifungal agents as well as pyelography to confirm success of drainage (Chitale et al. 2004). Once access is achieved, clinical specimens should be collected for microbiological analysis. Instillation of amphotericin B deoxycholate (50 mg/L of sterile water) via the PCN tube can be considered as adjunctive therapy; the volume and rate of infusion should be patient-specific, with rates of 5–45 mL per hour twice daily reported (summarized in Bisht and VanDer Voort 2011). The local use of amphotericin B bladder irrigations and through nephrostomy tubes is generally safe but should be reserved for collecting-system and unique bladder infections; it is unlikely that they are effective in routine treatment for candiduria (Arthur et al. 2004; Drew et al. 2005). Fluconazole irrigation has been used successfully in some cases but the dosing is not well established (Chung et al. 2001). Local irrigation with saline, fibrinolytics (Kabaalıoglu et al. 2001; Babu and Hutton 2004), and methylene blue have been used (Aktug et al. 1998; Ofoegbu et al. 2007), but the number of cases is still too small to draw any substantive conclusions. Further mechanical debulking techniques for fungal bezoars, infected stones, and biofilms containing yeasts that have been successfully used including guidewire fragmentation, mechanical thrombectomy, stone basket extraction, and suction irrigation (Doemeny et al. 1988; Bell et al. 1993; Langenstroer et al. 2000; Morello et al. 2002; Campbell et al. 2004). In general, these patients are treated with antifungals for three to six weeks. Most experts recommend retention of upper tract access and continued treatment until consecutive cultures are negative. The use of radiography to guide treatment duration is controversial, as some reports have suggested that cessation of antifungal therapy at the time of microbiological clearance, but in advance of radiographic resolution, does not unfavourably affect outcomes or relapse potential (Benjamin and Fisher 1999). Open pyelotomy or nephrectomy is rarely required (Raghunath et al. 2013). A proposed algorithm is outlined in Figure 29.1.

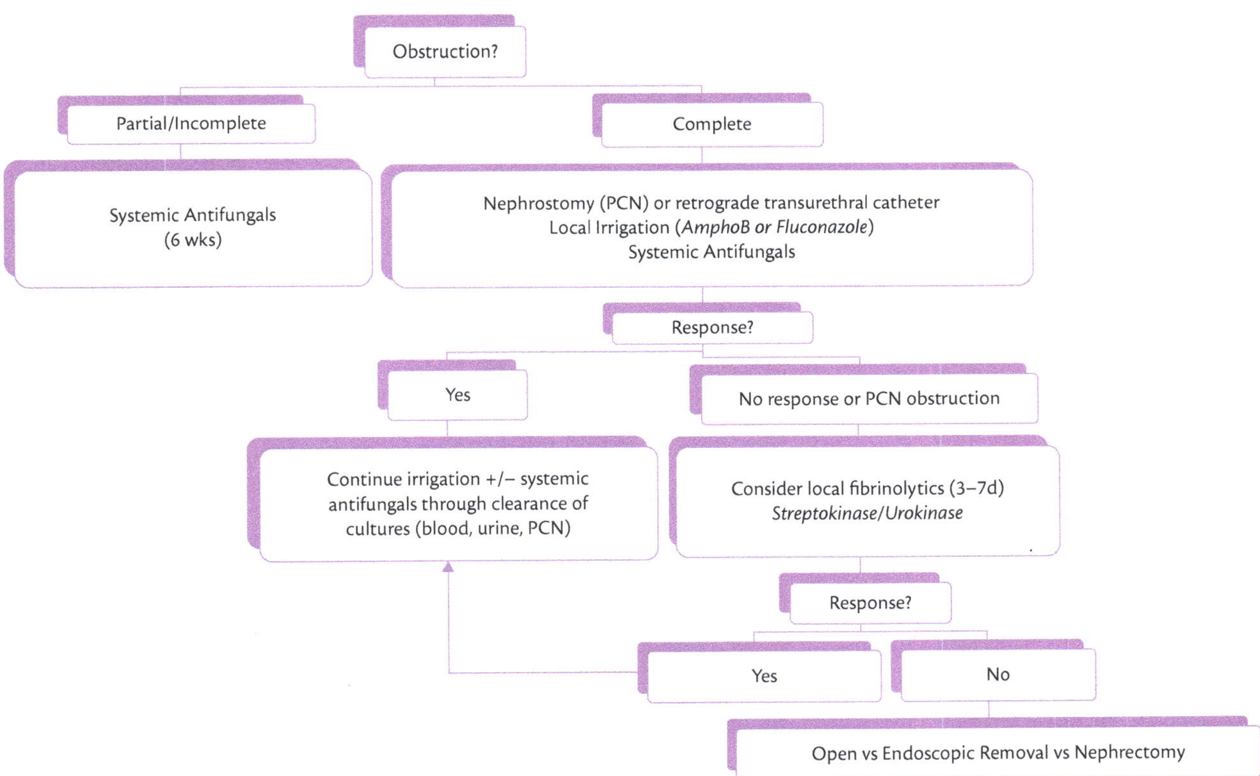

Figure 29.1 Suggested management of obstructive renal candidiasis.

PCN = percutaneous nephrostomy.

Adapted with permission from Bisht V & Voort JV, 'Obstructive renal candidiasis in infancy', *European Journal of Pediatrics*, Volume 170, pp. 1227–35, Copyright © 2011 Springer-Verlag, doi: 10.1007/s00431-011-1514-6

Fungal infections associated with chronic renal failure

Patients with chronic renal failure have a higher incidence of infection, including fungal infection, than those with normal renal function. Infection remains the second leading cause of death, behind cardiovascular disease, in patients with chronic renal failure and end-stage renal disease (United States Renal Data System 2015). While the majority of invasive fungal infections in this group of patients are related to complications of dialysis vascular access sites (see Chapters 21 and 25), several other factors contribute to this risk, which are seen in patients with pre-dialysis chronic renal failure (Wang et al. 2011). These include the multifaceted immune dysregulation related to the uraemic state, vitamin D deficiency, iron overload and treatment with desferrioxamine and comorbid and underlying conditions including malnutrition, diabetes mellitus and collagen vascular disorders (Box 29.1).

End-stage renal disease is a state of concomitant systemic inflammation and marked alteration in immune function that results in increased susceptibility to infection and inadequate response to vaccinations. The impaired immune response in uraemia is multifaceted, caused by accumulation of toxic metabolites and resulting in a chronic state of oxidative stress. The end result is impairment in both innate and adaptive immunity. Phagocytic function is defective owing to inappropriate priming of granulocytes and monocytes as well as increased leucocyte apoptosis; in addition, antigen presentation is impaired owing to depletion and dysfunction of dendritic cells. Cellular-mediated immunity is diminished via depletion of both naïve and central T-cell subsets, and humoral defects observed are likely due to both impaired helper T-cell function as well as B-cell depletion and dysfunction. Chronic renal failure represents a state of premature immune senescence, with expansion of the myeloid lineage similar to that observed in elderly patients. Some immune changes are not reversed with dialysis or renal transplantation, suggesting that the inflammatory milieu is not completely responsible for the immune deficits seen in these patients. In patients with severe proteinuria, the excretion of large proteins, including immunoglobulins, contributes to an increased susceptibility to infection as well (Vanholder and Ringoir 1993; Vanholder et al. 1996; Cohen and Hörl 2012; Vaziri et al. 2012; Betjes 2013; Kurts et al. 2013).

Box 29.1 Risk factors for fungal infection in patients with chronic renal failure

- Intravascular catheters for haemodialysis
- Intraperitoneal catheters for peritoneal dialysis
- Impaired host defence due to uraemic state
- Iron overload
- Treatment with desferrioxamine*
- Protein calorie malnutrition
- Vitamin D deficiency
- Comorbid conditions (diabetes mellitus, systemic lupus erythematosus, other rheumatological conditions)

*Less commonly used and now an uncommon risk factor for fungal disease.

Desferrioxamine and risk of invasive fungal infection

Iron is an essential element for the growth and success of certain micro-organisms. Iron overload states represent a risk factor for mucormycosis, as discussed in Chapter 18. Availability of host iron stores is increased in certain states, such as severe acidaemia or exposure to the chelating agent desferrioxamine. This iron- and aluminium-chelator was once commonly used to treat the aluminium toxicity of renal failure. Several cases of invasive mucormycosis have been observed in dialysis patients receiving desferrioxamine, with mortality approaching 90% (Boelaert et al. 1991). The iron-desferrioxamine chelate (ferrioxamine) acts as a xenosiderophore, facilitating iron uptake by these fungi and permitting fungal growth and dissemination (Boelaert et al. 1993; Ibrahim et al. 2012). Aluminium toxicity in patients with chronic renal failure is now rare, owing to enhanced water purification techniques and the availability of non-aluminium-based phosphate binders. However, the risk of invasive mucormycosis with ferrioxamine, when used for iron overload syndromes, should be appreciated. Other iron chelators do not act as exogenous siderophores or increase the risk of mucormycosis (Boelaert et al. 1994); importantly, one agent, deferasirox, can take iron from members of the Mucorales, and has been used as adjunctive therapy in mucormycosis (Spellberg et al. 2012).

Fungal infections associated with peritoneal dialysis

Peritoneal dialysis (PD) is an effective and practical alternative to haemodialysis for patients with end-stage renal disease. Peritonitis is one of the major complications of PD and cause of significant morbidity, including a major cause of peritoneal membrane failure and PD discontinuation. Fungal infections account for 1–15% of all peritonitis episodes related to PD and carry higher rates of morbidity and mortality than bacterial peritonitis (Prasad and Gupta 2005; Li et al. 2010).

Pathogenesis and causative pathogens

PD uses a semi-closed system in which bags of dialysate solutions are connected via tubing to an indwelling peritoneal catheter. The dialysate is allowed to dwell in the peritoneal cavity for a period of time, and is then drained back into the bags. The most common route of infection is thought to be related to improper sterile technique resulting in periluminal infection, although cutaneous exit site infection, secondary peritonitis from intestinal perforation (Suh et al. 1996), and peritoneovaginal communication are other recognized modes of infection (Li et al. 1993).

A number of risk factors for fungal peritonitis among PD patients have been identified in multiple series, including recent antibiotic exposure and recent and/or frequent episodes of bacterial peritonitis (Cheng et al. 1989; Michel et al. 1994; Bordes et al. 1995; Goldie et al. 1996; Miles et al. 2009). There are several plausible explanations for these observations, which have been demonstrated in both early and contemporary reports. These include: disruption of normal flora of the skin and gut, allowing for fungal overgrowth, inflammatory sequelae of prior peritonitis, leading to impaired defence mechanisms and, potentially, common risks associated with technical aspects of catheter manipulation. Other risk factors identified include immunosuppression—including HIV (human immunodeficiency virus) infection (Tebben et al. 1993) and use of immunosuppressive agents (Michel et al. 1994; Huang et al. 2000)—protein calorie malnutrition, and compulsory PD use due to comorbid conditions (Oygar et al. 2009). Environmental risk factors have also been implicated, including seasonal differences in infection rates (Bordes et al. 1995), outbreaks of mould infection associated with natural disasters (Torres et al. 2014), and reports of outbreaks of *Candida* peritonitis associated with contaminated water baths used to warm dialysate solutions (Yuen et al. 1992). Age, sex, underlying aetiology of renal failure, and comorbid conditions, including diabetes mellitus, have not been shown to be specific risk factors for fungal peritonitis in PD (Michel et al. 1994; Goldie et al. 1996).

Candida spp. cause the majority of episodes, accounting for more than 70% of fungal peritonitis episodes in most large series. Historically, the majority of episodes were due to *C. albicans;* more recently, however, a shift toward non-*albicans* species has been reported at many centres, accounting for more than half of fungal peritonitis episodes (Michel et al. 1994; Goldie et al. 1996; Wang et al. 2000; Prasad et al. 2004). Although *Candida* spp. remain the predominant cause of fungal peritonitis complicating PD, many fungi have been reported to cause disease (Prasad and Gupta 2005), including *Aspergillus* spp. (Nguyen and Muder 1994), other hyalohypomycetes including *Paecilomyces, Fusarium,* and *Acremonium* spp. (Landay et al. 1982; Rippon et al. 1988; Chiaradia et al. 1990; Lye 1990), Mucorales spp. (Polo et al. 1989), dermatophytes including *Trichosporon* spp. (Carr et al. 1987; Yuen et al. 1990) and *Cryptococcus* spp. (Yinnon et al. 1993), as well as the dimorphic fungi *Coccidioides* and *Histoplasma* spp. (Ampel et al. 1988; Lopes et al. 1994).

Clinical features and diagnosis

Clinical symptoms of fungal peritonitis in PD patients are indistinguishable from those seen in bacterial peritonitis episodes, including cloudy dialysate, abdominal pain, fever, and nausea. Peritoneal signs with rebound tenderness and rigidity may be seen. Patients should be examined for evidence of superficial fungal infections and vaginal candidiasis as these may represent sources of infection. Particulate matter may be identified in the effluent fluid, corresponding to fungal elements, but this is not a routine finding (Charlton et al. 2010). Poor dialysate return due to obstruction of the catheter by fungal elements may be reported, and can occur in the absence of peritonitis (DeVault et al. 1985; Huang et al. 2000; Jeloka et al. 2011).

In patients presenting with compatible symptoms (cloudy dialysate, abdominal pain with or without fever), a sample of dialysate should be obtained and sent for cell count with differential, Gram stain, and culture. The peritoneal white blood cell (WBC) count should be greater than 100 cells per millilitre, with more than 50% polymorphonuclear (PMN) cells. Shorter dwell times, as with automated PD or recent peritoneal lavage, may lead to low peritoneal WBC or falsely negative culture results, though the PMN predominance usually persists; in equivocal cases, repeat sampling after a dwell time of at least two hours can be recommended. While certain observations have been made, including the association of peritoneal eosinophilia with certain mould infections (Sridhar et al 1990; Nankivell et al 1991), neither the absolute peritoneal WBC nor the differential accurately discriminate the offending pathogen (Keane et al. 2000; Chavada et al. 2011). Gram stain of dialysate fluid may reveal yeasts, allowing for prompt initiation of antifungal therapy, but additional fungal stains are required for identification of the other causative fungi. The presence of multiple organisms on Gram stain should prompt evaluation for a source of secondary peritonitis. A high index of suspicion is necessary for prompt detection of fungal peritonitis and initiation of appropriate therapy; patients with recent bacterial peritonitis episodes and antibiotic treatment are at increased risk. It is recommended that 10 mL of peritoneal fluid be sent for fungal culture. While *Candida* spp. often grow quickly in culture, other fungi may grow more slowly; as such, the microbiology lab should be alerted to hold plates for a minimum of three weeks. In cases of culture-negative PD-associated peritonitis—particularly in those patients failing to improve on appropriate antibacterial coverage at 96 hours—repeated assessment and consideration of fungal peritonitis are strongly warranted (Keane et al. 2000). Furthermore, if fungal cultures are negative but fungal disease is suspected, it may be necessary to use lipid-enriched culture media to facilitate growth of *Malassezia* spp., which may cause disease in the PD setting. While there may be an emerging role for non-culture-based diagnostics, such as the (1→3)-β-D-glucan test, in the evaluation of patients with suspected PD-related fungal peritonitis (Worasilchai et al. 2015), their role at this time is not well defined.

Treatment and prevention

An optimal approach to the patient with suspected or confirmed fungal peritonitis aims to reduce mortality as well as minimize morbidity, including the long-term complications of peritoneal adhesions and sclerosing peritonitis and their sequelae, and to allow for successful resumption of PD.

Historically, there was no established consensus regarding the treatment of fungal peritonitis, and at times the recommendations appeared as murky as the initial effluent fluid encountered. There have been no randomized controlled trials related to the management of fungal peritonitis in PD, and small single-centre studies have demonstrated success with catheter removal alone (Nagappan et al. 1992) as well as with antifungal therapy alone with catheter retention (Corbella et al. 1991; Tsai et al. 1991). Eradication of infection in the setting of foreign bodies colonized with fungi is exquisitely challenging without their removal. However, in some cases, sterilization of peritoneal fluid has been accomplished despite persistent dense colonization of peritoneal catheters (Kerr et al. 1983), which likely explains relapses observed when the catheter is retained (Miles et al. 2009). Figure 29.2 shows an electron micrograph of a fungal biofilm involving a PD catheter infected with *Fusarium* spp. Based on these observations as well as findings from multiple large single-centre studies, consistently demonstrating excess mortality associated with catheter retention (Goldie et al. 1996; Wang et al. 2000; Prasad et al. 2004), contemporary guidelines recommend immediate catheter removal upon identification of fungi in microscopy or culture, with haemodialysis bridge until the infection is successfully eradicated (Li et al. 2010). Early catheter removal has been associated with improved survival compared with delayed removal (Chang et al. 2011).

Systemic antifungal therapy should commence as soon as fungal peritonitis is diagnosed, in conjunction with plans for immediate catheter removal. Peritoneal lavage can be considered prior to removal if the dialysate is particularly turbid. In many cases, initial therapy is initiated without knowledge of the specific pathogen.

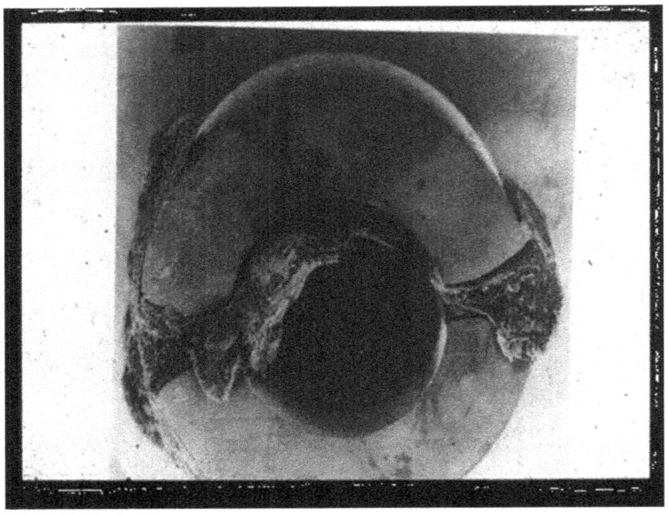

Figure 29.2 Electron micrograph of a peritoneal dialysis catheter tip showing a *Fusarium* species within the lumen of the catheter during a case of chronic fungal peritonitis.
Reproduced courtesy of John Perfect.

For patients without significant azole exposure or limited suspicion of mould infection, oral fluconazole is a preferred up-front agent. Fluconazole has excellent bioavailability and achieves comparable concentrations in the peritoneal fluid to those in plasma (Debruyne and Ryckelynck 1992; Wong et al. 1997; Blowey et al. 1998). It has been used in conjunction with catheter removal to successfully treat these infections for nearly 25 years (Levine et al. 1989).

When mould infection is suspected on the basis of the initial microscopy, or when a patient has significant prior azole exposure, up-front therapy with intravenous amphotericin B (with or without flucytosine) or an intravenous echinocandin is recommended (Table 29.2). There are very limited data regarding the peritoneal penetration of the echinocandins (Yamada et al. 2011) and some *in vitro* data to suggest that their fungicidal activity may be impaired by dialysate fluid (Tobudic et al. 2013). They have, however, been used successfully in fungal PD peritonitis, both as monotherapy and in combination with other antifungal agents (Madriaga et al. 2003; Fourtounas et al. 2006). Owing to the risk of resistance when used as monotherapy, flucytosine should only be used in combination with another agent, and therapeutic drug monitoring is recommended (Li 2010). Intraperitoneal amphotericin B should be avoided as it has been associated with abdominal pain, chemical peritonitis, and peritoneal fibrosis, and may affect an individual patient's ability to resume PD (Hogg et al. 1982; Struijk et al. 1987; Coronel et al. 1993), without a substantive impact on outcome.

Antifungal susceptibility testing should be requested once the pathogen is identified in culture. Therapy should be tailored based on culture and susceptibility results. In general, susceptible *Candida* spp. can be treated for 10–14 days following catheter removal. Fluconazole-resistant *Candida* spp. and mould infections will often require longer courses of therapy. These patients often

Table 29.2 Dosing and spectrum of antifungal agents in PD-associated fungal peritonitis

Agent	Route	Dosage	Spectrum*
Fluconazole	Oral	200 mg/day	*C. albicans* *C. parapsilosis* *C. tropicalis*
Amphotericin B**	IV IP#	0.6–1 mg/kg/day NA	*C. krusei* and *C. glabrata* *Cryptococcus* spp. Susceptible moulds including *Mucorales* spp.
Echinocandins			
Micafungin	IV	100 mg/day	Resistant *Candida* spp. including
Caspofungin	IV	70 mg LD, then 50 mg/day	*C. krusei* and *C. glabrata*
Anidulafungin	IV	200 mg LD, then 100 mg/day	
Voriconazole	Oral	400 mg b.i.d. LD, then 200 mg b.i.d.***	Susceptible moulds including *Aspergillus* and phaeohyphomycetes
Posaconazole	Oral	300 mg/day (extended release tablet)*** 400 mg b.i.d. (solution)***	Susceptible moulds including *Aspergillus*, phaeohyphomycetes, and *Mucorales* spp.
Flucytosine	Oral	2 g LD, then 1 g/day***	Used as adjunctive therapy for synergy for *Candida* spp., *Cryptococcus* spp., and some phaeohyphomycetes. Monotherapy promotes resistance.

Not recommended (see text)

* Review of antifungal susceptibility testing recommended in selecting optimal agent for specific pathogen.

** Liposomal products can be used for patients with residual renal function.

*** Therapeutic drug monitoring advised for optimal dosing and to minimize adverse effects.

IV = intravenous; IP = intraperitoneal; LD = loading dose

Reproduced with permission from Prasad N. and Gupta A., 'Fungal peritonitis in peritoneal dialysis patients', *Peritoneal Dialysis International*, Volume 25, pp. 207–22, Copyright © 2005 Multimedia Inc require treatment for at least four weeks, and should have resolution of symptoms prior to discontinuation. Dosing recommendations are provided in Table 29.2. The optimal timing of catheter re-insertion has not been systematically studied in cases of fungal peritonitis. Immediate replacement is not recommended given the risks of colonizing the new catheter. Most experts agree that attempts at catheter re-insertion should be deferred for four to six weeks and following successful completion of an antifungal course (Prasad and Gupta 2005; Li et al. 2010).

Given the excess mortality and high morbidity associated with fungal peritonitis in PD, including PD drop-out, and the strong association between prior antibacterial use and bacterial peritonitis episodes, consideration of targeted antifungal prophylaxis in high-risk patients has been evaluated. An early report of nystatin prophylaxis found a significant decrease in fungal peritonitis rates (Zaruba et al. 1991), while other reports have demonstrated conflicting results, with some studies showing no effect of prophylaxis (Thodis et al. 1998; Williams et al. 2000) and others demonstrating a reduction in antibiotic-related fungal peritonitis episodes (Wong et al. 2007). The mixed findings in these reports may be related to the use of historical controls and variable rates of fungal peritonitis at different centres. In the only randomized controlled trial of nystatin prophylaxis, the authors found a reduction in overall fungal peritonitis rates but no significant impact on antibiotic-related fungal peritonitis episodes (Lo et al. 1996). Based on these findings, most experts agree that nystatin prophylaxis (500,000 IU orally three to four times per day) during courses of antibiotic treatment may be considered based on fungal peritonitis rates in an individual programme (Prasad and Gupta 2005; Li et al. 2010). Fluconazole is not recommended owing to the potential for emerging resistance, and routine prophylaxis in the absence of concomitant antibiotic use is discouraged. Finally, every effort should be made to reinforce adherence to best practices and techniques to reduce the overall infection risk, as this will influence an individual's risk for fungal peritonitis.

Fungal infections associated with renal transplantation

Renal transplantation is an established therapy for patients with chronic renal failure and end-stage renal disease. Owing to advances in surgical techniques and immunosuppressive therapy, overall graft survival rates have improved over recent decades. This translates into a significant survival advantage for patients compared with survival on dialysis, with five-year patient survival rates approaching 85% for transplant recipients compared with 36% for dialysis patients (NIDDK Health Statistics). Despite advances in immunosuppressive strategies and prophylaxis regimens, infection remains a considerable cause of morbidity and a major cause of death after renal transplantation, behind cardiovascular disease (Briggs 2001). Incidence rates of fungal infection after kidney transplant have remained relatively stable at 5.3 infections per 100-patient years over the first three post-transplant years, and are considerably lower than rates of bacterial or viral infections (Snyder et al. 2009). However, given the significant morbidity and mortality associated with invasive mycoses following kidney transplant, a high index of suspicion for these diagnoses and prompt institution of appropriate antifungal therapy (sometimes empirically) are imperative for a successful outcome.

Epidemiology and causative fungi

Compared with other solid organ transplant (SOT) recipients, renal transplant patients have the lowest overall incidence of invasive fungal infection (IFI) following solid organ transplantation, with an estimated incidence of 1.3% in the largest surveillance study to date (Pappas et al. 2010). Invasive candidiasis is the most common IFI in SOT recipients (49% of all IFIs), followed by cryptococcosis (15%), aspergillosis (14%), endemic mycoses (10%), and other/unspecified mould infections (5.1%). The epidemiology of post-transplant infections is heavily influenced by the environment, however, and in certain settings, mould infections predominate (Einollahi et al. 2008). This bears particular relevance in the context of commercial transplantation or 'transplant tourism', an increasingly popular phenomenon which has been complicated by high rates of invasive and particularly devastating mould infections (primarily due to *Aspergillus* and *Mucorales* spp.) in multiple case series (Shoham et al. 2010; Babik and Chin-Hong 2015). Invasive fungal infections following transplantation can be categorized by the presumed mode of acquisition: nosocomial, including unrecognized donor-derived infection; reactivation or disseminated infection due to 'true pathogens' (either from recipient or donor); and opportunistic infection due to pathogens that uncommonly cause disease in the normal host (Tolkoff-Rubin and Rubin 1992). Particularly devastating cases of donor-derived mould infections in the transplanted kidneys have been reported, resulting in both allograft loss and death (Alexander et al. 2010).

The mycology of invasive fungal infections in renal transplant recipients is partially dependent upon the time from transplant, which has been well-characterized in SOT recipients and is influenced by individual patient risk factors (Fishman 2007). With the exception of perioperative *Candida* infections, the majority of invasive fungal infections complicating organ transplantation are, in general, late-onset infections, occurring more than 90 days after transplant (Pappas et al. 2010) (see also Chapter 34).

Causative fungi: clinical features and diagnosis

Candiduria is not an uncommon finding in renal transplant patients, occurring in up to 11% of patients. Generally speaking, this is an asymptomatic finding, observed more commonly in female patients, in diabetics, in those with neurogenic bladder, and in the setting of recent antibiotic use, bladder catheters, or ureteral stents. Isolation of *Candida* from urine cultures in a renal transplant recipient should prompt evaluation for evidence of systemic disease. Once systemic infection is excluded, management of asymptomatic candiduria in renal transplant patients is controversial in the absence of planned urological manipulation or neutropenia (Pappas et al. 2009). Similar to non-transplant patients, candiduria is associated with decreased survival in renal transplant recipients, but treatment of asymptomatic patients has not been shown to improve survival or reduce recurrence rates (Safdar et al. 2005; Delgado et al. 2010). Moreover, non-*albicans Candida* spp., in particular *C. glabrata*, are more likely to affect transplant recipients, and therapeutic decisions about treating fluconazole-resistant organisms should weigh the benefits of therapy with the potential toxicities of the required antifungal agents. A prudent approach to the renal transplant patient with asymptomatic candiduria includes: verification of infection by repeat urinalysis and urine culture; removal or exchange of bladder catheter, where appropriate;

and—in cases of critical illness or localizing symptoms—dedicated imaging of the genitourinary tract to evaluate for fungal bezoars or pyelonephritis (Kauffman et al. 2011).

Disseminated *Candida* infections in renal transplant recipients often occur early in the post-transplant period. Risk factors for candidaemia are similar to those for non-transplant patients, including intravascular catheters, prolonged antibacterial treatment, heavy yeast colonization, and prolonged hospitalization (Kullberg and Arendrup 2015). Mortality is high for these infections and the diagnosis is challenging owing to both the limits of culture-based diagnostics (Clancy and Nguyen 2013) and the potential for attenuated host responses to infection in these immunocompromised patients.

Early-onset candidiasis in renal transplant patients has also been reported as due to contamination of preservation fluid at the time of multi-organ procurement as well as untreated candidaemia in the donor. The spectrum of disease includes fungal urinomas, infected perinephric haematomas and surgical site infections, candidaemia, obstructive uropathy secondary to fungal bezoars, and highly morbid (and often fatal) vascular complications including fungal arteritis and rupture of mycotic aneurysms (Figure 29.3) (Albano et al. 2009; Veroux et al. 2009; Dębska-Ślizień et al. 2015). Graft arteritis due to *Aspergillus* as well as *Mucorales* spp. has also been reported, with a similar mode of transmission suspected (Garrido et al. 2003; Zhan et al. 2008). Vascular anastomotic involvement can be catastrophic and may require nephrectomy for successful management (Mai et al. 2006). At this time, however, routine culture of preservation fluid and/or antifungal prophylaxis is not recommended in the absence of suspected contamination at the time of organ procurement. When recognized, however, prompt initiation of antifungal therapy and vigilant surveillance with serial imaging have successfully averted the need for pre-emptive graft nephrectomy (Matignon et al. 2008). Donor candiduria is not regarded as a contraindication to renal transplantation, but it is generally recommended that the recipient be treated with an appropriate antifungal agent to minimize post-transplant complications (Singh et al. 2012).

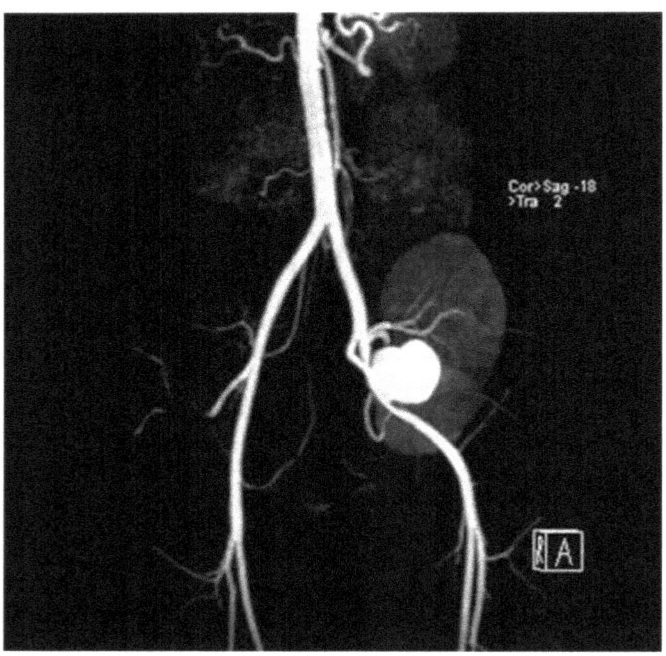

Figure 29.3 Magnetic resonance arteriogram demonstrating pseudoaneurysm of anastomosis of external iliac artery to allograft renal artery.

Reprinted from *Kidney International*, Volume 72, Issue 6, Henderson A., Pall A. A., Chakraverty S., 'Unsuspected mycotic aneurysm of renal transplant artery', pp. 775–5, Copyright © 2007 with permission from International Society of Nephrology, http://www.sciencedirect.com/science/article/pii/S0085253815527129.

Cryptococcal infection in renal transplant recipients most commonly presents as disseminated disease or meningoencephalitis due to *Cryptococcus neoformans* (Singh et al. 2008). While both primary infection and reactivation of latent infection occur, it is thought that the majority of cases are due to reactivation of latent disease, which manifests significantly earlier in the post-transplant course (Saha et al. 2007). Patients with central nervous system (CNS) disease can present with headache, fever, or altered mentation; the clinical presentation, however, can vary based on host factors and extent of disease. Serum cryptococcal antigen testing is positive in up to 90% of SOT patients with cryptococcal meningitis, and up to 39% of patients will have positive blood cultures (Wu et al. 2002). Transplant recipients on the calcineurin-inhibitor tacrolimus seem to be more likely to develop pulmonary, skin and soft tissue, and osteoarticular infections due to *Cryptococcus*, potentially related to the anti-cryptococcal activity of this agent at high temperatures (Singh et al. 1997; Odom et al. 2007; Singh et al. 2007). All SOT recipients with diagnosed or suspected cryptococcal infection, irrespective of site of infection, should undergo thorough evaluation to exclude CNS involvement, including a lumbar puncture with opening pressure, given the implications for management (Baddley et al. 2013). The severity of disease in renal transplant recipients with cryptococcal infection influences mortality rates, which approach 15% in contemporary studies (Singh et al. 2007).

While early infection with *Aspergillus* spp. can occur in renal transplant recipients, invasive aspergillosis remains a late-onset infection in this group of patients, similar to that which is described in other SOT groups (Pappas et al. 2010; Heylen et al. 2015). The vast majority of infections are pulmonary, though dissemination to the CNS can occur. The primary mode of acquisition is considered to be inhalation of infectious spores, and nosocomial outbreaks in renal transplant recipients have been described in association with hospitals under construction (Panackal et al. 2003). Classical risk factors for invasive aspergillosis identified for other SOT groups are not typically seen in renal transplant recipients (Hoyo et al. 2014); leucopenia is associated with increased risk of aspergillosis following renal transplantation, whereas the duration of pre-transplant renal replacement therapy and donor CMV (cytomegalovirus) seropositivity are associated with early-onset and late-onset disease, respectively (Heylen et al. 2015). Crude mortality for invasive aspergillosis in renal transplant patients is consistent with other SOT groups and has been reported to be as high as 39% in the current era. Renal insufficiency, CNS involvement, and treatment with either amphotericin B or caspofungin are associated with increased risk of death in SOT recipients with invasive aspergillosis (Baddley et al. 2010).

A history of travel to, or residence in, areas endemic for *Histoplasma capsulatum*, *Blastomyces dermatitidis*, *Coccidioides immitis/posadasii*, and *Paracoccidioides brasiliensis* should be part of the standard preoperative evaluation of potential transplant candidates. While the endemic mycoses account for only a small minority of IFIs following SOT, disseminated disease is common, particularly in cases of histoplasmosis and coccidioidomycosis, and early mortality approaches 15%. Reactivation of latent infection and primary infection both occur, which likely explains the bimodal distribution observed with respect to onset of infection and the potential for late-onset cases, decades following transplantation (Assi et al. 2013; Kauffman et al. 2014).

Histoplasmosis in renal transplant patients commonly presents with fever, weight loss, and pulmonary symptoms. Pulmonary involvement is seen in up to 80% of cases, and multi-organ dissemination—including bone marrow involvement—is common, particularly in severe cases (Assi et al. 2013); cases of thrombotic microangiopathy and haemophagocytic lymphohistiocytosis in renal transplant patients with histoplasmosis have been reported (Dwyre et al. 2006; Lo et al. 2010). Diagnostic modalities include: culture of blood or sterile sites, serum and urine antigen testing, histopathology, and antibody-based testing. Urine and serum antigen testing are the most sensitive tests for disseminated histoplasmosis in SOT recipients, whereas antibody-based tests perform poorly in isolation. Blood culture positivity correlates with disease severity (Assi et al. 2013).

Historically, *Pneumocystis jirovecii* pneumonia (PJP) occurred in up to 5% of renal transplant recipients, primarily during the first post-transplant year. It is now a relatively uncommon cause of IFI in contemporary cohorts, accounting for 1% of all IFIs in kidney transplant recipients, likely due to the routine use of trimethoprim-sulfamethoxazole prophylaxis for the duration of most intensive immune suppression (Martin et al. 2013).

Organ transplant recipients are at risk for rare infections transmitted via the allograft itself. While extensive discussion regarding the transmission of invasive mycoses via renal transplantation is beyond the scope of this chapter, a few points should be emphasized. In general, donor-derived fungal infections are uncommon events; however, the transmission of both true pathogenic and opportunistic fungi through organ transplantation has been reported, including that due to *Candida, Cryptococcus, Histoplasma, Coccidioides, Aspergillus*, zygomycetes, and many other filamentous fungi (Limaye et al. 2000; Wright et al. 2003; Mueller et al. 2010; Baddley et al. 2011; Dierberg et al. 2012; Gomez and Singh 2013). The potential for donor-derived infection should be considered in the following scenarios: infection occurring earlier than expected based on the recognized timeline of post-transplant infections (Fishman 2007; Pappas et al. 2010); isolation of organism from atypical sites, including the allograft or surgical site; diagnosis of invasive mycoses outside of an area of endemicity; and diagnosis of the same infection in multiple organ recipients from the same donor. Prompt recognition of potential donor-derived infection, notification of appropriate parties, and intervention to further mitigate risk can be life-saving in some cases (Alexander et al. 2010).

Treatment

The management of invasive fungal infections after renal transplantation presents considerable challenge to the treating clinician. While the treatment of specific infections will be reviewed elsewhere in this text, several unique considerations for the renal transplant patient on chronic immunosuppression (often inclusive of a calcineurin inhibitor) should be emphasized. First, owing to the nephrotoxic effects of conventional amphotericin B products, lipid formulations are often preferred to limit nephrotoxicity. Close monitoring of renal function is implicit in these patients to monitor for drug toxicity, and in cases where immunosuppression is reduced to aid in disease control, signs of early allograft rejection and/or immune reconstitution inflammatory syndrome (IRIS) may occur. Second, disease response may be delayed in these patients and longer treatment courses may be required. In the case of cryptococcal meningitis, a longer course of induction therapy is indicated if CSF cultures remain positive at two weeks, as this scenario is associated with increased six-month mortality (Singh et al. 2005). Third, drug–drug interactions are an important consideration in these patients and the importance of therapeutic drug monitoring cannot be overemphasized. Azole compounds vary in their inhibitory effects on cytochrome P450 enzymes (in particular CYP 3A4 and CYP 2C19) and serve as both substrates and inhibitors of P-glycoprotein, key enzymes involved in the metabolism of calcineurin inhibitors (both cyclosporine and tacrolimus) as well as sirolimus (Saad et al. 2006), and will increase drug levels of these immunosuppressive agents when initiated. Pre-emptive dose reduction of these agents and close therapeutic drug monitoring of both the immunosuppressant and antifungal agents are recommended upon initiation of azole therapy. In addition, flucytosine should be dose-adjusted for renal dysfunction, with therapeutic monitoring performed to mitigate its primary side effect of bone marrow suppression (Drew and Perfect 1997). Management of immunosuppression in the setting of invasive fungal infections requires recognition of the increased risk of IRIS in some situations. While classically described in the setting of cryptococcal infection, IRIS has been associated with increased rates of allograft loss in renal transplant recipients (Singh et al. 2005). In such cases, an alteration in reduction of immunosuppression is recommended, although the approach should be individualized for each patient.

Prevention

An ounce of prevention is worth a pound of cure. This is true in many aspects of medicine and is particularly true with respect to invasive mycoses in transplant recipients, given the significant morbidity and mortality associated with these infections, implications for allograft function, and potential toxicities associated with antifungal therapy. However, universal systemic antifungal prophylaxis carries its own risks, including the very real problem of emerging resistance in *Candida* and other fungi, and is not recommended for the majority of IFIs encountered after renal transplantation, given the overall low incidence of these infections. Oral and oesophageal *Candia* prophylaxis with either nystatin or clotrimazole for one to three months after transplant is recommended and is a standard practice at most transplant centres (KDIGO Transplant Work Group 2009). General measures regarding hand hygiene, limiting high-risk exposures including areas of new construction and high soil turnover, and use of gloves when gardening can be advised but have not been proven to reduce the risk of IFIs in transplant patients. Additionally, patients should be counselled prior to travel to areas endemic for the geographically restricted dimorphic fungi.

PJP prophylaxis, in contrast, is recommended for all renal transplant recipients for three to six months following transplant and during episodes of acute rejection requiring intensification of the immunosuppressive regimen (KDIGO Transplant Work Group 2009). Prophylaxis has been associated with a 91% reduction in risk of PJP infection and a decrease in infection-related mortality in non-HIV-infected immunocompromised hosts (Green et al. 2007).

While reactivation of latent infection with the endemic mycoses is an important mode of acquisition following organ transplantation, prior infection itself is not a contraindication to transplantation. Prior to transplantation, patients should be queried regarding history of travel to, or residence in, these areas of endemicity; even remote exposures are potentially important. All patients should be screened for active disease and treated according to accepted guidelines; the goal is quiescent disease prior to initiation of immunosuppression (Singh et al. 2012; Len et al. 2014). In renal transplant candidates who can be bridged on haemodialysis, this is often achievable. For histoplasmosis, the risk of subsequent infection is low (Vail et al. 2002) and screening for latent infection (either radiographically or serologically) is not recommended. If infection occurred or was treated within two years prior to anticipated transplant, prophylaxis can be considered (Miller et al. 2013). Given the excess mortality associated with disseminated *Coccidioides* infection after SOT early studies (Cohen et al. 1982), targeted fluconazole prophylaxis is recommended for patients with prior history of coccidioidomycosis undergoing organ transplantation, with duration dependent upon serological and disease status at the time of transplant (Blair 2007).

References

Agustin J, Lacson S, Raffalli J, et al. (1999) Failure of lipid amphotericin B preparation to eradicate candiduria: preliminary findings based on three cases. *Clin Infect Dis* 29: 686–7.

Aktug T, Olguner M, Akgur FM, et al. (1998) A new ancient irrigation therapy for childhood renal candidiasis. *Int Urol Nephrol* 30: 127–32.

Albano L, Bretagne S, Mamzer-Bruneel M, et al. (2009) Evidence that graft-site candidiasis after kidney transplantation is acquired during organ recovery: a multicenter study in France. *Clin Infect Dis* 48: 194–202.

Alexander BD, Schell WA, Siston AM, et al. (2010) Fatal *Apophysomyces elegans* infection transmitted by deceased donor renal allografts. *Am J Transplant* 10: 2161–7.

Ampel NM, White JD, Varanasi UR, et al. (1988) Coccidioidal peritonitis associated with peritoneal dialysis. *Am J Kidney Dis* 11: 512–14.

Ang BSP, Telenti A, King B, et al. (1993) Candidemia from a urinary tract source: microbiological aspects and clinical significance. *Clin Infect Dis* 17: 662–6.

Arthur RR, Drew RH and Perfect JR (2004) Novel models of antifungal drug administration. *Expert Opin Investig Drugs* 13: 903–32.

Assi M, Martin S, Wheat J, et al. (2013) Histoplasmosis after solid organ transplant. *Clin Infect Dis* 57: 1542–9.

Babik JM and Chin-Hong P (2015) Transplant tourism: understanding the risks. *Curr Infect Dis Rep* 17: 473.

Babu R and Hutton KAR (2004) Renal fungal balls and pelvi-ureteric junction obstruction in a very low birth weight infant: treatment with streptokinase. *Pediatr Surg Int* 20: 804–5.

Baddley JW, Andes DR, Marr KA, et al. (2010) Factors associated with mortality in transplant patients with invasive aspergillosis. *Clin Infect Dis* 50: 1559–67.

Baddley JW, Forrest GN and the AST Infectious Diseases Community of Practice (2013) Cryptococcosis in solid organ transplantation. *Am J Transpl* 13: 242–9.

Baddley JW, Schain DC, Gupte AA, et al. (2011) Transmission of *Cryptococcus neoformans* by organ transplantation. *Clin Infect Dis* 52: e94–8.

Bell DA, Rose SC, Starr NK, et al. (1993) Percutaneous nephrostomy for nonoperative management of fungal urinary tract infections. *J Vasc Interv Radiol* 4: 311–15.

Benjamin DK Jr, Fisher RG, McKinney RE Jr, et al. (1999) Candidal mycetoma in the neonatal kidney. *Pediatrics* 104: 1126–9.

Berman LH, Stringer DA, St Onge O, et al. (1989) An assessment of sonography in the diagnosis and management of neonatal renal candidiasis. *Clin Radiol* 40: 577–81.

Betjes M (2013) Immune cell dysfunction and inflammation in end-stage renal disease. *Nat Rev Nephrol* 9: 255–65.

Bisht V and VanDer Voort J (2011) Obstructive renal candidiasis in infancy. *Eur J Pediatr* 170: 1227–35.

Blair JE (2007) Coccidioidomycosis in patients who have undergone transplantation. *Ann N Y Acad Sci* 1111: 365–76.

Blowey DL, Garg UC, Kearns GL and Warady BA (1998) Peritoneal penetration of amphotericin B lipid complex and fluconazole in a pediatric patient with fungal peritonitis. *Adv Perit Dial* 14: 247–50.

Boelaert JR, de Locht M, Van Cutsem J, et al. (1993) Mucormycosis during deferoxamine therapy is a siderophore-mediated infection. In vitro and in vivo animal studies. *J Clin Invest* 91: 1979–86.

Boelaert JR, Fenves AZ and Coburn JW (1991) Deferoxamine therapy and mucormycosis in dialysis patients: report of an international registry. *Am J Kidney Dis* 18: 660–7.

Boelaert JR, Van Cutsem J, de Locht M, et al. (1994) Deferoxamine augments growth and pathogenicity of Rhizopus, while hydroxypyridinone chelators have no effect. *Kidney Int* 45: 667–71.

Bordes A, Campos-Herrera MI, Fernandez A, et al. (1995) Predisposing and prognostic factors of fungal peritonitis in peritoneal dialysis. *Perit Dial Int* 15: 275–6.

Brieland J, Essig D, Jackson C, et al. (2001) Comparison of pathogenesis and host immune responses to *Candida glabrata* and *Candida albicans* in systemically infected immunocompetent mice. *Infect Immun* 69: 5046–55.

Briggs JD (2001) Causes of death after renal transplantation. *Nephrol Dial Transplant* 16: 1545–9.

Bryant K, Maxfield C and Rabalais G (1999) Renal candidiasis in neonates with candiduria. *Pediatr Infect Dis J* 18: 959–63.

Campbell JB, Seidel FG and Gonzales ET Jr (2004) Use of a mechanical thrombectomy catheter for percutaneous extraction of renal fungal bezoars in a premature infant. *Urol* 64: 589.

Carr ME, O'Brien AA, Moore D and Keogh JA (1987) *Trichosporon cutaneum* C.A.P.D. peritonitis. *Postgrad Med J* 63: 1008.

Chang TI, Kim HW and Park JT (2011) Early catheter removal improves patient survival in peritoneal dialysis patients with fungal peritonitis: results of ninety-four episodes of fungal peritonitis at a single center. *Perit Dial Int* 31: 60–6.

Charlton JR, Barcia JP and Norwood VF (2010) Black specks in dialysis fluid: an unusual case of peritonitis in a pediatric patient on peritoneal dialysis. *Dial Transplant* 39: 445–8.

Chavada R, Kok J, van Hal S and Chen S (2011) Seeking clarity within cloudy effluents: differentiating fungal from bacterial peritonitis in peritoneal dialysis patients. *PLoS One* 6: e28247.

Cheng IKP, Fang G, Chan T, et al. Fungal peritonitis complicating peritoneal dialysis: report of 27 cases and review of treatment. *Q J Med* 71: 407–16.

Chiaradia V, Shcinella D, Pascioli L, et al. *Fusarium* peritonitis in peritoneal dialysis: report of two cases. *Microbiologica* 13: 77–8.

Chitale SV, Shaida N, Burtt G, et al. (2004) Endoscopic management of renal candidiasis. *J Endourol* 18: 865–6.

Chung BH, Chang SY, Kim SI, et al. (2001) Successfully treated renal fungal ball with continuous irrigation of fluconazole. *J Urol* 166: 1835–6.

Clancy CJ and Nguyen MH (2013) Finding the 'missing 50%' of invasive candidiasis: how nonculture diagnostics will improve understanding of disease spectrum and transform patient care. *Clin Infect Dis* 56: 1284–92.

Cohen IM, Galgiani JN, Potter D and Ogden DA (1982) Coccidioidomycosis in renal replacement therapy. *Arch Intern Med* 142: 489–94.

Cohen G and Hörl WH (2012) Immune dysfunction in uremia—an update. *Toxins* 4: 962–90.

Corbella X, Sirvent JM and Carratala J (1991) Fluconazole treatment without catheter removal in *Candida albicans* peritonitis complicating peritoneal dialysis. *Am J Med* 90: 277.

Coronel F, Martin-Rabadan P and Romero J (1993) Chemical peritonitis after intraperitoneal administration of amphotericin B in a fungal infection of the catheter subcutaneous tunnel. *Perit Dial Int* 13: 161–2.

Cotter G and Kavanagh K (2000) Adherence mechanisms of *Candida albicans. Br J Biomed Sci* 57: 241–9.

Debruyne D and Ryckelynck JP (1992) Fluconazole serum, urine, and dialysate levels in CAPD patients. *Perit Dial Int* 12: 328–9.

Dębska-Ślizień, Chrobak L, Bzoma B, et al. (2015) *Candida* arteritis in kidney transplant recipients: case report and review of the literature. *Transpl Infect Dis* 17: 449–55.

Delgado J, Calvo N, Gomis A, et al. (2010) Candiduria in renal transplant recipients: incidence, clinical repercussion and treatment indication. *Transplant Proc* 42: 2944–6.

DeVault GA, Brown ST 3rd, King JW, et al. (1985) Tenckhoff catheter obstruction resulting from invasion by *Curvularia lunata* in the absence of peritonitis. *Am J Kidney Dis* 6: 124–7.

Dierberg KL, Marr KA, Subramanian A, et al. (2012) Donor-derived organ transplant transmission of coccidioidomycosis. *Transpl Infect Dis* 14: 300–4.

Doemeny JM, Banner MP, Shapiro MJ, et al. (1988) Percutaneous extraction of renal fungus ball. *AJR Am J Roentgenol* 150: 1331–2.

Drew RH, Arthur RR and Perfect JR (2005) Is it time to abandon the use of amphotericin B bladder irrigations? *Clin Infect Dis* 40: 1465–70.

Drew RH and Perfect JR (1997) Flucytosine, *in*: V Yu, R Weber and D Raoult, eds, *Antimicrobial Therapy and Vaccines* (New York: Apple Trees Productions), 656–7.

Dwyre DM, Bell AM, Siecher S, et al. (2006) Disseminated histoplasmosis presenting as thrombotic microangiopathy. *Transfusion* 46: 1221–5.

Einollahi B, Lessan-Pezeshki M, Pourfarziani V, et al. (2008) Invasive fungal infections following renal transplantation: a review of 2410 recipients. *Ann Transplant* 13: 55–8.

Fisher JF, Kavanagh K, Sobel JD, et al. (2011) *Candida* urinary tract infection: pathogenesis. *Clin Infect Dis* 52 (Suppl. 6): S437–51.

Fishman JA (2007) Infection in solid-organ transplant recipients. *N Engl J Med* 357: 2601–14.

Fourtounas C, Marangos M, Kalliakmani P, et al. (2006) Treatment of peritoneal dialysis related fungal peritonitis with caspofungin plus amphotericin B combination therapy. *Nephrol Dial Transplant* 21: 236–7.

Garrido J, Lerma JL, Heras M, et al. (2003) Pseudoaneurysm of the iliac artery secondary to Aspergillus infection in two recipients of kidney transplants from the same donor. *Am J Kidney Dis* 41: 488–92.

Goldie SJ, Kiernan-Tridle L, Torres C, et al. (1996) Fungal peritonitis in a large chronic peritoneal dialysis population: a report of 55 episodes. *Am J Kidney Dis* 28: 86–91.

Gomez CA and Singh N (2013) Donor-derived filamentous fungal infections in solid organ transplant recipients. *Curr Opin Infect Dis* 26: 309–16.

Green H, Paul M, Vidal L and Leibovici L (2007) Prophylaxis of Pneumocystis pneumonia in immunocompromised non-HIV-infected patients: systematic review and meta-analysis of randomized controlled trials. *Mayo Clin Proc* 82: 1052–9.

Heylen L, Maertens J, Naesens M, et al. (2015) Invasive aspergillosis after kidney transplant: a case-control study. *Clin Infect Dis* 60: 1505–11.

Hogg RJ, Arant BS Jr and Houser MT (1982) Candida peritonitis in children on continuous ambulatory peritoneal dialysis. *Int J Pediatr Nephrol* 3: 287–91.

Hoyo I, Sanclemente G, Puig de la Bellacasa J, et al. (2014) Epidemiology, clinical characteristics, and outcome of invasive aspergillosis in renal transplant recipients. *Transpl Infect Dis* 16: 951–7.

Huang JW, Chu TS, Wu MS, et al. (2000) Visible *Penicillium* spp. colonization plaques on a Tenckhoff catheter without resultant peritonitis in a peritoneal dialysis patient. *Nephrol Dial Transplant* 15: 1872–3.

Huang JW, Hung KY, Wu KD, et al. (2000) Clinical features of and risk factors for fungal peritonitis in peritoneal dialysis patients. *J Formos Med Assoc* 99: 544–8.

Hurley R and Winner HI (1963) Experimental renal moniliasis in the mouse. *J Pathol Bacteriol* 86: 75–82.

Hurtrel B, Lagrange PH and Michel JC (1980) Systemic candidiasis in mice. I.—Correlation between kidney infection and mortality rate. *Ann Immunol (Paris)* 131C: 93–104.

Ibrahim A, Spellberg B, Walsh TJ and Kontoyiannis DP (2012) Pathogenesis of mucormycosis. *Clin Infect Dis* 54 (Suppl. 1): S16–22.

Irby PB, Stoller ML and McAninch JW (1990) Fungal bezoars of the upper urinary tract. *J Urol* 143: 447–51.

Jeloka TK, Shrividya S and Wagholikar G (2011) Catheter outflow obstruction due to an Aspergilloma. *Perit Dial Int* 31: 211–12.

Kabaalioğlu A, Bahat E and Boneval C (2001) Renal candidiasis in a 2-month-old infant. *AJR Am J Roentgenol* 176: 511–12.

Kauffman CA, Fisher JF, Sobel JD and Newman CA (2011) *Candida* urinary tract infections—diagnosis. *Clin Infect Dis* 52: S452–6.

Kauffman CA, Freifeld AG, Andes DR, et al. (2014) Endemic fungal infections in solid organ and hematopoietic cell transplant recipients enrolled in the Transplant-Associated Infection Surveillance Network (TRANSNET). *Transpl Infect Dis* 16: 213–24.

Kauffman CA and Tan JS (1974) *Torulopsis glabrata* renal infection. *Am J Med* 57: 217–24.

Kauffman CA, Vazquez JA, Sobel JD, et al. (2000) Prospective multicenter surveillance study of funguria in hospitalized patients. *Clin Infect Dis* 30: 14–18.

Keane WF, Bailie GR, Boeschoten E, et al. (2000) Adult peritoneal dialysis-related peritonitis treatment recommendations: 2000 update. *Perit Dial Int* 20: 396–411.

Kerr CN, Perfect JR, Craven PC, et al. (1983) Fungal peritonitis in patients on continuous ambulatory dialysis. *Ann Intern Med* 99: 334–7.

Kidney Disease: Improving Global Outcomes (KDIGO) Transplant Work Group (2009) KDIGO clinical practice guideline for the care of kidney transplant recipients. *Am J Transplant* 9 (Suppl. 3): S1–155.

Kobayashi C, Fernandes O, Miranda K, et al. (2004) Candiduria in hospital patients: a study prospective. *Mycopathologica* 158: 49–52.

Kullberg BJ and Arendrup MC (2015) Invasive candidiasis. *N Engl J Med* 373: 1445–56.

Kurts C, Panzer U, Anders H and Rees AJ (2013) The immune system and kidney disease: basic concepts and clinical implications. *Nat Rev Immunol* 13: 738–53.

Landay ME, Greenwald JH, Stemer AA and Ashbach DL (1982) *Cephalosporium* (*Acremonium*) in dialysis-connected peritonitis. *J Indiana State Med Assoc* 75: 391.

Langenstroer P, Balcom AH and Klinko C (2000) Laparoscopic suction irrigator for percutaneous removal of renal pelvic bezoar. *J Urol* 164: 2002–3.

Lehner T (1964) Systemic candidiasis and renal involvement. *Lancet* 283: 1414–16.

Len O, Garzoni C, Grossi P, et al. (2014) Recommendations for screening of donor and recipient prior to solid organ transplantation and to minimize transmission of donor-derived infections. *Clin Microbiol Infect* 20: 10–18.

Levine J, Bernard DB, Idelson BA, et al. (1989) Fungal peritonitis complicating continuous ambulatory peritoneal dialysis: successful treatment with fluconazole, a new orally active antifungal agent. *Am J Med* 86: 825–7.

Levinson ME and Pitsakis PG (1987) Susceptibility to experimental *Candida albicans* urinary tract infections in the rat. *J Infect Dis* 155: 841–6.

Li PK, Leung CB, Leung AK, Luk WK and Lai KN (1993) Post hysteroscopy fungal peritonitis in a patient on continuous ambulatory peritoneal dialysis. *Am J Kidney Dis* 21: 446–8.

Li PK, Szeto CC, Piraino B, et al. (2010) Peritoneal dialysis-related infections recommendations: 2010 update. *Perit Dial Int* 30: 393–423.

Limaye AP, Connolly PA, Sagar M, et al. (2000) Transmission of *Histoplasma capsulatum* by organ transplantation. *N Engl J Med* 343: 1163–6.

Lo MM, Mo JQ, Dixon BP and Czech KA (2010) Disseminated histoplasmosis associated with hemophagocytic lymphohistiocytosis in kidney transplant recipients. *Am J Transpl* 10: 687–91.

Lo W, Chan CY, Cheng SW, et al. (1996) A prospective randomized control study of oral nystatin prophylaxis for Candida peritonitis complicating continuous ambulatory peritoneal dialysis. *Am J Kidney Dis* 28: 549–52.

Lopes JO, Alves SH, Benevenga JP and Rosa AC (1994) The second case of peritonitis due to *Histoplasma capsulatum* during continuous ambulatory peritoneal dialysis in Brazil. *Mycoses* 37: 161–3.

Louria DB, Stiff DP and Bennett B (1962) Disseminated moniliasis in the adult. *Medicine (Baltimore)* 41: 307–37.

Luyckx VA, Cairo LV, Compston CA, Phan WL and Mueller TF (2009) The oncostatin M pathway plays a major role in the renal acute phase response. *Am J Physiol Renal Physiol* 296: F875–83.

Lye WC (1990) *Paecilomyces* peritonitis in a patient on continuous ambulatory peritoneal dialysis. *Nephrol Dial Transplant* 5: 1053–4.

MacCallum DM (2009) Massive induction of innate immune response to *Candida albicans* in the kidney in a murine intravenous challenge model. *FEMS Yeast Res* 9: 1111–22.

MacCallum D and Odds F (2005) Temporal events in the intravenous challenge model for experimental Candida albicans infections in female mice. *Mycoses* 48: 151–61.

Madriaga MG, Tenorio A and Proia L (2003) *Trichosporon inkin* peritonitis treated with caspofungin. *J Clin Microbiol* 41: 5827–9.

Mai H, Champion L, Quali N, et al. (2006) *Candida albicans* arteritis transmitted by conservative liquid after renal transplantation; a report of four cases and review of the literature. *Transplantation* 82: 1163–7.

Martin SI, Fishman JA and the AST Infectious Diseases Community of Practice (2013) Pneumocystis pneumonia in solid organ transplantation. *Am J Transpl* 13: 272–9.

Matignon M, Botterel F, Audard V, et al. (2008) Outcome of renal transplantation in eight patients with *Candida* sp. contamination of preservation fluid. *Am J Transplant* 8: 697–700.

Michel C, Courdavault L, al Khayat R, Viron B, Roux P and Mignon F (1994) Fungal peritonitis in patients on peritoneal dialysis. *Am J Nephrol* 14: 113–20.

Miles R, Hawley CM, McDonald S, et al. (2009) Predictors and outcomes of fungal peritonitis in peritoneal dialysis patients. *Kidney Int* 76: 622–8.

Miller R, Assi M and the AST Infectious Diseases Community of Practice (2013) Endemic fungal infections in solid organ transplantation. *Am J Transplant* 13: 250–61.

Morello FA, Mansilla AV and Wallace MJ (2002) Removal of renal fungus balls using a mechanical thrombectomy device. *AJR Am J Roentgenol* 178: 1191–3.

Mueller NJ, Weisser M, Fehr T, et al. (2010) Donor-derived aspergillosis from use of a solid organ recipient as a multiorgan donor. *Transpl Infect Dis* 12: 54–9.

Nagappan R, Collins JF and Lee WT (1992) Fungal peritonitis in continuous ambulatory peritoneal dialysis—the Auckland experience. *Am J Kidney Dis* 20: 492–6.

Nair RG and Samaranayake LP (1996) The effect of oral commensal bacteria on candidal adhesion to human buccal epithelial cells in vitro. *J Med Microbiol* 45: 179–85.

Nankivell BJ, Pacey D and Gordon DL (1991) Peritoneal eosinophilia associated with *Paecilomyces variotii* infection in continuous ambulatory peritoneal dialysis. *Am J Kidney Dis* 18: 603–5.

National Institute of Diabetes and Digestive and Kidney Diseases, Kidney Disease Statistics for the United States, http://www.niddk.nih.gov/health-information/health-statistics/Pages/kidney-disease-statistics-united-states.aspx#11, accessed 19 May, 2017.

Nguyen MH and Muder R (1994) *Aspergillus* peritonitis in a continuous ambulatory peritoneal dialysis patient: case report and review of the literature. *Diagn Microbiol Infect Dis* 20: 99–103.

Nobile CJ and Johnson AD (2015) *Candida albicans* biofilms and human disease. *Annu Rev Microbiol* 69: 71–92.

Odom A, Muir S, Lim E, Toffaletti D, Perfect J and Heitman J (2007) Calcineurin is required for virulence of *Cryptococcus neoformans. EMBO J* 16: 2576–89.

Ofoegbu BN, Agarwal RP and Lewis MA (2007) Methylene blue irrigation—treatment of renal fungal balls causing acute renal failure in a preterm infant. *Acta Paediatr* 96: 939–40.

Oygar DD, Altiparmak MR, Murtezaoglu A, et al. (2009) Fungal peritonitis in peritoneal dialysis: risk factors and prognosis. *Ren Fail* 31: 25–8.

Panackal A, Dahlman A, Keil K, et al. (2003) Outbreak of invasive aspergillosis among renal transplant recipients. *Transplantation* 75: 1050–3.

Pappas, PG, Alexander, BD, Andes DR, et al. (2010) Invasive fungal infections among organ transplant recipients: results of the Transplant-Associated Infection Surveillance Network (TRANSNET). *Clin Infect Dis* 50: 1101–11.

Pappas PG, Kauffman CA, Andes D, et al. (2009) Clinical practice guidelines for the management of candidiasis: 2009 update by the Infectious Diseases Society of America. *Clin Infect Dis* 48: 503–35.

Parkash C, Chugh TD, Gupta SP and Thanik KD (1970) Candida infection of the urinary tract-an experimental study. *J Assoc Physicians India* 18: 497–502.

Perfect JR, Dismukes WE, Dromer F, et al. (2010) Clinical Practice Guidelines for the Management of Cryptococcal Disease: 2010 update by the Infectious Disease Society of America. *Clin Infect Dis* 50: 291–322.

Polo JR, Luno J, Menarguez C, et al. (1989) Peritoneal mucormycosis in a patient receiving continuous ambulatory peritoneal dialysis. *Am J Kidney Dis* 13: 237–9.

Prasad KN, Prasad N, Gupta A, Sharma RK, Verma AK and Ayyagari A (2004) Fungal peritonitis in patients on continuous ambulatory peritoneal dialysis: a single centre Indian experience. *J Infect* 48: 96–101.

Prasad N and Gupta A (2005) Fungal peritonitis in peritoneal dialysis patients. *Perit Dial Int* 25: 207–22.

Quaia E, Martiingano P, Cavallaro M, et al. (2014) Chronic renal infections and renal fungal infections, *in*: E Quaia, L Giarraputo, P Martingano, et al., eds, *Radiological Imaging of the Kidney* (2nd edn, Heidelberg: Springer), 437–67.

Raghunath BV, Gowrishankar BC, Narendrababu M and Ramesh S (2013) Successful management of a renal fungal ball in a premature neonate: a case report and review of the literature. *J Indian Assoc Pediatr Surg* 18: 121–3.

Rippon JW, Larson RA, Rosenthal DM and Clayman J (1988) Disseminated cutaneous and peritoneal hyalohypomycosis caused by *Fusarium* species: three cases and review of the literature. *Mycopathologica* 101: 105–11.

Robinson JL, Davies HD, Barton M, et al. (2009) Characteristics and outcome of infants with candiduria in neonatal intensive care—a Paediatric Investigators Collaborative Network on Infections in Canada (PICNIC) Study. *BMC Infect Dis* 9: 183.

Ryley JF and Ryley NG (1990) *Candida albicans—do mycelia matter? J Med Vet Mycol* 28: 225–39.

Saad AH, DePestel DD and Carver PL (2006) Factors influencing the magnitude and clinical significance of drug interactions between azole antifungals and select immunosuppressants. *Pharmacotherapy* 26: 1730–44.

Sadegi BJ, Patel BK, Wilbur AC, et al. (2009) Primary renal candidiasis: importance of imaging and clinical history in diagnosis and management. *J Ultrasound Med* 28: 507–14.

Safdar N, Slattery WR, Knasinski V, et al. (2005) Predictors and outcomes of candiduria in renal transplant recipients. *Clin Infect Dis* 40: 1413–21.

Saha DC, Goldman DL, Shao X, et al. (2007) Serologic evidence for reactivation of cryptococcosis in solid-organ transplant recipients. *Clin Vaccine Immunol* 12: 1550–4.

Scerpella EG and Alhalel R (1994) An unusual cause of acute renal failure: bilateral ureteral obstruction due to *Candida tropicalis*. *Clin Infect Dis* 18: 440–2.

Schmid J, Hunter P, White G, et al. (1995) Physiological traits associated with success of *Candida albicans* strains as commensal colonisers and pathogens. *J Clin Microbiol* 33: 2920–26.

Shoham S, Hinestrosa F, Moore J, et al. (2010) Invasive filamentous fungal infections associated with renal transplant tourism. *Transpl Infect Dis* 12: 371–4.

Singh N, Alexander BD, Lortholary O, et al. (2007) Cryptococcus neoformans in organ transplant recipients: impact of calcineurin-inhibitor agents on mortality. *J Infect Dis* 195: 756–64.

Singh N, Dromer F, Perfect JR and Lortholary O (2008) Cryptococcosis in solid organ transplant recipients: current state-of-the-science. *Clin Infect Dis* 47: 1321–7.

Singh N, Gayowski T, Wagener MM and Marino IR (1997) Clinical spectrum of invasive cryptococcosis in liver transplant recipients receiving tacrolimus. *Clin Transplant* 11: 66–70.

Singh N, Huprikar S, Burdette SD, et al. (2012) Donor-derived fungal infections in organ transplant recipients: guidelines of the American Society of Transplantation, Infectious Diseases Community of Practice. *Am J Transplant* 12: 2414–28.

Singh N, Lortholary O, Alexander BD, et al. (2005a) Antifungal management practices and evolution of infection in organ transplant recipients with *Cryptococcus neoformans* infection. *Transplantation* 80: 1033–9.

Singh N, Lortholary O, Alexander BD, et al. (2005b) Allograft loss in renal transplant recipients with *Cryptococcus neoformans* associated immune reconstitution syndrome. *Transplantation* 80: 1131–3.

Snyder JJ, Israni AK, Peng Yi, Zhang L, Simon T and Kasiske BL (2009) Rates of first infection following kidney transplant in the United States. *Kidney Int* 75: 317–26.

Sobel JD, Bradshaw SK, Lipka CJ and Kartsonis NA (2007) Caspofungin in the treatment of symptomatic candiduria. *Clin Infect Dis* 44: e46–49.

Sobel JD, Fisher JF, Kauffman CA and Newman CA (2011) *Candida* urinary tract infections—epidemiology. *Clin Infect Dis* 52 (Suppl. 6): S433–36.

Sobel JD, Kauffman CA, McKinsey D, et al. (2000) Candiduria: a randomized, double-blind study of treatment with fluconazole and placebo. *Clin Infect Dis* 30: 19–24.

Song Z, Papanicolaou N, Dean S and Bing Z (2012) Localized candidiasis in kidney presented as a mass mimicking renal cell carcinoma. *Case Rep Infect Dis* 2012; Article ID 953590. doi: 10.1155/2012/953590

Spellberg B, Ibrahim AS, Chin-Hong PV, et al. (2012) The Deferasirox-AmBisome Therapy for Mucormycosis (DEFEAT Mucor) study: a randomized, double-blinded, placebo-controlled trial. *J Antimicrob Chemother* 67: 715–22.

Spellberg B, Ibrahim AS, Edwards JE Jr, et al. (2005) Mice with disseminated candidiasis die of progressive sepsis. *J Infect Dis* 192: 336–43.

Spellberg B, Johnston D, Phan Q, et al. (2003) Parenchymal organ, and not splenic, immunity correlates with host survival during disseminated candidiasis. *Infect Immun* 71: 5756–64.

Sridhar R, Thornley-Brown D and Shashi Rant R (1990) Peritonitis due to *Aspergillus niger*: the diagnostic importance of peritoneal eosinophilia. *Perit Dial Int* 10: 100–1.

Struijk DG, Krediet RT, Boeschoten EW, et al. (1987) Antifungal treatment of *Candida* peritonitis in CAPD patients. *Am J Kidney Dis* 9: 66–70.

Suh H, Wadhwa NK, Cabralda T and Sorrento J (1996) Endogenous peritonitis and related outcome in peritoneal dialysis patients. *Adv Perit Dial* 12: 192–5.

Sultana SR, McNeill SA, Phillips G and Byrne DJ (1998) Candidal urinary tract infection as a cause of pneumaturia. *J R Coll Surg Edinb* 43: 198–9.

Tebben JA, Rigsby MO, Selwyn PA, et al. (1993) Outcome of HIV infected patients on continuous ambulatory peritoneal dialysis. *Kidney Int* 44: 191–8.

Tennant FS Jr, Remmers Jr AR and Perry JE (1968) Primary renal candidiasis. *Arch Intern Med* 122: 435–40.

Thodis E, Vas SI, Bargman JM, et al. (1998) Nystatin prophylaxis: its inability to prevent fungal peritonitis in patients on continuous ambulatory peritoneal dialysis. *Perit Dial Int* 18: 583–9.

Tobudic S, Forstner C, Schranz H, et al. (2013) Comparative *in vitro* fungicidal activity of echinocandins against *Candida albicans* in peritoneal dialysis fluids. *Mycoses* 56: 623–30.

Tolkoff-Rubin NE and Rubin RH (1992) Opportunistic fungal and bacterial infection in the renal transplant recipient. *J Am Soc Nephrol* 2 (Suppl. 12): S264–9.

Torres R, Gonzalez M, Sanhueza M, et al. (2014) Outbreak of *Paecilomyces variotii* peritonitis in peritoneal dialysis patients after the 2010 Chilean earthquake. *Perit Dial Int* 34: 322–5.

Tsai TJ, Chen YM, Hsieh BS, et al. (1991) Can intracatheter retention of antifungal agents cure fungal peritonitis? Two cases successfully treated without catheter removal. *Perit Dial Int* 11: 355–6.

United States Renal Data System (2015) *USRDS Annual Data Report: Epidemiology of Kidney Disease in the United States* (Bethesda, MD: National Institutes of Health, National Institute of Diabetes and Digestive and Kidney Diseases, 2015), https://www.usrds.org/2015/view/v2_06.aspx, accessed 10 June 2017.

Vail GM, Young RS, Wheat LJ et al. (2002) Incidence of histoplasmosis following allogeneic bone marrow transplant or solid organ transplant in a hyperendemic area. *Transpl Infect Dis* 148–51.

Vanholder R and Ringoir S (1993) Infectious morbidity and defects of phagocytic function in end-stage renal disease: a review. *J Am Soc Nephrol* 3: 1541–54.

Vanholder R, Van Loo A, Dhondt AM, et al. (1996) Influence of uraemia and haemodialysis on host defence and infection. *Nephrol Dial Transplant* 11: 593–8.

Vaziri ND, Pahl MV, Crum A and Norris K (2012) Effect of uremia on structure and function of immune system. *J Ren Nutr* 22: 149–56.

Veroux M, Corona D, Giuffrida G, et al. (2009) Acute renal failure due to ureteral obstruction in a kidney transplant recipient with *Candida albicans* contamination of preservation fluid. *Transpl Infect Dis* 11: 266–8.

Wang AY, Yu AW, Li PK, et al. (2000) Factors predicting outcome of fungal peritonitis in peritoneal dialysis: analysis of a 9-year experience of fungal peritonitis in a single center. *Am J Kidney Dis* 36: 1183–92.

Wang HE, Gamboa C, Warnock DG and Muntner P (2011) Chronic kidney disease and risk of death from infection. *Am J Nephrol* 34: 330–6.

Whiteway M and Oberholzer V (2004) *Candida* morphogenesis and host-pathogen interactions. *Curr Opin Microbiol* 7: 350–7.

Williams PF, Moncrieff N and Marriott J (2000) No benefit in using nystatin prophylaxis against fungal peritonitis in peritoneal dialysis patients. *Perit Dial Int* 20: 352–3.

Wong PM, Lo KY, Tong GMW, et al. (2007) Prevention of fungal peritonitis with nystatin prophylaxis in patients receiving CAPD. *Perit Dial Int* 27: 531–6.

Wong SF, Leung MP and Chan MY (1997) Pharmacokinetics of fluconazole in children requiring peritoneal dialysis. *Clin Ther* 19: 1039–47.

Worasilchai N, Leelahavanichkul A, Kanjanabuch T, et al. (2015) (1→3)-β-D-glucan and galactomannan testing for the diagnosis of fungal peritonitis in peritoneal dialysis patients, a pilot study. *Med Mycol* 53: 338–46.

Wright PW, Pappagianis D, Wilson M, et al. (2003) Donor-related coccidioidomycosis in organ transplant recipients. *Clin Infect Dis* 37: 1265–9.

Wu G, Vichez RA, Eidelman B, et al. (2002) Cryptococcal meningitis: an analysis among 5521 consecutive organ transplant recipients. *Transpl Infect Dis* 4: 183–8.

Yamada N, Kumada K, Kishino S, et al. (2011) Distribution of micafungin in the tissue fluids of patients with invasive fungal infections. *J Infect Chemother* 17: 731–4.

Yinnon AM, Solages A and Treanor JJ (1993) Cryptococcal peritonitis: report of a case developing during continuous ambulatory peritoneal dialysis and review of the literature. *Clin Infect Dis* 17: 736–41.

Yuen KY, Seto WH, Ching TY, et al. (1992) An outbreak of *Candida tropicalis* peritonitis in patients on intermittent peritoneal dialysis. *J Hosp Infect* 22: 65–72.

Yuen KY, Seto WH, Li KS and Leung R (1990) Trichosporon beigelii peritonitis in continuous ambulatory peritoneal dialysis. *J Infect* 20: 178–80.

Zaruba K, Peters J and Jungblut H (1991) Successful prophylaxis for fungal peritonitis in patients on continuous ambulatory peritoneal dialysis: six years' experience. *Am J Kidney Dis* 17: 43–6.

Zhan HX, Lv Y, Zhang Y, et al. (2008) Hepatic and renal artery rupture due to Aspergillus and Mucor mixed infection after combined liver and kidney transplantation: a case report. *Transpl Proc* 1771–3.

CHAPTER 30

Fungal diseases of the respiratory tract

Samantha E. Jacobs, Catherine B. Small, and Thomas J. Walsh

Introduction to fungal diseases of the respiratory tract

Fungal infections of the respiratory tract are important causes of morbidity and mortality in immunocompromised patients. Among such patients are those receiving cytotoxic chemotherapy for neoplastic diseases, those undergoing haematopoietic stem cell transplantation (HSCT), those who have undergone organ transplantation, and those infected with human immunodeficiency virus (HIV). Invasive aspergillosis remains the most common invasive fungal infection among an expanding population of immunocompromised patients. Other filamentous fungi, such as *Fusarium* spp., Mucorales, and *Scedosporium* spp., are reported with increasing frequency, particularly in patients with quantitative or qualitative defects in neutrophils. Endemic mycoses, including those due to *Histoplasma capsulatum* var. *capsulatum*, *Coccidioides* spp., and *Talaromyces* (*Penicillium*) *marneffei*, are also increasingly prevalent in immunocompromised hosts in respective geographic regions (Box 30.1).

This chapter will review the current approaches to the diagnosis, treatment, and prevention of fungal diseases of the respiratory tract.

Causative fungi and epidemiology

Moulds

The causative filamentous fungi include *Aspergillus* spp., and among neutropenic hosts, the emerging moulds: Mucorales, *Fusarium* spp., and *Scedosporium* spp. *Aspergillus* spp. are ubiquitous in the environment and cause invasive disease in hosts with structural lung disease or defects in immune function that allow germination of spores into tissue-invasive hyphae. The most common species of *Aspergillus* recovered from patients are *Aspergillus fumigatus*, *Aspergillus flavus*, and *Aspergillus niger*.

Pulmonary mucormycosis most commonly occurs in profoundly neutropenic patients and in HSCT recipients with graft-versus-host disease. Other risk factors are listed in Box 30.2. Breakthrough infection in neutropenic patients receiving voriconazole is an increasingly recognized risk factor for mucormycosis (Marty et al. 2004). *Rhizopus*, *Mucor*, and *Rhizomucor* spp. account for up to 75% of mucormycosis infections in haematological malignancy patients.

Fusarium and *Scedosporium* spp. and other hyaline moulds may cause pneumonia and disseminated infection. The most clinically prevalent *Fusarium* spp. include: *Fusarium solani* species complex, *F. oxysporum* species complex, *Gibberella* (*Fusarium*) *fujikuroi* species complex, and *F. dimerum* species complex. Historically, the most commonly encountered *Scedosporium* spp. are *S. apiospermum* and *S. prolificans* (now termed *Lomentospora prolificans*). Moreover, *Scedosporium aurantiacum* is now recognized as an important cause of *Scedosporium* infections in Australia.

Dimorphic fungi

The dimorphic fungi include the agents of histoplasmosis, blastomycosis, coccidioidomycosis, sporotrichosis, talaromycosis (penicilliosis), and paracoccidioidomycosis. With the exception of *Sporothrix schenckii*, these fungi have a characteristic geographic distribution. They primarily affect normal hosts but may cause severe disease in immunocompromised patients. *Histoplasma capsulatum* is classically found in the Midwest United States, including the Ohio and Mississippi River Valleys. *Blastomyces dermatitidis* is endemic in North America, including the Canadian province of Manitoba, the Kenora region of Ontario, and the south-central and upper midwestern United States. *Coccidioides* spp., *C. immitis*, and *C. posadasii* are endemic in the desert of the south-western United States, adjacent northern Mexico, and parts of Central and South America. *Paracoccidioides brasiliensis* is endemic in Brazil and other parts of South America. *Talaromyces* (*Penicillium*) *marneffei* is endemic in Southeast Asia.

Yeasts

The most common yeasts causing respiratory infections are *Cryptococcus* spp., *Candida* spp., and *Trichosporon* spp. *Cryptococcus neoformans*, followed by *C. albidus* and *C. laurentii*, most commonly causes clinical disease in patients with defects in cell-mediated immunity. Infections due to *C. gattii* have been reported in immunocompetent hosts, predominantly in tropical and subtropical areas as well as in outbreaks in Vancouver and the north-western United States.

Box 30.1 Common and emerging fungal pathogens causing respiratory mycoses

Opportunistic fungi

Hyaline moulds

Aspergillus spp.
Fusarium spp.
Mucorales
Scedosporium spp.

Yeasts

Cryptococcus neoformans/gattii
Candida spp.
Trichosporon asahii

Pathogenic dimorphic fungi

Histoplasma capsulatum
Coccidioides spp.
Blastomyces dermatitidis
Paracoccidioides brasiliensis
Talaromyces (Penicillium) marneffei
Sporothrix schenckii

Candida albicans and non-*albicans* spp. are normal human commensals found in sputum, the gastrointestinal tract, the female genital tract, and on skin. Primary *Candida* bronchopneumonia may occur in severely debilitated patients with solid tumours, neutropenic patients with extensive chemotherapy-induced oral mucositis, and very low birthweight infants. Haematogenous pulmonary candidiasis may cause lung infection in neutropenic patients with disseminated infection (Masur et al. 1977).

Trichosporon spp. are opportunistic pathogens in immunocompromised hosts, particularly neutropenic patients or those receiving corticosteroids. While relatively uncommon, occurring in 0.4% of patients with acute leukaemia in one study (Girmenia et al. 2005), they may cause life-threatening fungaemia and disseminated infection similar to that caused by *Candida* spp.

Pneumocystis jirovecii is an opportunistic pathogen that colonizes the airways of approximately 20% of normal hosts. *Pneumocystis jirovecii* can lead to severe disease in immunocompromised patients, including those with HIV infection and other defects in cell-mediated immunity, and those receiving corticosteroids.

Box 30.2 Risk factors associated with the development of sinopulmonary mucormycosis

- Diabetic ketoacidosis
- Other forms of chronic metabolic acidosis (rare)
- Corticosteroid therapy
- Neutropenia
- Iron overload states

Clinical features

Moulds

Aspergillosis

Allergic aspergillosis

Extrinsic allergic alveolitis due to *Aspergillus* spp. occurs after repeated exposure—in non-atopic workers—to *Aspergillus* antigen in mouldy hay or grain, hence the terms 'farmer's lung' or 'malt-worker's lung'. Symptoms include cough, dyspnoea, fever, chills, and myalgias within eight hours of exposure.

The process of allergic bronchopulmonary aspergillosis (ABPA) involves an allergic response to *Aspergillus* hyphae without direct tissue invasion by the organism. Bronchospasm is thought to be mediated by an IgE (type I reaction) immediate hypersensitivity, whereas the bronchial and peribronchial inflammation in ABPA appears to be induced by immune complex formation (type III reaction). ABPA most often presents in children and young adults with asthma and evanescent, unexplained pulmonary infiltrates. Allergic *Aspergillus* sinusitis is found in atopic patients with a history of nasal polyps. These patients often have repeated bouts of sinus congestion with tenacious mucoid impaction.

Chronic pulmonary aspergillosis

Chronic pulmonary aspergillosis encompasses a spectrum of conditions: aspergilloma, chronic cavitary pulmonary aspergillosis, and chronic necrotizing pulmonary aspergillosis (CNPA). Saprophytic involvement of the respiratory tract involves the development of a mass of hyphae amidst a proteinaceous matrix to form a fungus ball known as an aspergilloma. This process develops within pre-existing cavities or ectatic bronchi, such as in cavitary tuberculosis, sarcoidosis, or cystic fibrosis. Typically, aspergilloma of the respiratory tract is a clinically occult process until the patient complains of haemoptysis. Filamentous fungi other than *Aspergillus*, such as *Scedosporium* spp. and Mucorales, may also cause intracavitary fungus balls and simulate an aspergilloma.

CNPA is an indolent infection associated with subtle defects in systemic host defence due to malnutrition, alcoholism, diabetes mellitus, or low-dose corticosteroids. It presents as a chronic refractory bronchopneumonia with fever, weight loss, cough, progressive infiltrates, and evidence of invasive aspergillosis on biopsy. This infection may progress to cavitation and formation of an aspergilloma or may develop from an aspergilloma as the initial focus.

Acute invasive pulmonary aspergillosis

Acute invasive pulmonary aspergillosis in immunocompromised patients has several manifestations: pneumonia, haemoptysis, invasion of contiguous intrathoracic structures, and dissemination. Other opportunistic fungi also cause angio-invasion, thrombosis, and infarction and may have similar findings (Box 30.3). A common clinical scenario is that of persistent fever, despite broad-spectrum antibiotics, in a neutropenic patient with pulmonary infiltrates. The most common radiographic manifestations of invasive pulmonary aspergillosis and other pathogenic fungi are described in Table 30.1 and Figure 30.1.

Mucormycosis

The clinical manifestations of pulmonary mucormycosis reflect its pathophysiology. An initial bronchopneumonia progresses to pulmonary vascular invasion, thrombosis, and infarction, with late dissemination to extrapulmonary tissues. The characteristics of the

Box 30.3 Patterns of invasive pulmonary infection due to angio-invasive fungi

Aspergillus spp., Mucorales, *Scedosporium* spp., *Fusarium* spp.

- Nodules
- Halo sign
- Bronchopneumonia
- Segmental or lobar consolidation
- Cavity formation
- Pleural effusion
- Pulmonary vascular invasion, thrombosis, and infarction
- Dissemination to extrapulmonary tissues
- Invasion of chest wall, diaphragm, pericardium, and myocardium
- Involvement of trachea to cause airway obstruction
- Acute Pancoast's syndrome
- Haemoptysis
- Fistulae:
  - broncho-arterial
  - bronchopleural
  - bronchocutaneous
- Chronic necrotizing infection*
- Necrotizing tracheobronchitis*

* Best described with *Aspergillus* spp.

pulmonary infiltrates on chest imaging are indistinguishable from those of invasive aspergillosis.

Fusariosis and scedosporiosis

Invasive infections due to *Fusarium* and *Scedosporium* spp. produce a pattern similar to that of invasive aspergillosis (Anaissie et al. 1989). *Fusarium* infections in neutropenic patients are characterized by pulmonary infiltrates, cutaneous lesions, positive blood cultures, and sinusitis. Unlike *Aspergillus* spp., *Fusarium* spp. are frequently detected by conventional blood culture detection systems. Patients with haematological malignancy and neutropenia appear more susceptible to infection with *L. prolificans* than to infection with *S. apiospermum,* perhaps owing to differences in virulence in the lower respiratory tract. In neutropenic patients, mortality ranges from 57% to 85%.

Dimorphic fungi

Histoplasmosis

Acute primary pulmonary histoplasmosis (APPH) may develop in a normal, immunocompetent host exposed to a heavy inoculum. The symptoms of APPH, which resemble an influenza-type illness, are usually self-limiting and managed with general supportive care. Chronic cavitary pulmonary histoplasmosis is an indolent but progressive respiratory infection of patients with underlying chronic obstructive pulmonary disease. Disseminated histoplasmosis may develop in immunocompromised patients with cellular immunodeficiencies, including HIV infection (Wheat et al. 1990). In these patients, signs of disseminated infection (hepatosplenomegaly, pancytopenia, hypoadrenalism, and disseminated intravascular coagulation) may overshadow pulmonary involvement.

Coccidioidomycosis

Clinical manifestations of coccidioidomycosis have been classified into three general groups: (1) initial pulmonary infection, which is usually self-limiting; (2) pulmonary complications; and (3) extrapulmonary disease (Knoper and Galgiani 1988). Primary pulmonary infection may evolve into pulmonary nodules, thin-walled cavities, progressive pneumonia, pyopneumothorax, and bronchopleural fistula.

Dissemination to extrapulmonary sites may result in cutaneous and soft tissue infection, osteomyelitis, arthritis, and meningitis.

Blastomycosis

The manifestations of infection with *Blastomyces dermatitidis* include: asymptomatic disease; a brief influenza-like illness; self-limited, localized pneumonia in immunocompetent patients; subacute to chronic respiratory illness; and fulminant infection with acute respiratory distress syndrome. Among patients with chronically progressive infection, complications include dissemination to one or more organs, including the skin, genitourinary tract, bone, or central nervous system (CNS) in immunocompromised patients (Bradsher 1997).

Paracoccidioidomycosis

Paracoccidioidomycosis has three patterns of infection: acute pneumonia, chronic pneumonia, and disseminated infection. Fever, cough, sputum production, chest pain, dyspnoea, haemoptysis, malaise, and weight loss may occur with pneumonia and disseminated infection. Extrapulmonary lesions often develop on the face and oral mucosa. Other sites include lymph nodes, spleen, liver, gastrointestinal tract, and adrenal glands.

Talaromycosis (Penicilliosis)

Increasingly recognized as a cause of disseminated infection in HIV-infected patients from Southeast Asia and, to a lesser extent, in patients with haematological malignancy, *T. marneffei* has emerged as an important endemic pathogen. Little is reported about the pulmonary manifestations of disseminated infection; however, the infection has a striking resemblance to disseminated histoplasmosis in HIV-infected patients with fungaemia and multiple disseminated cutaneous lesions.

Sporotrichosis

Pulmonary sporotrichosis is an unusual infection, principally observed in older males with a chronic cavitary pneumonia typically in an upper lobe distribution (Pluss and Opal 1986). Patients often have a history of alcohol use or diabetes mellitus, which may further contribute to immune impairment. The initial manifestations of pulmonary sporotrichosis include productive cough, fever, weight loss, anorexia, dyspnoea, and haemoptysis.

Yeasts

Cryptococcosis

Pulmonary cryptococcosis is usually a limited pulmonary infection in patients with chronic obstructive pulmonary disease. Fever, cough, dyspnoea, and pleural pain are common symptoms. Disseminated cryptococcal disease, including meningoencephalitis and cutaneous lesions, may develop in immunocompromised patients.

Table 30.1 Characteristics of radiographic pulmonary infiltrates and differential diagnosis of pathogenic fungi by host*

Host population	Neutropenia (ANC <500 cells/μL)	Post-engraftment HSCT recipient with chronic GVHD	Solid organ transplant recipient	HIV/AIDS	Normal host**
LOCALIZED					
Nodules	*Aspergillus* spp. *Fusarium* spp. Mucorales *Scedosporium* spp.	*Aspergillus* spp. *Fusarium* spp. Mucorales *Scedosporium* spp.	*Cryptococcus neoformans*	*Cryptococcus neoformans* *Talaromyces marneffei*	*Cryptococcus gattii*
Nodules with halo	*Aspergillus* spp. *Fusarium* spp. Mucorales *Scedosporium* spp.	*Aspergillus* spp. Mucorales *Scedosporium* spp.	*Aspergillus* spp. (especially lung transplant)		
Segmental pneumonia	*Aspergillus* spp. *Fusarium* spp. Mucorales *Scedosporium* spp.	*Aspergillus* spp. Mucorales *Scedosporium* spp.		*Talaromyces marneffei*	*Blastomyces dermatitidis*
Bronchopneumonia	*Aspergillus* spp. *Fusarium* spp. Mucorales *Scedosporium* spp.	*Aspergillus* spp. Mucorales *Scedosporium* spp.	*Aspergillus* spp. (especially lung transplant) *Cryptococcus neoformans*	*Cryptococcus neoformans*	*Blastomyces dermatitidis* *Histoplasma capsulatum****
Cavities	*Aspergillus* spp. *Fusarium* spp. Mucorales *Scedosporium* spp.	*Aspergillus* spp. *Fusarium* spp. Mucorales *Scedosporium* spp.			*Aspergillus* spp. (Aspergilloma) Chronic necrotizing pulmonary aspergillosis Chronic cavitary pulmonary aspergillosis *Histoplasma capsulatum* *Coccidioides* spp. (thin-walled cavities)
Bronchiectasis					Allergic bronchopulmonary aspergillosis
DIFFUSE					
	Haematogenous pulmonary candidiasis	*Pneumocystis jirovecii* *Coccidioides* spp.	*Pneumocystis jirovecii*	*Histoplasma capsulatum* *Pneumocystis jirovecii* *Coccidioides* spp.	*Histoplasma capsulatum* *Coccidioides* spp.

* This table summarizes the most common patterns of radiographic pulmonary infiltrates with common pathogenic fungi according to host immune status.

** 'Normal' host in this context includes those patients with more subtle immunodysregulation and impairments of innate host defence.

*** Chronic cavitary.

AIDS = acquired immunodeficiency syndrome; ANC = absolute neutrophil count; GVHD = graft-versus-host disease; HIV = human immunodeficiency virus; HSCT = haematopoietic stem cell transplantation

Pulmonary candidiasis

Among profoundly immunocompromised hosts such as neutropenic patients with chemotherapy-induced mucositis and very low birthweight infants, aspiration of infected oral secretions into the tracheobronchial tree with extension into pulmonary parenchyma is the primary route of infection for *Candida* bronchopneumonia. Haematogenous pulmonary candidiasis may occur in neutropenic patients with disseminated infection.

Trichosporonosis

Invasive *Trichosporon* infections are uncommon, but frequently fatal, infections in neutropenic patients or those receiving corticosteroids (Walsh et al. 1993). Clinical manifestations are characterized by refractory fungaemia, funguria, renal dysfunction, cutaneous lesions, chorioretinitis, and pneumonia.

Pneumocystis jirovecii pneumonia

In immunocompromised patients without HIV infection, *Pneumocystis* pneumonia often presents as fulminant respiratory failure associated with fever and dry cough. This may occur in the setting of tapering corticosteroids, or following receipt of immunosuppressive drugs affecting cell-mediated immunity. In contrast, the clinical presentation may be indolent in HIV-infected patients (Huang et al. 2011).

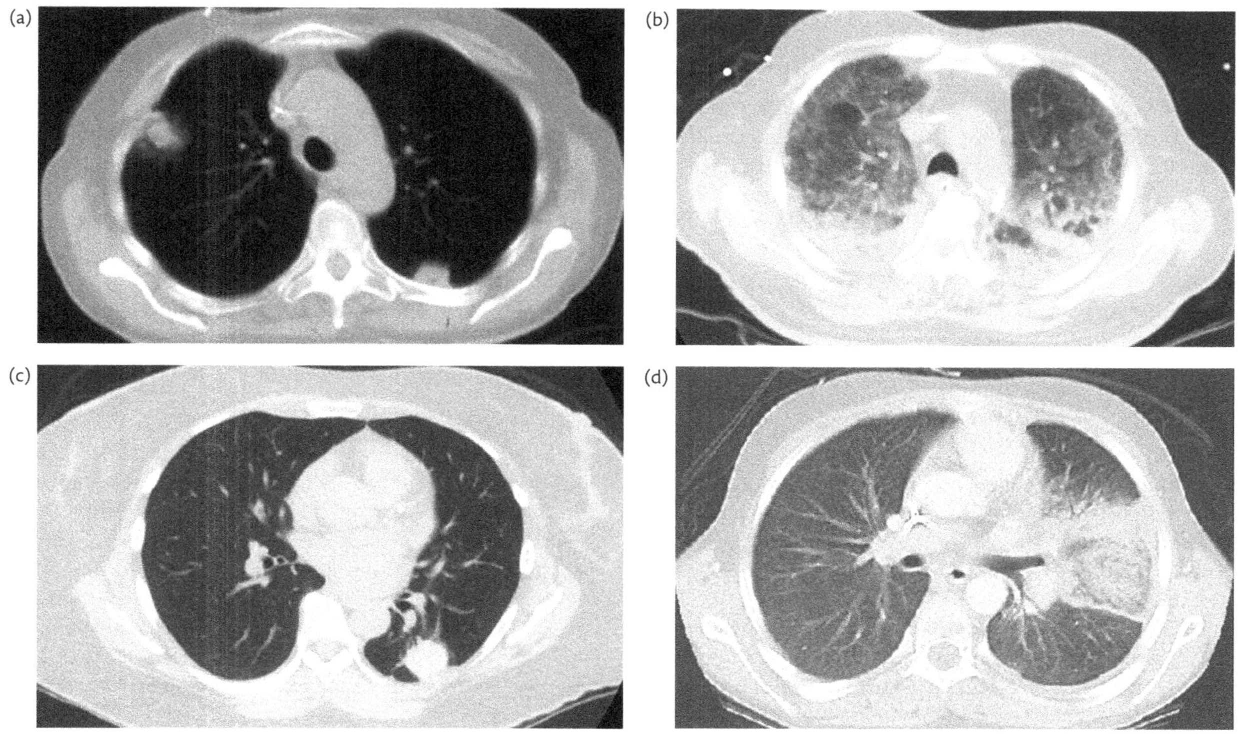

Figure 30.1 Common patterns of radiographic pulmonary infiltrates in patients with fungal pneumonia.

a A 14-year-old male patient with pre-B-cell acute lymphocytic leukaemia and acute invasive pulmonary aspergillosis. Left and right upper lobe dense nodules with surrounding ground glass representing haemorrhage ('halo' sign).

b A 76-year-old male patient with follicular lymphoma and *Pneumocystis jirovecii* pneumonia. Diffuse bilateral ground-glass infiltrates with consolidative changes posteriorly.

c A 48-year-old female kidney transplant recipient with pulmonary cryptococcosis. Round, well-circumscribed, dense left lower lobe nodule.

d A 12-year-old female with pre-B-cell acute lymphocytic leukaemia and pulmonary mucormycosis. Left lower lobe consolidation with central lucency and increased surrounding opacification ('reverse halo' sign).

Diagnosis

Diagnosis of fungal infections of the respiratory tract may be challenging owing to non-specific clinical symptoms and challenges in diagnostic methods. Invasive diagnostic tests are typically warranted, including fine-needle aspirate, thoracoscopic lung biopsy, or open lung biopsy, depending on local expertise and pace of the illness. However, diagnostic yield may be limited by previous antifungal therapy, sampling error, or inadequate recovery of pathogen from infected tissues. For these reasons, non-invasive diagnostic tests, such as the serum sandwich EIA (enzyme immunoassay) for detecting galactomannan, the (1→3)-β-D-glucan assay, and molecular amplification methods to improve the diagnosis and identification of clinically relevant fungal organisms have been developed.

Galactomannan (GM), a component of fungal cell wall that can be detected by a sandwich-type ELISA (enzyme-linked immunosorbent assay), is used as a diagnostic adjunct for invasive aspergillosis. Depending upon the patient population, sensitivity ranges from 50% to 95% and specificity ranges from 87% to 99% for diagnosis of invasive aspergillosis. The revised international definitions of invasive fungal disease state that in the appropriate host, a positive serum GM assay combined with a CT (computed tomography) scan characteristic of invasive pulmonary aspergillosis are sufficient to diagnose probable invasive disease (de Pauw et al. 2008). Additional studies in animal models and patients indicate that serial serum GM antigen levels permit therapeutic monitoring and have prognostic implications including clinical response and survival at 12 weeks (Chai et al. 2012). GM testing in bronchoalveolar lavage (BAL) fluid has also been evaluated. In one study of patients with haematological malignancy, using a cut-off of 0.5, BAL GM showed improved sensitivity compared with serum GM for diagnosis of invasive pulmonary aspergillosis. Limitations to the utility of GM include false-negative results in the setting of previous antifungal therapy. False-positive results due to therapy with piperacillin-tazobactam are now uncommon with improved fermentation and drug purification techniques (Mikulska et al. 2012). Serum GM may also be elevated in patients with disseminated fusariosis (Tortorano et al. 2012) and histoplasmosis (Vergidis et al. 2012).

Real-time PCR (polymerase chain reaction) for diagnosis of invasive fungal infection has been studied most extensively with *Aspergillus* spp. Most studies test for a pan-*Aspergillus* PCR that targets ribosomal RNA common to all *Aspergillus* spp.; however, primers that are used vary from laboratory to laboratory, raising issues of standardization. Clinical reports of sensitivities and specificities range from 43% to 100% and 64% to 100%, respectively (Arvanitis et al. 2014). Studies comparing the diagnostic performance of PCR and GM assays for *Aspergillus* spp. show similar performance in both serum and BAL fluid. The current status of PCR in the diagnosis of invasive aspergillosis is discussed in more detail in Chapter 43.

(1→3)-β-D-glucan is a major component of the cell wall in many fungi, including *Candida* spp., *Aspergillus* spp., *Fusarium* spp., and *Pneumocystis jirovecii* (but not *Cryptococcus* spp. and the Mucorales). The (1→3)-β-D-glucan assay is a useful adjunctive diagnostic test; a cutoff value of 60 pg/mL for the Fungitell assay has been shown to be optimal in distinguishing patients with invasive fungal infections from those without invasive fungal infection (mainly due to *Candida* and *Aspergillus* spp.) (He et al. 2015). Among patients with haematological malignancy, the (1→3)-β-D-glucan assay is more sensitive than the GM assay, but less specific in detecting invasive aspergillosis and other mould infections (Hachem et al. 2009). Serum (1→3)-β-D-glucan levels may be a useful diagnostic adjunct in suspected *Pneumocystis* pneumonia, where sensitivity and specificity are 94.8% and 86.3% in a recent meta-analysis involving immunocompromised hosts with compatible clinical features (Karageorgopoulos et al. 2013). Of note, false-positive (1→3)-β-D-glucan results are seen in patients undergoing haemodialysis with cellulose membranes, patients treated with immunoglobulin, albumin, or other blood products filtered through cellulose depth filters containing (1→3)-β-D-glucan, and patients with serosal exposure to glucan-containing gauze (Marty et al. 2006).

Diagnostic procedures and approaches for pulmonary mucormycosis, fusariosis, scedosporiosis, and trichosporonosis—including thoracic CT scan, BAL, and lung biopsy—are also similar to those for invasive pulmonary aspergillosis. Direct examination of BAL fluid may reveal distinctive broad, non-septate hyphae of Mucorales versus slender dichotomously branching septate hyphae of *Fusarium*, *Scedosporium*, and other hyaline moulds. Pulmonary trichosporonosis may be detected in immunocompromised patients with compatible pulmonary infiltrates and positive blood cultures, BAL, or lung biopsy. BAL fluid from patients with suspected pulmonary mycoses should be processed both by clinical microbiology and by cytopathology laboratories. BAL fluid may be processed by centrifugation, direct examination, and special stains, including fluorescent dyes (Fungi-Fluor®, Calcofluor®, Blankofluor®), periodic acid Schiff (PAS) stain, and Gomori methenamine silver (GMS) stain.

BAL and/or biopsy and culture of pulmonary lesions are similarly needed to confirm a diagnosis of pulmonary cryptococcosis. Detection of organisms in biopsy specimens can be enhanced by use of mucicarmine or Alcian blue stains of the capsular acid mucopolysaccharide (glucuronoxylomannan). Cryptococcal antigen detection by latex agglutination, lateral flow assay, or EIA in the serum may suggest a diagnosis of pulmonary cryptococcosis in a patient with compatible clinical features. However, serum cryptococcal antigen titres may be negative in up to 40% of HIV-uninfected patients with pulmonary cryptococcosis (Pappas et al. 2001). The serum cryptococcal latex agglutination test may also be false positive owing to shared antigens and resultant cross-reactivity between *Trichosporon asahii* and *Cryptococcus neoformans*.

Pulmonary candidiasis is most reliably diagnosed by biopsy of lung tissue. Growth of *Candida* spp. in a BAL of a patient with pulmonary infiltrates is non-specific given the frequency of *Candida* colonization of the upper respiratory tract in critically ill patients and those receiving mechanical ventilation. Other serological tests for invasive candidiasis are the mannan antigen and anti-mannan antibody tests (Marchetti et al. 2012).

The gold standard for diagnosis of the endemic fungi is culture from a clinical specimen; however, growth may be slow, particularly for *Histoplasma capsulatum* and *Blastomyces dermatitidis*. Various diagnostic tests, including histopathology using stains for fungi, antigen detection, and/or serological tests for organism-specific antibodies, may be employed to diagnose pulmonary or disseminated histoplasmosis, blastomycosis, or coccidioidomycosis. The *Histoplasma* antigen detection EIA using urine, blood, or BAL fluid is particularly useful for diagnosis in severely ill patients. An antigen detection assay is also available for blastomycosis. Other serum tests commonly used to diagnose coccidioidomycosis include complement fixation and immunodiffusion tests of either tube precipitin antibodies (IgM) or complement-fixing antibodies (IgG). The lysis-centrifugation technique (Isolator; Wampole Laboratories, Cranberry, NJ) is a highly sensitive method by which *H. capsulatum* can be rapidly recovered from blood specimens. *Paracoccidioides brasiliensis* may be identified by direct examination of sputum or BAL, scrapings from mucocutaneous ulcers, or tissue biopsies to reveal variations of the characteristic thick-walled 'pilot's wheel' or 'mariner's wheel' configuration of the yeast form. The diagnosis of *T. marneffei* is readily established by direct smear and culture of umbilicated centrally necrotic lesions, bone marrow aspirate, or peripheral lymph node.

Pneumocystis jirovecii cannot be cultured; therefore, the most common method of diagnosis relies on visualization of *Pneumocystis* cysts or trophozoites by use of direct fluorescent antibody staining on expectorated or induced sputum specimens, BAL fluid, or lung tissue biopsy specimens. The cell wall of cysts can also be seen with stains, including GMS, toluidine blue, and Calcofluor White. PCR assays may be useful in non-HIV-infected patients, in whom the sensitivity of microscopy with staining is reduced as compared with that in HIV-infected patients (Azoulay et al. 2009); however, the optimal cutoff to distinguish colonization from infection is unknown.

Treatment

Among immunocompromised patients with fungal respiratory infections, successful therapy depends upon early initiation of antifungal agents and reversal of immunosuppression. The administration of recombinant cytokines granulocyte colony-stimulating factor (G-CSF) and granulocyte-macrophage colony-stimulating factor (GM-CSF) to patients receiving myelosuppressive chemotherapy and HSCT recipients has reduced the degree and duration of neutropenia and diminished the frequency of infections (Brandt et al. 1988; Sung et al. 2007). Reducing or temporarily withholding corticosteroids or other immunosuppressive drugs until the infection has stabilized or improved may also improve outcome (Box 30.4). Surgical management may be required in patients with angio-invasive fungal infections, particularly those with life-threatening haemoptysis or lesions contiguous with the pericardium. Approaches to treatment of pulmonary mycoses are summarized in Table 30.2.

Aspergillosis

Voriconazole is recommended for the primary treatment of invasive aspergillosis in most patients. In the largest randomized controlled trial of therapy for invasive aspergillosis, voriconazole was associated with significantly improved survival compared with amphotericin B (71% vs 58%, respectively) (Herbrecht et al. 2002). In a recent phase 3 clinical trial of adults with invasive aspergillosis and other filamentous fungi, isavuconazole was non-inferior to voriconazole on the primary endpoint of all-cause mortality at day 42 (Falci and Pasqualatto 2013). Isavuconazole was safer and better

Box 30.4 Reversal of immunosuppression: immunological adjuncts to prevention and treatment of pulmonary fungal infections

- Recombinant cytokines:
  - granulocyte colony-stimulating factor (G-CSF)
  - granulocyte-macrophage colony-stimulating factor (GM-CSF)
  - interferon-gamma
- Stem cell reconstitution
- Immune reconstitution
- Granulocyte transfusions
- Adoptive immunotherapy
- Discontinuation of corticosteroids

tolerated than voriconazole, thus offering an emerging alternative. Liposomal amphotericin B is another alternative to voriconazole, particularly in those patients with concomitant hepatic transaminase elevation. Agents for salvage therapy include posaconazole, itraconazole, caspofungin, or micafungin. The role of combination therapy with voriconazole and anidulafungin in the treatment of invasive aspergillosis as primary or salvage therapy is suggested by preclinical data and by a recent prospective, controlled clinical trial (Petraitis et al. 2009; Marr et al. 2015).

ABPA is managed with a combination of antifungal therapy (itraconazole or voriconazole) and corticosteroids. Early aggressive therapy may attenuate progression to an irreversible bronchiectatic and fibrotic phase. Allergic *Aspergillus* sinusitis is managed by corticosteroids and possibly itraconazole; refractory cases with inflammatory masses may require drainage. Chronic *Aspergillus* sinusitis is managed with drainage and antifungal therapy.

Treatment of aspergilloma is individualized according to the severity of symptoms and the underlying chronic lung disease. Current therapeutic approaches include conservative management (e.g. pulmonary toilet), antifungal therapy, and surgical resection. Patients with CNPA may respond to voriconazole. Isavuconazole, posaconazole, or itraconazole may also be considered. The dose and duration of therapy should be tailored to patient response. Recurrent or life-threatening haemoptysis, despite antifungal therapy, is a relative indication for bronchial artery embolization or surgical intervention.

Mucormycosis

Lipid formulations of amphotericin B have replaced amphotericin B as the antifungal agents of choice for treatment of mucormycosis in high-resource environments (Cornely et al. 2014). Based on *in vivo* and *in vitro* data, the initial dosage is 5.0–7.5 mg/kg/day. Isavuconazole is the first antifungal agent to receive FDA (Food and Drug Administration) approval in nearly 50 years for primary treatment of mucormycosis (FDA Jan 22 2015). Data from case reports and large case series suggest a role for posaconazole as salvage therapy in some patients who are refractory to, or intolerant of, amphotericin B and its lipid derivatives (Gameletsou et al. 2012). Surgical excision of infected lesions is also important in the management of pulmonary mucormycosis. As much devitalized tissue and necrotic debris should be removed as possible.

Fusariosis

Invasive fusariosis is treated with a lipid formulation of amphotericin B or voriconazole (Nucci and Anaissie 2007). However, since antifungal susceptibility varies by species, and there may also be inter-strain variation with a given species complex, initial treatment with the combination of amphotericin B and voriconazole pending susceptibility profiles is reasonable. *Fusarium solani* species complex and *Fusarium verticillioides* may be resistant to triazoles and exhibit higher amphotericin B minimum inhibitory concentrations than other *Fusarium* spp. Small studies have described the use of voriconazole or posaconazole as salvage therapy with response rates (complete or partial cure) of up to 45% (Campo et al. 2010).

Scedosporiosis

Scedosporium spp. are generally intrinsically resistant to antifungal agents, and their optimal treatment remains elusive. *In vitro* resistance and clinical resistance to amphotericin B have often been reported. In disease due to *S. apiospermum*, clinical response has been reported with voriconazole alone (Walsh et al. 2002; Tortorano et al. 2014). *L. prolificans* is resistant to all currently approved triazoles. *In vitro* synergy has been demonstrated with the combination of terbinafine and triazoles; however, correlations of *in vivo* and clinical data are needed (Meletiadis et al. 2003).

Endemic fungal infections

Treatment of respiratory infection due to the endemic fungi depends upon the host and patterns of disease. Immunocompetent patients with acute pulmonary histoplasmosis and coccidioidomycosis usually have self-limiting disease, which may be managed with supportive care, while stable patients with advanced infection or those who are immunocompromised may be treated with itraconazole. Fluconazole may also be used in patients with pulmonary coccidioidomycosis. Disseminated infection with *Coccidioides* spp. may require intravenous voriconazole or lipid formulation of amphotericin B. Patients with pulmonary blastomycosis and paracoccidioidomycosis typically require treatment with itraconazole or voriconazole. Those with infection due to Talaromyces (Penicillium) marnefii should receive induction therapy with a formulation of amphotericin B followed by maintenance therapy with itraconazole or voriconazole (Le et al. 2017). Trimethoprim-sulphamethoxazole may be used for paracoccidioidomycosis, although it requires a longer duration of therapy.

Profoundly immunocompromised patients or those with severe pulmonary infection due to endemic fungi are treated with liposomal amphotericin B as initial therapy followed by itraconazole. The duration of liposomal amphotericin B ranges from at least one week to four weeks, depending on the severity and extent of disease. Duration of triazole therapy is usually at least 12 months and possibly lifelong if immunosuppression cannot be reversed. Detection in the serum and urine of a carbohydrate antigen of *H. capsulatum* is a valuable tool in therapeutic monitoring of disseminated histoplasmosis, particularly in HIV-infected patients (Hage et al. 2011).

Pulmonary sporotrichosis is treated with lipid formulations of amphotericin B. Medical therapy alone is likely sufficient for non-cavitary disease, while early surgery should be considered for cavitary primary pulmonary sporotrichosis (Aung et al. 2013).

Cryptococcosis

The treatment of pulmonary cryptococcosis in patients with mild to moderate symptoms and no extrapulmonary disease is fluconazole

Table 30.2 Summary of approaches to treatment of fungal diseases of the respiratory tract

Allergic aspergillosis Extrinsic allergic alveolitis Extrinsic asthma Allergic bronchopulmonary aspergillosis (ABPA)	Removal of patients from exposure to antigen Bronchodilators Corticosteroids Itraconazole or voriconazole (primarily used in ABPA)
Chronic aspergillosis Pulmonary aspergilloma Chronic necrotizing aspergillosis Chronic cavitary aspergillosis	Observation (may be appropriate for pulmonary aspergilloma) Itraconazole or voriconazole Bronchial artery embolization for haemoptysis Surgical resection (usually indicated for intractable haemoptysis and pain)
Invasive aspergillosis Bronchopneumonia Necrotizing tracheobronchitis Local extension to intrathoracic structures Invasive sinusitis Disseminated aspergillosis	Voriconazole (consider combination therapy with an echinocandin in patients with hematological malignancy) Isavuconazole (primary alternative to voriconazole) Lipid formulation amphotericin B Reversal of immunosuppression (refer to Box 30.4) Surgery (indications): (1) haemoptysis from a single cavitary lesion (2) progression of a cavitary lesion despite antifungal therapy (3) infiltration into pericardium, great vessels, bone, or thoracic soft tissue while receiving antifungal therapy (4) progressive sinusitis
Mucormycosis Rhinocerebral Pulmonary	Lipid formulation amphotericin B Isavuconazole (primary alternative to lipid formulation amphotericin B) Salvage therapy: posaconazole Surgical debridement of rhinocerebral infection down to viable tissue Surgical indications for sinopulmonary infection (see 'Invasive aspergillosis' above) Reversal of immunosuppression Correction of metabolic acidosis
Fusarium infection	Voriconazole or lipid formulation amphotericin B (consider combination pending susceptibilities) Alternative: posaconazole Reversal of immunosuppression Obtain susceptibilities because resistance is common
Scedosporium infection	Voriconazole Alternative: posaconazole Consider combination terbinafine-triazole therapy Reversal of immunosuppression
Pulmonary histoplasmosis	Observation in selected normal hosts Mild to moderate: itraconazole Alternative: posaconazole or voriconazole Severe or immunocompromised: lipid formulation amphotericin B Reversal of immunosuppression
Pulmonary coccidioidomycosis	Observation in selected normal hosts Mild to moderate: itraconazole, fluconazole, voriconazole, or posaconazole Severe or immunocompromised: lipid formulation amphotericin B Reversal of immunosuppression
Pulmonary blastomycosis	Mild to moderate: itraconazole or voriconazole Severe or immunocompromised: lipid formulation amphotericin B
Pulmonary paracoccidioidomycosis	Itraconazole Voriconazole Trimethoprim-sulphamethoxazole
Pulmonary Talaromycosis (Penicilliosis)	Initial therapy with a formulation of amphotericin B followed by itraconazole
Pulmonary sporotrichosis	Lipid formulation amphotericin B
Pulmonary cryptococcosis	Mild to moderate: fluconazole Severe or disseminated disease: Lipid formulation amphotericin B plus flucytosine

Table 30.2 (Continued)

Pulmonary candidiasis	Echinocandin Alternatives: lipid formulation amphotericin B or fluconazole Reversal of immunosuppression
Trichosporon infection	Voriconazole Alternative: posaconazole Reversal of immunosuppression
Pneumocystis jirovecii	Trimethoprim-sulphamethoxazole Alternatives: Intravenous pentamidine in severe disease and atovaquone, trimethoprim-dapsone, or clindamycin-primaquine in mild to moderate infection

for 6–12 months. Patients with severe pneumonia and/or disseminated disease (e.g. CNS infection) should be treated with an initial course of amphotericin B with flucytosine, followed by maintenance therapy with fluconazole (Perfect et al. 2010).

Pulmonary candidiasis

An echinocandin should be used for initial treatment of *Candida* bronchopneumonia or haematogenous disseminated candidiasis. Fluconazole may be used once the patient is stabilized and once susceptibilities are known.

Trichosporonosis

The composite of preclinical and clinical data supports antifungal triazoles for the treatment of invasive trichosporonosis, particularly voriconazole. Itraconazole and fluconazole demonstrate reduced *in vitro* susceptibility compared with voriconazole and may be considered as alternatives. Amphotericin B and echinocandins are not effective for treating invasive disease. Similar antifungal susceptibility profiles have been found across all *Trichosporon* spp.

Pneumocystis jirovecii pneumonia

The treatment of choice for *Pneumocystis jirovecii* pneumonia is trimethoprim-sulphamethoxazole (TMP 15–20 mg and SMX 75–100 mg/kg/day intravenously or orally) in divided doses. Alternative therapies include intravenous pentamidine in severely ill patients and atovaquone, trimethoprim-dapsone, or clindamycin-primaquine in patients with mild to moderate infection. Duration of therapy is 21 days. In HIV-infected patients with severe infection, defined as an alveolar–arterial oxygen gradient of ≥35 mmHg or a partial pressure of arterial oxygen of <70 mmHg, adjunctive corticosteroids reduce morbidity and mortality (Gagnon et al. 1990). In non-HIV-infected immunocompromised hosts, no randomized trials have evaluated the role of adjunctive corticosteroids, but it is generally the favoured approach (Pareja et al. 1998).

Prevention

Control of the environmental transmission of conidia can be an important adjunct in managing an outbreak of nosocomial aspergillosis. The capacity of *Aspergillus fumigatus* to establish a pulmonary infection in an immunocompromised host depends upon the level of inoculum (Dixon et al. 1989). Consistent with these findings are the observations that large pulses of conidia from contaminated environmental sources appear to present a particularly high risk for development of pulmonary aspergillosis in immunocompromised patients (Rhame et al. 1984). A review of nosocomial invasive aspergillosis found that the most common environmental sources of *Aspergillus* in hospital outbreaks were contaminated air-conditioning units and construction sites (Walsh and Dixon 1989). Air conditioning systems should be microbiologically monitored, especially during periods of repair or malfunction. High-efficiency particulate air (HEPA) filters should be utilized, when possible, in hospital areas accommodating patients with profound protracted neutropenia. Appropriate environmental and infection control measures should be implemented in cooperation with hospital infection control authorities, hospital engineering staff, and physicians caring for immunocompromised patients when air-conditioning repairs or construction are performed within a medical facility.

Among specific immunocompromised patient populations, antifungal agents are administered for prophylaxis of invasive fungal infections. As an example, neutropenic hosts, such as patients with acute leukaemia undergoing induction chemotherapy and allogeneic HSCT recipients, routinely receive antifungal prophylaxis with voriconazole or posaconazole. Furthermore, many transplant centres routinely administer nebulized amphotericin B or systemic voriconazole to prevent pulmonary mould infections in lung transplant recipients. Guidelines for these high-risk groups have been published by the Infectious Diseases Society of America, the European Society of Clinical Microbiology and Infectious Diseases, and the European Conference on Infections in Leukaemia (see Chapter 49), and there are many national guidelines available.

References

Anaissie E, Bodey GP, Kantarjian H, et al. (1989) New spectrum of fungal infections in patients with cancer. *Rev Infect Dis* 11: 369–78.

Arvanitis M, Anagnostou T, Fuchs BB, Caliendo AM and Mylonakis E (2014) Molecular and nonmolecular diagnostic methods for invasive fungal infections. *Clin Microbiol Rev* 27: 490–526.

Aung AK, Teh BM, McGrath C and Thompson PJ (2013) Pulmonary sporotrichosis: case series and systematic analysis of literature on clinico-radiological patterns and management outcomes. *Med Mycol* 51: 534–44.

Azoulay E, Bergeron A, Chevret S, Bele N, Schlemmer B and Menotti J (2009) Polymerase chain reaction for diagnosing *pneumocystis* pneumonia in non-HIV immunocompromised patients with pulmonary infiltrates. *Chest* 135: 655–61.

Bradsher RW (1997) Clinical features of blastomycosis. *Semin Respir Infect* 12: 229–34.

Brandt SJ, Peters WP, Atwater SK, et al. (1988) Effect of recombinant human granulocyte-macrophage colony-stimulating factor on hematopoietic

reconstitution after high-dose chemotherapy and autologous bone marrow transplantation. *N Engl J Med* 318: 869–76.
Campo M, Lewis RE and Kontoyiannis DP (2010) Invasive fusariosis in patients with hematologic malignancies at a cancer center: 1998–2009. *J Infect* 60: 331–7.
Chai LY, Kullberg BJ and Johnson EM (2012) Early serum galactomannan trend as a predictor of outcome of invasive aspergillosis. *J Clin Microbiol* 50: 2330–6.
Cornely OA, Arikan-Akdagli S, Dannaoui E, et al. (2014) ESCMID and ECMM joint clinical guidelines for the diagnosis and management of mucormycosis 2013. *Clin Microbiol Infect* 20 (Suppl. 3): 5–26.
De Pauw B, Walsh TJ, Donnelly JP, et al. (2008) Revised definitions of invasive fungal disease from the European Organization for Research and Treatment of Cancer/Invasive Fungal Infections Cooperative Group and the National Institute of Allergy and Infectious Diseases Mycoses Study Group (EORTC/MSG) Consensus Group. *Clin Infect Dis* 46: 1813–21.
Dixon DM, Polak A and Walsh TJ (1989) Fungus dose-dependent primary pulmonary aspergillosis in immunosuppressed mice. *Infect Immun* 57: 1452–6.
Falci DR and Pasqualatto AC (2013) Profile of isavuconazole and its potential in the treatment of severe invasive fungal infections. *Infect Drug Resist* 6: 163–74.
Food and Drug Administration Anti-Infection Drug Advisory Committee January 22, 2015, http://www.fda.gov/downloads/AdvisoryCommittees/CommitteesMeetingMaterials/Drugs/Anti-InfectiveDrugsAdvisoryCommittee/UCM431846.pdf, accessed 20 May 2017.
Gagnon S, Boota AM, Fischl MA, Baier H, Kirksey OW and La Voie L (1990) Corticosteroids as adjunctive therapy for severe *Pneumocystis carinii* pneumonia in the acquired immunodeficiency syndrome. A double-blind, placebo-controlled trial. *N Engl J Med* 323: 1444–50.
Gameletsou MN, Sipsas NV, Roilides E and Walsh TJ (2012) Rhino-orbital-cerebral mucormycosis. *Curr Infect Dis Rep* 14: 423–34.
Girmenia C, Pagano L, Martino B, et al. (2005) Invasive infections caused by *Trichosporon* species and *Geotrichum capitatum* in patients with hematological malignancies: a retrospective multicenter study from Italy and review of the literature. *J Clin Microbiol* 43: 1818–28.
Hachem RY, Kontoyiannis DP, Chemaly RF, Jiang Y, Reitzel R and Raad I (2009) Utility of galactomannan enzyme immunoassay and (1,3) beta-D-glucan in diagnosis of invasive fungal infections: low sensitivity for *Aspergillus fumigatus* infection in hematologic malignancy patients. *J Clin Microbiol* 47: 129–33.
Hage CA, Kirsch EJ, Stump TE, et al. (2011) *Histoplasma* antigen clearance during treatment of histoplasmosis in patients with AIDS determined by quantitative antigen enzyme immunoassay. *Clin Vaccine Immunol* 18: 661–6.
He S, Hang JP, Zhang L, Wang F, Zhang DC and Gong FH (2015) A systematic review and meta-analysis of diagnostic accuracy of serum 1,3-β-D-glucan for invasive fungal infection: focus on cutoff levels. *J Microbiol Immunol Infect* 48: 351–61.
Herbrecht R, Denning DW, Patterson TF, et al. (2002) Voriconazole versus amphotericin B for primary therapy of invasive aspergillosis. *N Engl J Med* 347: 408–15.
Huang L, Cattamanchi A, Davis JL, et al. (2011) HIV-associated *Pneumocystis* pneumonia. *Proc Am Thorac Soc* 8: 294–300.
Karageorgopoulos DE, Qu JM, Korbila IP, Zhu YG, Vasileiou VA and Falagas ME (2013) Accuracy of β-D-glucan for the diagnosis of *Pneumocystis jirovecii* pneumonia: a meta-analysis. *Clin Microbiol Infect* 19: 39–49.
Knoper SR and Galgiani JN (1988) Systemic fungal infections: diagnosis and treatment. I. Coccidioidomycosis. *Infect Dis Clin North Am* 2: 861–75.
Le T, Van Kinh N, Cuc N TK, et al. (2017) A trial of itraconazole or amphotericin B for HIV-associated talaromycosis. *New Eng J Med* 376: 2329–40.
Marchetti O, Lamoth F and Mikulska M (2012) ECIL recommendations for the use of biological markers for the diagnosis of invasive fungal diseases in leukemic patients and hematopoietic SCT recipients. *Bone Marrow Transplant* 47: 846–54.
Marr KA, Schlamm HT, Herbrecht R, et al. (2015) Combination antifungal therapy for invasive aspergillosis: a randomized trial. *Ann Intern Med* 162: 81–9.
Marty FM, Cosimi LA and Baden LR (2004) Breakthrough zygomycosis after voriconazole treatment in recipients of hematopoietic stem-cell transplants. *N Engl J Med* 350: 950–2.
Marty FM, Lowry CM, Lempitski SJ, Kubiak DW, Finkelman MA and Baden LR (2006) Reactivity of (1→3)-beta-D-glucan assay with commonly used intravenous antimicrobials. *Antimicrob Agents Chemother* 50: 3450–3.
Masur H, Rosen PR and Armstrong D (1977) Pulmonary disease caused by *Candida* species. *Am J Med* 63: 914–25.
Meletiadis J, Mouton JW, Meis JF and Verweij PE (2003) *In vitro* drug interaction modeling of combinations of azoles with terbinafine against clinical *Scedosporium prolificans* isolates. *Antimicrob Agents Chemother* 47: 106–17.
Mikulska M, Furfaro E, Del Bono V, et al. (2012) Piperacillin/tazobactam (Tazocin™) seems to be no longer responsible for false-positive results of the galactomannan assay. *J Antimicrob Chemother* 67: 1746–8.
Nucci M and Anaissie E (2007) Fusarium infections in immunocompromised patients. *Clin Microbiol Rev* 20: 695–704.
Pappas PG, Perfect JR, Cloud GA, et al. (2001) Cryptococcosis in human immunodeficiency virus-negative patients in the era of effective azole therapy. *Clin Infect Dis* 33: 690–9.
Pareja JG, Garland R and Koziel H (1998) Use of adjunctive corticosteroids in severe adult non-HIV *Pneumocystis carinii* pneumonia. *Chest* 113: 1215–24.
Perfect JR, Dismukes WE, Dromer F, et al. (2010) Clinical Practice Guidelines for the Management of Cryptococcal Disease: 2010 update by the Infectious Diseases Society of America. *Clin Infect Dis* 50: 291–322.
Petraitis V, Petraitiene R, Hope W, et al. (2009) Combination therapy in treatment of experimental pulmonary aspergillosis: *in vitro* and *in vivo* correlation of the concentration and dose dependent interaction between anidulafungin and voriconazole by Bliss independence drug interaction analysis. *Antimicrob Agents Chemother* 53: 2382–91.
Pluss JL and Opal SM (1986) Pulmonary sporotrichosis: review of treatment and outcome. *Medicine (Baltimore)* 65: 143–53.
Rhame FS, Streifel AJ, Kersey JH Jr and Glave PB (1984) Extrinsic risk factors for pneumonia in the patient at high risk of infection. *Am J Med* 76: 42–52.
Sung L, Nathan PC, Alibhai SM, Tomlinson GA and Beyene J (2007) Meta-analysis: effect of prophylactic hematopoietic colony-stimulating factors on mortality and outcomes of infection. *Ann Intern Med* 147: 400–11.
Tortorano AM, Esposto MC, Prigitano A, et al. (2012) Cross-reactivity of *Fusarium* spp. in the *Aspergillus* Galactomannan enzyme-linked immunosorbent assay. *J Clin Microbiol* 50: 1051–3.
Tortorano AM, Richardson M, Roilides E, et al. (2014) ESCMID and ECMM joint guidelines on diagnosis and management of hyalohyphomycosis: *Fusarium* spp., *Scedosporium* spp. and others. *Clin Microbiol Infect* 20 (Suppl. 3): 27–46.
Vergidis P, Walker RC, Kaul DR, et al. (2012) False-positive *Aspergillus* galactomannan assay in solid organ transplant recipients with histoplasmosis. *Transpl Infect Dis* 14: 213–17.
Walsh TJ and Dixon DM (1989) Nosocomial Aspergillosis: environmental microbiology, hospital epidemiology, diagnosis, and treatment. *Eur J Epidemiol* 5: 131–42.
Walsh TJ, Lutsar I, Driscoll T, et al. (2002) Voriconazole in the treatment of aspergillosis, scedosporiosis, and other invasive fungal infections in children. *Pediatr Infect Dis J* 21: 240–8.
Walsh TJ, Melcher GP, Lee JW and Pizzo PA (1993) Infections due to *Trichosporon* species: new concepts in mycology, pathogenesis, diagnosis, and treatment. *Curr Top Med Mycol* 5: 79–113.
Wheat LJ, Connolly-Springfield PA, Baker RL, et al. (1990) Disseminated histoplasmosis in the acquired immune deficiency syndrome: clinical findings, diagnosis, and treatment, and review of the literature. *Medicine (Baltimore)* 69: 361–4.

CHAPTER 31

Fungal toxin-mediated disease

Christopher C. Kibbler

Introduction to toxin-mediated disease

Fungi produce many different metabolic products, and increasing numbers of these have been shown to have pathogenic effects in humans. Mycotoxins may cause organ failure, or have carcinogenic, mutagenic, immunosuppressive, or oestrogenic effects, and their clinical impact depends upon the quantity and duration of exposure and their interaction with other compounds or agents which may be present.

Exposure may occur via three main routes:

1. Contamination ('spoilage') of food or infection of cereals with toxin-producing fungi, the production of toxin(s) *in situ*, and the subsequent ingestion of toxin in the foodstuff
2. Ingestion of mushrooms or toadstools containing significant quantities of toxin ('mycetism')
3. Inhalation of airborne toxins from fungi growing in damp environments ('damp building related illness').

Food-borne toxins

Outbreaks of ergotism, following the ingestion of cereal grain contaminated with *Claviceps purpurea,* have been reported for centuries as St Anthony's fire, named after the St Anthony monks who were thought to be expert in the treatment of the disease. However, ergot-contaminated rye has been discovered in the stomach contents of a 2,000-year-old bog mummy (Stokilde-Jorgensen et al. 2008) and it is likely that other grain-associated mycotoxin diseases have occurred in man since the advent of agriculture.

Causative fungi

More than 300 food-borne mycotoxins have been described (Abrunhosa et al. 2016). However, the majority thought to be pathogenic in humans are produced by five main genera: *Aspergillus, Penicillium, Fusarium, Byssochlamys* (anamorph *Paecilomyces)*, and *Claviceps.* Some of these are produced by more than one genus, and they are found in a wide variety of foodstuffs—from cereals, spices, and coffee, to nuts and even wine and beer (Table 31.1).

Food-borne mycotoxins

Aflatoxins

Aflatoxins are difuranocoumarins (Figure 31.1) produced by *Aspergillus* spp.; there are approximately 20 compounds classified in several series. B1, B2, G1, G2, and M1 are amongst the most important, with B1 being the most prevalent in food. The International Agency for Research on Cancer (IARC) has classified them as Group 1 carcinogens—that is, proven to cause cancer (IARC 2017)—and they are particularly associated with hepatocellular cancer (Wild et al. 2015). There appears to be an additive interaction with hepatitis B virus for increasing the risk of liver cancer (Wu et al. 2009). Other associations with aflatoxin exposure include hepatotoxicity and child growth stunting, and these compounds have been shown to impair fetal development, immune function, and gut function in animal models (Wild et al. 2015).

Aflatoxin B1 has been shown to undergo epoxidation via the cytochrome P450 complex to a number of products including aflatoxin B1-8-9-epoxide, which is the most toxic. This is able to form molecular adducts such as aflatoxin B1-N7-guanine, which is capable of causing point mutations in a variety of genes, primarily through G to T transversions (Levy et al. 1992; Iyer et al. 1994). Hepatocellular carcinoma in areas of high aflatoxin exposure is strongly associated with mutations in the p53 tumour suppressor gene (Bressac et al. 1991), whereas no point mutations were found in areas of low aflatoxin exposure in the study by Aguilar et al. (1994). Other potential causes of cell toxicity include the formation of protein adducts and stimulation of reactive oxygen species formation (Guindon et al. 2007).

Aflatoxins have a major impact on animal husbandry. The first report of mass poisoning, from contaminated peanut meal, and the consequent death of more than 100,000 turkeys in the UK, in 1960, led to the discovery of these compounds (Goldblatt 1969). In man, the clinical features of acute aflatoxin poisoning include vomiting, abdominal pain, liver necrosis, and pulmonary oedema, and there have been many reports of multiple deaths since the 1970s. An outbreak in western India resulted in at least 97 deaths following ingestion of contaminated maize (Krishnamachari et al. 1975). In Malaysia, where aflatoxicosis resulted in a number of cases of acute hepatic encephalopathy, as much as 3 mg of toxin were detected in a single portion of the responsible noodles (Lye et al. 1995). One of the largest mass episodes followed the consumption of home-grown maize in Kenya, resulting in 317 cases and 125 deaths (CDC 2004). Treatment of acute aflatoxicosis is largely supportive, but a number of compounds (such as chlorophyll, chlorophyllin, smectite clays, and lactobacilli) have been shown to sequester these molecules in the gut and help reduce their absorption (Wild et al. 2015).

The worldwide incidence of hepatocellular cancer is 780,000 per year (Ferlay et al. 2015), and aflatoxins are thought to increase the risk of this condition by up to 59.4-fold, when associated

Table 31.1 Mycotoxin-producing fungi and examples of contaminated foodstuffs

Genus	Example species	Toxins	Foodstuffs	Geographic area(s) affected
Aspergillus	*A. flavus* *A. nomius* *A. parasiticus* *A. ochraceoroseus* *A. toxicarius*	Aflatoxins (B1, B2, G1, G2)	Cereals, nuts, seeds, spices dried fruit, dairy products, eggs, meat	Africa, South Asia
		Ochratoxin A	Coffee, tea, cocoa, rice, wheat, dried fruit, spices, wine, beer, meat	North and South America, Europe, Africa, South Asia
		Patulin	Fruit (especially apples), cereal	North and South America, Europe, Africa, South Asia, Australasia
	A. niger	Fumonisins (B2)	Coffee, grapes	North America, Europe, Southeast Asia
Penicillium	*P. verrucosum* *P. nordicum*	Ochratoxin A	Coffee, tea, cocoa, rice, wheat, dried fruit, spices, wine, beer, meat	North and South America, Europe, Africa, South Asia
	P. expansum	Patulin	Fruit (especially apples), cereal	North and South America, Europe, Africa, South Asia, Australasia
Byssochlamys (anamorph: Paecilomyces)	*B. nivea*	Patulin	Fruit (especially apples), cereal	North and South America, Europe, Africa, South Asia, Australasia
Fusarium	*F. graminearum* *F. sporotrichioides*	Trichothecenes	Cereals	North America, Europe, Asia
	F. proliferatum *F. verticillioides*	Fumonisins	Cereals	Europe, Africa
	F. graminearum *F. sporotrichioides*	Zearalenone	Cereals, bananas	North America, Europe, Asia
	F. proliferatum *F. sporotrichioides*	Beauvericin	Cereals	Europe
	F. verticillioides *F. sporotrichioides*	Moniliformin	Cereals	Europe
Claviceps	*C. purpurea*	Ergotamine	Cereals	North and South America, Europe, Africa, South Asia, Australasia

Source: data from Bryden, 2012; Marin, Ramos, Cano-Sancho, & Sanchis, 2013; Da Rocha, Da Freire, Maia, Guedes, Rondina, 2014; Bosco & Mollea, 2012; Creppy, 2002; Ficheux, Sibiril, Le Garrec, & Parent-Massin, 2012; Filazi & Sireli, 2013; Filazi & Tansel Sireli, 2014; Glenn, 2007; Logrieco et al., 2009; Logrieco et al., 1998; Oliveira, Zannini, & Arendt, 2014; Pitt, 2000; Yazar & Omurtag, 2008; Mogensen, Frisvad, Thrane & Nielsen, 2010.

with hepatitis B virus infection (Ross et al. 1992). The impact of aflatoxins on other aspects of human health, such as childhood growth, is more difficult to quantify, but a number of studies in Africa have shown a significant effect in areas of high exposure (Wild et al. 2015).

The Food and Drug Administration (FDA) and the EU have set limits for aflatoxins in food and animal feeds, but there is much discrepancy, with the US limits being much higher than the European ones. Preventative measures to reduce the content of crops and foodstuffs involve simple agricultural modifications (such as the use of fungicides, insecticides, and fungal-resistant crops) and storage improvements (such as the use of palettes to prevent contact of harvested crops with soil). Sorting and removal of contaminated crops are carried out in all countries and help to reduce toxin content. A number of other methods (such as the addition of toxin binders) have been shown to reduce aflatoxin levels (Wild et al. 2015).

Ochratoxin A

Ochratoxin A is a di-hydroisocoumarin (Figure 31.1) which is produced by *Aspergillus* and *Penicillium* spp. and is nephrotoxic and carcinogenic in animals. The International Agency for Research on Cancer (IARC) has classified it as belonging to Group 2B (possible human carcinogens), as there is no firm clinical evidence for carcinogenicity in humans (IARC 2017). In addition, although it has been suggested that the toxin is responsible for several different renal diseases (such as Balkan endemic nephropathy and chronic interstitial nephropathy), a systematic review has found no evidence to support this (Stiborová et al. 2016).

In cellular and animal models, ochratoxin A has been shown to be genotoxic, forming DNA adducts via oxidation and hydroxyquinone metabolites. It also induces oxidative stress in a variety of cells and may induce apoptosis (Pfohl-Leszkowicz and Manderville 2007).

The EU has set limits for food content, but the FDA has not.

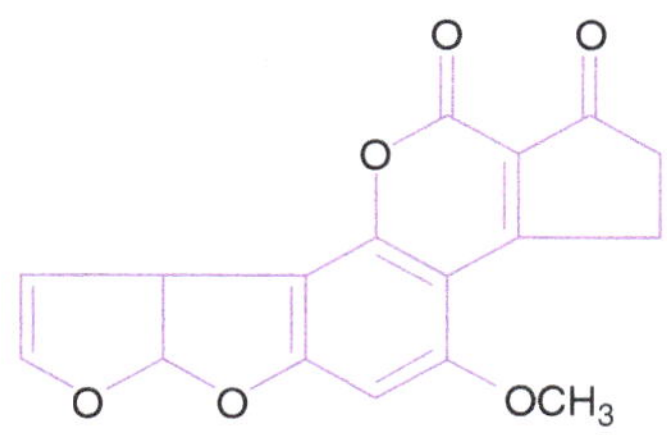

Aflatoxin B1

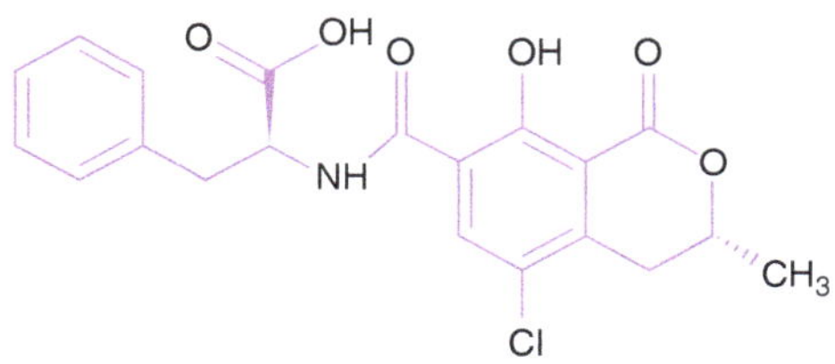

Ochratoxin A

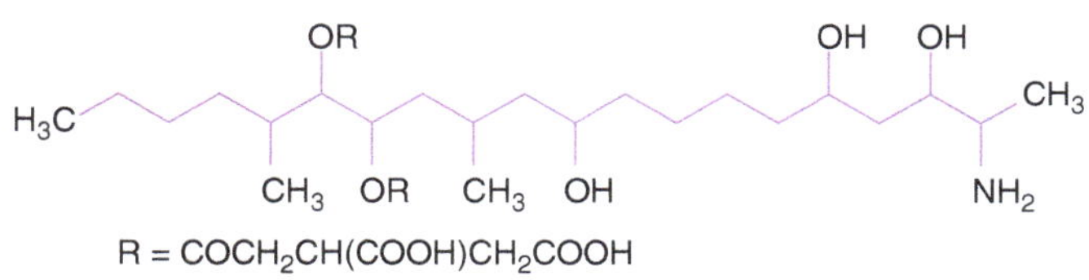

Fumonisin B1

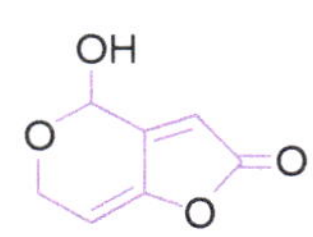

Patulin

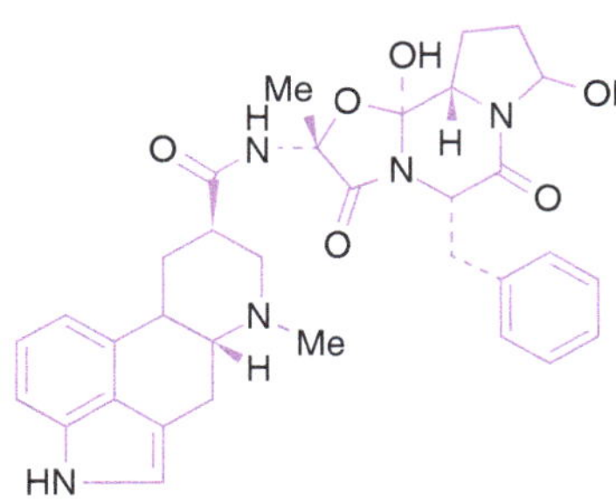

Ergotamine

Figure 31.1 Structure of common food mycotoxins.

Patulin

Patulin is a polyketide lactone (Figure 31.1) produced by *Aspergillus*, *Penicillium* (especially *P. expansum*), and *Byssochlamys* spp. It is destroyed by fermentation and so, although found in fruit juices, alcoholic beverages are usually patulin-free. The compound binds strongly to sulfhydryl groups, resulting in enzyme inhibition and gene mutations.

Animal models have demonstrated acute toxicity in the form of convulsions, pulmonary oedema, gastrointestinal ulceration in the rat, and renal toxicity in monkeys (Puel et al. 2010). More chronic exposure has been shown to be neuro-, nephro-, immuno- and geno-toxic, as well as teratogenic and carcinogenic (Moake et al. 2005). IARC has given it a Group 3 classification (unclassifiable as a cause of human cancer), although the World Health Organization (WHO) considers it to be genotoxic.

The FDA and the EU have set limits for patulin in food, but not animal feed.

Fumonisins

Fumonisins are long, highly polar molecules (Figure 31.1) with a similar structure to sphingosine and sphinganine, precursors of complex sphingolipids important for cell membrane structure and function. They are produced by *Fusarium* spp. and *Aspergillus niger.* There are at least 28 fumonisins, classified into four groups—A, B, C, and P—with B1 and B2 being the most important. They inhibit ceramide synthase, reducing sphingolipid biosynthesis, disrupting cell growth, and inducing apoptosis (Voss et al. 2007).

In animals, fumonisins have been reported to cause equine leucoencephalomalacia and porcine pulmonary oedema. In humans, studies have shown an association with oesophageal carcinoma, and IARC has classified them as belonging to Group 2B (possible human carcinogens) (IARC 2017). Other reported effects in animals include renal and liver toxicity.

There are EU and FDA limits for fumonisins for animal feed and foodstuffs.

Other *Fusarium* mycotoxins

There are more than 170 trichothecenes, which form two main groups: Type A (e.g. T-2 toxin, HT-2 toxin) and Type B (deoxynivalenol, nivalenol), based on solubility. Food trichothecene mycotoxins are mainly produced by *Fusarium* spp., but these compounds are also produced by other environmental fungi such as *Stachybotrys* (see 'Environmental toxin exposure'). They are sesquiterpene molecules which bind to polysomes and ribosomes, inhibiting protein and nucleic acid synthesis. Deoxynivalenol is also known as vomitoxin, and trichothecene acute toxicity is characterized by vomiting in humans and animals (Rotter 1996). Other adverse effects in animals include immunosuppression, blood dyscrasias, anorexia, and skin lesions (Rotter 1996). IARC classifies trichothecenes as belonging to Group 3 (unclassifiable as a cause of cancer).

Zearalenone is a lactone, with a steroid-like structure, which, following bioactivation, behaves in a similar fashion to oestradiol and exerts effects through oestrogen-binding receptors. This results in reduced fertility and other reproductive tract effects in animals (Zinedine et al. 2007). IARC has classified this as a Group 3 carcinogen.

Beauvericin and moniliformin are other mycotoxins produced by *Fusarium* spp. and have been found in a variety of foodstuffs and animal feeds. Beauvericin has been shown to produce a variety of effects on peripheral blood cells, but its human pathogenicity is unclear.

The FDA has published limits for deoxynivalenol in foodstuffs and animal feed, and the EU also regulates zearalenone.

Ergot alkaloids

There are more than 40 ergot alkaloids, of which ergotamine is the most well-studied. They are produced by many *Claviceps* spp. (especially *C. purpurea*) and exert their effects through vasoconstriction and neurotoxicity. Different biosynthetic gene clusters are responsible for the products of the different species. *C. purpurea* has been found to possess a gene cluster which encodes for enzymes catalysing the synthesis of ergotamine and ergopeptines via a branching pathway from the intermediary compound D-lysergic acid (Gerhards et al. 2014). These ergopeptines (such as ergocryptine) are characterized by a lactam ring but are more complex than the naturally occurring penicillins and cephalosporins produced by other fungi and have dopaminergic activity. Such a branching pathway, dependent on the interaction of two non-ribosomal peptide synthetase subunits, is thought to be unique amongst fungi (Gerhards et al. 2014). Hence, these fungi are capable of producing many different neuroactive compounds. Ergotamine (Figure 31.1) has a similar structure to adrenaline, dopamine, and 5-hydroxytryptamine (5-HT) and interacts with the receptors for these molecules within blood vessels and the central nervous system (Walkembach et al. 2005).

Human toxicity is characterized by abdominal pain, vomiting, convulsions, hallucinations, burning sensation in the skin ('St Anthony's fire'), and severe gangrene and death in high doses. Outbreaks of ergotism largely ceased, once the link with cereal infection was established, but they were once widespread and documented from the ninth century. Indeed, it has been suggested that ergotism may have been responsible for the behaviour of the so-called Salem witches, causing the convulsions and psychosis which led to their arrests and subsequent trials (Caporael 1976). However, this is controversial (Spanos and Gottlieb 1976).

Treatment of acute toxicity is primarily supportive, combined in cases of severe gangrene with the use of vasodilators, such as prostacycline, prostaglandin E2, nitroprusside, and prazocin, and, if necessary, surgical intervention (Garcia et al. 2000).

Mushroom poisoning

Mushroom poisoning, or mycetism, is usually the result of the ingestion of mushrooms misidentified as edible. Occasionally, it is the result of deliberate action, either for recreational use, such as the use of so-called 'magic mushrooms' containing psilocybin and related compounds, or intentional poisoning, as may have occurred in the case of the Emperor Claudius and Pope Clement VII. Indeed, mushrooms such as *Amanita muscaria* (fly agaric) have been used over the centuries by a number of religions to achieve hallucinogenic trance-like states.

What follows is intended to give some background and understanding of a spectrum of conditions about which there is a high level of ignorance amongst healthcare professionals. The reader should not consider this to be an exhaustive text and should refer to more detailed literature and seek expert help for the management of clinical cases.

Causative fungi

There are approximately 100 species of mushroom capable of poisoning humans (Graeme 2014). However, only a few species have been reported to cause fatalities. Most of these belong to the *Amanita, Cortinarius, Clitocybe*, and *Galerina* genera, and the majority of deaths are due to *Amanita phalloides* (the death cap mushroom; Figure 31.2) and closely related species *A. bisporigera, A. ocreata*, and *A. virosa* (collectively called 'destroying angels') (Table 31.2).

Epidemiology

The majority of cases occur in the spring and autumn, when most fungi are fruiting. It is likely that many episodes of poisoning are unreported, but in 1998, 1,675 cases of mushroom poisoning were reported in France and 8–10,000 cases are currently estimated to occur in Brazil every year (Lima et al. 2012). Between 1976 and 1981, 16 outbreaks—including 44 cases—were reported to the US Centres for Disease Control and Prevention (Rattanvilay et al. 1982). Between 1994 and 2002, 706 cases of *Gyromitra esculenta* poisoning were reported in Sweden, 135 cases of poisoning with *Cortinarius orellanus* were recorded in Poland between 1953 and 1962, and 237 cases of possible mushroom poisoning were discussed with the UK National Poisons Information Service in 2013 (Public Health England 2014: https://www.gov.uk/government/news/take-care-when-picking-mushrooms-poisons-experts-warn).

The American Association of Poison Control Centres (AAPCC) has kept a surveillance database for more than 25 years and has found that the exact species responsible for each case of poisoning was unidentified in more than 95% of cases (Trestrail 1991). More recent data from the AAPCC has shown that 67% of affected individuals were less than 6 years old, 6% experienced minor toxicity, 0.3% experienced major toxicity, and only one (of more than 6,000 cases) died—from an unidentified species (Nordt and Clark 2000).

There is evidence that mushroom poisoning is increasing in frequency in many countries, particularly amongst adolescent and adult males, when foraging for uncultivated species (Diaz 2005a).

Major mushroom toxins

There are several important neurotoxins. Muscarine acts on muscarinic receptors, producing a rapid-onset cholinergic syndrome, but is not inactivated by cholinesterase, resulting in a prolonged effect. Typically, vasodilatation, bradycardia (and possible syncope), bronchorrhoea, bronchospasm, abdominal pain, vomiting and diarrhoea, and tremor are seen, and this may progress to shock and confusion and, rarely, respiratory failure (Lima et al. 2012).

Gyromitrin is metabolized to monomethylhydrazine, which inhibits pyridoxal phosphate. Hence, this impacts on gamma-aminobutyric acid (GABA) production and produces rapid onset of vomiting, ataxia, tremor, and convulsions, progressing to loss of consciousness and death in about 10% of cases (Michelot and Toth 1991).

Ibotenic acid and muscimol interact with N-methyl-D-aspartate and GABA receptors, respectively, to produce an inebriation syndrome, characterized by excitatory or depressive effects, including hysteria, drowsiness, and alteration of perception (Lima et al. 2012; Graeme 2014). Rarely, loss of consciousness and death occur.

Table 31.2 Examples of fungi from the main genera associated with human fatalities

Species	Common name	Toxin	Main organ/system involvement	Region
Amanita bisporigera and *Amanita ocreata*	North American destroying angels	Amatoxins	Liver	North America
Amanita phalloides	Death cap	α-Amanitin	Liver	Europe, North Africa, North America, Australia, New Zealand
Amanita smithiana	Smith's Lepidella	Uncharacterized (previously thought to be amino-hexadienoic acid)	Kidney (and liver)	Japan and Northwest America and Canada
Amanita verna	Fool's mushroom	Amatoxins	Liver	Europe
Amanita virosa	European destroying angel	Amatoxins	Liver	Europe
Clitocybe dealbata	Ivory funnel	Muscarine	CNS	Europe, North America
Clitocybe rivulosa	False champignon	Muscarine	CNS	Europe, North America
Cortinarius orellanus	Fool's webcap	Orellanine	Kidney	Europe
Cortinarius rubellus	Deadly webcap	Orellanine	Kidney	Europe
Galerina marginata	Autumn skullcap	Amatoxins	Liver	Europe, North America, Asia, Australia
Gyromitra esculenta	False morel	Gyromitrin	Multiple	Europe, North America
Inocybe erubescens	Red-staining inocybe	Muscarine	CNS	Europe
Lepiota castanea	Chestnut dapperling	Amatoxins	Liver	Europe
Lepiota subincarnata	Deadly parasol	Amatoxins	Liver	Europe, North America, Asia
Pholiotina rugosa (*Conocybe filaris*)	Fool's conecap	amatoxins	liver	Europe, North America and Asia

Source: data from Graeme, 2014; Lima, Costa Fortes, Carvalho Garbi Novaes, & Percário, 2012; West, Lindgren, & Horowitz, 2009; Diaz, 2005a,b; Trestrail, 1991.

Psilocybin is metabolized to psilocin, which is structurally similar to 5-HT and produces a variety of central nervous system effects, such as hallucinations, altered perception, and other mind-altering effects (Passie et al. 2002; Lima et al. 2012).

Amatoxins, of which there are at least nine (including α-amanitin, the main toxin in *Amanita phalloides* poisoning), are cyclic octapeptides which inhibit RNA polymerase II and result in cytotoxicity (Wieland et al. 1981; Lima et al. 2012). Their main impact is on the liver, causing centrilobular necrosis and fatty degeneration, although renal acute tubular necrosis is also seen (Graeme 2014). Phallotoxins, which accompany amatoxins in *Amanita phalloides* poisoning, are poorly absorbed from the gastrointestinal tract and are thought to play little part in *Amanita* toxicity (Santi et al. 2012).

Orellanine is a bipyridine molecule which inhibits RNA polymerase B and alkaline phosphatase, producing its primary cytotoxic effect on the renal tubular epithelium, as a result of concentration within the kidneys (Frank et al. 2009).

Other toxins may produce significant disease, such as coprine, an inhibitor of acetaldehyde dehydrogenase which causes disulfiram-like reactions (flushing, tachycardia, malaise, dyspnoea, and hypotension) in association with alcohol, and the uncharacterized toxin of *Tricholoma* spp., which is associated with severe rhabdomyolysis (Graeme 2014).

Clinical features of mushroom poisoning

As already discussed, the majority (over 90% in more recent data) of individuals do not experience any symptoms after accidental consumption of poisonous fungi (Nordt and Clark 2000).

The clinical syndromes associated with mushroom poisoning have been classified by toxin, by end-organ involvement, or by time of onset. Diaz (2005b) proposed a three-phase time of onset classification, extending previous two-phase systems, based on the premise that this was more helpful to the clinician as it facilitated diagnosis in situations where the causative mushroom could not be identified.

Early-onset toxicity is defined as occurring within six hours and includes cholinergic (e.g. from *Clitocybe* spp.), glutaminergic (e.g. caused by *A. muscaria)*, epileptogenic (e.g. due to *Gyromitra* spp.), and allergic & gastrointestinal syndromes. Late onset is between 6 and 24 hours, where the liver and renal clinical features of *Amanita* and other amatoxin-producing species commence. Delayed-onset toxicity is defined as occurring after more than 24 hours. The features of orellanine poisoning (e.g. due to *Cortinarius* spp.), as well as some other less commonly produced toxins, typically begin then.

Diagnosis

The diagnosis of mushroom poisoning depends on the clinical presentation (which is usually non-specific initially), a history of

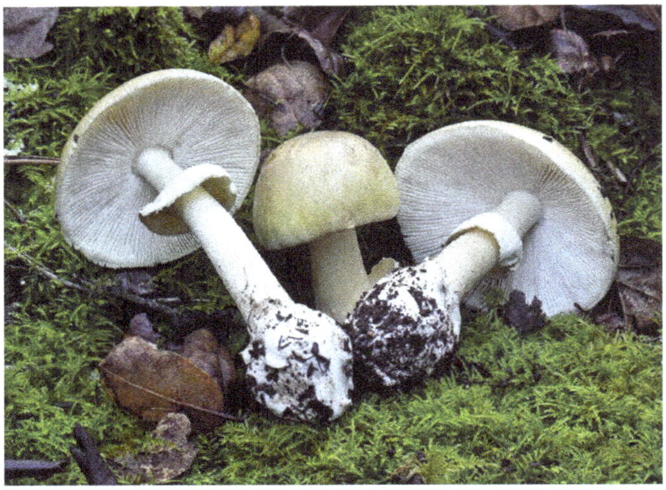

Figure 31.2 *Amanita phalloides* (http://www.discoverlife.org).

The 'death cap' is responsible for the majority of fatal episodes of mushroom poisoning. The creamy brown cap is 5–15 cm in diameter. Note the white gills, which turn cream with age, the annulus which is retained on the stem, and the bag-like volvulus which is important for identification. These fungi are almost always found in association with tree roots.

See the British Mycological Society webpage for useful identification keys: http://www.britmycolsoc.org.uk

Image reproduced courtesy of Michael Wood.

recent mushroom ingestion, and the precise identification of the mushroom species by an expert mycologist. As previously noted, the timing of the onset of symptoms, with respect to the mushroom consumption, can be helpful in narrowing down the likely cause. If the fungi are no longer available for identification, a description, or a naming of the species intended for consumption (the edible 'look-alike'), is very helpful to the mycologist. There is, of course, a wide differential diagnosis in the early stages, which includes gastroenteritis and other forms of poisoning.

Amatoxins may be detected by a variety of methods in the mushroom source, in urine and plasma, including radioimmunoassay, high-performance liquid chromatography, and ELISA (enzyme-linked immunosorbent assay). Positive urinary assays may be found up to 96 hours post ingestion, but detection rates fall with time (Jaeger et al. 1993). Assays for other mushroom toxins are not available, although the uncharacterized *A. smithiana* nephrotoxin has been detected by thin-layer chromatography in source material (Apperley et al. 2013).

Gastric contents should also be sent for toxicological and spore analysis (by an expert mycologist), and urea, creatinine, electrolytes, coagulation, liver function, amylase, and urine should be monitored where later onset syndromes are suspected.

Treatment

Fewer than 25% of cases require or receive treatment (Trestrail 1991), but all management should be undertaken in conjunction with expert toxicological advice. Initial treatment is mainly supportive, with fluid resuscitation and gastric lavage (if presenting early and where the individual is not vomiting) on admission. Early-onset neurotoxic syndromes may require atropine to control cholinergic symptoms in cases of muscarine poisoning, and seizure control (usually with benzodiazepines) in cases of gyromitrin, muscimol, and ibotenic acid toxicity (Diaz 2005b).

Suspected amatoxin poisoning should be managed in a facility with expertise in fulminant liver failure and renal support. Activated charcoal is usually recommended, although there are no supporting data. Benzyl penicillin, thioctic acid, and cimetidine have not been shown to be of benefit. N-acetyl cysteine has conflicting evidence for its use, but silbinin (from the milk thistle) is probably the best agent for combatting the effects of amatoxins by inhibiting specific uptake transporter molecules and reducing intrinsic and extrinsic apoptosis (Lacombe and St-Onge 2016). An open multicentre trial is currently ongoing and is scheduled for completion in December 2018.

There are no known antidotes for orellanine poisoning and management is supportive, with renal replacement therapy forming the mainstay for those with severe toxicity; 40–60% of cases will achieve full recovery of renal function, with the remainder requiring chronic haemodialysis or renal transplantation (Karlson-Stiber and Persson 2003).

Environmental toxin exposure

Individuals living or working in damp conditions, on farms, or in buildings ventilated by means of air conditioning are exposed to airborne mycotoxins. The majority of these are products of *Aspergillus, Penicillium, Alternaria, Cladosporium, Chaetomium*, and *Stachybotrys* spp. (Fromme et al. 2016), many of which have already been discussed as food-borne mycotoxins (Table 31.1).

The World Health Organization published a report in 2009 reviewing the evidence for a causal effect between damp building environments and poor health, and concluded that '... there is sufficient evidence of an association between indoor dampness-related factors and a wide range of respiratory health effects, including asthma development, asthma exacerbation, current asthma, respiratory infections, upper respiratory tract symptoms, cough, wheeze and dyspnoea' (WHO 2009). However, the report also states that, '... although it is plausible that heavy exposure to indoor mould or other microbial agents plays a causal role, this has not been established conclusively'.

This effectively summarizes the current difficulty in assessing the significance of air-borne mycotoxins. On the one hand, these toxins have been shown to produce pathological effects in animal and cell models, as noted earlier in this chapter, and they can be detected in human environments. On the other, they are not consistently found in high concentrations in the setting of human disease. For example, a series of studies of residential air and dust found mycotoxin levels to be near or below the level of quantification in most cases and no significant differences between damp buildings and control ones (without water damage) (Fromme et al. 2016). Indeed, the issue is exacerbated by the fact that there are no agreed standards for sampling and assay methods and few reliable data on human inhalation toxicity and the mycotoxin concentrations actually inhaled in these environments.

There are many case reports suggesting a causal relationship between the trichothecenes produced by *Stachybotrys chartarum* (the so-called 'toxic black mould') and a variety of conditions. An initial investigation of a cluster of eight infant cases of pulmonary haemorrhage in Cleveland, Ohio, concluded that there was an association with exposure to *S. chartarum* (CDC 1997). However, a subsequent review of the methodology and analysis of data by external experts criticized these conclusions. It was found that there were errors in the measurements of airborne *S. chartarum* spores, that locations of cases were not blinded (and twice as many samples were taken from the homes of cases), and that in water-damaged homes *S. chartarum* was present in the same percentage of control homes as case homes, suggesting that the fungus was more of a marker of a damp environment than a cause of the disease (CDC 2000).

Nevertheless, it is clear that *S. chartarum* causes stachybotryotoxicosis (a severe, life-threatening disease) in farm animals fed mouldy straw or heavily contaminated feed, via trichothecene toxicity (Fromme et al. 2016), and it seems rational to reduce potential human exposure to such compounds to a minimum. The WHO has published guidelines for reducing mould exposure, based on the avoidance of dampness on internal walls and structures, through the design of well-constructed, well-ventilated, and well-maintained buildings (WHO 2009). It is to be hoped that future studies will clarify exposure levels for toxicity for all of these mycotoxins.

References

Abrunhosa L, Morales H, Soares C, et al. (2016) A review of mycotoxins in food and feed products in Portugal and estimation of probable daily intakes. *Crit Rev Food Sci Nutr* 56: 249–65.

Aguilar F, Harris CC, Sun T, Hollstein M and Cerutti P (1994) Geographic variation of p53 mutational profile in nonmalignant human liver. *Science* 264: 1317–19.

Apperley S, Kroeger P, Kirchmair M, Kiaii M, Holmes DT and Garber I (2013) Laboratory confirmation of Amanita smithiana mushroom poisoning. *Clin Toxicol (Phila)* 51: 249–51.

Bosco F and Mollea C (2012) Mycotoxins in food, *in*: B Valdez, ed., *Food Industrial Processes—Methods and Equipment* (Torino, Italy: InTech), 169–200.

Bressac B, Kew M, Wands J and Ozturk M (1991) Selective G to T mutations of p53 gene in hepatocellular carcinoma from southern Africa. *Nature* 350: 429–31.

Bryden WL (2012) Mycotoxin contamination of the feed supply chain: implications for animal productivity and feed security. *Anim Feed Sci Technol* 173: 134–58.

Caporael LR (1976) Ergotism: the satan loosed in Salem? *Science* 192: 21–6.

Centers for Disease Control and Prevention (CDC) (1997) Pulmonary hemorrhage/hemosiderosis among infants—Cleveland, Ohio, 1993-1996. *MMWR Morb Mortal Wkly Rep* 46: 33–5.

Centers for Disease Control and Prevention (CDC) (2000) **Update**: pulmonary hemorrhage/hemosiderosis among infants—Cleveland, Ohio, 1993–1996. *MMWR Morb Mortal Wkly Rep* 49: 180–4.

Centers for Disease Control and Prevention (CDC) (2004) Outbreak of aflatoxin poisoning—Eastern and Central Provinces, Kenya, January–July 2004. *MMWR* 53: 790–3.

Creppy EE (2002) Update of survey, regulation and toxic effects of mycotoxins in Europe. *Toxicol Lett* 127: 19–28.

Da Rocha MEB, da Freire FCO, Maia FEF, Guedes MIF and Rondina D (2014) Mycotoxins and their effects on human and animal health. *Food Control* 36: 159–65.

Diaz JH (2005a) Evolving global epidemiology, syndromic classification, general management, and prevention of unknown mushroom poisonings. *Crit Care Med* 33: 419–26.

Diaz JH (2005b) Syndromic diagnosis and management of confirmed mushroom poisonings. *Crit Care Med* 33: 427–36.

Ferlay J, Soerjomataram I, Dikshit R, et al. (2015) Cancer incidence and mortality worldwide: sources, methods and major patterns in GLOBOCAN 2012. *Int J Cancer* 136: E359–86.

Ficheux AS, Sibiril Y, le Garrec R and Parent-Massin D (2012) In vitro myelotoxicity assessment of the emerging mycotoxins Beauvericin, Enniatin b and Moniliformin on human hematopoietic progenitors. *Toxicon* 59: 182–91.

Filazi A and Sireli UT (2013) Occurrence of aflatoxins in food, *in*: M Razzaghi-Abyaneh, ed., *Aflatoxins—Recent Advances and Future Prospects* (Ankara, Turkey: InTech). doi: 10.5772/51031

Frank H, Zilker T, Kirchmair M, et al. (2009) Acute renal failure by ingestion of Cortinarius species confounded with psychoactive mushrooms: a case series and literature survey. *Clin Nephrol* 71: 557–62.

Fromme H, Gareis M, Völkel W and Gottschalk C (2016) Overall internal exposure to mycotoxins and their occurrence in occupational and residential settings—an overview. *Int J Hyg Environ Health* 219: 143–65.

Garcia GD, Goff JM, Hadro NC, O'Donnell SD and Greatorex PS (2000) Chronic ergot toxicity: a rare cause of lower extremity ischemia. *J Vasc Surg* 31: 1245–7.

Gerhards N, Neubauer L, Tudzynski P and Li SM (2014) Biosynthetic pathways of ergot alkaloids. *Toxins (Basel)* 6: 3281–95.

Glenn AE (2007) Mycotoxigenic Fusarium species in animal feed. *Anim Feed Sci Technol* 137: 213–40.

Goldblatt L (ed.) (1969) *Aflatoxin: Scientific background, control, and implications* (New York: Academic Press).

Graeme KA (2014) Mycetism: a review of the recent literature. *J Med Toxicol* 10: 173–89.

Guindon KA, Bedard LL and Massey TE (2007) Elevation of 8-hydroxydeoxyguanosine in DNA from isolated mouse lung cells following in vivo treatment with aflatoxin B1. *Toxicol Sci* 98: 57–62.

IARC (International Agency for Research on Cancer), IARC Monographs on the Evaluation of Carcinogenic Risks to Humans, http://monographs.iarc.fr/ENG/Classification/latest_classif.php, accessed 10 June 2017.

Iyer RS, Voehler MW and Harris TM (1994) Adenine adduct of aflatoxin B1 epoxide. *J Am Chem Soc* 116: 8863–9.

Jaeger A, Jehl F, Flesch F, Sauder P and Kopferschmitt J (1993) Kinetics of amatoxins in human poisoning: therapeutic implications. *J Toxicol* 31: 63–80.

Karlson-Stiber C and Persson H (2003) Cytotoxic fungi—an overview. *Toxicon* 42: 339–49.

Krishnamachari KA, Bhat RV, Nagarajan V and Tilak TB (1975) Hepatitis due to aflatoxicosis. An outbreak in Western India. *Lancet* 1: 1061–3.

Lacombe G and St-Onge M (2016) Best evidence topic reports. BET 1: Silibinin in suspected amatoxin-containing mushroom poisoning. *Emerg Med J* 33: 76–7.

Levy DD, Groopman, JD, Lim SE, Seidman MM and Kraemer KH (1992) Sequence specificity of aflatoxin B1-induced mutations in a plasmid replicated in xeroderma pigmentosum and DNA repair proficient human cells. *Cancer Res* 52: 5668–73.

Lima AD, Costa Fortes R, Carvalho Garbi Novaes MR and Percário S (2012) Poisonous mushrooms: a review of the most common intoxications. *Nutr Hosp* 27: 402–8.

Logrieco A, Ferracane R, Haidukowsky M, Cozzi G, Visconti A and Ritieni A (2009) Fumonisin B(2) production by Aspergillus niger from grapes and natural occurrence in must. *Food Addit Contam Part A Chem Anal Control Expo Risk Assess* 26: 1495–500.

Logrieco A, Moretti A, Castella G, et al. (1998) Beauvericin production by Fusarium species. *Appl Environ Microbiol* 64: 3084–8.

Lye MS, Ghazali AA, Mohan J, Alwin N and Nair RC (1995) An outbreak of acute hepatic encephalopathy due to severe aflatoxicosis in Malaysia. *Am J Trop Med Hyg* 53: 68–72.

Marin S, Ramos AJ, Cano-Sancho G and Sanchis V (2013) Mycotoxins: occurrence, toxicology, and exposure assessment. *Food Chem Toxicol* 60: 218–37.

Martinović T, Andjelković U, Gajdošik MŠ, Rešetar D and Josić D (2016) Foodborne pathogens and their toxins. *Proteomics* 147: 226–35.

Michelot D and Toth B (1991) Poisoning by Gyromitra esculenta—a review. *J Appl Toxicol* 11: 235–43.
Moake MM, Padilla-Zakour OI and Worobo RW (2005) Comprehensive review of patulin control methods in foods. *Compre Rev Food Sci Food Saf* 4: 8–21.
Mogensen JM, Frisvad JC, Thrane U and Nielsen KF (2010) Production of Fumonisin B2 and B4 by Aspergillus niger on grapes and raisins. *J Agric Food Chem* 58: 954–8.
Nordt SP and Clark RF (2000) 5-year analysis of mushroom exposures in California. *West J Med* 173: 314–17.
Oliveira PM, Zannini E and Arendt EK (2014) Cereal fungal infection, mycotoxins, and lactic acid bacteria mediated bioprotection: from crop farming to cereal products. *Food Microbiol* 37: 78–95.
Passie T, Seifert J, Schneider U and Emrich HM (2002) The pharmacology of psilocybin. *Addict Biol* 7: 357–64.
Pfohl-Leszkowicz A and Manderville RA (2007) Ochratoxin A: an overview on toxicity and carcinogenicity in animals and humans. *Mol Nutr Food Res* 51: 61–99.
Pitt JI (2000) Toxigenic fungi and mycotoxins. *Br Med Bull* 56: 184–92.
Public Health England (2014) https://www.gov.uk/government/news/take-care-when-picking-mushrooms-poisons-experts-warn, accessed 20 May 2017.
Puel O, Galtier P and Oswald IP (2010) Biosynthesis and toxicological effects of patulin. *Toxins* 2: 613–31.
Rattanvilay K, Tavares N, Eliaser G, et al. (1982) Mushroom poisoning among Laotian refugees—1981. *MMWR Morb Mortal Wkly Rep* 31: 287–8.
Ross RK, Yuan JM, Yu MC, et al. (1992) Urinary aflatoxin biomarkers and risk of hepatocellular carcinoma. *Lancet* 339: 943–6.
Rotter BA (1996) Invited review: toxicology of deoxynivalenol (vomitoxin). *J Toxicol Environ Health* 48: 1–34.
Santi L, Maggioli C, Mastroroberto M, Tufoni M, Napoli L and Caraceni P (2012) Acute liver failure caused by Amanita phalloides poisoning. *Int J Hepatol* 2012: 1–6.
Spanos N and Gottlieb J (1976) Ergotism and the Salem Village witch trials. *Science* 194: 1390–4.
Stiborová M, Arlt VM and Schmeiser HH (2016) Balkan endemic nephropathy: an update on its aetiology. *Arch Toxicol.* 90: 2595–615.
Stokilde-Jorgensen H, Jacobson N, Warncke E and Heinemeier J (2008) The intestines of a more than 2000 years old peat-bog man: microscopy, magnetic resonance imaging and ^{14}C-dating. *J Archaeol Sci* 35: 530–4.
Trestrail JH 3rd (1991) Mushroom poisoning in the United States: an analysis of 1989 United States Poison Center data. *J Toxicol Clin Toxicol* 45: 459–65.
Voss KA, Smith GW and Haschek WM (2007) Fumonisins: toxicokinetics, mechanism of action and toxicity. *Anim Feed Sci Technol* 137: 299–325.
Walkembach J, Brüss M, Urban BW and Barann M (Oct 2005) Interactions of metoclopramide and ergotamine with human 5-HT3A receptors and human 5-HT reuptake carriers. *Br J Pharmacol* 146: 543–52.
West PL, Lindgren J and Horowitz BZ (2009) Amanita smithiana mushroom ingestion: a case of delayed renal failure and literature review. *J Med Toxicol* 5: 32–8.
WHO (2009) *WHO Guidelines for Indoor Air Quality: Dampness and Mould* (Geneva: World Health Organization).
Wieland T, Gotzendorfer C, Zanotti G and Vaisius AC (1981) The effect of the chemical nature of the side chains of amatoxins in the inhibition of eukaryotic RNA polymerase B. *Eur J Biochem* 117: 161–4.
Wild CP, Miller JD and Groopman JD (eds) (2015) *Mycotoxin Control in Low and Middle-Income Countries* (Lyon, France: International Agency for Research on Cancer).
Wu HC, Wang Q, Yang HI, et al. (2009) Aflatoxin B1 exposure, hepatitis B virus infection, and hepatocellular carcinoma in Taiwan. *Cancer Epidemiol Biomarkers Prev* 18: 846–53.
Yazar S and Omurtag GZ (2008) Fumonisins, trichothecenes and zearalenone in cereals. *Int J Mol Sci* 9: 2062–90.
Zinedine A, Soriano JM, Molto JC and Manes J (2007) Review on the toxicity, occurrence, metabolism, detoxification, regulations and intake of zearalenone: an oestrogenic mycotoxin. *Food Chem Toxicol* 45: 1–18.

SECTION 4

Fungal infections in specific patient groups

CHAPTER 32

Fungal infections in haemato-oncology

Philipp Koehler and Oliver A. Cornely

Introduction to fungal infections in haemato-oncology

A wide variety of strategies for the prevention and management of fungal infections arise from the lack of reliable diagnostics for invasive fungal diseases and for different patient cohorts. Each invasive fungal disease has a typical set of varying risk factors defining a high-risk patient population. However, the challenge in managing invasive fungal disease in everyday patient care is predominantly found on haematology wards (Wisplinghoff et al. 2004; Maschmeyer et al. 2015). There are three major entities—invasive candidiasis, invasive aspergillosis (IA), and mucormycosis—which account for the vast majority of fungal infections in haematology and oncology (Maschmeyer et al. 2007; Pfaller and Diekema 2007; Lewis et al. 2013; Wisplinghoff et al. 2014; Koehler et al. 2016a).

Epidemiology

The daily candidaemia incidence in Europe is 63 (95% confidence interval [CI], range 60–64), of which 22 (95% CI, range 21–23) have a fatal outcome (Koehler et al. 2016b). The incidence increases from patients with solid tumours to haematopoietic stem cell transplantation (HSCT) recipients. In addition, indications for immunosuppressive therapy and HSCT are expanding (Gyurkocza et al. 2010). Recent studies report an involvement of rare yeast pathogens in up to 5% of patients with fungaemia (Cuenca-Estrella et al. 2012), and discussion as to whether there is a shift to non-*albicans Candida* species remains unanswered (Playford et al. 2008; Andes et al. 2012).

The incidence of IA in patients with acute leukaemia ranges from 5% to 12% (Pagano et al. 2007b; Cornely et al. 2014b; Koehler et al. 2016b). For allogeneic HSCT recipients, the cumulative incidence 12 months after transplantation is 3.9–16.4% with an unrelated donor, 3.2–8.1% with a human leucocyte antigen (HLA)-mismatched related donor, and 2.3–11.3% with an HLA-matched related donor (Morgan et al. 2005; Kontoyiannis et al. 2010; Nucci et al. 2013). In autologous stem cell transplant recipients, the incidence of IA is 0.4–1.2% (Morgan et al. 2005; Pagano et al. 2007a; Kontoyiannis et al. 2010).

Mucormycosis is the third most common entity (Petrikkos et al. 2012) and comes with particularly high morbidity and mortality (Roden et al. 2005). Among patients undergoing chemotherapy or allogeneic HSCT, an incidence of 7% was found (Neofytos et al. 2009).

Immunosuppression

Patients at risk for invasive fungal disease usually have a compromised immune system. Patients with acute leukaemia, myelodysplastic syndrome, or aplastic anaemia develop bone marrow failure due to underlying disease (Kume et al. 2003; Pagano et al. 2006; Dohner et al. 2010; Cornely et al. 2014b). In addition, intensive chemotherapy causes prolonged neutropenia. Patients receiving HSCT have three at-risk periods: first, when they undergo conditioning chemotherapy with prolonged neutropenia; second, after engraftment, immunosuppression often relying on glucocorticosteroids, T-cell depletion, and tumour necrosis factor-α inhibition for acute graft-versus-host disease (GvHD) (Marty et al. 2003; Lewis et al. 2013); and third, in cases of chronic GvHD, defined as occurring more than 100 days post HSCT (Marty and Rubin 2006). Risk for IA varies throughout these three periods and also according to the extent of HLA discordance between donor and recipient (Morgan et al. 2005). Both the duration and degree of neutropenia determine the risk of developing invasive fungal disease.

Specific host and therapeutic factors predisposing to invasive fungal disease

Well-known risk factors and conditions for invasive candidiasis are neutropenia, indwelling central venous catheters, (number of) broad-spectrum antibiotics, the extremes of age, mucosal *Candida* colonization, recent gastrointestinal surgery, prolonged intensive care unit (ICU) stay, and renal failure (Wey et al. 1989; Almirante et al. 2005; Ruping et al. 2008; Andes et al. 2012). In HSCT recipients, there is a complex relationship between GvHD, cytomegalovirus (CMV) reactivation, ganciclovir exposure, and development of IA. Both CMV infection and ganciclovir administration cause myelosuppression and consequently increase the risk for IA (Thursky et al. 2004). Respiratory virus infections per se increase the risk for IA (Marr et al. 2002; Vehreschild et al. 2012).

Predisposing conditions for mucormycosis are diabetes mellitus and ketoacidosis along with iron-overload, some iron chelators, and glucocorticosteroids (Petrikkos et al. 2012; Rammaert et al. 2012). A series of 41 patients with invasive mucormycosis included malignancies as the predominant underlying condition in 63%, followed by diabetes mellitus (17%) and solid organ transplantations (10%) (Ruping et al. 2010).

Clinical presentation

Invasive candidiasis is typically diagnosed by isolation of a *Candida* species in a blood culture, following disruption of the mucosal barrier after chemotherapy (Cornely and Schirmacher 2001). Features of candidaemia are non-specific, and include fever, tachypnoea, sepsis syndrome, and septic shock irresponsive to broad-spectrum antimicrobials (Cornely et al. 2015b). In cases of dissemination, clinical presentation varies according to the affected organ system.

IA typically involves the respiratory tract as ubiquitous *Aspergillus* spores are inhaled by the patient. Non-specific signs of IA include fever, cough, and dyspnoea. Pleuritic chest pain may occur, but is likely to resolve as soon as pleural effusion occurs. Involvement of the paranasal sinuses may result in local clinical signs and symptoms such as epistaxis, cranial-nerve dysfunctions, proptosis and asymmetric facial swelling. Rare manifestations such as skin, bone, and gastrointestinal involvement may occur (Koehler et al. 2014a). In rare cases of disseminated infection, the presentation can be highly variable, as any organ may be involved.

The most common clinical forms of mucormycosis are, in order of decreasing frequency: pulmonary, rhinocerebral, cutaneous, disseminated, and gastrointestinal disease (Petrikkos et al. 2012). Uncommon conditions e.g. endocarditis or osteomyelitis (Koehler et al. 2014b) may also occur. A considerable number of patients are not overtly immunosuppressed (Torres-Narbona et al. 2007) and usually have cutaneous involvement after trauma, inoculation of contaminated material or burns (Skiada and Petrikkos 2009; Neblett Fanfair et al. 2012). Typically, extensive tissue necrosis results from angioinvasion and vessel occlusion. Pulmonary mucormycosis occurs mostly in haematology patients.

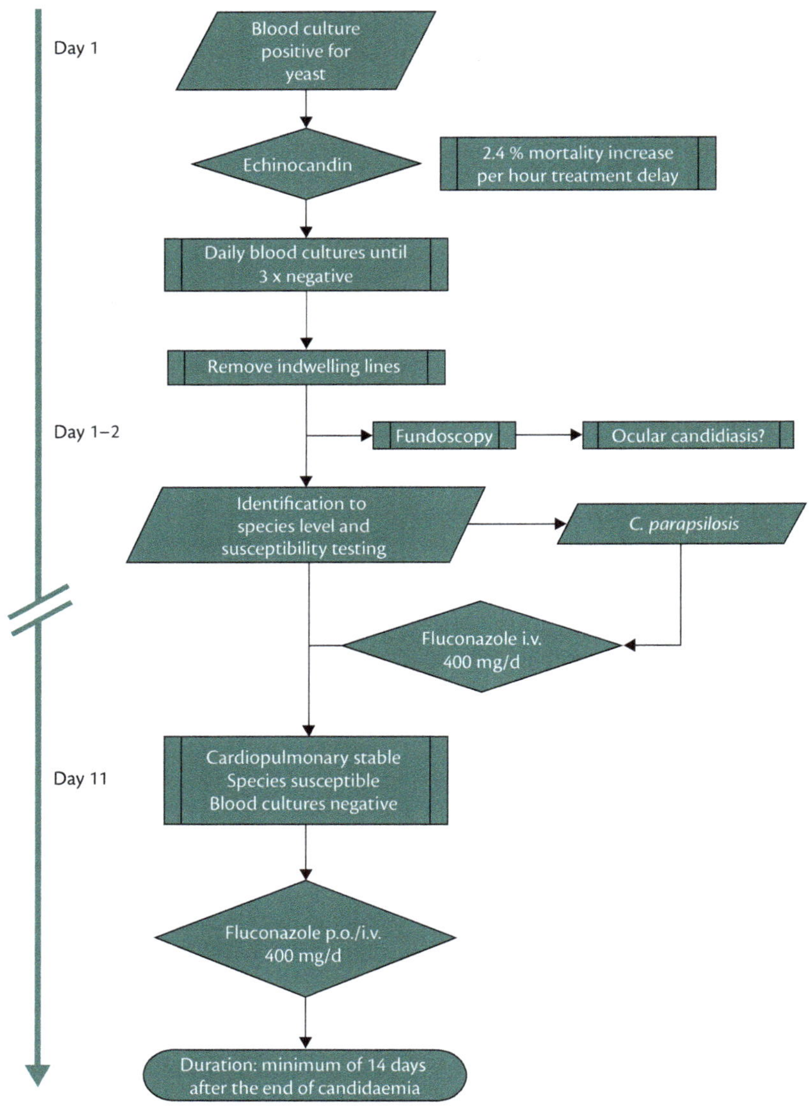

Figure 32.1 *Candida* diagnosis and treatment algorithm.

Reproduced with permission from Koehler P., Tacke D., Cornely O. A., 'Our 2014 approach to candidaemia', *Mycoses*, Volume 57, Issue 10, pp. 581–3, Copyright © 2014 Blackwell Verlag GmbH. DOI: 10.1111/myc.12207.

The clinical presentation is non-specific and similar to IA. Due to angioinvasion, haemoptysis may occur and tissue destruction can result in lung collapse and airway obstruction (Gupta et al. 1998). Invasive growth may spread beyond organ boundaries, e.g. splenic, mediastinal or chest wall invasion (Asai et al. 2003). Rhinocerebral involvement is predominantly observed in patients with diabetes mellitus (Roden et al. 2005), although this has been described in the haematological setting as well (Vehreschild et al. 2013).

Diagnosis

Candidaemia is diagnosed by growth of *Candida* species from peripheral and central line blood cultures, with a sensitivity of 50-75% (De Pauw et al. 2008; Cuenca-Estrella et al. 2012). After establishing the diagnosis, daily blood cultures should be taken until at least two consecutive samples are negative (Ullmann et al. 2012a). Ocular candidiasis should be ruled out by fundoscopy and may require prolonged treatment courses (Oude Lashof et al. 2011; Ullmann et al. 2012a) (Figure 32.1). If candidemia persists more than 5 days into targeted treatment, an endovascular source needs to be ruled out by trans-oesophageal echocardiography for *Candida* endocarditis (Tacke et al. 2013), and vessel ultrasound to search for thrombosis (Cornely et al. 2012; Ullmann et al. 2012a). When only fever persists, in particular beyond recovery from neutropenia, computed tomography (CT) or (contrast enhanced) abdominal ultrasound should be performed to look for hepatosplenic candidiasis (Figure 32.2) (Cornely et al. 2015a).

In patients with fever during neutropenia, which is unresponsive to antibiotic treatment and persists for 72-96 hours, CT of the chest is highly sensitive and rules out pneumonia and pulmonary aspergillosis or mucormycosis (Figure 32.3). Infiltrates of macronodular shape surrounded by a perimeter of ground-glass opacity is suggestive of IA (Figure 32.4). Halos correspond to alveolar haemorrhage and angio-invasion. An inverse halo (a.k.a. reverse halo or atoll sign) should draw clinical suspicion towards the possibility of mucormycosis (Figure 32.5). Additional neurological findings, facial asymmetries, or swellings should trigger head and brain imaging to rule out sinus and bony erosion, specifically of orbits and the skull base.

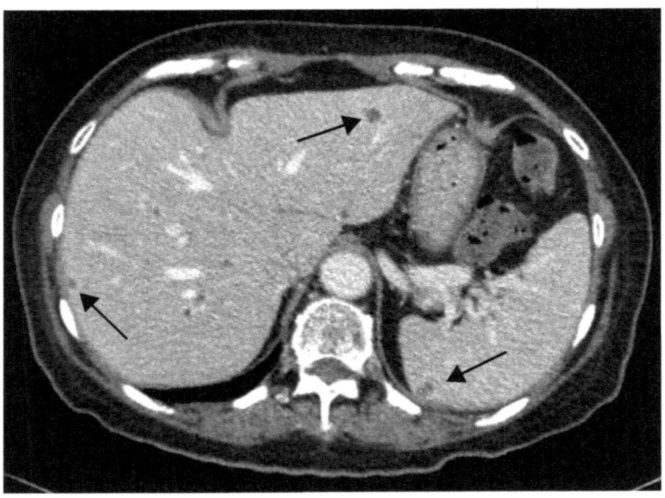

Figure 32.2 Computed tomography image reveals disseminated lesions in liver and spleen in hepatosplenic candidiasis.

However, none of the findings is pathognomonic (Figures 32.3–32.5). Rather further diagnostic work-up should be initiated immediately, including broncho-alveolar lavage and the fluid should be cultured and tested for the presence of galactomannan (GM). Fungal disease is proven only by culture from physiologically sterile material (blood, cerebrospinal fluid or biopsy) or histopathological evidence of tissue invasion (De Pauw et al. 2008). Unfortunately this has not changed since the nineteenth century (Virchow 1856; Paltauf 1885).

Radiographic imaging, changes with the administration of antifungal medication and recovery from neutropenia. The development of crescent shaped gas collection within the area of consolidation indicates the recovery of white blood cell function and is called the air crescent sign (Figure 32.6). This finding heralds a favourable outcome, whereas an increase in lung infiltrates beyond day 7 places patients at very high risk (Brodoefel et al. 2006; Caillot et al. 2010) (Figure 32.3).

Prophylaxis and Treatment Strategies

Invasive Candidiasis

Prophylaxis

Candida-directed prophylaxis is of differential benefit for allogeneic HSCT, autologous HSCT and severe, prolonged neutropenic patients. Azoles, in particular fluconazole (Goodman et al. 1992; Slavin et al. 1995; Morgenstern et al. 1999; Marr et al. 2000; Marr et al. 2004) and voriconazole (Wingard et al. 2010) are recommended during neutropenia following conditioning chemotherapy for allogeneic HSCT (Ullmann et al. 2012a). For invasive candidiasis, micafungin and posaconazole have yielded similar results to fluconazole (van Burik et al. 2004; Ullmann et al. 2007).

In the remaining settings of autologous HSCT and prolonged neutropenia, data specific to prophylaxis for invasive candidiasis is lacking. One reason for this is that all antifungals active against *Aspergillus* are active against *Candida*, too, so there is an inherent overlap of preventative strategies. However, autologous HSCT patients are not at high-risk for invasive candidiasis (Ullmann et al. 2012a). For patients with prolonged neutropenia only one trial has demonstrated improved survival rates (with posaconazole prophylaxis), but the benefit was not attributed to invasive candidiasis (Cornely et al. 2007b).

Fever/diagnostic driven approach (empiric/pre-emptive)

Following chemotherapy with associated prolonged neutropenia, fever is very frequent. With a first fever, broad-spectrum antibacterial treatment is usually commenced. When fever persists for 72-96 hours, antifungal therapy may be added. Such empiric antifungal treatment is usually directed towards invasive yeast and mould diseases; however, different kinds of filamentous fungi have to be considered. Liposomal amphotericin B (Walsh et al. 1999) and caspofungin (Walsh et al. 2004; Maertens et al. 2010) have been recommended for broad-spectrum antifungal efficacy. For pre-emptive therapy, no randomized clinical trials have been performed. Detection of *Candida* species in respiratory, urine or stool samples of asymptomatic neutropenic patients suggests colonisation and should not be treated in isolation (Cornely et al. 2012).

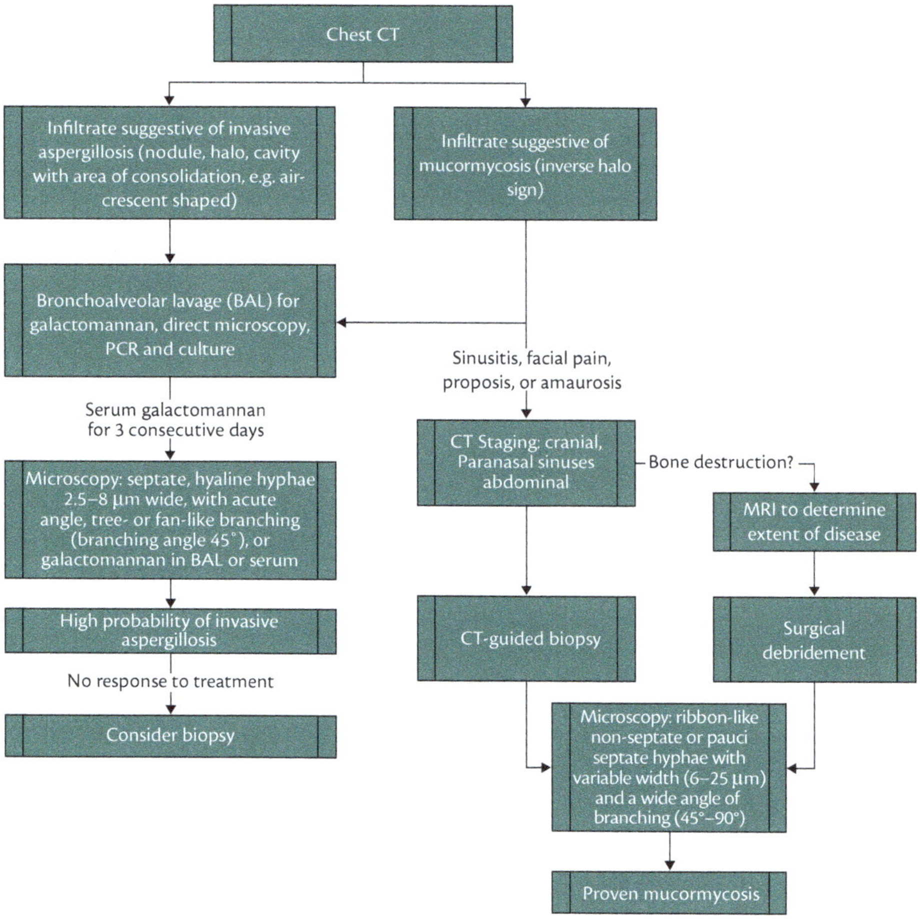

Figure 32.3 Diagnostic algorithm for suspected invasive aspergillosis or mucormycosis.

Adapted with permission from Liss B. et al., 'Our 2015 approach to invasive pulmonary aspergillosis', *Mycoses*, Volume 58, pp. 375–82, Copyright © 2015 Blackwell Verlag GmbH, DOI: 10.1111/myc.319 and Tacke D., Koehler P., Markiefka, M., Cornely A., 'Our 2014 approach to mucormycosis', *Mycoses*, Volume 57, pp. 519–24, Copyright © 2014 Blackwell Verlag GmbH, DOI: 10.1111/myc.12203.

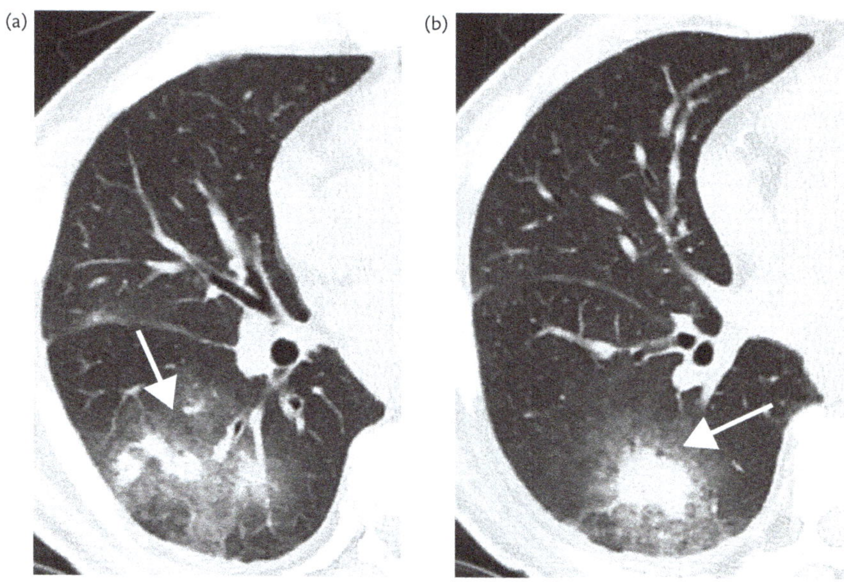

Figure 32.4 Computed tomography images with a dense nodule surrounded by ground-glass opacity as a sign of angio-invasion: the 'halo' sign.
a Slice through outer portion of the lesion; **b** Slice through the centre of the lesion.

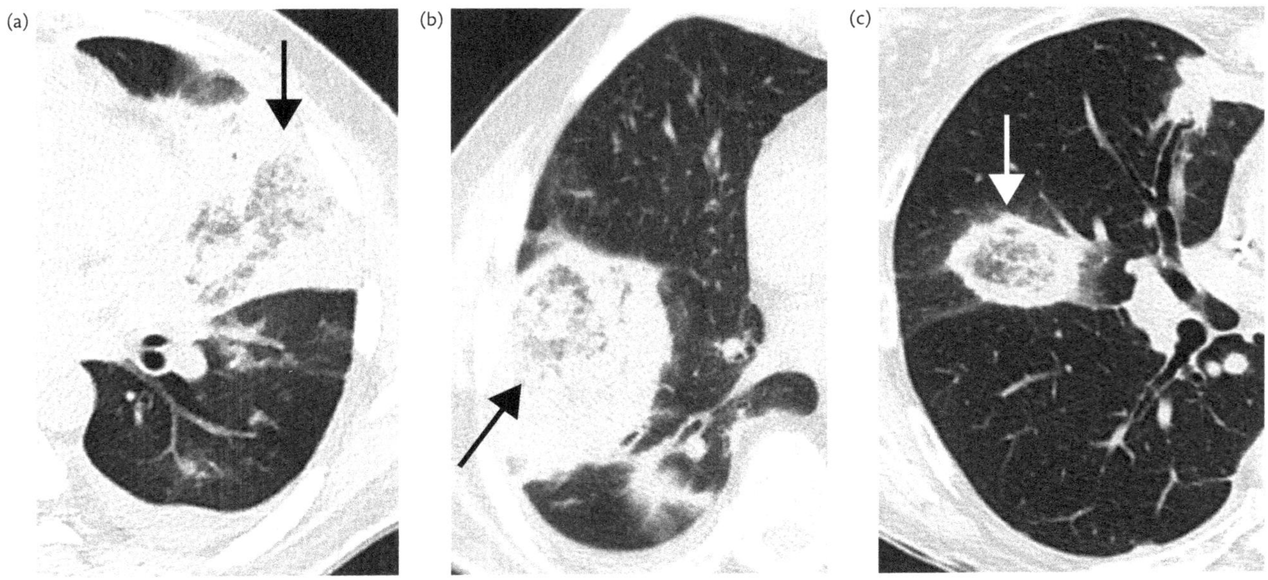

Figure 32.5 Computed tomography images with large areas of consolidation surrounding an area of ground-glass opacity: the 'inverse halo' sign.
a,b,c Different examples of this phenomenon.

Targeted treatment

Echinocandins are the drugs of choice (Mora-Duarte et al. 2002; Kuse et al. 2007; Pappas et al. 2007; Reboli et al. 2007) for candidaemia (Figure 32.1). Since candidaemia increases mortality by 20-49%, delays in commencing antifungal therapy need to be avoided (Blot et al. 2002; Gudlaugsson et al. 2003; Oude Lashof et al. 2003; Morrell et al. 2005; Garey et al. 2006; Taur et al. 2010; Cuenca-Estrella et al. 2012; Ullmann et al. 2012a). Species identification and susceptibility testing are essential to guide treatment (Cornely et al. 2012; Cuenca-Estrella et al. 2012; Ullmann et al. 2012b; Arendrup et al. 2014). If *Candida parapsilosis* complex (*Candida parapsilosis, C. metapsilosis* or *C. orthopsilosis*) is detected, the initial echinocandin regimen should be changed to fluconazole (Cornely et al. 2012). Patients on antifungal prophylaxis may need a class change depending on fungal susceptibility. Fluconazole is a common step down treatment option if susceptibility of isolates is proven (Rex et al. 1994; Anaissie et al. 1996; Ullmann et al. 2012a). Treatment is recommended for at least 14 days after the last positive blood culture (Ullmann et al. 2012a). A step-down to oral formulation is possible, usually after ten days (Koehler et al. 2014c). Complicated or disseminated candidiasis requires prolonged treatment (Ullmann et al. 2012a). Removal of indwelling intravascular catheters is crucial as it increases survival rates (Andes et al. 2012). If removal is not feasible, echinocandins or liposomal amphotericin B will slow biofilm activity (Kuhn et al. 2002; Bernhardt et al. 2011).

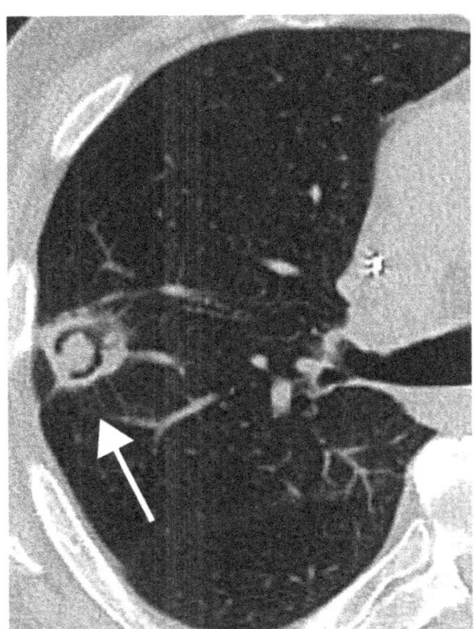

Figure 32.6 Air crescent sign—a crescent-shaped collection of air within the area of consolidation in the left lung indicating recovery from neutropenia.

Invasive Aspergillosis

Prophylaxis

Echinocandins, polyenes and most azoles (but not fluconazole) are active against *Aspergillus* (Tacke et al. 2014a). Allogeneic HSCT recipients and patients with prolonged neutropenia are at high risk for invasive aspergillosis. In the early phase of allogeneic HSCT, micafungin, posaconazole or voriconazole have successfully been used (van Burik et al. 2004; Cornely et al. 2007b; Wingard et al. 2010; Marks et al. 2011; Huang et al. 2012; Tacke et al. 2014a). In the post engraftment period, especially during episodes of GvHD, posaconazole is preferable (Ullmann et al. 2007). For patients with AML, MDS or severe aplastic anaemia and chemotherapy induced neutropenia, posaconazole is the drug of choice (Cornely et al. 2007b; Tacke et al. 2014a). If oral bioavailability of posaconazole liquid formulation appears unreliable in cases of nausea, vomiting or gastrointestinal GvHD, posaconazole tablets are a well-tolerated alternative with more reliable pharmacokinetics (Duarte et al. 2014).

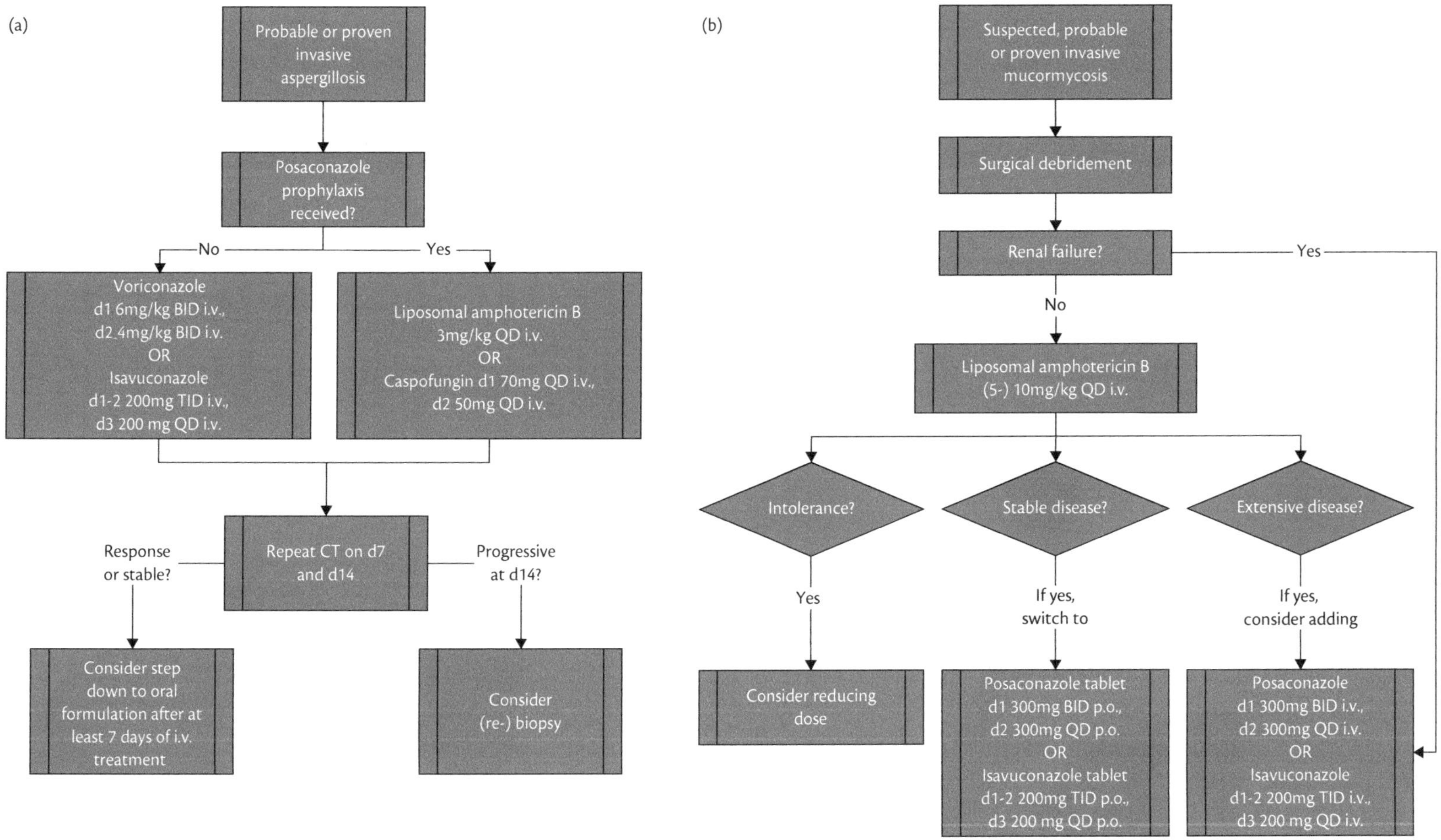

Figure 32.7 Treatment algorithm for **a** invasive aspergillosis and **b** mucormycosis.

Fever/diagnostic driven approach (empiric/pre-emptive)

Fever driven/empiric treatment approaches are mostly based on liposomal amphotericin B, voriconazole and caspofungin (Walsh et al. 1999; Walsh et al. 2002; Walsh et al. 2004). The latest development and clinical data on isavuconazole show non-inferiority in comparison to voriconazole, but improved tolerability for the treatment of invasive aspergillosis (Maertens et al. 2016) Diagnostic driven approaches (pre-emptive) were developed as the true incidence of invasive fungal diseases was estimated to be much lower than the number of patients receiving empiric treatment. Detection of invasive fungal disease is improved by the use of diagnostic tests that enhance sensitivity e.g. CT imaging, serial GM measurements or *Aspergillus* PCR assays (Maertens et al. 2005; Cordonnier et al. 2009; Girmenia et al. 2009; Hebart et al. 2009; Pagano et al. 2011).

Targeted treatment

Targeted therapy for invasive aspergillosis is based on four major trials. Voriconazole is the drug of choice as it showed improved responses and survival, with less side effects, in comparison with amphotericin B deoxycholate (Herbrecht et al. 2002) (Figure 32.7a). Liposomal amphotericin B demonstrated efficacy in highly immunocompromised patients at standard dose, although the compound has not been directly compared to voriconazole (Cornely et al. 2007a). Caspofungin showed inferior response rates for targeted treatment of invasive aspergillosis in several studies (Viscoli et al. 2009; Herbrecht et al. 2010), but similar rates in another trial (Cornely et al. 2011).

Mucormycosis

Prophylaxis

Very few drugs are active against Mucorales, and currently posaconazole is the drug of choice for use in prophylaxis (Cornely et al. 2014a).

Targeted Treatment

For targeted treatment of mucormycosis, no well-designed trial has been published. Surgical debridement is associated with decreased mortality (Tedder et al. 1994) and is an integral part of the treatment concept, as is immediate treatment with liposomal amphotericin B or isavuconazole. (Tedder et al. 1994; Cornely et al. 2014a; Koehler and Cornely 2016; Maertens et al. 2016; Marty et al. 2016). For salvage therapy, posaconazole is strongly recommended (Figure 32.7b) (Cornely et al. 2014a). The combination of isavuconazole or posaconazole with liposomal amphotericin B is a further option in patients with extensive disease (Pagano et al. 2013; Cornely et al. 2014a; Koehler and Cornely 2016).

References

Almirante B, Rodriguez D, Park BJ, et al. (2005) Epidemiology and predictors of mortality in cases of Candida bloodstream infection: results from population-based surveillance, Barcelona, Spain, from 2002 to 2003. *J Clin Microbiol* 43: 1829–35.

Anaissie EJ, Darouiche RO, Abi-Said D, et al. (1996) Management of invasive candidal infections: results of a prospective, randomized, multicenter study of fluconazole versus amphotericin B and review of the literature. *Clin Infect Dis* 23: 964–72.

Andes DR, Safdar N, Baddley JW, et al. (2012) Impact of treatment strategy on outcomes in patients with candidemia and other forms of invasive candidiasis: a patient-level quantitative review of randomized trials. *Clin Infect Dis* 54: 1110–22.

Arendrup MC, Boekhout T, Akova M, et al. (2014) ESCMID and ECMM joint clinical guidelines for the diagnosis and management of rare invasive yeast infections. *Clin Microbiol Infect* 20 (Suppl. 3): 76–98.

Asai K, Suzuki K, Takahashi T, Ito Y, Kazui T and Kita Y (2003) Pulmonary resection with chest wall removal and reconstruction for invasive pulmonary mucormycosis during antileukemia chemotherapy. *Jpn J Thorac Cardiovasc Surg* 51: 163–6.

Bernhardt H, Knoke M and Bernhardt J (2011) Efficacy of anidulafungin against biofilms of different Candida species in long-term trials of continuous flow cultivation. *Mycoses* 54: e821–7.

Blot SI, Vandewoude KH, Hoste EA and Colardyn FA (2002) Effects of nosocomial candidemia on outcomes of critically ill patients. *Am J Med* 113: 480–5.

Brodoefel H, Vogel M, Hebart H, et al. (2006) Long-term CT follow-up in 40 non-HIV immunocompromised patients with invasive pulmonary aspergillosis: kinetics of CT morphology and correlation with clinical findings and outcome. *AJR Am J Roentgenol* 187: 404–13.

Caillot D, Latrabe V, Thiebaut A, et al. (2010) Computer tomography in pulmonary invasive aspergillosis in hematological patients with neutropenia: an useful tool for diagnosis and assessment of outcome in clinical trials. *Eur J Radiol* 74: e172–5.

Cordonnier C, Pautas C, Maury S, et al. (2009) Empirical versus preemptive antifungal therapy for high-risk, febrile, neutropenic patients: a randomized, controlled trial. *Clin Infect Dis* 48: 1042–51.

Cornely OA, Arikan-Akdagli S, Dannaoui E, et al. (2014a) ESCMID and ECMM joint clinical guidelines for the diagnosis and management of mucormycosis 2013. *Clin Microbiol Infect* 20 (Suppl. 3): 5–26.

Cornely OA, Bangard C and Jaspers NI (2015a) Hepatosplenic candidiasis. *Clin Liver Dis (Hoboken)* 6: 47–50.

Cornely OA, Bassetti M, Calandra T, et al. (2012) ESCMID* guideline for the diagnosis and management of Candida diseases 2012: non-neutropenic adult patients. *Clin Microbiol Infect* 18 (Suppl. 7): 19–37.

Cornely OA, Gachot B, Akan H, et al. (2015b) Epidemiology and outcome of fungemia in a cancer Cohort of the Infectious Diseases Group (IDG) of the European Organization for Research and Treatment of Cancer (EORTC 65031). *Clin Infect Dis* 61: 324–31.

Cornely OA, Leguay T, Maertens J, et al. (2014b) A Double-Blind, Multicentre, Randomised, Placebo-Controlled Study to Assess the Efficacy, Safety and Tolerability of Prophylactic Liposomal Amphotericin B (AmBisome®) for the Prevention of Invasive Fungal Infections in Subjects Receiving Remission-Induction Chemotherapy for Acute Lymphoblastic Leukaemia (AmBiGuard trial). *Poster session presented at: American Society of Hematology. 56th ASH Annual Meeting and Exposition; 2014 Dec 6-9; San Francisco, CA.*

Cornely OA, Maertens J, Bresnik M, et al. (2007) Liposomal amphotericin B as initial therapy for invasive mold infection: a randomized trial comparing a high-loading dose regimen with standard dosing (AmBiLoad trial). *Clin Infect Dis* 44: 1289–97.

Cornely OA, Maertens J, Winston DJ, et al. (2007b) Posaconazole vs. fluconazole or itraconazole prophylaxis in patients with neutropenia. *N Engl J Med* 356: 348–59.

Cornely OA and Schirmacher P (2001) Clinical picture: bacterial translocation in neutropenic sepsis. *Lancet* 358: 1842.

Cornely OA, Vehreschild JJ, Vehreschild MJ, et al. (2011) Phase II dose escalation study of caspofungin for invasive Aspergillosis. *Antimicrob Agents Chemother* 55: 5798–803.

Cuenca-Estrella M, Verweij PE, Arendrup MC, et al. (2012) ESCMID* guideline for the diagnosis and management of Candida diseases 2012: diagnostic procedures. *Clin Microbiol Infect* 18 (Suppl. 7): 9–18.

De Pauw B, Walsh TJ, Donnelly JP, et al. (2008) Revised definitions of invasive fungal disease from the European Organization for Research and Treatment of Cancer/Invasive Fungal Infections Cooperative Group and the National Institute of Allergy and Infectious Diseases Mycoses Study Group (EORTC/MSG) Consensus Group. *Clin Infect Dis* 46: 1813–21.

Dohner H, Estey EH, Amadori S, et al. (2010) Diagnosis and management of acute myeloid leukemia in adults: recommendations from an international expert panel, on behalf of the European LeukemiaNet. *Blood* 115: 453–74.

Duarte RF, Lopez-Jimenez J, Cornely OA, et al. (2014) Phase 1b study of new posaconazole tablet for prevention of invasive fungal infections in high-risk patients with neutropenia. *Antimicrob Agents Chemother* 58: 5758–65.

Garey KW, Rege M, Pai MP, et al. (2006) Time to initiation of fluconazole therapy impacts mortality in patients with candidemia: a multi-institutional study. *Clin Infect Dis* 43: 25–31.

Girmenia C, Barosi G, Aversa F, et al. (2009) Prophylaxis and treatment of invasive fungal diseases in allogeneic stem cell transplantation: results of a consensus process by Gruppo Italiano Trapianto di Midollo Osseo (GITMO). *Clin Infect Dis* 49: 1226–36.

Goodman JL, Winston DJ, Greenfield RA, et al. (1992) A controlled trial of fluconazole to prevent fungal infections in patients undergoing bone marrow transplantation. *N Engl J Med* 326: 845–51.

Gudlaugsson O, Gillespie S, Lee K, et al. (2003) Attributable mortality of nosocomial candidemia, revisited. *Clin Infect Dis* 37: 1172–7.

Gupta KL, Khullar DK, Behera D, Radotra BD and Sakhuja V (1998) Pulmonary mucormycosis presenting as fatal massive haemoptysis in a renal transplant recipient. *Nephrol Dial Transplant* 13: 3258–60.

Gyurkocza B, Rezvani A and Storb RF (2010) Allogeneic hematopoietic cell transplantation: the state of the art. *Expert Rev Hematol* 3: 285–99.

Hebart H, Klingspor L, Klingebiel T, et al. (2009) A prospective randomized controlled trial comparing PCR-based and empirical treatment with liposomal amphotericin B in patients after allo-SCT. *Bone Marrow Transplant* 43: 553–61.

Herbrecht R, Denning DW, Patterson TF, et al. (2002) Voriconazole versus amphotericin B for primary therapy of invasive aspergillosis. *N Engl J Med* 347: 408–15.

Herbrecht R, Maertens J, Baila L, et al. (2010) Caspofungin first-line therapy for invasive aspergillosis in allogeneic hematopoietic stem cell transplant patients: an European Organisation for Research and Treatment of Cancer study. *Bone Marrow Transplant* 45: 1227–33.

Huang X, Chen H, Han M, et al. (2012) Multicenter, randomized, open-label study comparing the efficacy and safety of micafungin versus itraconazole for prophylaxis of invasive fungal infections in patients undergoing hematopoietic stem cell transplant. *Biol Blood Marrow Transplant* 18: 1509–16.

Koehler P and Cornely OA (2016) Contemporary strategies in the prevention and management of fungal infections. *Infect Dis Clin North Am* 30: 265–75.

Koehler P, Cornely OA, Tacke D, Vehreschild MJGT, Wissplinghoff H and Vehreschild J-J (2016a) P1559—meta-analysis of incidence and mortality of candidaemia in Europe. *ECCMID 2016—Amsterdam, The Netherlands. Poster presentation.*

Koehler P, Hamprecht A, Bader O, et al. (2016b) Epidemiology of invasive aspergillosis and azole resistance in patients with acute leukaemia: the SEPIA Study. *Int J Antimicrob Agents* 49: 218–23.

Koehler P, Tacke D and Cornely OA (2014a) Aspergillosis of bones and joints—a review from 2002 until today. *Mycoses* 57: 323–35.

Koehler P, Tacke D and Cornely OA (2014b) Bone and joint infections by Mucorales, Scedosporium, Fusarium and even rarer fungi. *Crit Rev Microbiol*: 42: 158–171.

Koehler P, Tacke D and Cornely OA (2014c) Our 2014 approach to candidaemia. *Mycoses* 57: 581–3.

Kontoyiannis DP, Marr KA, Park BJ, et al. (2010) Prospective surveillance for invasive fungal infections in hematopoietic stem cell transplant recipients, 2001–2006: overview of the Transplant-Associated Infection Surveillance Network (TRANSNET) Database. *Clin Infect Dis* 50: 1091–100.

Kuhn DM, George T, Chandra J, Mukherjee PK and Ghannoum MA (2002) Antifungal susceptibility of Candida biofilms: unique efficacy of amphotericin B lipid formulations and echinocandins. *Antimicrob Agents Chemother* 46: 1773–80.

Kume H, Yamazaki T, Abe M, Tanuma H, Okudaira M and Okayasu I (2003) Increase in aspergillosis and severe mycotic infection in patients with leukemia and MDS: comparison of the data from the Annual of the Pathological Autopsy Cases in Japan in 1989, 1993 and 1997. *Pathol Int* 53: 744–50.

Kuse ER, Chetchotisakd P, Da Cunha CA, et al. (2007) Micafungin versus liposomal amphotericin B for candidaemia and invasive candidosis: a phase III randomised double-blind trial. *Lancet* 369: 1519–27.

Lewis RE, Cahyame-Zuniga L, Leventakos K, et al. (2013) Epidemiology and sites of involvement of invasive fungal infections in patients with haematological malignancies: a 20-year autopsy study. *Mycoses* 56: 638–45.

Liss B, Vehreschild JJ, Bangard C, et al. (2015) Our 2015 approach to invasive pulmonary aspergillosis. *Mycoses* 58: 375–82.

Maertens JA, Madero L, Reilly AF, et al. (2010) A randomized, double-blind, multicenter study of caspofungin versus liposomal amphotericin B for empiric antifungal therapy in pediatric patients with persistent fever and neutropenia. *Pediatr Infect Dis J* 29: 415–20.

Maertens JA, Raad II, Marr KA, et al. (2016) Isavuconazole versus voriconazole for primary treatment of invasive mould disease caused by Aspergillus and other filamentous fungi (SECURE): a phase 3, randomised-controlled, non-inferiority trial. *Lancet* 387: 760–9.

Maertens J, Theunissen K, Verhoef G, et al. (2005) Galactomannan and computed tomography-based preemptive antifungal therapy in neutropenic patients at high risk for invasive fungal infection: a prospective feasibility study. *Clin Infect Dis* 41: 1242–50.

Marks DI, Pagliuca A, Kibbler CC, et al. (2011) Voriconazole versus itraconazole for antifungal prophylaxis following allogeneic haematopoietic stem-cell transplantation. *Br J Haematol* 155: 318–27.

Marr KA, Carter RA, Boeckh M, Martin P and Corey L (2002) Invasive aspergillosis in allogeneic stem cell transplant recipients: changes in epidemiology and risk factors. *Blood* 100: 4358–66.

Marr KA, Crippa F, Leisenring W, et al. (2004) Itraconazole versus fluconazole for prevention of fungal infections in patients receiving allogeneic stem cell transplants. *Blood* 103: 1527–33.

Marr KA, Seidel K, Slavin MA, et al. (2000) Prolonged fluconazole prophylaxis is associated with persistent protection against candidiasis-related death in allogeneic marrow transplant recipients: long-term follow-up of a randomized, placebo-controlled trial. *Blood* 96: 2055–61.

Marty FM, Lee SJ, Fahey MM, et al. (2003) Infliximab use in patients with severe graft-versus-host disease and other emerging risk factors of non-Candida invasive fungal infections in allogeneic hematopoietic stem cell transplant recipients: a cohort study. *Blood* 102: 2768–76.

Marty FM, Ostrosky-Zeichner L, Cornely OA, et al. (2016) Isavuconazole treatment for mucormycosis: a single-arm open-label trial and case-control analysis. *Lancet Infect Dis* 16: 828–37.

Marty FM and Rubin RH (2006) The prevention of infection post-transplant: the role of prophylaxis, preemptive and empiric therapy. *Transpl Int* 19: 2–11.

Maschmeyer G, Carratala J, Buchheidt D, et al. (2015) Diagnosis and antimicrobial therapy of lung infiltrates in febrile neutropenic patients (allogeneic SCT excluded): updated guidelines of the Infectious Diseases Working Party (AGIHO) of the German Society of Hematology and Medical Oncology (DGHO). *Ann Oncol* 26: 21–33.

Maschmeyer G, Haas A and Cornely OA (2007) Invasive aspergillosis: epidemiology, diagnosis and management in immunocompromised patients. *Drugs* 67: 1567–601.

Mora-Duarte J, Betts R, Rotstein C, et al. (2002) Comparison of caspofungin and amphotericin B for invasive candidiasis. *N Engl J Med* 347: 2020–9.

Morgan J, Wannemuehler KA, Marr KA, et al. (2005) Incidence of invasive aspergillosis following hematopoietic stem cell and solid organ transplantation: interim results of a prospective multicenter surveillance program. *Med Mycol* 43 (Suppl. 1): S49–58.

Morgenstern GR, Prentice AG, Prentice HG, Ropner JE, Schey SA and Warnock DW (1999) A randomized controlled trial of itraconazole

versus fluconazole for the prevention of fungal infections in patients with haematological malignancies. U.K. Multicentre Antifungal Prophylaxis Study Group. *Br J Haematol* 105: 901–11.
Morrell M, Fraser VJ and Kollef MH (2005) Delaying the empiric treatment of candida bloodstream infection until positive blood culture results are obtained: a potential risk factor for hospital mortality. *Antimicrob Agents Chemother* 49: 3640–5.
Neblett Fanfair R, Benedict K, Bos J, et al. (2012) Necrotizing cutaneous mucormycosis after a tornado in Joplin, Missouri, in 2011. *N Engl J Med* 367: 2214–25.
Neofytos D, Horn D, Anaissie E, et al. (2009) Epidemiology and outcome of invasive fungal infection in adult hematopoietic stem cell transplant recipients: analysis of Multicenter Prospective Antifungal Therapy (PATH) Alliance registry. *Clin Infect Dis* 48: 265–73.
Nucci M, Garnica M, Gloria AB, et al. (2013) Invasive fungal diseases in haematopoietic cell transplant recipients and in patients with acute myeloid leukaemia or myelodysplasia in Brazil. *Clin Microbiol Infect* 19: 745–51.
Oude Lashof AM, Donnelly JP, Meis JF, et al. (2003) Duration of antifungal treatment and development of delayed complications in patients with candidaemia. *Eur J Clin Microbiol Infect Dis* 22: 43–8.
Oude Lashof AM, Rothova A, Sobel JD, et al. (2011) Ocular manifestations of candidemia. *Clin Infect Dis* 53: 262–8.
Pagano L, Caira M, Candoni A, et al. (2006) The epidemiology of fungal infections in patients with hematologic malignancies: the SEIFEM-2004 study. *Haematologica* 91: 1068–75.
Pagano L, Caira M, Nosari A, et al. (2007a) Fungal infections in recipients of hematopoietic stem cell transplants: results of the SEIFEM B-2004 study—Sorveglianza Epidemiologica Infezioni Fungine Nelle Emopatie Maligne. *Clin Infect Dis* 45: 1161–70.
Pagano L, Caira M, Nosari A, et al. (2011) The use and efficacy of empirical versus pre-emptive therapy in the management of fungal infections: the HEMA e-Chart Project. *Haematologica* 96: 1366–70.
Pagano L, Caira M, Picardi M, et al. (2007b) Invasive Aspergillosis in patients with acute leukemia: update on morbidity and mortality—SEIFEM-C Report. *Clin Infect Dis* 44: 1524–5.
Pagano L, Cornely OA, Busca A, et al. (2013) Combined antifungal approach for the treatment of invasive mucormycosis in patients with hematologic diseases: a report from the SEIFEM and FUNGISCOPE registries. *Haematologica* 98: e127–30.
Paltauf AP (1885) Mycosis mucorina. *Virchows Arch* 102: 543–64.
Pappas PG, Rotstein CM, Betts RF, et al. (2007) Micafungin versus caspofungin for treatment of candidemia and other forms of invasive candidiasis. *Clin Infect Dis* 45: 883–93.
Petrikkos G, Skiada A, Lortholary O, Roilides E, Walsh TJ and Kontoyiannis DP (2012) Epidemiology and clinical manifestations of mucormycosis. *Clin Infect Dis* 54 (Suppl. 1): S23–34.
Pfaller MA and Diekema DJ (2007) Epidemiology of invasive candidiasis: a persistent public health problem. *Clin Microbiol Rev* 20: 133–63.
Playford EG, Marriott D, Nguyen Q, et al. (2008) Candidemia in nonneutropenic critically ill patients: risk factors for non-albicans Candida spp. *Crit Care Med* 36: 2034–9.
Rammaert B, Lanternier F, Poiree S, Kania R and Lortholary O (2012) Diabetes and mucormycosis: a complex interplay. *Diabetes Metab* 38: 193–204.
Reboli AC, Rotstein C, Pappas PG, et al. (2007) Anidulafungin versus fluconazole for invasive candidiasis. *N Engl J Med* 356: 2472–82.
Rex JH, Bennett JE, Sugar AM, et al. (1994) A randomized trial comparing fluconazole with amphotericin B for the treatment of candidemia in patients without neutropenia. Candidemia Study Group and the National Institute. *N Engl J Med* 331: 1325–30.
Roden MM, Zaoutis TE, Buchanan WL, et al. (2005) Epidemiology and outcome of zygomycosis: a review of 929 reported cases. *Clin Infect Dis* 41: 634–53.
Ruping MJ, Heinz WJ, Kindo AJ, et al. (2010) Forty-one recent cases of invasive zygomycosis from a global clinical registry. *J Antimicrob Chemother* 65: 296–302.
Ruping MJ, Vehreschild JJ and Cornely OA (2008) Patients at high risk of invasive fungal infections: when and how to treat. *Drugs* 68: 1941–62.
Skiada A and Petrikkos G (2009) Cutaneous zygomycosis. *Clin Microbiol Infect* 15 (Suppl. 5): 41–5.
Slavin MA, Osborne B, Adams R, et al. (1995) Efficacy and safety of fluconazole prophylaxis for fungal infections after marrow transplantation—a prospective, randomized, double-blind study. *J Infect Dis* 171: 1545–52.
Tacke D, Buchheidt D, Karthaus M, et al. (2014a) Primary prophylaxis of invasive fungal infections in patients with haematologic malignancies. 2014 update of the recommendations of the Infectious Diseases Working Party of the German Society for Haematology and Oncology. *Ann Hematol* 93: 1449–56.
Tacke D, Koehler P and Cornely OA (2013) Fungal endocarditis. *Curr Opin Infect Dis* 26: 501–7.
Tacke D, Koehler P, Markiefka B and Cornely OA (2014b) Our 2014 approach to mucormycosis. *Mycoses* 57: 519–24.
Taur Y, Cohen N, Dubnow S, Paskovaty A and Seo SK (2010) Effect of antifungal therapy timing on mortality in cancer patients with candidemia. *Antimicrob Agents Chemother* 54: 184–90.
Tedder M, Spratt JA, Anstadt MP, Hegde SS, Tedder SD and Lowe JE (1994) Pulmonary mucormycosis: results of medical and surgical therapy. *Ann Thorac Surg* 57: 1044–50.
Thursky K, Byrnes G, Grigg A, Szer J and Slavin M (2004) Risk factors for post-engraftment invasive aspergillosis in allogeneic stem cell transplantation. *Bone Marrow Transplant* 34: 115–21.
Torres-Narbona M, Guinea J, Martinez-Alarcon J, Munoz P, Gadea I and Bouza E (2007) Impact of zygomycosis on microbiology workload: a survey study in Spain. *J Clin Microbiol* 45: 2051–3.
Ullmann AJ, Akova M, Herbrecht R, et al. (2012a) ESCMID* guideline for the diagnosis and management of Candida diseases 2012: adults with haematological malignancies and after haematopoietic stem cell transplantation (HCT). *Clin Microbiol Infect* 18 (Suppl. 7): 53–67.
Ullmann AJ, Cornely OA, Donnelly JP, et al. (2012b) ESCMID* guideline for the diagnosis and management of Candida diseases 2012: developing European guidelines in clinical microbiology and infectious diseases. *Clin Microbiol Infect* 18 (Suppl. 7): 1–8.
Ullmann AJ, Lipton JH, Vesole DH, et al. (2007) Posaconazole or fluconazole for prophylaxis in severe graft-versus-host disease. *N Engl J Med* 356: 335–47.
Van Burik JA, Ratanatharathorn V, Stepan DE, et al. (2004) Micafungin versus fluconazole for prophylaxis against invasive fungal infections during neutropenia in patients undergoing hematopoietic stem cell transplantation. *Clin Infect Dis* 39: 1407–16.
Vehreschild JJ, Birtel A, Vehreschild MJ, et al. (2013) Mucormycosis treated with posaconazole: review of 96 case reports. *Crit Rev Microbiol* 39: 310–24.
Vehreschild JJ, Brockelmann PJ, Bangard C, et al. (2012) Pandemic 2009 influenza A(H1N1) virus infection coinciding with invasive pulmonary aspergillosis in neutropenic patients. *Epidemiol Infect* 140: 1848–52.
Virchow R (1856) Beiträge zur Lehre von den beim Menschen vorkommenden pflanzlichen Parasiten. *Virchows Arch A Pathol Pathol Anat* 9: 557–93.
Viscoli C, Herbrecht R, Akan H, et al. (2009) An EORTC Phase II study of caspofungin as first-line therapy of invasive aspergillosis in haematological patients. *J Antimicrob Chemother* 64: 1274–81.
Walsh TJ, Finberg RW, Arndt C, et al. (1999) Liposomal amphotericin B for empirical therapy in patients with persistent fever and neutropenia. National Institute of Allergy and Infectious Diseases Mycoses Study Group. *N Engl J Med* 340: 764–71.
Walsh TJ, Pappas P, Winston DJ, et al. (2002) Voriconazole compared with liposomal amphotericin B for empirical antifungal therapy in patients with neutropenia and persistent fever. *N Engl J Med* 346: 225–34.

Walsh TJ, Teppler H, Donowitz GR, et al. (2004) Caspofungin versus liposomal amphotericin B for empirical antifungal therapy in patients with persistent fever and neutropenia. *N Engl J Med* 351: 1391–402.

Wey SB, Mori M, Pfaller MA, Woolson RF and Wenzel RP (1989) Risk factors for hospital-acquired candidemia. A matched case-control study. *Arch Intern Med* 149: 2349–53.

Wingard JR, Carter SL, Walsh TJ, et al. (2010) Randomized, double-blind trial of fluconazole versus voriconazole for prevention of invasive fungal infection after allogeneic hematopoietic cell transplantation. *Blood* 116: 5111–18.

Wisplinghoff H, Bischoff T, Tallent SM, et al. (2004) Nosocomial bloodstream infections in US hospitals: analysis of 24,179 cases from a prospective nationwide surveillance study. *Clin Infect Dis* 39: 309–17.

Wisplinghoff H, Ebbers J, Geurtz L, et al. (2014) Nosocomial bloodstream infections due to Candida spp. in the USA: species distribution, clinical features and antifungal susceptibilities. *Int J Antimicrob Agents* 43: 78–81.

CHAPTER 33

Fungal infections among patients with AIDS

Blandine Denis, Fanny Lanternier, and Olivier Lortholary

Introduction

Fungal infections, which are usually controlled by cellular immunity, are the most frequent opportunistic diseases occurring during the course of HIV (human immunovirus) infection. *Pneumocystis jirovecii, Candida albicans* (which is responsible for mucosal candidiasis), and *Cryptococcus neoformans* (the most frequent cause of meningitis) are the three major fungal pathogens in patients with AIDS. In endemic areas, infections due to dimorphic fungi are also an important group. *Histoplasma capsulatum, Coccidioides* spp., and *Talaromyces marneffei* infection are the most important endemic pathogens. In some patients with AIDS, mycotic disease is often the consequence of reactivation several years after a primary infection. Fungal diseases can be the initial sign of HIV infection, are a good marker of the severity of the immune deficit, and have prognostic value. The global burden of HIV infection is shown in Figures 33.1 and 33.2.

Candidiasis

Since the advent of combination antiretroviral therapy (cART) there has been a dramatic decline in all forms of candidiasis in HIV-infected patients. Refractory mucosal candidiasis is now a rare event and observed in patients without restoration of immunity, with CD4 counts often below 50/μL.

Oropharyngeal candidiasis

Thrush, or acute pseudomembranous candidiasis, is the most common clinical form and classifies the patient as having symptomatic HIV disease.

Treatment

Fluconazole, 100 mg daily for 7–14 days, should be initiated for oropharyngeal candidiasis (Lortholary et al. 2012). The oral solution of itraconazole, 100–200 mg daily, or miconazole mucoadhesive tablets are an effective alternative.

Oesophageal candidiasis

Oesophageal candidiasis, typically observed in patients with more advanced immunosuppression, classifies the patient as having AIDS.

Clinical presentation

Most patients have odynophagia. Nausea, vomiting, or oesophageal bleeding may be observed as well as fever and occasionally posterior thoracic pain. In a patient with oral thrush and retrosternal odynophagia, a systemic antifungal agent can be used as a diagnostic test.

Treatment

For oesophageal candidiasis, oral fluconazole 200 mg daily for two to three weeks is the drug of choice (Pappas et al. 2009; Lortholary et al. 2012). Itraconazole solution is an alternative (Lortholary et al. 2012).

Cryptococcosis

Cryptococcus neoformans var. *grubii* (serotype A) is responsible for most of the cryptococcosis cases in patients with AIDS and will be referred to as *C. neoformans* in this section.

Epidemiology

While the incidence of cryptococcosis has dramatically declined in HIV-infected patients in industrialized countries with the availability of cART, cryptococcosis is of increasing concern in Africa and Southeast Asia. It is encountered in up to 15–20% of hospitalized patients with AIDS in sub-Saharan Africa (Micol et al. 2007; Jarvis et al. 2008). Many countries in Africa and Asia have limited access to antifungal agents, and in low-resource countries a mortality rate of ≥50% within the first 15 days has been observed (Loyse et al. 2013a, b). In France, mortality remains at 17% (Dromer et al. 2007).

Pathogenesis

CD4 T-cell quantitative and/or qualitative deficiency is a major risk factor for cryptococcosis, and HIV infection represents the most prevalent underlying disease. The median CD4 cell count at the time of diagnosis is 20/μL (Dromer et al. 2007). The portal of entry is mainly pulmonary and the interaction of *C. neoformans* with alveolar macrophages is a determinant for pulmonary infection and subsequent systemic dissemination.

Clinical presentation

Meningoencephalitis is the most frequent presentation of cryptococcosis in HIV-infected patients. Neurological symptoms are most often subacute; fever and headache are common, but meningeal symptoms are not consistently noted. Cerebral imaging is abnormal in 50% of cases and magnetic resonance imaging is more sensitive than computed tomography (CT) (Charlier et al. 2008). Measurement of cerebrospinal fluid (CSF) opening pressure is

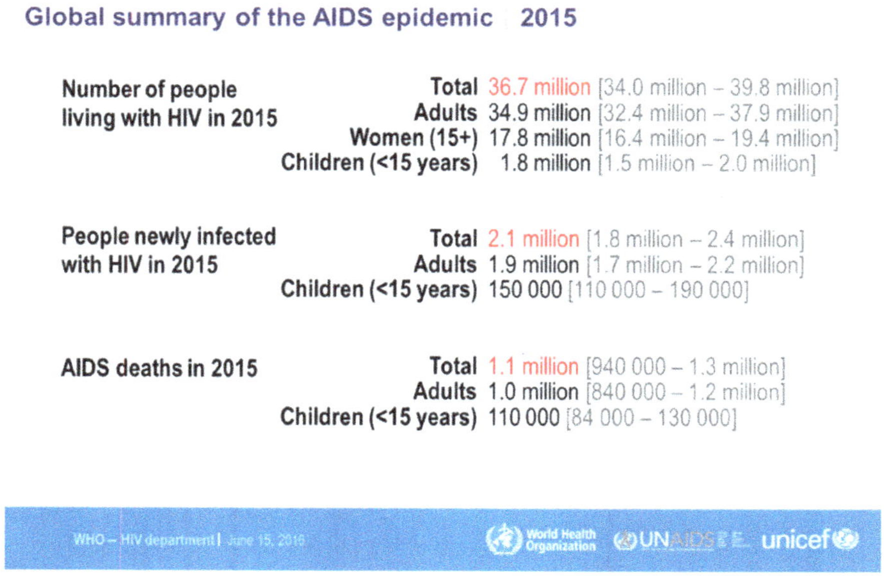

Figure 33.1 Global summary of the AIDS epidemic in 2015.

Reprinted from 'Global summary of the HIV/AIDS epidemic, December 2015', WHO—HIV department, World Health Organisation, Copyright © 2016. Accessed on 09 March 2017, Available from http://www.who.int/hiv/data/epi_core_2016.png

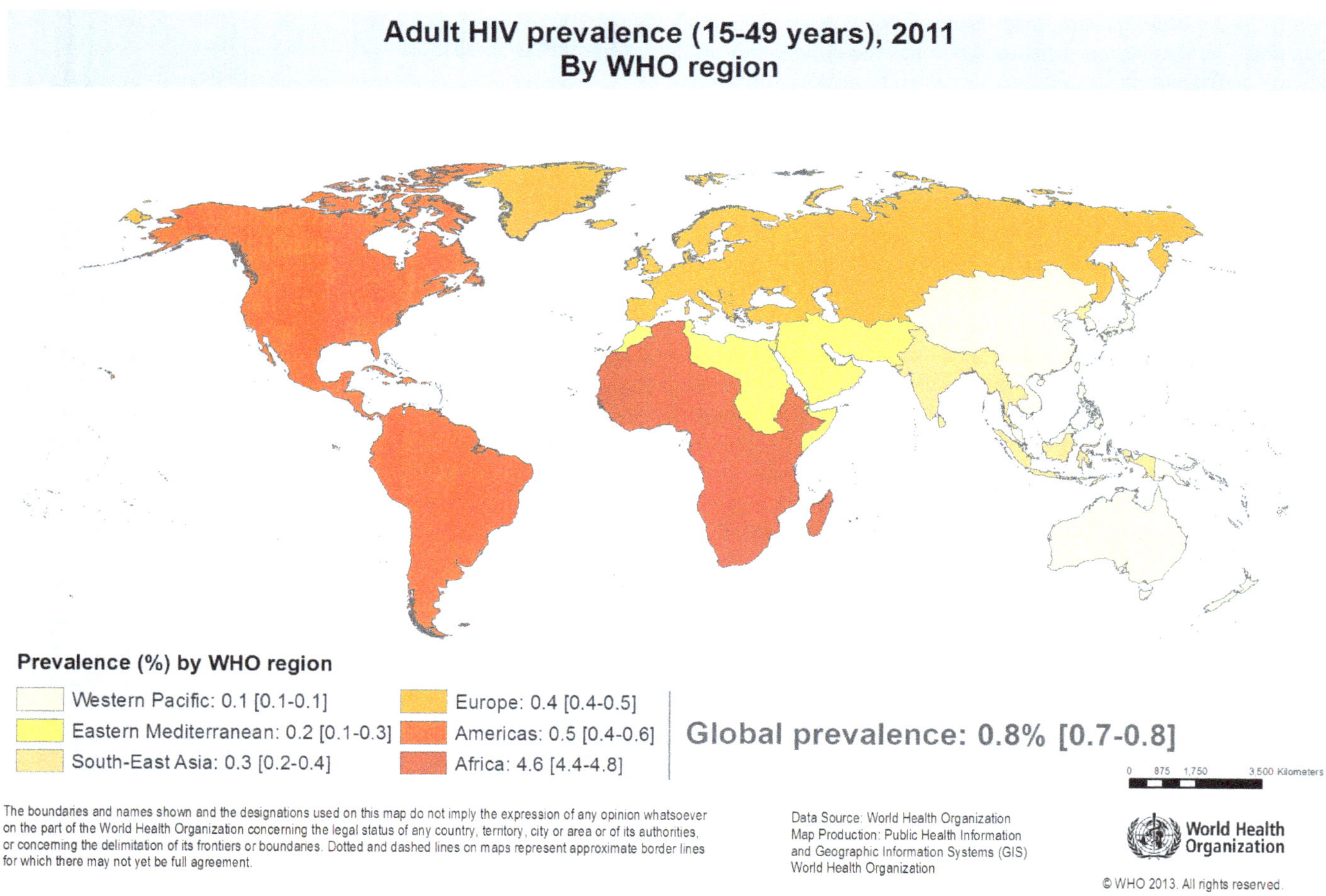

Figure 33.2 Estimation of adult HIV prevalence.

Reprinted from 'Global Health Observatory (GHO) data: HIV/AIDS', Global Health Observatory, World Health Organisation, Copyright © 2017. Accessed on 09 March 2017, Available from http://www.who.int/gho/hiv/en/

mandatory, since prognosis is highly associated with the magnitude of the increased intracranial pressure.

Pneumonia with cough and dyspnoea, and less commonly chest pain and haemoptysis, may also occur. Acute respiratory distress syndrome is associated with a poor prognosis. Chest radiographs and CT scans show interstitial infiltrates, nodules, pleural effusions, mediastinal lymphadenopathy, or cavitary lesions. Disseminated cryptococcosis should be suspected in febrile HIV-infected patients who present with skin lesions. Urinary tract involvement occurs commonly in men and is usually asymptomatic, and the prostate can serve as a sanctuary for *C. neoformans*.

Diagnosis

Analysis of CSF with India ink preparation shows encapsulated yeasts in more than 80% of HIV-infected patients with cryptococcal infection. Samples should be incubated for at least four weeks at 35–37°C and the yield is improved by using larger volumes of CSF. Blood and urine cultures should be obtained for all patients.

Cryptococcal antigen (CRAG) assays should be performed on serum and CSF (see Chapters 22 and 42). Commercially available tests are sensitive (≥95%) and specific (≥95%). A high serum CRAG titre is associated with a higher mycological failure rate, but a lack of decrease is not predictive of a worse outcome. New CRAG detection methods, such as CRAG lateral flow assays (LFAs), particularly the method developed by Immy, are easy to use and have improved diagnosis of cryptococcal meningitis in Africa (Binnicker et al. 2012; Boulware et al. 2014b; Kabanda et al. 2014). A recent study demonstrated that baseline CSF CRAG LFA titres predicted survival at two and ten weeks (Kabanda et al. 2014). More recently, a new LFA has been developed by Biosynex with the advantage of simultaneously providing a diagnostic and semi-quantitative approach.

Treatment

Antifungal agents used to treat cryptococcosis include amphotericin B and its liposomal formulation, flucytosine (5-fluorocytosine) and fluconazole. For initial therapy, the combination of amphotericin B (0.7–1.0 mg/kg daily) and flucytosine (100 mg/kg daily), for at least 14 days, has been shown to be superior to monotherapy, and flucytosine use is an independent predictor of early mycological outcome (van der Horst et al. 1997; Dromer et al. 2007; Perfect et al. 2010; Day et al. 2013).

If clinical outcome is favourable and CSF culture has become negative, therapy can be switched to oral fluconazole 400 mg daily, for a duration of eight to ten weeks. Maintenance therapy with fluconazole, 200 mg daily, should be given until persistent immune restoration is obtained. If the patient has renal failure, liposomal amphotericin B 3–5 mg/kg daily, can be used.

The appropriate management of elevated CSF opening pressure (≥25 cm H_20) strongly influences early mortality, and repeated lumbar punctures with evacuation of up to 20 ml of fluid should be performed every one to three days until the pressure returns to a normal value (Perfect et al. 2010; Boulware et al. 2014a). In cases of persistently increased intracranial pressure, a ventriculo-peritoneal shunt or a lumbar drain should be placed. Mannitol, acetazolamide, and steroids have not been proven to be helpful (Graybill et al. 2000).

In the case of an isolated positive serum CRAG titre, an exhaustive workup should be performed to search for a site of infection, and if none is found and the patient has a CD4 count <200/μL, therapy with fluconazole should be initiated.

Maintenance therapy can be safely withdrawn in patients who have been treated for cryptococcosis for at least one year, are on cART, have a CD4 cell count >100/μL and an undetectable viral load for at least three months and an Ag titre <1:512 (Vibhagool et al. 2003; Lortholary et al. 2006).

Primary prophylaxis is not recommended in industrialized countries. Cryptococcal antigen screening and pre-emptive therapy for those who are CRAG positive and asymptomatic is recommended by the World Health Organization in patients with a CD4 count <100 μL in areas where there is a high prevalence of cryptococcal antigenaemia. Screening and pre-emptive treatment for cryptococcal infection could reduce mortality in HIV-infected patients in Africa (Mfinanga et al. 2015).

Pneumocystosis

Pneumocystis jirovecii pneumonia

During the early years of the AIDS epidemic, *Pneumocystis* pneumonia (PCP) accounted for two-thirds of AIDS-defining illness in patients in the USA, and an estimated 75% of HIV individuals developed PCP during their lifetime (Hay et al. 1988; Morris et al. 2004a); rates of PCP were as high as 20 per 100 person-years among those with a CD4 count <200/mm^3. The first decline in the incidence of PCP occurred after the introduction of anti-*Pneumocystis* prophylaxis in 1989. The advent of cART resulted in a dramatic decline in rates of PCP, with incidence rates reduced by more than ten times (Mocroft et al. 2000), and an increased three-year survival from 51% in the pre-cART era to 87% in 2001–2003 was observed (Grabar et al. 2008). However, PCP remains one of the most common AIDS-defining illnesses (ADIs) in industrialized countries and was the second most frequent ADI in France in 2001–2003 (Kaplan et al. 2000; Morris et al. 2004b; Grabar et al. 2008). A study of 1,259 PCP cases in HIV-infected individuals in France during the 2004–2011 period showed that, in the context of a decreasing risk of PCP, almost half of PCP diagnoses occurred in patients already in care, mainly with a previous cART prescription but with waning adherence to care (Denis et al. 2014).

Dimorphic (endemic) fungal infections

Among fungal infections due to dimorphic fungi, only three—histoplasmosis, coccidioidomycosis, and penicilliosis—are frequently found in patients with AIDS (see Chapter 16).

Histoplasmosis

Histoplasmosis due to *H. capsulatum* var. *capsulatum* is endemic in the United States, the Caribbean, and Central and South America, and occurs with much less frequency in Africa and Southeast Asia. In HIV-infected patients living in endemic areas in the midwestern United States, the incidence of histoplasmosis varied from 1% to 25% historically (Wheat et al. 1990). It is a major threat in areas such as French Guyana and Surinam (Nacher et al. 2013) and more generally in South American countries. Outside endemic areas, infection usually represents reactivation occurring several years after the primary infection (Warnock et al. 1998). Histoplasmosis generally occurs in patients with CD4 counts <100 cells/μL and is an AIDS-defining illness in its disseminated form.

Clinical presentation

In patients with AIDS, histoplasmosis is usually disseminated and presents with fever (84%), weight loss, fatigue, and night sweats. Pneumonia is present in over half of the cases, and hepatomegaly (40%), splenomegaly (40%), and lymphadenopathy (63%) are common findings. Septic shock and respiratory failure are seen in about 10% of cases and are associated with a poor prognosis (Wheat et al. 2000). Central nervous system involvement—either meningitis or a space-occupying lesion—occurs in approximately 15% of patients (Wheat et al. 1990). Various cutaneous lesions are seen, including maculopapular rashes, pustules, papules, and ulcers, and mucosal ulcers are typical. Gastrointestinal involvement is fairly frequent. Mediastinal granuloma and chronic cavitary lung disease are unusual in this population. Death is associated with a low CD4 count and absence of antiretroviral treatment (Nacher et al. 2013).

Histoplasmosis due to *H. capsulatum* var. *duboisii* is rarely observed in patients with AIDS and is usually seen amongst patients living in, or who have travelled to, Central and West Africa and Madagascar.

Diagnosis

In histoplasmosis, pancytopenia is common at presentation. The chest radiograph demonstrates patchy infiltrates or diffuse interstitial pneumonitis in more severe cases. Microscopic examination of biopsy specimens or body fluid aspirates is the fastest diagnostic approach, but the sensitivity varies. The greatest yield is from bone marrow, skin, and mucosal lesions. The classic 2–4 μm budding yeasts, visualized best by periodic acid-Schiff or methenamine silver stains, should be sought (see Chapter 40). Material for culture should be obtained from blood, bone marrow, bronchoalveolar lavage fluid, and tissue samples.

Histoplasma antigen detection in blood, urine, or CSF is a specific and sensitive test among patients with disseminated disease. Antigenuria correlates well with response to therapy and is useful for detecting relapsing histoplasmosis (Wheat et al. 2007). Serum galactomannan antigen can also be a diagnostic and follow-up marker when *Histoplasma* antigen is negative (Rivière et al. 2012). More recently, specific PCR (polymerase chain reaction) assays have been developed.

Treatment

Amphotericin B and itraconazole are effective against both *H. capsulatum* and *H. capsulatum* var. *duboisii* (Wheat et al. 2007). Among patients with severe disease, initial treatment should be with liposomal amphotericin B, 3 mg/kg daily. When patients have improved, generally after several weeks, the regimen can be switched to oral itraconazole 400 mg daily, for 12 months. Milder illness can be treated initially with itraconazole, beginning with a loading dose of 200 mg thrice daily for three days, then 400 mg daily for 12 months (Wheat et al. 2007). Monitoring of serum itraconazole levels is mandatory in patients with AIDS. Fluconazole is less effective than itraconazole, but can be given at a dosage of 400–800 mg daily if itraconazole is not tolerated. The role of newer azoles has not been established.

Itraconazole can be withdrawn in patients who have been treated for at least 12 months, have at least two measurements of CD4 cell counts >150/μL in the preceding six months, and have received cART for at least six months (Goldman et al. 2004). Maintenance therapy should be restarted when CD4 cells fall below 100/μL. Primary prophylaxis can be considered in areas in which the incidence of histoplasmosis is highest. IRIS (immune response inflammatory syndrome) is reported after antiretroviral initiation.

Coccidioidomycosis

Coccidioides immitis and *Coccidioides posadasii* are dimorphic fungi found in semi-arid areas in the southwestern United States, Mexico, and Central and South America. The disease is acquired by inhalation of arthroconidia present in the soil. Disease can occur following reactivation or as a primary infection. Extrathoracic coccidioidomycosis involving sites other than the respiratory tract is an AIDS-defining illness.

Clinical presentation

The most common symptoms of coccidioidomycosis in patients with AIDS are fever, cough, and weight loss. Chest radiography reveals a variety of abnormalities, including focal pulmonary alveolar infiltrates, discrete nodules, hilar lymphadenopathy, and pleural effusions in more than 60% of patients. In 40% of those with radiographic findings, a diffuse reticulonodular infiltrate is present. Approximately 12% of patients develop meningitis. Lymphadenopathy, cutaneous lesions, and subcutaneous abscesses are common. Fungaemia, thyroiditis, peritonitis, adrenal involvement, osteoarticular disease, and prostatic involvement have also been reported (Fish et al. 1990).

Diagnosis

In diagnosing coccidioidomycosis, the CD4 cell count is usually <200 cells/μL and often <50 cells/μL. Definitive diagnosis relies on visualization of the typical large spherules containing numerous endospores in clinical specimens and isolation of *Coccidioides* species in culture. *Coccidioides* cultures should not be handled in clinical microbiology laboratories which are not equipped with a containment Level 3 facility. In the case of meningitis, CSF analysis typically shows leucocytic pleocytosis with the presence of eosinophils in some cases, decreased glucose, and increased protein values. Culture for *Coccidioides* species in CSF is often negative, but if serology is positive (see Chapter 42), it can establish the diagnosis of coccidioidal meningitis. Specific PCR assays have been developed more recently.

Treatment

The drug of choice for severe life-threatening coccidioidal infection is a lipid formulation of amphotericin B, 3–5 mg/kg daily (Galgiani et al. 2005). When the disease is controlled, generally after two to three weeks, switching to an oral triazole drug should be considered. Fluconazole 400 mg daily is a good alternative, particularly in patients with meningitis; itraconazole 400 mg daily has also given good results, especially in patients with skeletal disease (Galgiani et al. 2005). Lifelong maintenance therapy with a triazole—either fluconazole 400 mg daily or itraconazole 400 mg daily—is necessary to avoid relapse in patients with AIDS (Kaplan et al. 2009).

Talaromyces (Penicillium) marneffei infection

Talaromyces (Penicillium) marneffei is a dimorphic fungus present in soil in Southeast Asia. Cases may be imported into Europe, and the US *Talaromyces marneffei* is associated with several species of bamboo rats; however, contact with soil seems to be the most important risk factor regarding exposure to this fungus. In northern Thailand, penicilliosis is the third most common AIDS-defining opportunistic disease, following tuberculosis and cryptococcosis (Supparatpinyo et al. 1994). The condition is frequent in South China, with 4.8% of AIDS-related hospital admissions having *T. marneffei* infection.

Clinical presentation

Disseminated *T. marneffei* infection is very common at presentation and CD4 counts are usually below 50 cells/μL. In one study of 92 patients with disseminated *T. marneffei* infection seen at Chiang Mai University Hospital in Thailand, 86 (93%) were HIV infected (Supparatpinyo et al. 1994); most patients were young men, with fever (93%), anaemia (78%), pronounced weight loss (76%), skin lesions (68%), generalized lymphadenopathy (58%), hepatomegaly (51%), cough (49%), diarrhoea (31%), splenomegaly (16%), and jaundice (8%). Skin lesions, especially a generalized papular rash, are very suggestive of the diagnosis of *T. marneffei* infection in at-risk patients. Some of the papules with central umbilication mimic lesions caused by molluscum contagiosum. Subcutaneous nodules, acne-like lesions, and folliculitis may also be present. Genital ulcers and palatal papules have also been reported. Chest radiography is abnormal in almost 30% of patients with disseminated *T. marneffei* infection. *T. marneffei* infection was found to be responsible for 11% of mucocutaneous lesions in Chinese HIV patients in Guangxi (Han et al. 2013), and 16.5% of all positive blood cultures in Ho Chi Minh City in 2005 (Nga et al. 2012). IRIS has also been reported.

Diagnosis

Fever, with or without pancytopenia, skin, and/or lung lesions could suggest a diagnosis of leishmaniasis or disseminated histoplasmosis. For any HIV-positive patient, a history of living in, or previous travel to, Southeast Asia is the first clue towards considering a diagnosis of penicilliosis (Warnock et al. 1998).

In the Chiang Mai series, diagnosis of *T. marneffei* infection was made by culture of the fungus from blood (76%), skin lesions (90%), bone marrow aspirate (100%), and sputum. The galactomannan test for the detection of *Aspergillus* antigen has the ability to detect *T. marneffei*, because of cross-reactivity, hence enabling diagnosis in HIV-infected patients with a travel history to Southeast Asia (Zheng et al. 2015). A presumptive diagnosis of *T. marneffei* infection can be made by examination of sputum or from biopsy material from bone marrow, skin, or lymph node.

Treatment

Itraconazole and amphotericin B are the mainstays of therapy for *T. marneffei* infection in all patients, regardless of their immune status. Induction treatment with amphotericin B 0.6 mg/kg daily for approximately two weeks, followed by itraconazole 400 mg daily for ten weeks, is the treatment of choice (Sirisanthana et al. 1998). Voriconazole has also been shown to be effective. Suppressive therapy with itraconazole, 200 mg daily, is recommended for all patients with a persistently low CD4 cell count (Supparatpinyo et al. 1998). In geographic areas in which *T. marneffei* is endemic, primary prophylaxis with itraconazole 200 mg daily was recommended before the antiretroviral therapy era (Chariyalertsak et al. 2002).

Paracoccidioidomycosis

Paracoccidioidomycosis is not commonly reported in patients with AIDS, a fact that remains unexplained. Almost all reported cases of AIDS-associated paracoccidioidomycosis have occurred in Brazil, with only one case reported from Venezuela. Most of the reported patients had advanced AIDS with CD4 cell counts well below 200/μL, with disseminated disease.

Diagnosis of paracoccidioidomycosis is usually made by direct microscopic examination and culture of clinical specimens, most commonly skin and lymph nodes. Cultures of blood, bone marrow, and sputum may also be positive. An assay for *P. brasiliensis* antigen and PCR for *P. brasiliensis* DNA are promising diagnostic tools in these patients.

Therapeutic options include trimethoprim-sulphamethoxazole, amphotericin B, and itraconazole as primary treatment. Lifelong maintenance therapy with trimethoprim-sulphamethoxazole or itraconazole is recommended (Paniago et al. 2005).

Blastomycosis

Blastomycosis is also uncommon among HIV-infected patients. Several cases of blastomycosis have been reported in patients with AIDS, and most had CD4 cell counts well below 200/μL. Amphotericin B is considered the initial treatment of choice for patients with severe disease and for all immunosuppressed patients (Chapman et al. 2008). For patients who improve after two to four weeks of therapy with amphotericin B, it is reasonable to switch to oral itraconazole 200 mg twice daily, and to maintain chronic suppressive therapy with itraconazole indefinitely in those patients who remain severely immunosuppressed.

Sporotrichosis

A systematic review of sporotrichosis (see Chapter 23) cases in HIV-infected patients found the majority to be reported from Brazil and the United States. Males predominated in 84.5% of cases, and the overall mortality was 30%. The median CD4+ cell count was 97 cells/mm^3 (Moreira et al. 2015). All patients presented with diffuse ulcerative skin lesions. Other sites of disease included the central nervous system, joints, eyes, spleen, and bone marrow. *Sporothrix schenckii* fungaemia was noted in two patients.

Examination of tissue biopsies or material aspirated from skin lesions usually leads to the diagnosis when the typical cigar-shaped yeast forms are seen. Culture of tissue or body fluids at 25°C reveals the mould form of *S. schenckii*.

The optimal therapy for disseminated sporotrichosis in HIV-infected patients has not been determined. Amphotericin B for the most severe cases followed by itraconazole appears to be the most reasonable approach to therapy. Itraconazole should be considered for long-term maintenance therapy amongst those patients who remain immunosuppressed (Kauffman et al. 2007).

Emmonsiosis

Emmonsia sp. are novel dimorphic fungi recently reported as responsible for disseminated infections in HIV-infected patients in South Africa. Patients have very low CD4 cell counts (16/mm^3). All patients have disseminated infections involving skin and lung in most cases. Emmonsiosis is diagnosed by visualization of yeasts on pathological examination (Schwartz et al. 2015). Studies have revealed that most patients are treated with liposomal amphotericin B (71%) and that the mortality rate is ~48% (Kenyon et al. 2013; van Hougenhouck-Tulleken et al. 2014; Schwartz et al. 2015) (see Chapter 16).

Other opportunistic mould and yeast infections

Invasive aspergillosis

Before the advent of cART, invasive aspergillosis (IA) in HIV-infected individuals occurred mainly at CD4 cell counts below 100/mm^3 and median survival after diagnosis was less than four months. Up to 50% of individuals with IA do not have the classical predisposing host factors. The lungs are involved in >70% of cases, showing nodular lesions, cavitary infiltrates, and bilateral interstitial infiltrates (Denning et al. 1991; Lortholary et al. 1993; Khoo and Denning 1994). Invasive necrotizing tracheobronchitis is also seen in patients with AIDS. *A. fumigatus* is the main species found in culture. Serum galactomannan assay is considered unreliable in this population. In a recent study of 242 cases of IA in HIV-infected patients over a 20-year period in France, classical risk factors were still uncommonly observed, with only half of validated IA cases fulfilling the EORTC/MSG (European Organization for Research and Treatment of Cancer/Mycoses Study Group) criteria (Denis et al. 2015). Median CD4 cell count at IA diagnosis was 82 (12–327) cells/mm^3 in 2002–2011. The majority of patients (74%) had pulmonary involvement, and 28 patients (10%) had disseminated disease. The incidence decreased over time, with rates of 30 cases per 10,000 person-years in 2002–2011. The three-month survival rate improved after the advent of cART (38% before cART *vs* 69% after), with a median survival of 29 months (interquartile range 2.2–98.2) in 2002–2011. Voriconazole exposure decreased mortality between 2002 and 2011 (hazard ratio 0.1 [range 0.01–0.6]) and should be considered as the first-line drug in this setting (Denis et al. 2015).

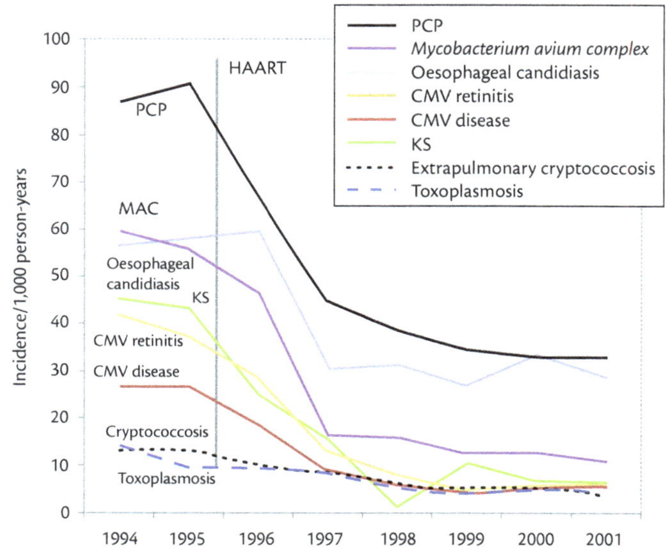

Figure 33.3 Yearly opportunistic infection rates per 1,000 person-years, Centers for Disease Control and Prevention (CDC) Adult and Adolescent Spectrum of Disease Project, 1994–2001.

CMV = cytomegalovirus; HAART = highly active antiretroviral therapy; KS = Kaposi's sarcoma; MAC = *Mycobacterium avium* complex; PCP = *Pneumocystis* pneumonia. Data are standardized to the population of AIDS cases reported nationally in the same year by age, sex, race, HIV exposure mode, country of origin, and CD4+ lymphocyte count.

Reproduced from Morris, A. et al. 'Current Epidemiology of Pneumocystis Pneumonia', *Emerging Infectious Diseases*, Volume 10, Issue 10, pp. 1713–1720. Centers for Disease Control and Prevention, U.S. Department of Health & Human Services, DOI: 10.3201/eid1010.030985.

Impact of antiretroviral therapy on fungal infections

cART has resulted in dramatic declines in morbidity and mortality among HIV-infected patients with advanced immune dysfunction (Figure 33.3) (Palella et al. 1998) A successful response to cART is characterized by a marked reduction in viral load and a subsequent increase in CD4 cell count. However, the partial restoration of cell-mediated immunity and possibly other immune effectors may facilitate the development of an inflammatory reaction at the site of previous infection, which can mimic reactivation of the opportunistic disease. IRIS has been reported in patients with AIDS with cryptococcosis and histoplasmosis (Lortholary et al. 2005; Shelburne et al. 2005; Breton et al. 2006; Sungkanuparph et al. 2009; Boulware et al. 2014a). In cases of IRIS reported during the course of histoplasmosis in patients with AIDS, uveitis, liver abscesses, arthritis, and necrotizing lymphadenopathy have been observed. In a prospective study of 101 patients with AIDS who had cryptococcal meningitis, IRIS developed in 13% (Sungkanuparph et al. 2009). For cryptococcosis, IRIS can present as aseptic meningitis with increased intracranial pressure. Other manifestations include necrotic lymphadenopathy, necrotizing pneumonia, and cerebral or medullary abscesses. Risk factors for development of IRIS that have been noted in various studies include early initiation of cART after the diagnosis of cryptococcosis, high CSF antigen titre, fungaemia, low CD4 cell count, and high viral load.

The symptoms and signs of IRIS raise the diagnostic challenge for the clinician to decide whether the patient is experiencing a relapse of the initial infection, a new infection, or IRIS. When an opportunistic infection occurs at low CD4 cell counts, studies have shown that starting early cART after treatment of the opportunistic infection improves overall survival except in cases of cryptococcal meningitis. In a recent randomized study of 500 HIV-infected individuals with cryptococcal meningitis, deferring cART for five weeks after the diagnosis of cryptococcal meningitis was associated with significantly improved survival, as compared with initiating cART at one to two weeks (Boulware et al. 2014a). In patients with cryptococcal meningitis, caution should be exercised in initiating cART, and waiting at least until CSF cultures have become negative is recommended (Kaplan et al. 2009; Boulware et al. 2014a). In cases of IRIS, treatment with anti-inflammatory agents, including corticosteroids, may be effective without necessitating a change in cART or the anti-infective treatment.

References

Binnicker MJ, Jespersen DJ, Bestrom JE and Rollins LO (2012) Comparison of four assays for the detection of cryptococcal antigen. *Clin Vaccine Immunol* 19: 1988–90. doi: 10.1128/CVI.00446-12

Boulware DR, Meya DB, Muzoora C, et al. (2014a) Timing of antiretroviral therapy after diagnosis of cryptococcal meningitis. *N Engl J Med* 370: 2487–98. doi:10.1056/NEJMoa1312884

Boulware DR, Rolfes MA, Rajasingham R, et al. (2014b) Multisite validation of cryptococcal antigen lateral flow assay and quantification by laser thermal contrast. *Emerg Infect Dis* 20: 45–53. doi:10.3201/eid2001.130906

Breton G, Adle-Biassette H, Therby A, et al. (2006) Immune reconstitution inflammatory syndrome in HIV-infected patients with disseminated histoplasmosis. *AIDS* 20: 119–21.

Chapman SW, Dismukes WE, Proia LA, et al. (2008) Clinical practice guidelines for the management of blastomycosis: 2008 update by the Infectious Diseases Society of America. *Clin Infect Dis* 46: 1801–12. doi:10.1086/588300

Chariyalertsak S, Supparatpinyo K, Sirisanthana T and Nelson KE (2002) A controlled trial of itraconazole as primary prophylaxis for systemic fungal infections in patients with advanced human immunodeficiency virus infection in Thailand. *Clin Infect Dis* 34: 277–84. doi:10.1086/338154

Charlier C, Dromer F, Lévêque C, et al. (2008) Cryptococcal neuroradiological lesions correlate with severity during cryptococcal meningoencephalitis in HIV-positive patients in the HAART era. *PLoS One* 3: e1950. doi:10.1371/journal.pone.0001950

Day JN, Chau TTH and Lalloo DG (2013) Combination antifungal therapy for cryptococcal meningitis. *N Engl J Med* 368: 2522–3. doi:10.1056/NEJMc1305981

Denis B, Guiguet M, de Castro N, et al. (2014) Critical importance of long-term adherence to care in HIV infected patients in the cART era: new insights from Pneumocystis jirovecii pneumonia cases over 2004-2011 in the FHDH-ANRS CO4 cohort. *PLoS One* 9: e94183. doi:10.1371/journal.pone.0094183

Denis B, Guiguet M, de Castro N, et al. (2015) Relevance of EORTC criteria for the diagnosis of invasive aspergillosis in HIV-infected patients, and survival trends over a 20-year period in France. *Clin Infect Dis* 61: 1273–80. doi:10.1093/cid/civ492

Denning DW, Follansbee SE, Scolaro M, Norris S, Edelstein H and Stevens DA (1991) Pulmonary aspergillosis in the acquired immunodeficiency syndrome. *N Engl J Med* 324: 654–62. doi:10.1056/NEJM199103073241003

Dromer F, Mathoulin-Pélissier S, Launay O and Lortholary O (2007) Determinants of disease presentation and outcome during cryptococcosis: the CryptoA/D study. *PLoS Med* 4: e21. doi:10.1371/journal.pmed.0040021

Fish DG, Ampel NM, Galgiani JN, et al. (1990) Coccidioidomycosis during human immunodeficiency virus infection. A review of 77 patients. *Medicine (Baltimore)* 69: 384–91.

Galgiani JN, Ampel NM, Blair JE, et al. (2005) Coccidioidomycosis. *Clin Infect Dis* 41: 1217–23. doi:10.1086/496991

Goldman M, Zackin R, Fichtenbaum CJ, et al. (2004) Safety of discontinuation of maintenance therapy for disseminated histoplasmosis after immunologic response to antiretroviral therapy. *Clin Infect Dis* 38: 1485–9. doi: 10.1086/420749

Grabar S, Lanoy E, Allavena C, et al. (2008) Causes of the first AIDS-defining illness and subsequent survival before and after the advent of combined antiretroviral therapy. *HIV Med* 9: 246–56. doi:10.1111/j.1468-1293.2008.00554.x

Graybill JR, Sobel J, Saag M, et al. (2000) Diagnosis and management of increased intracranial pressure in patients with AIDS and cryptococcal meningitis. The NIAID Mycoses Study Group and AIDS Cooperative Treatment Groups. *Clin Infect Dis* 30: 47–54. doi: 10.1086/313603

Han J, Lun WH, Meng ZH, et al. (2013) Mucocutaneous manifestations of HIV-infected patients in the era of HAART in Guangxi Zhuang Autonomous Region, China. *J Eur Acad Dermatol Venereol* 27: 376–82. doi: 10.1111/j.1468-3083.2011.04429.x

Hay JW, Osmond DH and Jacobson MA (1988) Projecting the medical costs of AIDS and ARC in the United States. *J Acquir Immune Defic Syndr* 1: 466–85.

Jarvis JN, Dromer F, Harrison TS and Lortholary O (2008) Managing cryptococcosis in the immunocompromised host. *Curr Opin Infect Dis* 21: 596–603. doi: 10.1097/QCO.0b013e3283177f6c

Kabanda T, Siedner MJ, Klausner JD, Muzoora C and Boulware DR (2014) Point-of-care diagnosis and prognostication of cryptococcal meningitis with the cryptococcal antigen lateral flow assay on cerebrospinal fluid. *Clin Infect Dis* 58: 113–16. doi: 10.1093/cid/cit641

Kaplan JE, Benson C, Holmes KK, et al. (2009) Guidelines for prevention and treatment of opportunistic infections in HIV-infected adults and adolescents: recommendations from CDC, the National Institutes of Health, and the HIV Medicine Association of the Infectious Diseases Society of America. *MMWR Recomm Rep* 58(RR-4): 1–207.

Kaplan JE, Hanson D, Dworkin MS, et al. (2000) Epidemiology of human immunodeficiency virus-associated opportunistic infections in the United States in the era of highly active antiretroviral therapy. *Clin Infect Dis* 30 (Suppl. 1): S5–14. doi: 10.1086/313843

Kauffman CA, Bustamante B, Chapman SW, Pappas PG and Infectious Diseases Society of America (2007) Clinical practice guidelines for the management of sporotrichosis: 2007 update by the Infectious Diseases Society of America. *Clin Infect Dis* 45: 1255–65. doi: 10.1086/522765

Kenyon C, Bonorchis K, Corcoran C, et al. (2013) A dimorphic fungus causing disseminated infection in South Africa. *N Engl J Med* 369: 1416–24. doi: 10.1056/NEJMoa1215460

Khoo SH and Denning DW (1994) Invasive aspergillosis in patients with AIDS. *Clin Infect Dis* 19 (Suppl. 1): S41–8.

Lortholary O, Fontanet A, Mémain N, Martin A, Sitbon K and Dromer F (2005) Incidence and risk factors of immune reconstitution inflammatory syndrome complicating HIV-associated cryptococcosis in France. *AIDS* 19: 1043–9.

Lortholary O, Meyohas MC, Dupont B, et al. (1993) Invasive aspergillosis in patients with acquired immunodeficiency syndrome: report of 33 cases. French Cooperative Study Group on Aspergillosis in AIDS. *Am J Med* 95: 177–87.

Lortholary O, Petrikkos G, Akova M, et al. (2012) ESCMID* guideline for the diagnosis and management of Candida diseases 2012: patients with HIV infection or AIDS. *Clin Microbiol Infect* 18 (Suppl. 7): 68–77. doi: 10.1111/1469-0691.12042

Lortholary O, Poizat G, Zeller V, et al. (2006) Long-term outcome of AIDS-associated cryptococcosis in the era of combination antiretroviral therapy. *AIDS* 20: 2183–91. doi: 10.1097/01.aids.0000252060.80704.68

Loyse A, Dromer F, Day J, Lortholary O and Harrison TS (2013a) Flucytosine and cryptococcosis: time to urgently address the worldwide accessibility of a 50-year-old antifungal. *J Antimicrob Chemother* 68: 2435–44. doi: 10.1093/jac/dkt221

Loyse A, Thangaraj H, Easterbrook P, et al. (2013b) Cryptococcal meningitis: improving access to essential antifungal medicines in resource-poor countries. *Lancet Infect Dis* 13: 629–37. doi: 10.1016/S1473-3099(13)70078-1

Mfinanga S, Chanda D, Kivuyo SL, et al. (2015) Cryptococcal meningitis screening and community-based early adherence support in people with advanced HIV infection starting antiretroviral therapy in Tanzania and Zambia: an open-label, randomised controlled trial. *Lancet* 385: 2173–82. doi: 10.1016/S0140-6736(15)60164-7

Micol R, Lortholary O, Sar B, et al. (2007) Prevalence, determinants of positivity, and clinical utility of cryptococcal antigenemia in Cambodian HIV-infected patients. *J Acquir Immune Defic Syndr* 45: 555–9. doi: 10.1097/QAI.0b013e31811ed32c

Mocroft A, Katlama C, Johnson AM, et al. (2000) AIDS across Europe, 1994-98: the EuroSIDA study. *Lancet* 356: 291–6.

Moreira JAS, Freitas DFS and Lamas CC (2015) The impact of sporotrichosis in HIV-infected patients: a systematic review. *Infection* 43: 267–76. doi: 10.1007/s15010-015-0746-1

Morris A, Lundgren JD, Masur H, et al. (2004a) Current epidemiology of Pneumocystis pneumonia. *Emerging Infect Dis* 10: 1713–20. doi: 10.3201/eid1010.030985

Morris A, Lundgren JD, Masur H, et al. (2004b) Current epidemiology of Pneumocystis pneumonia. *Emerging Infect Dis* 10: 1713–20.

Nacher M, Adenis A, Mc Donald S, et al. (2013) Disseminated histoplasmosis in HIV-infected patients in South America: a neglected killer continues on its rampage. *PLoS Negl Trop Dis* 7: e2319. doi: 10.1371/journal.pntd.0002319

Nga TVT, Parry CM, Le T, et al. (2012) The decline of typhoid and the rise of non-typhoid salmonellae and fungal infections in a changing HIV landscape: bloodstream infection trends over 15 years in southern Vietnam. *Trans R Soc Trop Med Hyg* 106: 26–34. doi: 10.1016/j.trstmh.2011.10.004

Palella FJ Jr, Delaney KM, Moorman AC, et al. (1998) Declining morbidity and mortality among patients with advanced human immunodeficiency virus infection. HIV Outpatient Study Investigators. *N Engl J Med* 338: 853–60. doi: 10.1056/NEJM199803263381301

Paniago AMM, de Freitas ACC, Aguiar ESA, et al. (2005) Paracoccidioidomycosis in patients with human immunodeficiency virus: review of 12 cases observed in an endemic region in Brazil. *J Infect* 51: 248–52. doi: 10.1016/j.jinf.2005.01.010

Pappas PG, Kauffman CA, Andes D, et al. (2009) Clinical practice guidelines for the management of candidiasis: 2009 update by the Infectious Diseases Society of America. *Clin Infect Dis* 48: 503–35. doi: 10.1086/596757

Perfect JR, Dismukes WE, Dromer F, et al. (2010) Clinical practice guidelines for the management of cryptococcal disease: 2010 update by the infectious diseases society of america. *Clin Infect Dis* 50: 291–322. doi: 10.1086/649858

Rivière S, Denis B, Bougnoux M-E, Lanternier F, Lecuit M and Lortholary O (2012) Serum Aspergillus galactomannan for the management of disseminated histoplasmosis in AIDS. *Am J Trop Med Hyg* 87: 303–5. doi: 10.4269/ajtmh.2012.12-0119

Schwartz IS, Govender NP, Corcoran C, et al. (2015) Clinical characteristics, diagnosis, management, and outcomes of disseminated emmonsiosis: a retrospective case series. *Clin Infect Dis* 61: 1004–12. doi: 10.1093/cid/civ439

Shelburne SA, Darcourt J, White AC, et al. (2005) The role of immune reconstitution inflammatory syndrome in AIDS-related Cryptococcus neoformans disease in the era of highly active antiretroviral therapy. *Clin Infect Dis* 40: 1049–52. doi: 10.1086/428618

Sirisanthana T, Supparatpinyo K, Perriens J and Nelson KE (1998) Amphotericin B and itraconazole for treatment of disseminated Penicillium marneffei infection in human immunodeficiency virus-infected patients. *Clin Infect Dis* 26: 1107–10.

Sungkanuparph S, Filler SG, Chetchotisakd P, et al. (2009) Cryptococcal immune reconstitution inflammatory syndrome after antiretroviral therapy in AIDS patients with cryptococcal meningitis: a prospective multicenter study. *Clin Infect Dis* 49: 931–4. doi: 10.1086/605497

Supparatpinyo K, Khamwan C, Baosoung V, Nelson KE and Sirisanthana T (1994) Disseminated Penicillium marneffei infection in southeast Asia. *Lancet* 344: 110–13.

Supparatpinyo K, Perriens J, Nelson KE and Sirisanthana T (1998) A controlled trial of itraconazole to prevent relapse of Penicillium marneffei infection in patients infected with the human immunodeficiency virus. *N Engl J Med* 339: 1739–43. doi: 10.1056/NEJM199812103392403

van der Horst CM, Saag MS, Cloud GA, et al. (1997) Treatment of cryptococcal meningitis associated with the acquired immunodeficiency syndrome. National Institute of Allergy and Infectious Diseases Mycoses Study Group and AIDS Clinical Trials Group. *N Engl J Med* 337: 15–21. doi: 10.1056/NEJM199707033370103

van Hougenhouck-Tulleken WG, Papavarnavas NS, Nel JS, et al. (2014) HIV-associated disseminated emmonsiosis, Johannesburg, South Africa. *Emerging Infect Dis* 20: 2164–6. doi: 10.3201/eid2012.140902

Vibhagool A, Sungkanuparph S, Mootsikapun P, et al. (2003) Discontinuation of secondary prophylaxis for cryptococcal meningitis in human immunodeficiency virus-infected patients treated with highly active antiretroviral therapy: a prospective, multicenter, randomized study. *Clin Infect Dis* 36: 1329–31. doi: 10.1086/374849

Warnock DW, Dupont B, Kauffman CA and Sirisanthana T (1998) Imported mycoses in Europe. *Med Mycol* 36 (Suppl. 1): 87–94.

Wheat LJ, Chetchotisakd P, Williams B, Connolly P, Shutt K and Hajjeh R (2000) Factors associated with severe manifestations of histoplasmosis in AIDS. *Clin Infect Dis* 30: 877–81. doi: 10.1086/313824

Wheat LJ, Connolly-Stringfield PA, Baker RL, et al. (1990) Disseminated histoplasmosis in the acquired immune deficiency syndrome: clinical findings, diagnosis and treatment, and review of the literature. *Medicine (Baltimore)* 69: 361–74.

Wheat LJ, Freifeld AG, Kleiman MB, et al. (2007) Clinical practice guidelines for the management of patients with histoplasmosis: 2007 update by the Infectious Diseases Society of America. *Clin Infect Dis* 45: 807–25. doi: 10.1086/521259

Zheng J, Gui X, Cao Q, et al. (2015) A clinical study of acquired immunodeficiency syndrome associated Penicillium marneffei infection from a non-endemic area in China. *PLoS One* 10: e0130376. doi: 10.1371/journal.pone.0130376

CHAPTER 34

Fungal infections in solid organ transplantation

Darius Armstrong James, Anand Shah, and Anna Reed

Introduction to fungal infections in solid organ transplantation

Solid organ transplantation has emerged as a major life-saving treatment for end-stage organ failure. However, opportunistic infections have been a serious complication of organ transplantation that has limited the utility of this approach (Bell and Briggs 1973). The development of successive refinements to immunosuppressive strategies and an evolving understanding of strategies to induce transplant tolerance have significantly impacted on the severity, timing, and epidemiology of opportunistic fungal diseases in organ transplantation (Shoham 2013). It has become a fast-moving field in which successively more complex transplants such as multi-visceral, face, and hand transplants are now becoming routine. Furthermore, it has become a realistic therapy in many low- to middle-income countries with varying endemic mycoses. Immunosuppressive therapy in transplantation, complex organ transplants, new geographic challenges, and novel antifungal and immunotherapeutic approaches for fungal disease have all impacted on this rapidly evolving area of medicine. There is a pressing challenge to define the evolving epidemiology of fungal infections among organ transplant recipients, and to develop robust management strategies that integrate systematic surveillance, appropriate risk stratification, diagnostic approaches, targeted prophylaxis, and directed treatment algorithms to enable optimal outcomes and limit the development of antifungal drug resistance (Pappas et al. 2010).

Epidemiology

The epidemiology of invasive fungal diseases varies widely, both between continents and countries, as well as within cities. This is because most fungi are opportunistic pathogens that primarily exist within the environment, which is the major determinant of human exposure. Since organ transplantation became an established therapeutic modality, opportunistic infections with *Candida, Aspergillus*, or *Histoplasma* species have been well described (Karalakulasingam et al. 1976). For solid organ transplants there have been relatively few historical studies; however, significant progress has been made, particularly in North America, where the Transplant-Associated Infection Surveillance Network (TRANSNET) undertook systematic surveillance for fungal disease in both haematological stem cell transplant and solid organ transplant patients at multiple centres (Pappas et al. 2010). The solid organ transplant study encompassed 23 US centres surveyed between 2001 and 2006. TRANSNET demonstrated an overall cumulative incidence of proven or probable invasive fungal disease (IFD) across all organ transplants of 3.1% in the first 12 months. However, there was wide variation in the disease incidence dependent upon transplant type, with an 11.6% risk for small-bowel transplants, an 8.6% risk for lung and heart-lung transplants, a 4.6% risk for liver transplants, a 4.1% risk for pancreas and kidney-pancreas transplants, and a 1.3% risk for kidney transplant recipients. *Candida* accounted for the majority of infections (53%), followed by *Aspergillus* (19%), *Cryptococcus* (8%), other moulds (8%), and endemic mycoses (5%). In addition, the infecting species varied widely with transplant type, with small-bowel transplants strongly associated with candidiasis (85%), and lung transplants principally associated with aspergillosis (44%). The majority of infections occurred between 90 days and three years after transplantation, although there were a significant number of late infections consistent with the prolonged immunosuppressive regimes used in this group.

A seven-year study (2003–2010) in Italy, of 1,656 organ transplant recipients, revealed a 10% incidence of opportunistic pulmonary infections, of which 63% were due to pulmonary aspergillosis, followed by *Pneumocystis* pneumonia (15%) (Hoyo et al. 2012). A further Spanish study demonstrated a 4% overall incidence of candidaemia in organ transplantation (Moreno et al. 2007). European cryptococcosis studies indicate broadly similar incidences to the United States, at around 0–1.5%. These studies suggest no major differences in the epidemiology of the major fungal infections in transplantation between the USA and Europe.

Endemic mycoses are a significant issue in the Americas, where histoplasmosis, blastomycosis, and coccidioidomycosis are all prevalent. Data from TRANSNET indicate that these occur primarily in solid organ rather than haematological transplant recipients (Kauffman et al. 2014). The 12-month cumulative incidence for histoplasmosis was estimated to be 0.1%, with a bimodal incidence either in the first six months, or after two years post-transplant. The majority of infections occurred in renal or liver transplant recipients. Phaeohyphomycoses are a further emerging problem in solid organ transplant recipients, often occurring late post-transplant (greater than 2 years) and accounting for 2.5% of all IFD, with an overall mortality of 25% (McCarty et al. 2015). The epidemiology of IFD in the Asia-Pacific region is less well described. Pulmonary aspergillosis remains the most common mould infection overall, although *A. flavus* may be more common than *A. fumigatus* in tropical areas (Slavin and Chakrabarti 2012). Scedosporiosis and fusariosis also occur with significant frequency across a broad range of immunocompromised individuals. Whilst disseminated penicilliosis in organ transplantation is well described, the overall incidence has not been defined (Chakrabarti and Slavin 2011).

Transplant immunosuppressive drugs and susceptibility to IFD

Lifelong immunosuppressive therapy is required to limit graft rejection, and this carries the associated risk of increased susceptibility to infection (Halloran 2004). Hyper-acute rejection occurs hours after transplantation and is mediated by complement-fixing antibodies, mostly directed against MHC (major histocompatibility complex) class I. This leads to activation of complement and clotting cascades and rapid graft loss. Cross-matching to identify anti-donor antibodies has almost completely eliminated the risk of hyper-acute rejection. Acute rejection may occur weeks to months post-transplantation and is mediated by recipient allo-reactive T cells, leading to cytotoxic graft destruction and activation of innate immunity. Activated T cells may also precipitate B-cell antibody class switching, and subsequent antibody-mediated chronic rejection. Chronic rejection arises months to years after transplantation and is characterized by donor-specific antibody deposition, leading to innate immune activation and graft injury.

The primary goal of transplant immunosuppression is to suppress allograft rejection. Current immunosuppressive strategies target the three-signal model of allo-immune responses, which involve both naïve and memory lymphocytes (Halloran 2004). Presentation of antigen by host or allograft dendritic cells to T cells in secondary lymphoid organs leads to T-cell receptor activation. Dendritic cell co-stimulatory CD80/CD86 T-cell activation leads to engagement of CD28 on T cells. This leads to activation of the calcineurin-NFAT (nuclear factor of activated T cell), MAPK (mitogen-activated protein kinase), and NF (nuclear factor)-κB signalling pathways. Subsequent activation of interleukin 2 and interleukin 15 leads to activation of the mTOR (mammalian target of rapamycin) pathway and cellular proliferation. Subsequent generation of effector T cells leads to increased B-cell antigen presentation and allo-antibody production. Immunosuppressive drugs used in organ transplantation are classified as glucocorticoids, small-molecule inhibitors (e.g. calcineurin inhibitors, mTOR inhibitors), inhibitors of nucleotide synthesis (e.g. purine and pyrimidine inhibitors), and antibodies (e.g. antithymocyte globulin, anti-CD3, anti-CD28, anti-CD20, anti-CD25) (Halloran 2004). Glucocorticoids are glucocorticoid receptor agonists that primarily target transcription factors such as AP-1 and NF-κB. Small molecular inhibitors target the calcineurin and mTOR pathways. Most antibodies in use deplete T cells, B cells, or both. This reduces early rejection, but can lead to increased risk of infection. The major immunological determinants of fungal diseases in transplantation are illustrated in Figure 34.1.

Glucocorticoids are a major risk factor for fungal disease, both within the context of transplantation and more widely in clinical medicine (Baddley et al. 2010). Steroids directly enable fungal

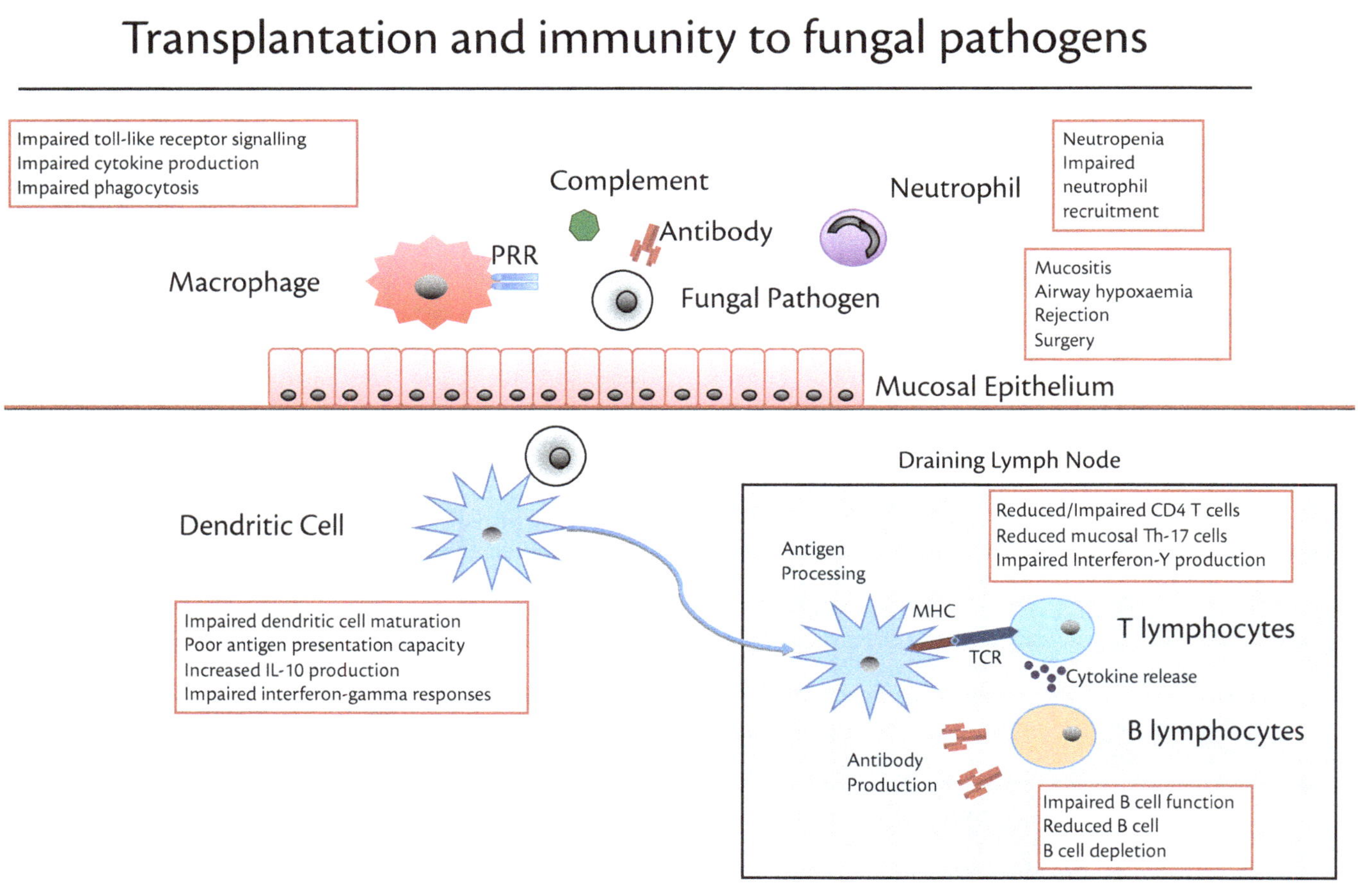

Figure 34.1 Transplantation and immunity to fungal pathogens.

growth, likely due to direct effects on glucocorticoid receptors in fungi, or metabolism of sterol nuclei by fungi (Ng et al. 1994). Furthermore, they impair innate immune responses to fungi, particularly in macrophages (Philippe et al. 2003). Whilst calcineurin inhibitors primarily inhibit T cell-based immunity, recent studies have revealed a major role of calcineurin in innate fungal immunity (Herbst et al. 2015). Notably, these drugs have natural and potent antifungal activity; however, an increasing body of evidence indicates that their immunosuppressive effects strongly outweigh any protective effect. Early unpublished trial data further suggest that sirolimus may have a significantly increased risk for fungal disease. Mycophenolate mofetil has significant antifungal effects against *Pneumocystis* pneumonia, and initial data suggested that it may be protective in clinical studies (Azevedo et al. 2005). However, more recent studies demonstrate a link between mycophenolate mofetil and risk for *Pneumocystis* pneumonia (Zhang and Zheng 2014). A major comparative study of lymphocyte-depleting agents indicated that whilst there were no significant differences in their risk of fungal infection, alemtuzumab had an increased risk of disseminated fungal disease and mortality (Safdar et al. 2010).

Specific host and therapeutic factors predisposing to IFD

Solid organ transplant recipients represent a diverse group of individuals with a number of clinical factors that lead to major differences in the type, location, and severity of fungal disease (Table 34.1). As organ transplant is performed primarily for end-stage organ dysfunction, understanding the underlying disease process that leads to graft failure, and whether this is likely to alter fungal disease susceptibility and outcome, is of critical importance. In addition, the organ type transplanted has a major impact on the risk, location, and type of IFD. This would appear to be, in part, due to a propensity for the transplanted organ to become the target for fungal disease as a function of its environmental exposure during and after transplantation. There is also variation in the degree of immunosuppressive therapy required for different organs and their degree of mismatch, in order to limit the likelihood of subsequent allograft rejection (Bodro et al. 2012). Thus, the degree of immunosuppression is also a major determinant of fungal disease susceptibility that also varies according to the transplant.

Renal allografts account for around 50% of all transplants performed (http://www.srtr.org). Whilst less than 1% of renal transplant recipients develop IFD per annum, because of the large number of kidney transplants performed there are numerically more cases of IFD in this group than in any other (Pappas et al. 2010). Invasive candidiasis is typical (in approximately 50% of cases), followed by invasive aspergillosis and disseminated cryptococcosis (both accounting for around 15% of cases) and endemic mycoses (10% overall) (Neofytos et al. 2010; Pappas et al. 2010; Gavalda et al. 2014).

Liver transplant recipients are at very high risk of IFD, with a 5% risk per annum in the first three years post-transplant. Invasive candidiasis accounts for 66% of infections, with invasive aspergillosis accounting for a further 10%. Small-bowel recipients have an even higher risk of IFD (approximately 10% per annum), and infection is dominated by invasive candidiasis in 85% of cases. Pancreatic transplantation carries around a 4% risk per annum, with 75% of cases due to invasive candidiasis. Lung transplant recipients are also at high risk of infection (approximately 8–9% per annum). In contrast to renal or liver transplants, invasive aspergillosis is the predominant infection, accounting for around 50% of infections. Other mould infections of the lung (20%) and invasive candidiasis (10%) are also prevalent. Heart transplantation is typified by invasive candidiasis in around half of cases and invasive aspergillosis in about a quarter.

Candidiasis in heart transplantation may be the consequence of biofilm formation on intravascular devices during the early post-transplant phase. The annual incidence is around 3–4%. Transplantation of abdominal organs is dominated by candidiasis, presumably due to the prevalence of *Candida* species in the gastrointestinal tract, whereas lung transplantation is associated with mould infection, probably because of inhalation of fungi into the target organ (Husain et al. 2003). The incidence of disseminated cryptococcosis is relatively low in the context of organ transplantation at less than 1.5%; however, this is slightly higher in heart or

Table 34.1 Fungal infection risk and prophylaxis strategies

Transplant type	Risk per annum	Principal fungal pathogens	Major risk factors	Prophylactic drug	Duration
Kidney	1–2%	*Candida, Aspergillus*	Urinary tract candidiasis	Not recommended	
Liver	4–5%	*Candida, Aspergillus*	Re-transplantation, fulminant hepatic failure, choledochojejunostomy, multi-site *Candida* spp. colonization, and high transfusion requirements	Fluconazole, liposomal amphotericin	1–4 weeks
Pancreas	4–5%	*Candida*	Surgical	Fluconazole	1–4 weeks
Small bowel	10–15%	*Candida*	Unknown	Fluconazole	1–4 weeks
Heart	4–5%	*Candida, Aspergillus*	Intravascular device	Itraconazole	3–6 months
Lung	8–9%	*Aspergillus*	Prior colonization, single lung transplant, cystic fibrosis	Mould-active drug plus nebulized lipid formulation amphotericin	3–6 months
Overall	4%	*Candida, Aspergillus*	Graft rejection, renal failure, cytomegalovirus viraemia, steroids		

kidney transplant recipients, and in particular in patients receiving high-dose steroids or monoclonal lymphocyte-depleting agents. Furthermore, it is important to note that whilst transplantation carries a significant risk of pneumocystosis, the risk is effectively reduced by the widespread use of co-trimoxazole prophylaxis (Perez-Ordono et al. 2014). However, late pneumocystosis may occur in the post-prophylaxis period.

In the wider context of transplantation, there are a number of factors that significantly increase the risk of developing IFD (Pappas et al. 2010; Bodro et al. 2012; Gavalda et al. 2014). One major risk is the development of allograft rejection, where causality for increased risk is complex and includes the degree of allograft mismatching, cytomegalovirus viraemia, and the requirement for increased immunosuppressive therapy (Brizendine et al. 2011). Within this context, the use of steroids as well as the absolute steroid dosage and duration appear to be critical in driving fungal immunosusceptibility (Lionakis and Kontoyiannis 2003). Another global risk factor in transplantation is severe renal failure. The mechanistic basis for this may relate to uraemic immune dysfunction (Pappas et al. 2010). Within the context of lung transplantation, prior colonization of the respiratory tract with pathogenic moulds, single lung transplant (where the native lung acts as a reservoir for fungal infection), and cystic fibrosis are risk factors for subsequent pulmonary mould infection (Brizendine et al. 2011). In addition, hypogammaglobulinaemia and use of induction monoclonal lymphocyte-depleting agents are further risk factors. For individuals undergoing heart or heart–lung transplantation, intravascular devices are a further risk factor for invasive candidiasis. In liver failure, re-transplantation, fulminant hepatic failure, choledochojejunostomy, multi-site *Candida* spp. colonization, and high transfusion requirements are all risk factors for subsequent IFD. Thus, in-depth knowledge of organ-specific factors is critical for prediction of risk and type of IFD.

Clinical presentation

Invasive candidiasis

In organ transplantation, invasive candidiasis generally accounts for around 50–60% of all cases of invasive fungal disease (Neofytos et al. 2010; Pappas et al. 2010; Bodro et al. 2012; Gavalda et al. 2014). Typical manifestations include candidaemia, peritonitis, and urinary tract infections. There is wide species variability between institutions, with *C. glabrata* in particular emerging as an important pathogen. Patients with abdominal organ transplants are particularly vulnerable. In addition, kidney and pancreatic transplant recipients are prone to recurrent urinary tract infection. Invasive candidiasis is common in the early post-transplant period, where it presents with fever and a typical systemic inflammatory response syndrome. Key clinical indicators include the presence of *Candida* colonization, thrush, fungal endophthalmitis, and urinary symptoms. All patients should be investigated for features of endocarditis and, in addition, vascular thrombophlebitis where a central venous catheter is involved.

Invasive aspergillosis and other mould infections

Invasive aspergillosis (IA) primarily occurs in lung transplant recipients, with major contributions from kidney, liver, and heart transplant recipients to the overall burden of disease (Baddley et al. 2010). Renal or hepatic failure, disseminated disease, CNS involvement, renal or hepatic transplant, organ rejection, and use of methylprednisolone are all adverse factors for outcome. Pulmonary involvement occurs in 90% of cases, with 20% being disseminated and a further 10% presenting with an extrapulmonary infection (Hoyo et al. 2012). Compared with haematological patients, there is a wider spectrum of disease, with aggressive angio-invasive infection less common, and semi-invasive disease more common. A number of patients present with life-threatening haemoptysis, where surgical intervention should be considered. Within the context of lung transplantation, a decline in FEV1 (forced expiratory volume in one second) is a typical trigger for investigation for pulmonary aspergillosis (Husain et al. 2011). In lung transplantation, nodular or ulcerative tracheobronchitis may occur, or bronchial anastomotic infection. Other features include solitary nodules, infiltrates, or consolidation. A number of non-*Aspergillus* moulds may also cause pulmonary and extrapulmonary infections in organ transplantation (Park et al. 2011). Principal amongst these are the mucormycetes *Scedosporium* and *Fusarium*. Within the context of lung transplantation, *Talaromyces (Penicillium)* species and *Paecilomyces* species also cause significant infections. Non-*Aspergillus* moulds also tend to present much later post-transplant. The infections are very difficult to distinguish clinically or radiologically from aspergillosis, and are usually diagnosed on culture.

Cryptococcosis

Cryptococcosis in organ transplant differs from advanced HIV in terms of distribution (Singh et al. 2008b). Only 40% of individuals present with CNS disease, with a further 30% having limited pulmonary disease. Pulmonary disease appears to be associated with calcineurin inhibitors, which have natural antifungal activity. Significant numbers present with extrapulmonary cryptococcomas, skin involvement (nodules, cellulitis), or cryptococcaemia. Of note, cryptococcosis tends to be a late complication, typically presenting at more than one year post-transplantation.

Endemic mycoses

The endemic mycoses histoplasmosis, coccidioidomycosis, penicilliosis, and blastomycosis are all well-recognized complications of organ transplantation (Slavin and Chakrabarti 2012; Kauffman et al. 2014). Usually these infections are associated with clear geographic exposure, but for histoplasmosis this may be less obvious. In addition, the potential for donor-organ-related transmission should be considered. In terms of post-transplant incidence, endemic mycoses may present at any stage, from as early as the immediate post-transplant period to a decade later. There is a bimodal distribution, with either the six-month or two-year post-transplant periods being most common. Presentation may be with either a pulmonary syndrome, or symptoms of disseminated infection.

Pneumocystosis

Before the use of universal prophylaxis for *Pneumocystis jirovecii* pneumonia (PCP) in organ transplantation, PCP was a significant problem, occurring in around 10–15% of individuals overall and up to 40% in lung transplantation. However co-trimoxazole prophylaxis reduces risk by 90%, and is generally used in the first 6–12 months post-transplant (Perez-Ordono et al. 2014). Therefore, the current risk period for PCP is in the post-prophylaxis period, from

12 months onwards. In contrast to HIV-PCP, mortality in organ transplantation is high at up to 60%. The clinical features of PCP are similar to those in HIV-AIDS, with the triad of dry cough, dyspnoea-hypoxaemia, and ground-glass shadowing radiographically.

Phaeohyphomycoses

Phaeohyphomycoses are a small but significant problem in organ transplant recipients, accounting for about 2.5% of all fungal infections (McCarty et al. 2015). These black moulds are able to cause diverse infections, ranging from skin nodules to pneumonia to CNS infection, for which these organisms appear to have a predilection. Dissemination occurs in 50% of patients and worsens outcome. The majority of infections occur late at more than one year post-transplant. The TRANSNET study suggests that most infections occur in lung transplant recipients, with cough, fever, and nodular or lobar abnormalities on computed tomography (McCarty et al. 2015). The skin and sinuses are also common sites, from which the organism can often be recovered. *Alternaria* species are by far the most common causative agents, although around 100 different phaeohyphomycetes have been reported to cause human disease.

Diagnosis

The European Organisation for Research and Treatment of Cancer/Mycoses Study Group criteria define IFD as proven, probable, and possible infection (De Pauw et al. 2008). However, it is recognized that the real world usage of these criteria, initially developed for clinical trials, will lead to misdiagnosis in many individuals.

For the diagnosis of candidiasis, blood culture has been the gold standard procedure across all patient groups; however, the sensitivity for candidaemia is only 50–75%, and even lower for deep-seated candidiasis. Two further assays—the combined mannan–anti-mannan assay and the 1,3 β-D glucan assay—also have utility for diagnosing candidiasis. The mannan–anti-mannan assay is considered specific for candidiasis; however, it is not widely used owing to its low sensitivity and specificity. The 1,3 β-D glucan assay is considered a pan-fungal assay and therefore will also detect other organisms such as *Aspergillus*, and PCP. However, it has excellent sensitivity and specificity, and is superior to blood culture for detecting deep-seated candidiasis. Finally, there is increasing data to support the use of blood *Candida* PCR (polymerase chain reaction) assays, which appear to have excellent specificity and sensitivity; however, there is no international consensus technique as yet.

For the diagnosis of IA, there are a number of differences in the organ transplant population when compared with those with haematological malignancies. Firstly, the radiological features of pulmonary aspergillosis tend to be more diverse, such that new infiltrates, progressive consolidation, endobronchial lesions, multiple nodules, or tree-in-bud infiltrates are all consistent with pulmonary aspergillosis in addition to the established macronodule, halo, and air crescent signs. Furthermore, whilst serum galactomannan has utility in diagnosing haematological malignancy, it performs poorly in organ transplant recipients (Mennink-Kersten et al. 2004; Pasqualotto et al. 2010). This is probably because frank angio-invasive aspergillosis is less common. Instead, bronchoalveolar lavage galactomannan measurement has emerged as a highly sensitive and specific technique for diagnosing pulmonary aspergillosis in a range of non-neutropenic hosts including organ transplant recipients. Furthermore, a recently licensed lateral flow device is showing great promise for aspergillosis (Hoenigl et al. 2014). Likewise, there are emerging data for the utility of *Aspergillus* PCR, and much international effort has been expended in establishing consensus approaches (Mengoli et al. 2009). A newer commercial assay is CE marked and is also able to detect azole resistance (White et al. 2015) (see Chapter 43).

For cryptococcal disease, culture and cryptococcal antigen detection are the standards for diagnosis, with no major differences compared with other groups such as advanced HIV patients (Singh et al. 2008a). A novel cryptococcal point-of-care test has shown excellent performance and is rapidly becoming the preferred assay owing to its ease of use (Lourens et al. 2014). For endemic mycoses and phaeohyphomycoses, diagnosis is based on culture, histopathology, and consistent clinical features in the context of an appropriate exposure history. Antigen-based assays are available for histoplasmosis and coccidioidomycosis (Durkin et al. 2008; Assi et al. 2013). For suspected disseminated histoplasmosis, bone-marrow culture and histopathology are important adjunctive investigations. Pneumocystosis is diagnosed on the basis of detection of cysts on induced sputum or BAL (bronchoalveolar lavage), or PCR (Maillet et al. 2014). *Pneumocystis* PCR is extremely sensitive and may also pick up colonization. Therefore, correlation with radiological and clinical features is essential.

For a number of fungal diseases, the clinical presentation may include mucosal or cutaneous manifestations. These may be indicative of disseminated infection, and therefore need to be urgently assessed in the context of the overall presentation. For example, skin nodules may be associated with cryptococcosis, phaeohyphomycosis, and endemic mycoses. Direct biopsy, culture, and Grocott or PAS (periodic acid-Schiff) staining will often reveal the infecting organism.

Treatment strategies

Prophylaxis

Whilst antifungal prophylaxis strategies have been clearly defined within the context of haematological malignancies through well-designed randomized controlled studies, the role of prophylaxis in solid organ transplantation is less rigorously defined (Cornely et al. 2007; Ullmann et al. 2007; Cadena et al. 2009; Eschenauer et al. 2009). The requirement for prophylaxis is further defined by the risk of IFD, which is highly variable depending on the transplant type and other independent risk factors (Brizendine et al. 2011; Winston et al. 2015) (Table 34.1). In addition, depending on whether the primary cause of IFD is *Candida* species or *Aspergillus* species, further consideration of whether to use mould-active prophylaxis is required. Another consideration is whether to adopt a universal or targeted prophylaxis strategy (Eschenauer et al. 2015). Currently, there is a lack of consensus on the approaches being followed, with high variability in practice between centres. Good understanding of local fungal epidemiology, drug resistance patterns, and variations in transplant protocols is critical for the development of appropriate institutional guidelines.

Liver transplants

In liver transplantation, invasive candidiasis is common, although significant numbers of cases of IA also occur. Consequently, the efficacy of fluconazole and also mould-active azoles, polyenes, and echinocandins has been assessed in this setting (Eschenauer et al.

2015; Winston et al. 2015). Additionally, the rationale for targeted prophylaxis is well established in liver transplantation, as a number of factors clearly contribute to risk of infection (Eschenauer et al. 2009). Patients with more than two contributory factors are generally considered high risk. Current consensus, on the basis of best available evidence, suggests that high-risk liver transplant recipients should receive antifungal prophylaxis with either fluconazole or liposomal amphotericin for one to four weeks post-transplantation, when the risk is highest.

Lung transplants

Lung transplant patients are at high risk for pulmonary aspergillosis and other mould infections (Drew et al. 2004; Pappas et al. 2010). Thus, mould-active agents are favoured. Most centres use either azoles, such as voriconazole or posaconazole, or alternatively systemic lipid amphotericin B formulations (Cadena et al. 2009). There is also evidence for the use of nebulized amphotericin B formulations as prophylaxis (Drew et al. 2004). Most studies support a universal approach, with a three- to six-month duration of therapy post-transplantation.

Small-bowel transplants

Patients undergoing small-bowel transplantation are at very high risk for invasive candidiasis in the immediate postoperative period (Pappas et al. 2010). Whilst objective clinical data are lacking, universal fluconazole prophylaxis—for one to four weeks post-transplantation—is the usual approach.

Pancreas transplants

There is a high risk of invasive candidiasis following pancreatic transplantation (Pappas et al. 2010), with well-defined surgical risk factors in the immediate postoperative period (Brizendine et al. 2011). Thus, prophylaxis with fluconazole for one to four weeks is generally used in most centres, primarily in high-risk patients.

Heart transplants

Heart transplantation is complicated by significant cases of invasive candidiasis, IA, and cryptococcosis (Pappas et al. 2010). There is a relative paucity of systematic data on prophylaxis in this setting. Targeted prophylaxis with itraconazole for three to six months in high-risk patients has been found to be useful (Munoz et al. 2013; Tissot et al. 2014). Inhaled amphotericin B formulations may also have a role. However, further studies are required before definitive recommendations can be made.

Kidney transplants

The risk of fungal infection in kidney transplant recipients is very low (Pappas et al. 2010). In addition, there is a paucity of data on antifungal prophylaxis in this setting. Therefore, antifungal prophylaxis is not generally recommended for kidney transplantation.

Treatment

Whilst the management of IFD in organ transplant recipients is broadly similar to that of other immunocompromised hosts, there are a number of aspects where the approaches differ.

Safe reduction in immunosuppressive therapy to a level that will maintain graft integrity, whilst optimizing immunological function, is highly desirable. In particular, corticosteroids are prone to worsen outcome from IFD, and should be reduced if safe in the short term (Lionakis and Kontoyiannis 2003). However, secondary fungal immune reconstitution inflammatory syndrome (IRIS) may occur as a consequence.

A major consideration in organ transplant IFD is the interaction between immunosuppressive therapy and fungi (Table 34.2). Calcineurin inhibitors are the mainstay of immunosuppressive therapy. However, they are nephrotoxic and interact with azoles and to a lesser extent caspofungin. The use of amphotericin B deoxycholate is not generally advisable in this group owing to risk of nephrotoxicity, and caution is required for prolonged use of intravenous

Table 34.2 Antifungal drug interactions in transplantation

	Tacrolimus	Cyclosporin	Prednisolone	Sirolimus	Everolimus
Fluconazole	Increases tacrolimus levels	Increases cyclosporin levels	Increases prednisolone levels	Severely increases sirolimus levels	Severely increases everolimus levels
Voriconazole	Increases tacrolimus levels	Increases cyclosporin levels	Increases prednisolone levels	Severely increases sirolimus levels	Severely increases everolimus levels
Itraconazole	Increases tacrolimus levels	Increases cyclosporin levels	Increases prednisolone levels	Severely increases sirolimus levels	Severely increases everolimus levels
Posaconazole	Increases tacrolimus levels	Increases cyclosporin levels	Increases prednisolone levels	Increases sirolimus levels	Increases everolimus levels
Caspofungin	Reduces tacrolimus levels	Possible hepatotoxicity	No effect	No effect	No effect
Micafungin	No effect	No effect	No effect	Slightly increases sirolimus levels	No effect
Anidulafungin	No effect	No effect	No effect	No effect	No effect
Amphotericin B	Renal toxicity risk	Renal toxicity risk	Hypokalaemia risk	Renal toxicity risk	No effect
Flucytosine (5-fluorocytosine)	No effect	No effect	No effect	No effect	No effect

voriconazole. In patients receiving voriconazole, the dose of calcineurin inhibitor should be reduced to a third. In addition, the combination of voriconazole and sirolimus should be carefully managed with therapeutic drug monitoring. For posaconazole, the dose of tacrolimus should be reduced to a third and cyclosporin to two-thirds. Caspofungin reduces the concentration of tacrolimus by 20%; however, this does not occur with anidulafungin or micafungin. In addition, under these circumstances it is very important to undertake regular monitoring of both azole and tacrolimus levels.

For invasive candidiasis, treatment with an echinocandin rather than fluconazole is advised, because of superior efficacy in clinical studies and the immunocompromised nature of transplant recipients (Reboli et al. 2007). For IA, treatment with either voriconazole or liposomal amphotericin B is advised (Walsh et al. 2008). In addition, in lung transplantation, *Aspergillus* colonization is treated with nebulized liposomal amphotericin B owing to the risk of conversion to invasive disease (Drew et al. 2004). Nebulized amphotericin B is also an important adjunctive treatment for ulcerative tracheobronchitis in combination with systemic therapy. For PCP, treatment with co-trimoxazole according to standard guidelines is recommended, with clindamycin-primaquine an alternative (Helweg-Larsen et al. 2009). The use of adjunctive steroids in severe PCP is not advised in organ transplantation, as most patients are already on steroids when they develop PCP. The management of cryptococcosis, other moulds, phaeohyphomycosis, and endemic mycoses is broadly along the lines of that for other patient groups. For further guidance, please refer to Sections 2 and 5.

References

Assi M, Martin S, Wheat LJ, et al. (2013) Histoplasmosis after solid organ transplant. *Clin Infect Dis* 57: 1542–9.

Azevedo LS, Castro MC, Paula FJ, Ianhez LE and David-Neto E (2005) Mycophenolate mofetil may protect against Pneumocystis carinii pneumonia in renal transplanted patients. *Rev Inst Med Trop Sao Paulo* 47: 143–5.

Baddley JW, Andes DR, Marr KA, et al. (2010) Factors associated with mortality in transplant patients with invasive aspergillosis. *Clin Infect Dis* 50: 1559–67.

Bell PR and Briggs JD (1973) Fungal and nocardial infections in renal-transplant recipients. *Lancet* 1: 324.

Bodro M, Sabe N, Gomila A, et al. (2012) Risk factors, clinical characteristics, and outcomes of invasive fungal infections in solid organ transplant recipients. *Transplant Proc* 44: 2682–5.

Brizendine KD, Vishin S and Baddley JW (2011) Antifungal prophylaxis in solid organ transplant recipients. *Expert Rev Anti Infect Ther* 9: 571–81.

Cadena J, Levine DJ, Angel LF, et al. (2009) Antifungal prophylaxis with voriconazole or itraconazole in lung transplant recipients: hepatotoxicity and effectiveness. *Am J Transplant* 9: 2085–91.

Chakrabarti A and Slavin MA (2011) Endemic fungal infections in the Asia-Pacific region. *Med Mycol* 49: 337–44.

Cornely OA, Maertens J, Winston DJ, et al. (2007) Posaconazole vs. fluconazole or itraconazole prophylaxis in patients with neutropenia. *N Engl J Med* 356: 348–59.

De Pauw B, Walsh TJ, Donnelly JP, et al. (2008) Revised definitions of invasive fungal disease from the European Organization for Research and Treatment of Cancer/Invasive Fungal Infections Cooperative Group and the National Institute of Allergy and Infectious Diseases Mycoses Study Group (EORTC/MSG) Consensus Group. *Clin Infect Dis* 46: 1813–21.

Drew RH, Dodds Ashley E, Benjamin DK Jr, Duane Davis R, Palmer SM and Perfect JR (2004) Comparative safety of amphotericin B lipid complex and amphotericin B deoxycholate as aerosolized antifungal prophylaxis in lung-transplant recipients. *Transplantation* 77: 232–7.

Durkin M, Connolly P, Kuberski T, et al. (2008) Diagnosis of coccidioidomycosis with use of the Coccidioides antigen enzyme immunoassay. *Clin Infect Dis* 47: e69–73.

Eschenauer GA, Kwak EJ, Humar A, et al. (2015) Targeted versus universal antifungal prophylaxis among liver transplant recipients. *Am J Transplant* 15: 180–9.

Eschenauer GA, Lam SW and Carver PL (2009) Antifungal prophylaxis in liver transplant recipients. *Liver Transpl* 15: 842–58.

Gavalda J, Meije Y, Fortun J, et al. (2014) Invasive fungal infections in solid organ transplant recipients. *Clin Microbiol Infect* 20 (Suppl. 7): 27–48.

Halloran PF (2004) Immunosuppressive drugs for kidney transplantation. *N Engl J Med* 351: 2715–29.

Helweg-Larsen J, Benfield T, Atzori C and Miller RF (2009) Clinical efficacy of first- and second-line treatments for HIV-associated Pneumocystis jirovecii pneumonia: a tri-centre cohort study. *J Antimicrob Chemother* 64: 1282–90.

Herbst S, Shah A, Mazon Moya M, et al. 2015. Phagocytosis-dependent activation of a TLR9-BTK-calcineurin-NFAT pathway co-ordinates innate immunity to Aspergillus fumigatus. *EMBO Mol Med* 7: 240–58.

Hoenigl M, Prattes J, Spiess B, et al. (2014) Performance of galactomannan, beta-d-glucan, Aspergillus lateral-flow device, conventional culture, and PCR tests with bronchoalveolar lavage fluid for diagnosis of invasive pulmonary aspergillosis. *J Clin Microbiol* 52: 2039–45.

Hoyo I, Sanclemente G, Cervera C, et al. (2012) Opportunistic pulmonary infections in solid organ transplant recipients. *Transplant Proc* 44: 2673–5.

Husain S, Alexander BD, Munoz P, et al. (2003) Opportunistic mycelial fungal infections in organ transplant recipients: emerging importance of non-Aspergillus mycelial fungi. *Clin Infect Dis* 37: 221–9.

Husain S, Mooney ML, Danziger-Isakov L, et al. (2011) A 2010 working formulation for the standardization of definitions of infections in cardiothoracic transplant recipients. *J Heart Lung Transplant* 30: 361–74.

Karalakulasingam R, Arora KK, Adams G, Serratoni F and Martin DG (1976) Meningoencephalitis caused by Histoplasma capsulatum: occurrence in a renal transplant recipient and a review of the literature. *Arch Intern Med* 136: 217–20.

Kauffman CA, Freifeld AG, Andes DR, et al. (2014) Endemic fungal infections in solid organ and hematopoietic cell transplant recipients enrolled in the Transplant-Associated Infection Surveillance Network (TRANSNET). *Transpl Infect Dis* 16: 213–24.

Lionakis MS and Kontoyiannis DP (2003) Glucocorticoids and invasive fungal infections. *Lancet* 362: 1828–38.

Lourens A, Jarvis JN, Meintjes G and Samuel CM (2014) Rapid diagnosis of cryptococcal meningitis by use of lateral flow assay on cerebrospinal fluid samples: influence of the high-dose 'hook' effect. *J Clin Microbiol* 52: 4172–5.

McCarty TP, Baddley JW, Walsh TJ, et al. (2015) Phaeohyphomycosis in transplant recipients: results from the Transplant Associated Infection Surveillance Network (TRANSNET). *Med Mycol* 53: 440–6.

Maillet M, Maubon D, Brion JP, et al. (2014) Pneumocystis jirovecii (Pj) quantitative PCR to differentiate Pj pneumonia from Pj colonization in immunocompromised patients. *Eur J Clin Microbiol Infect Dis* 33: 331–6.

Mengoli C, Cruciani M, Barnes RA, Loeffler J and Donnelly JP (2009) Use of PCR for diagnosis of invasive aspergillosis: systematic review and meta-analysis. *Lancet Infect Dis* 9: 89–96.

Mennink-Kersten MA, Donnelly JP and Verweij PE (2004) Detection of circulating galactomannan for the diagnosis and management of invasive aspergillosis. *Lancet Infect Dis* 4: 349–57.

Moreno A, Cervera C, Gavalda J, et al. (2007) Bloodstream infections among transplant recipients: results of a nationwide surveillance in Spain. *Am J Transplant* 7: 2579–86.

Munoz P, Valerio M, Palomo J, et al. (2013) Targeted antifungal prophylaxis in heart transplant recipients. *Transplantation* 96: 664–9.

Neofytos D, Fishman JA, Horn D, et al. (2010) Epidemiology and outcome of invasive fungal infections in solid organ transplant recipients. *Transpl Infect Dis* 12: 220–9.

Ng TT, Robson GD and Denning DW (1994) Hydrocortisone-enhanced growth of Aspergillus spp.: implications for pathogenesis. *Microbiology* 140 (Pt 9): 2475–9.

Pappas PG, Alexander BD, Andes DR, et al. (2010) Invasive fungal infections among organ transplant recipients: results of the Transplant-Associated Infection Surveillance Network (TRANSNET). *Clin Infect Dis* 50: 1101–11.

Park BJ, Pappas PG, Wannemuehler KA, et al. (2011) Invasive non-Aspergillus mold infections in transplant recipients, United States, 2001-2006. *Emerg Infect Dis* 17: 1855–64.

Pasqualotto AC, Xavier MO, Sanchez LB, et al. (2010) Diagnosis of invasive aspergillosis in lung transplant recipients by detection of galactomannan in the bronchoalveolar lavage fluid. *Transplantation* 90: 306–11.

Perez-Ordono L, Hoyo I, Sanclemente G, et al. (2014) Late-onset Pneumocystis jirovecii pneumonia in solid organ transplant recipients. *Transpl Infect Dis* 16: 324–8.

Philippe B, Ibrahim-Granet O, Prevost MC, et al. (2003) Killing of Aspergillus fumigatus by alveolar macrophages is mediated by reactive oxidant intermediates. *Infect Immun* 71: 3034–42.

Reboli AC, Rotstein C, Pappas PG, et al. (2007) Anidulafungin versus fluconazole for invasive candidiasis. *N Engl J Med* 356: 2472–82.

Safdar N, Smith J, Knasinski V, et al. (2010) Infections after the use of alemtuzumab in solid organ transplant recipients: a comparative study. *Diagn Microbiol Infect Dis* 66: 7–15.

Shoham S (2013) Emerging fungal infections in solid organ transplant recipients. *Infect Dis Clin North Am* 27: 305–16.

Singh N, Alexander BD, Lortholary O, et al. (2008a) Pulmonary cryptococcosis in solid organ transplant recipients: clinical relevance of serum cryptococcal antigen. *Clin Infect Dis* 46: e12–18.

Singh N, Dromer F, Perfect JR and Lortholary O (2008b) Cryptococcosis in solid organ transplant recipients: current state of the science. *Clin Infect Dis* 47: 1321–7.

Slavin MA and Chakrabarti A (2012) Opportunistic fungal infections in the Asia-Pacific region. *Med Mycol* 50: 18–25.

Tissot F, Pascual M, Hullin R, et al. (2014) Impact of targeted antifungal prophylaxis in heart transplant recipients at high risk for early invasive fungal infection. *Transplantation* 97: 1192–7.

Ullmann AJ, Lipton JH, Vesole DH, et al. (2007) Posaconazole or fluconazole for prophylaxis in severe graft-versus-host disease. *N Engl J Med* 356: 335–47.

Walsh TJ, Anaissie EJ, Denning DW, et al. (2008) Treatment of aspergillosis: clinical practice guidelines of the Infectious Diseases Society of America. *Clin Infect Dis* 46: 327–60.

White PL, Posso RB and Barnes RA (2015) Analytical and clinical evaluation of the PathoNostics AsperGenius® Assay for detection of Invasive Aspergillosis and resistance to azole antifungal drugs during testing of serum samples. *J Clin Microbiol* 53: 2115–21.

Winston DJ, Busuttil RW and Singh N (2015) Antifungal prophylaxis in liver transplant recipients. *Clin Infect Dis* 61: 1349–50.

Zhang Y and Zheng Y (2014) Pneumocystis jirovecii pneumonia in mycophenolate mofetil-treated patients with connective tissue disease: analysis of 17 cases. *Rheumatol Int* 34: 1765–71.

CHAPTER 35

Fungal infections in neonates

Adilia Warris

Introduction to neonatal fungal infections

The vast majority of fungal infections, both superficial and invasive, in the neonatal population are caused by *Candida* species. These species are responsible for a variety of disease entities in neonates ranging from mild oral thrush and diaper dermatitis in term healthy neonates to life-threatening nosocomial invasive fungal diseases (IFD) in prematurely born neonates. Infrequently, nosocomial infections caused by *Malassezia* species and moulds such as *Aspergillus* species and the Mucorales have been reported. *Malassezia* species are a group of lipid-dependent yeasts that easily colonize the skin and gastrointestinal tract (Leeming et al. 1995). *Malassezia furfur* infections in neonates are associated with the use of lipid infusions (e.g. in parenteral nutrition) combined with central vascular catheter (Stuart and Lane 1992). Occasionally, outbreaks may occur, such as the reported epidemic of *Malassezia pachydermatis* in an intensive care nursery associated with colonization of healthcare workers' pet-dogs (Chang et al. 1998). Infections caused by *Aspergillus* species and the Mucorales in neonates are often localized to the skin, affecting the most premature and extremely low birth weight (ELBW) neonates with an impaired and immature skin barrier function (Groll et al. 1998; Amod et al. 2000; Castagnola et al. 2011). These cutaneous infections were described in relation to the use of contaminated wooden tongue depressors, arm boards, and/or adhesive tapes. Owing to the sporadic nature of non-*Candida* IFD in neonates, this chapter will focus on infections caused by *Candida* species in the neonatal population.

Epidemiology

Among neonates, those born before 28 weeks of gestation and/or <1000 g birth weight (ELBW) have the highest risk of developing invasive candidiasis, while the risk is minimal in neonates born after 32 weeks of gestation and/or >1500 g birth weight. Reported incidences in neonates with a birth weight >1500 g is as low as 1%, increasing to >10% when born with a body weight <750 g (Stoll et al. 1996; Benjamin et al. 2003; Benjamin et al. 2010). Comparing the incidence of invasive candidiasis between adult patients, children, and neonates, the latter group has a three- to five-fold higher incidence per 100,000 admissions (30 [95% CI, range 26–34%] *vs* 47 [95% CI, range 40–54%] *vs* 150 [95% CI, range 130–160%], respectively) (Zaoutis et al. 2005, 2007). Incidences of neonatal candidiasis have clearly decreased since the late 1990s, with the largest decrease in absolute numbers of neonates affected occurring before the widespread use of fluconazole prophylaxis. Factors such as proper infection prevention and control measures, and a more rational antimicrobial prescribing behaviour leading to less antibiotic exposure, have had a positive effect on the incidence of neonatal candidiasis (Aliaga et al. 2014; Fisher et al. 2014).

Neonates can acquire *Candida* species by both vertical and horizontal transmission, leading to colonization and ultimately to infection depending on patient characteristics and associated risk factors. *Candida albicans* is the most common species transmitted vertically—that is, from mother to child—while horizontal transmission (e.g. by the hands of healthcare workers) will usually lead to colonization with *Candida parapsilosis* (Saiman et al. 2001a). Colonization with *Candida* species occurs early after birth, and of the neonates admitted to a neonatal intensive care unit (NICU), the majority of those becoming colonized will acquire *Candida* species before the third week of life (Farmaki et al. 2007).

C. albicans and *C. parapsilosis* are the most commonly encountered species causing IFD in neonates (Fridkin et al. 2006). Within the *C. parapsilosis* complex, consisting of *C. parapsilosis* sensu stricto, *C. orthopsilosis*, and *C. metapsilosis, C. parapsilosis* sensu stricto is the main species causing candidaemia in neonates (Cantón et al. 2011). *C. glabrata* and *C. krusei*, being (partially) resistant to fluconazole, are only sporadically reported as causing invasive disease in neonates (Roilides et al. 2004; Dotis et al. 2012).

Crude mortality rates for invasive candidiasis in ELBW infants are as high as 26%, with an attributable risk of 11.9% (95% CI, range 5.4–18.3%) (Zaoutis et al. 2005, 2007), although better outcome rates have recently been reported (Steinbach et al. 2012). Morbidity with respect to neurodevelopmental impairment in ELBW neonates with candidaemia, even when antifungal treatment has been prompt and appropriate, is of serious concern and has been observed in 57% of infants, which is clearly higher than in those with no septicaemia (29%) or those with bacteraemia (45%) (Benjamin et al. 2014).

The *Candida* species causing invasive candidiasis in neonates aged less than three months are shown in Table 35.1.

Risk factors

Host related

The immature immune system and the impaired barrier function of the skin and mucosa of ELBW neonates significantly contribute to the increased risk of developing invasive candidiasis, and a clear inverse relationship has been shown between birth

Table 35.1 *Candida* species causing invasive candidiasis in neonates aged less than three months

	C. albicans (%)	*C. parapsilosis* (%)	*C. tropicalis* (%)	*C. glabrata* (%)	*C. krusei* (%)	Other (%)
Fridkin 2006 (US) (Fridkin et al. 2006)	58	34	4	2	0	0
Blyth 2009 (AUS)* (Blyth et al. 2009)	39	42	3	9	0	3
Peman 2011 (SPAIN) (Peman et al. 2011)	53	33	4	6	2	3
Steinbach 2012 (Int.) (Steinbach et al. 2012)	48	28	0	4	0	24
Oeser 2014 (UK) (Oeser et al. 2014)	63	23	1	2	–	11

* Neonates aged less than one month.
Int. = international study

weight and the incidence of invasive candidiasis in neonates admitted to the NICU (Evans and Rutter 1986; Levy 2007; Basha et al. 2014) (Box 35.1). Antifungal effector mechanisms normally displayed by neutrophils, dendritic cells, and macrophages are reported to be either absent or diminished in premature neonates (Bektas et al. 1990; Kaufman et al. 1999; Schefold et al. 2015).

Treatment related

Changes in the microbiome of the gastrointestinal tract due to the use of broad-spectrum antibiotics (e.g. cephalosporins, carbapenems) will select for *Candida* colonization and consequently increase the risk of invasive infection (Kennedy and Volz 1985; Saiman et al. 2000, 2001b) (Box 35.1). The detection of *Candida* colonization at two or more body sites increases the risk of IFD (Kaufman et al. 2001). H_2-blockers increasing the pH of the stomach interfere with non-specific microbial defence mechanisms in the gut and lead to enhanced *Candida* intestinal colonization (Saiman et al. 2001b). Indwelling catheters facilitate the adherence and growth of *Candida* species evolving to a biofilm in which antifungals hardly penetrate (Adam et al. 2002). Administration of parenteral nutrition and the presence of hyperglycaemia will provide additional substrates for *Candida* growth.

Box 35.1 Host- and treatment-related risk factors for invasive candidiasis in neonates admitted to a neonatal intensive care unit

Extreme prematurity (<28 weeks' gestational age)
Extremely low birth weight (<1,000 g)
Immature immune system
Impaired barrier function of skin and mucosa
Indwelling catheters
Broad-spectrum antibiotics
Parenteral nutrition (lipid emulsions)
H_2 blockers
Steroids
Hyperglycaemia
Abdominal surgery
Multiple-site *Candida* colonization

Clinical presentation

Mucocutaneous infections

Oral thrush and diaper rash are benign diseases in otherwise healthy and term neonates and can develop within the first three months of life. Clinical features of oral thrush are a white coating of the tongue and/or with patches of oral mucosa which cannot be rubbed off easily and sometimes lead to feeding difficulties. Diaper rash caused by *Candida* species leads to dark red areas of the skin with or without raised yellow, fluid-filled pustules and satellite lesions (Ravanfar et al. 2012). In ELBW infants, mucocutaneous candidiasis is an additional risk factor for developing IFD (Faix et al. 1989; Kucinskiene et al. 2014; Manzoni et al. 2015).

A separate disease entity is congenital cutaneous candidiasis, present immediately after birth or which develops in the first day of life. This skin disease consists of a generalized eruption of erythematous macules, papules, and/or pustules in term neonates (Tieu et al. 2012). Development of a more widespread desquamating and/or erosive dermatitis may occur in preterm infants (Darmstadt et al. 2000; Aldana-Valenzuela et al. 2005).

Invasive infections

Candidaemia, single organ candidiasis, and disseminated candidiasis are the three main manifestations of invasive disease in neonates. IFD presents around the third week of life in the majority of ELBW infants. Clinical signs and symptoms of neonatal candidaemia are non-specific in nature and do not differ from neonatal sepsis caused by bacteria (Kaufman and Fairchild 2004). The occurrence of thrombocytopenia and hyperglycaemia is strongly associated with neonatal candidaemia (Warris et al. 2001; Guida et al. 2003). Candidaemia in premature neonates is associated with a meningo-encephalitis in almost 25% of cases, even when no overt neurological symptoms are present (Xia et al. 2014). Dissemination to the kidney (5%), eye (3%), and heart (5%) is a relatively frequent observation particularly in neonates with persistent candidaemia (Noyola et al. 2001; Benjamin et al. 2003). Single organ infections are reported in the CNS in the presence of indwelling devices (Jans et al. 2013) and in the kidneys (Ben Ameur et al. 2014), heart (Pana et al. 2015), and bones and joints (Evdoridou et al. 1997). *Candida* infection of the kidneys in neonates may be complicated by the development of a fungal bezoar (fungal ball), leading to urinary tract obstruction (Visser et al. 1998).

Diagnosis

Culture

Diagnosis of candidaemia in neonates is challenging owing to the issues related to blood sampling in ELBW neonates and the difficulties in obtaining a sufficient amount of blood to be cultured (Arendrup et al. 2009). The same holds true for obtaining samples from other normally sterile sites such as cerebrospinal fluid. The likelihood of false-negative cultures is high, and therefore empiric antifungal treatment is often initiated based on host- and treatment-related risk factors. Positive cultures from skin, mucosa, and respiratory lavages do not differentiate between colonization and infection, but should be considered as an additional risk factor in a susceptible ELBW neonate.

Separate attention is needed for a positive urine culture. Isolation of *Candida* species from the urine has been shown to be indicative of invasive candidiasis in a significant proportion of premature neonates and should prompt systemic evaluation and initiation of antifungal treatment (Phillips and Karlowicz 1997). Results from the Neonatal Research Network *Candida* study—the largest cohort of comprehensively studied ELBW infants with candiduria—showed comparable mortality rates and neurodevelopmental impairment between ELBW neonates with only a positive urine culture and those with positive blood cultures. These findings underscore the clinical relevance of a positive urine culture with *Candida* species in premature neonates (Wynn et al. 2012).

Non-culture-based methods

Non-culture-based methods which detect fungal antigens or DNA appear to be promising alternative methods, considering the high rate of false-negative blood cultures.

Detection of β-D-glucan in serum samples may offer an advantage, as reflected in studies performed in adults. Limited data are available for children, and uncertainties about the optimal cut-off in children have been raised (Koltze et al. 2015). Only one retrospective study has been performed in neonates suspected of invasive candidiasis, and this revealed significantly higher β-D-glucan levels in infected neonates ($n = 18$) than in uninfected neonates ($n=43$). Using a cut-off of 125 pg/mL, the test had a sensitivity of 84% and a specificity of 75% (Goudjil et al. 2013).

Use of *Candida* PCR (polymerase chain reaction) shows promising results in adults and children, but data are still awaited for the neonatal population. A small study in which a multiplex nested PCR was performed on 54 children and neonates admitted to an intensive care unit suspected of candidaemia increased the detection of *Candida* species by 10% compared with blood culture alone (Taira et al. 2014).

Imaging

Owing to the high frequency of disseminated infections, end-organ localization of *Candida* infections should be investigated by imaging or functional testing. Ultrasound of the abdominal organs, a cardiac ultrasound, and a fundoscopy should be performed when *Candida* is isolated from a normally sterile site. Imaging of

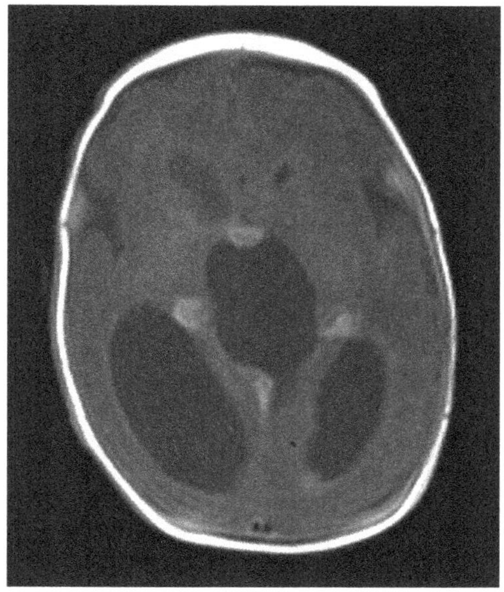

Figure 35.1 Magnetic resonance image of brain of neonate showing *Candida*-infected thrombo-emboli.

Reproduced with permission from Jans J., Brüggemann R. J. M., Christmann V., Verweij P. E., & Warris A., 'Favorable Outcome of Neonatal Cerebrospinal Fluid Shunt-Associated Candida Meningitis with Caspofungin', *Antimicrobial Agents and Chemotherapy*, Volume 57, Issue 5, pp. 2391–3, Copyright © 2013 American Society for Microbiology. DOI: 0.1128/AAC.02085-12

the brain should be considered if *Candida* is detected in the CSF to assess potential metastatic infectious foci in brain parenchyma (Figure 35.1). Positive findings of specific organ involvement will directly influence the choice of antifungal drug and duration of therapy.

Treatment strategies

Treatment of superficial and mucocutaneous candidiasis in the healthy term neonate consists of topical nystatin or miconazole (Hoppe 1997). Topical antifungals may be sufficient for the treatment of mucocutaneous candidiasis in premature neonates, although in the presence of several risk factors for invasive candidiasis, systemic antifungal treatment is indicated. Congenital cutaneous candidiasis should be treated with systemic antifungal treatment (either orally in the healthy term neonate or intravenously in premature neonates) owing to the risk of dissemination.

The treatment of neonatal invasive candidiasis is difficult because of the high likelihood of dissemination—in particular to the central nervous system—scarce pharmacokinetic data available, and the absence of phase III clinical trials in the neonatal population. Nevertheless, prompt treatment is critical to improving outcomes for ELBW neonates (Greenberg et al. 2012). Both conventional and lipid formulations of amphotericin B, fluconazole, micafungin, and caspofungin can be used to treat invasive candidiasis in neonates. The predominant *Candida* species causing invasive disease in neonates, *C. albicans* and *C. parapsilosis*, are equally susceptible to those antifungals. Although higher minimum inhibitory concentrations to echinocandins are reported for *C. parapsilosis*, this does not appear to be clinically relevant

(Peman et al. 2011; Pfaller et al. 2011). *C. krusei* is inherently resistant to fluconazole and *C. glabrata* shows variable susceptibility to fluconazole, but both are infrequent causes of invasive candidiasis in neonates. Therefore, fluconazole remains an option for the treatment of neonatal candidiasis, except in neonates with prior azole exposure (prophylaxis) (Pappas et al. 2009; Manzoni et al. 2015). *In vitro* susceptibility should be performed on all *Candida* species isolated when invasive candidiasis is suspected, to ensure appropriate antifungal treatment.

The use of amphotericin B, fluconazole, micafungin, and caspofungin in neonates is supported by neonatal pharmacokinetic studies and supportive evidence for efficacy and safety (Starke et al. 1987; Driessen et al. 1996, 1997; Fernandez et al. 2000; Juster-Reicher et al. 2000, 2003; Schwarze et al. 2000; Odio et al. 2004; Wurthwein et al. 2005; Heresi et al. 2006; Manzar et al. 2006; Queiroz-Telles et al. 2008; Wade et al. 2008, 2009; Saez-Llorens et al. 2009; Hope et al. 2010; Piper et al. 2011). Although the use of conventional amphotericin B has more or less been abandoned owing to its toxicity profile in children and adults, toxicity is hardly observed in neonates and it is considered to be reasonably safe in the treatment of neonatal candidiasis.

Only two clinical randomized controlled trials of antifungal therapy have been published in which neonates were included. Paediatric data from the international clinical trial in which liposomal amphotericin B was compared with micafungin included 19 premature neonates, and this subgroup analysis showed no differences in efficacy (although it was not powered for this purpose) (Queiroz-Telles et al. 2008). One single-centre randomized study comparing caspofungin with conventional amphotericin B, including 32 neonates with invasive candidiasis, suggested that caspofungin was more effective (Mohamed and Ismail 2012).

The European Society of Clinical Microbiology and Infectious Diseases has published a management guideline for *Candida* infections in neonates and children (Hope et al. 2012) in which recommendations for treatment are summarized. Conventional amphotericin B, liposomal amphotericin B, fluconazole, and micafungin are being graded identically (BII) and no evidence exists to consider one of those four agents to be superior or more efficacious than the others. Differences in the fungal epidemiology, pharmaco-kinetics and -dynamics, toxicity profiles, and costs will determine the choice of a particular antifungal agent in a particular NICU setting (Manzoni et al. 2015).

The duration of targeted antifungal therapy for candidaemia is 14 days after the last positive blood culture, and a minimum of six weeks for localized disease. Treatment duration for localized disease is determined by normalization of imaging and/or functional abnormalities.

Removal of indwelling catheters, in particular intravascular catheters, is an important part of the treatment owing to the high likelihood of *Candida* biofilm formation. Fluconazole in particular, and azole antifungal drugs in general, are poorly active in biofilms. Preclinical studies suggest that echinocandins may perform better (Katragkou et al. 2008; Kucharikova et al. 2010).

Surgical treatment may need to be considered for localized disease such as *Candida* endocarditis, osteomyelitis, and abscesses in visceral organs. Fungal bezoars caused by *Candida* species may either be treated conservatively, or will require surgical drainage and/or local irrigation with amphotericin B (50 mg/L) via percutaneously inserted nephrostomy catheters (Visser et al. 1998; Schilperoort et al. 2014; de Wall et al. 2015).

Prevention

Antifungal prophylaxis may be an appropriate strategy depending on the incidence of invasive candidiasis among ELBW neonates in an individual NICU. An important part of a preventive management strategy is the avoidance of transmission, which requires strict infection prevention and control measures. Rational use of broad-spectrum antibiotics (antimicrobial stewardship) and the implementation of intravascular catheter care bundles will lower the risk of invasive candidiasis (Aliaga et al. 2014; Fisher et al. 2014).

The use of fluconazole as a prophylactic antifungal agent has been extensively studied, including six randomized controlled trials (Kaufman et al. 2001, 2005; Kicklighter et al. 2001; Manzoni et al. 2007; Aydemir et al. 2011; Benjamin et al. 2014). Based on a systematic review, the use of fluconazole 3–6 mg/kg per dose (either intravenously or orally) twice weekly decreases colonization with *Candida* species, resulting in a 91% decrease in invasive candidiasis among ELBW neonates, with a reduction in mortality, although the latter is not statistically significant compared with no antifungal prophylaxis (Clerihew et al. 2008). It has to be noted that those findings were observed in studies performed in neonatal patient populations with an incidence of invasive candidiasis >10%, while most NICUs have an incidence of <5% of invasive candidiasis in ELBW neonates (Benjamin et al. 2010). Based on the results of the randomized controlled trials, a threshold of a 10% incidence to consider fluconazole prophylaxis seems to be reasonable, as fluconazole prophylaxis did not result in a significantly lower incidence of invasive candidiasis in settings with a baseline incidence <10% (Benjamin et al. 2014). Concerns have been raised about the development of fluconazole resistance among *Candida* species and/or a shift in *Candida* species causing invasive neonatal infections. To date, NICUs where fluconazole prophylaxis has been used for over ten years have not reported emergence of fluconazole-resistant *Candida* species or an increase in inherently fluconazole-resistant *Candida* species (Manzoni et al. 2008; Kaufman et al. 2011).

Nystatin is an orally administered non-absorbable antifungal which has been shown to be able to prevent colonization and infection with *Candida* species (reduction of 50–60%). The evidence comes from less robust studies than the fluconazole trials, but there is a good level of evidence to support the use of nystatin as an antifungal agent to prevent invasive neonatal candidiasis (Ganesan et al. 2009; Howell et al. 2009; Austin et al. 2015).

Lactoferrin and *Lactobacillus rhamnosus* act at the enteric level and are thought to be beneficial to a healthy gut microbiome by either directly or indirectly improving local host defences. In studies in which lactoferrin with or without *L. rhamnosus* was administered to neonates at <1500 g, a significant reduction in the incidence of late-onset sepsis including invasive candidiasis was shown (Manzoni et al. 2009, 2012). Administration of *L. rhamnosus* alone prevented enteric colonization with *Candida* species, but no effect was seen on the incidence of invasive candidiasis (Manzoni et al. 2006).

Table 35.2 summarizes the recommended dosing regimens for antifungals in the prophylaxis and treatment of invasive candidiasis in neonates.

Table 35.2 Recommended dosing regimens for antifungals in the prophylaxis and treatment of invasive candidiasis in neonates

	Prophylaxis	**Treatment**
ABLC	–	2.5–5 mg/kg/day
Amphotericin B deoxycholate	–	1 mg/kg/day
Liposomal amphotericin B	–	2.5–7 mg/kg/day
Caspofungin	–	25 mg/m²/day
Fluconazole	3–6 mg/kg twice weekly	12 mg/kg/day Consider loading dose 25 mg/kg
Micafungin	–	4–10 mg/kg/day
Nystatin (oral gel)	100.000 IU in three divided doses	–

ABLC = amphotericin B lipid complex

Source: data from Pappas et al., 2009; Hope et al., 2012; Ericson et al., 2013.

References

Adam B, Baillie GS and Douglas LJ (2002) Mixed species biofilms of Candida albicans and Staphylococcus epidermidis. *J Med Microbiol* 51: 344–9.

Aldana-Valenzuela C, Morales-Marquec M, Castellanos-Martinez J and Deanda-Gómez M (2005) Congenital candidiasis: a rare and unpredictable disease. *J Perinatol* 25: 680–2.

Aliaga S, Clark RH, Laughon M, et al. (2014) Changes in the incidence of candidiasis in neonatal intensive care units. *Pediatrics* 133: 236–42.

Amod FC, Coovadia YM, Pillay T and Ducasse G (2000) Primary cutaneous aspergillosis in ventilated neonates. *Pediatr Infect Dis J* 19: 482–3.

Arendrup MC, Fisher BT and Zaoutis TE (2009) Invasive fungal infections in the paediatric and neonatal population: diagnostics and management issues. *Clin Microbiol Infect* 15: 613–24.

Austin N, Cleminson J, Darlow BA and McGuire W (2015) Prophylactic oral/topical non-absorbed antifungal agents to prevent invasive fungal infection in very low birth weight infants. *Cochrane Database Syst Rev* 10: CD003478.

Aydemir C, Oguz SS, Dizdar EA, et al. (2011) Randomised controlled trial of prophylactic fluconazole versus nystatin for the prevention of fungal colonisation and invasive fungal infection in very low birth weight infants. *Arch Dis Child Fetal Neonatal Ed* 96: F164–8.

Basha S, Surendran N and Pichichero M (2014) Immune responses in neonates. *Expert Rev Clin Immunol* 10: 1171–84.

Bektas S, Goetze B and Speer CP (1990) Decreased adherence, chemotaxis and phagocytic activities of neutrophils from preterm neonates. *Acta Paediatr Scand* 79: 1031–8.

Ben Ameur S, Hentati Y, Ben Dhaoui M, et al. (2014) Neonatal renal candidiasis: a case report. *Arch Pediatr* 21: 287–90.

Benjamin DK Jr, Garges H and Steinbach WJ (2003) Candida bloodstream infection in neonates. *Semin Perinatol* 27: 375–83.

Benjamin DK Jr, Hudak ML, Duara S, et al. (2014) Effect of fluconazole prophylaxis on candidiasis and mortality in premature infants: a randomized clinical trial. *JAMA* 311: 1742–9.

Benjamin DK Jr, Poole C, Steinbach WJ, Rowen JL and Walsh TJ (2003) Neonatal candidemia and end-organ damage: a critical appraisal of the literature using meta-analytic techniques. *Pediatrics* 112 (Pt 1): 634–40.

Benjamin DK Jr, Stoll BJ, Gantz MG, et al. (2010) Neonatal candidiasis: epidemiology, risk factors, and clinical judgment. *Pediatrics* 126: e865–73.

Blyth CC, Chen SC, Slavin MA, et al. (2009) Not just little adults: candidemia epidemiology, molecular characterization, and antifungal susceptibility in neonatal and pediatric patients. *Pediatrics* 123: 1360–8.

Cantón E, Peman J, Quindos G, et al. (2011) Prospective multicenter study of the epidemiology, molecular identification, and antifungal susceptibility of Candida parapsilosis, Candida orthopsilosis, and Candida metapsilosis isolated from patients with candidemia. *Antimicrob Agents Chemother* 55: 5590–6.

Castagnola E, Faraci M, Fioredda F, et al. (2011) Invasive mould infections in newborns and children. *Early Hum Dev* 87 (Suppl. 1): S67–9.

Chang HJ, Miller HL, Watkins N, et al, (1998) An epidemic of Malassezia pachydermatis in an intensive care nursery associated with colonization of health care workers' pet dogs. *N Engl J Med* 338: 706–11.

Clerihew L, Austin N and McGuire W (2008) Systemic antifungal prophylaxis for very low birthweight infants: a systematic review. *Arch Dis Child Fetal Neonatal Ed* 93: F198–200.

Darmstadt GL, Dinulos JG and Miller Z (2000) Congenital cutaneous candidiasis: clinical presentation, pathogenesis, and management guidelines. *Pediatrics* 105: 438–44.

de Wall LL, van den Heijkant MM, Bokenkamp A, Kuijper CF, van der Horst HJ and de Jong TP (2015) Therapeutic approach to Candida bezoar in children. *J Pediatr Urol* 11: 81.e1–7.

Dotis J, Prasad PA, Zaoutis T and Roilides E (2012) Epidemiology, risk factors and outcome of Candida parapsilosis bloodstream infection in children. *Pediatr Infect Dis J* 31: 557–60.

Driessen M, Ellis JB, Cooper PA, et al. (1996) Fluconazole vs. amphotericin B for the treatment of neonatal fungal septicemia: a prospective randomized trial. *Pediatr Infect Dis J* 15: 1107–12.

Driessen M, Ellis JB, Muwazi F and De Villiers FP (1997) The treatment of systemic candidiasis in neonates with oral fluconazole. *Ann Trop Paediatr* 17: 263–71.

Ericson J, Manzoni P and Benjamin DK Jr (2013) Old and new: appropriate dosing for neonatal antifungal drugs in the nursery. *Early Hum Dev* 89 (Suppl. 1): S25–7.

Evans NJ and Rutter N (1986) Development of the epidermis in the newborn. *Biol Neonate* 49: 74–80.

Evdoridou J, Roilides E, Bibashi E and Kremenopoulos G (1997) Multifocal osteoarthritis due to Candida albicans in a neonate: serum level monitoring of liposomal amphotericin B and literature review. *Infection* 25: 112–16.

Faix RG, Kovarik SM, Shaw TR and Johnson RV (1989) Mucocutaneous and invasive candidiasis among very low birth weight (less than 1,500 grams) infants in intensive care nurseries: a prospective study. *Pediatrics* 83: 101–7.

Farmaki E, Evdoridou J, Pouliou T, et al. (2007) Fungal colonization in the neonatal intensive care unit: risk factors, drug susceptibility, and association with invasive fungal infections. *Am J Perinatol* 24: 127–35.

Fernandez M, Moylett EH, Noyola DE and Baker CJ (2000) Candidal meningitis in neonates: a 10-year review. *Clin Infect Dis* 31: 458–63.

Fisher BT, Ross RK, Localio AR, Prasad PA and Zaoutis TE (2014) Decreasing rates of invasive candidiasis in pediatric hospitals across the United States. *Clin Infect Dis* 58: 74–7.

Fridkin SK, Kaufman D, Edwards JR, Shetty S and Horan T (2006) Changing incidence of Candida bloodstream infections among NICU patients in the United States: 1995-2004. *Pediatrics* 117: 1680–7.

Ganesan K, Harigopal S, Neal T and Yoxall CW (2009) Prophylactic oral nystatin for preterm babies under 33 weeks' gestation decreases fungal colonisation and invasive fungaemia. *Arch Dis Child Fetal Neonatal Ed* 94: F275–8.

Goudjil S, Kongolo G, Dusol L, et al. (2013) (1-3)-beta-D-glucan levels in candidiasis infections in the critically ill neonate. *J Matern Fetal Neonatal Med* 26: 44–8.

Greenberg RG, Benjamin DK Jr, Gantz MG, et al. (2012) Empiric antifungal therapy and outcomes in extremely low birth weight infants with invasive candidiasis. *J Pediatr* 161: 264–9.e2.

Groll AH, Jaeger G, Allendorf A, Herrmann G, Schloesser R and von Loewenich V (1998) Invasive pulmonary aspergillosis in a critically ill neonate: case report and review of invasive aspergillosis during the first 3 months of life. *Clin Infect Dis* 27: 437–52.

Guida JD, Kunig AM, Leef KH, McKenzie SE and Paul DA (2003) Platelet count and sepsis in very low birth weight neonates: is there an organism-specific response? *Pediatrics* 111 (Pt 1): 1411–15.

Heresi GP, Gerstmann DR, Reed MD, et al. (2006) The pharmacokinetics and safety of micafungin, a novel echinocandin, in premature infants. *Pediatr Infect Dis J* 25: 1110–15.

Hope WW, Castagnola E, Groll AH, et al. (2012) ESCMID* guideline for the diagnosis and management of Candida diseases 2012: prevention and management of invasive infections in neonates and children caused by Candida spp. *Clin Microbiol Infect* 18 (Suppl. 7): 38–52.

Hope WW, Smith PB, Arrieta A, et al. (2010) Population pharmacokinetics of micafungin in neonates and young infants. *Antimicrob Agents Chemother* 54: 2633–7.

Hoppe JE (1997) Treatment of oropharyngeal candidiasis and candidal diaper dermatitis in neonates and infants: review and reappraisal. *Pediatr Infect Dis J* 16: 885–94.

Howell A, Isaacs D, Halliday R and Australasian Study Group For Neonatal Infections (2009) Oral nystatin prophylaxis and neonatal fungal infections. *Arch Dis Child Fetal Neonatal Ed* 94: F429–33.

Jans J, Bruggemann RJ, Christmann V, Verweij PE and Warris A (2013) Favorable outcome of neonatal cerebrospinal fluid shunt-associated Candida meningitis with caspofungin. *Antimicrob Agents Chemother* 57: 2391–3.

Juster-Reicher A, Flidel-Rimon O, Amitay M, Even-Tov S, Shinwell E and Leibovitz E (2003) High-dose liposomal amphotericin B in the therapy of systemic candidiasis in neonates. *Eur J Clin Microbiol Infect Dis* 22: 603–7.

Juster-Reicher A, Leibovitz E, Linder N, et al. (2000) Liposomal amphotericin B (AmBisome) in the treatment of neonatal candidiasis in very low birth weight infants. *Infection* 28: 223–6.

Katragkou A, Chatzimoschou A, Simitsopoulou M, et al. (2008) Differential activities of newer antifungal agents against Candida albicans and Candida parapsilosis biofilms. *Antimicrob Agents Chemother* 52: 357–60.

Kaufman D, Boyle R, Hazen KC, Patrie JT, Robinson M and Donowitz LG (2001) Fluconazole prophylaxis against fungal colonization and infection in preterm infants. *N Engl J Med* 345: 1660–6.

Kaufman D, Boyle R, Hazen KC, Patrie JT, Robinson M and Grossman LB (2005) Twice weekly fluconazole prophylaxis for prevention of invasive Candida infection in high-risk infants of <1000 grams birth weight. *J Pediatr* 147: 172–9.

Kaufman D and Fairchild KD (2004) Clinical microbiology of bacterial and fungal sepsis in very-low-birth-weight infants. *Clin Microbiol Rev* 17: 638–80, table of contents.

Kaufman D, Kilpatrick L, Hudson RG, et al. (1999) Decreased superoxide production, degranulation, tumor necrosis factor alpha secretion, and CD11b/CD18 receptor expression by adherent monocytes from preterm infants. *Clin Diagn Lab Immunol* 6: 525–9.

Kaufman DA, Cuff AL, Wamstad JB, et al. (2011) Fluconazole prophylaxis in extremely low birth weight infants and neurodevelopmental outcomes and quality of life at 8 to 10 years of age. *J Pediatr* 158: 759–65.e1.

Kennedy MJ and Volz PA (1985) Ecology of Candida albicans gut colonization: inhibition of Candida adhesion, colonization, and dissemination from the gastrointestinal tract by bacterial antagonism. *Infect Immun* 49: 654–63.

Kicklighter SD, Springer SC, Cox T, Hulsey TC and Turner RB (2001) Fluconazole for prophylaxis against candidal rectal colonization in the very low birth weight infant. *Pediatrics* 107: 293–8.

Koltze A, Rath P, Schoning S, et al. (2015) β-D-glucan screening for detection of invasive fungal disease in children undergoing allogeneic hematopoietic stem cell transplantation. *J Clin Microbiol* 53: 2605–10.

Kucharikova S, Tournu H, Holtappels M, Van Dijck P and Lagrou K (2010) In vivo efficacy of anidulafungin against mature Candida albicans biofilms in a novel rat model of catheter-associated Candidiasis. *Antimicrob Agents Chemother* 54: 4474–5.

Kucinskiene V, Sutkute A and Valiukeviciene S (2014) Cutaneous fungal infection in a neonatal intensive care unit patient: a case report and literature review. *Pediatr Dermatol* 31: 267–70.

Leeming JP, Sutton TM and Fleming PJ (1995) Neonatal skin as a reservoir of Malassezia species. *Pediatr Infect Dis J* 14: 719–21.

Levy O (2007) Innate immunity of the newborn: basic mechanisms and clinical correlates. *Nat Rev Immunol* 7: 379–90.

Manzar S, Kamat M and Pyati S (2006) Caspofungin for refractory candidemia in neonates. *Pediatr Infect Dis J* 25: 282–3.

Manzoni P, Leonessa M, Galletto P, et al. (2008) Routine use of fluconazole prophylaxis in a neonatal intensive care unit does not select natively fluconazole-resistant Candida subspecies. *Pediatr Infect Dis J* 27: 731–7.

Manzoni P, Mostert M and Castagnola E (2015) Update on the management of Candida infections in preterm neonates. *Arch Dis Child Fetal Neonatal Ed* 100: F454–9.

Manzoni P, Mostert M, Leonessa ML, et al. (2006) Oral supplementation with Lactobacillus casei subspecies rhamnosus prevents enteric colonization by Candida species in preterm neonates: a randomized study. *Clin Infect Dis* 42: 1735–42.

Manzoni P, Rinaldi M, Cattani S, et al. (2009) Bovine lactoferrin supplementation for prevention of late-onset sepsis in very low-birth-weight neonates: a randomized trial. *JAMA* 302: 1421–8.

Manzoni P, Stolfi I, Messner H, et al. (2012) Bovine lactoferrin prevents invasive fungal infections in very low birth weight infants: a randomized controlled trial. *Pediatrics* 129: 116–23.

Manzoni P, Stolfi I, Pugni L, et al. (2007) A multicenter, randomized trial of prophylactic fluconazole in preterm neonates. *N Engl J Med* 356: 2483–95.

Mohamed WA and Ismail M (2012) A randomized, double-blind, prospective study of caspofungin vs. amphotericin B for the treatment of invasive candidiasis in newborn infants. *J Trop Pediatr* 58: 25–30.

Noyola DE, Fernandez M, Moylett EH and Baker CJ (2001) Ophthalmologic, visceral, and cardiac involvement in neonates with candidemia. *Clin Infect Dis* 32: 1018–23.

Odio CM, Araya R, Pinto LE, et al. (2004) Caspofungin therapy of neonates with invasive candidiasis. *Pediatr Infect Dis J* 23: 1093–7.

Oeser C, Vergnano S, Naidoo R, et al. (2014) Neonatal invasive fungal infection in England 2004-2010. *Clin Microbiol Infect* 20: 936–41.

Pana ZD, Dotis J, Iosifidis E and Roilides E (2015) Fungal endocarditis in neonates: a review of seventy-one cases (1971-2013). *Pediatr Infect Dis J* 34: 803–8.

Pappas PG, Kauffman CA, Andes D, et al. (2009) Clinical practice guidelines for the management of candidiasis: 2009 update by the Infectious Diseases Society of America. *Clin Infect Dis* 48: 503–35.

Peman J, Canton E, Linares-Sicilia MJ, et al. (2011) Epidemiology and antifungal susceptibility of bloodstream fungal isolates in pediatric patients: a Spanish multicenter prospective survey. *J Clin Microbiol* 49: 4158–63.

Pfaller MA, Moet GJ, Messer SA, Jones RN and Castanheira M (2011) Candida bloodstream infections: comparison of species distributions and antifungal resistance patterns in community-onset and nosocomial isolates in the SENTRY Antimicrobial Surveillance Program, 2008-2009. *Antimicrob Agents Chemother* 55: 561–6.

Phillips JR and Karlowicz MG (1997) Prevalence of Candida species in hospital-acquired urinary tract infections in a neonatal intensive care unit. *The Pediatric Infectious Disease Journal* 16: 190–4.

Piper L, Smith PB, Hornik CP, et al. (2011) Fluconazole loading dose pharmacokinetics and safety in infants. *Pediatr Infect Dis J* 30: 375–8.

Queiroz-Telles F, Berezin E, Leverger G, et al. (2008) Micafungin versus liposomal amphotericin B for pediatric patients with invasive candidiasis: substudy of a randomized double-blind trial. *Pediatr Infect Dis J* 27: 820–6.

Ravanfar P, Wallace JS and Pace NC (2012) Diaper dermatitis: a review and update. *Curr Opin Pediatr* 24: 472–9.

Roilides E, Farmaki E, Evdoridou J, et al. (2004) Neonatal candidiasis: analysis of epidemiology, drug susceptibility, and molecular typing of causative isolates. *Eur J Clin Microbiol Infect Dis* 23: 745–50.

Saez-Llorens X, Macias M, Maiya P, et al. (2009) Pharmacokinetics and safety of caspofungin in neonates and infants less than 3 months of age. *Antimicrob Agents Chemother* 53: 869–75.

Saiman L, Ludington E, Dawson JD, et al. (2001a) Risk factors for Candida species colonization of neonatal intensive care unit patients. *Pediatr Infect Dis J* 20: 1119–24.

Saiman L, Ludington E, Dawson JD, et al. (2001b) Risk factors for Candida species colonization of neonatal intensive care unit patients. *Pediatr Infect Dis J* 20: 1119–24.

Saiman L, Ludington E, Pfaller M, et al. (2000) Risk factors for candidemia in Neonatal Intensive Care Unit patients. The National Epidemiology of Mycosis Survey study group. *Pediatr Infect Dis J* 19: 319–24.

Schefold JC, Porz L, Uebe B, et al. (2015) Diminished HLA-DR expression on monocyte and dendritic cell subsets indicating impairment of cellular immunity in pre-term neonates: a prospective observational analysis. *J Perinat Med* 43: 609–18.

Schilperoort JV, de Wall LL, van der Horst HJ, van Wijk JA, Verbeke JI and Bokenkamp A (2014) Anuria in a solitary kidney with Candida bezoars managed conservatively. *Eur J Pediatr* 173: 1623–25.

Schwarze R, Penk A and Pittrow L (2000) Treatment of candidal infections with fluconazole in neonates and infants. *Eur J Med Res* 5: 203–8.

Starke JR, Mason EO Jr, Kramer WG and Kaplan SL (1987) Pharmacokinetics of amphotericin B in infants and children. *J Infect Dis* 155: 766–74.

Steinbach WJ, Roilides E, Berman D, et al. (2012) Results from a prospective, international, epidemiologic study of invasive candidiasis in children and neonates. *Pediatr Infect Dis J* 31: 1252–7.

Stoll BJ, Gordon T, Korones SB, et al. (1996) Late-onset sepsis in very low birth weight neonates: a report from the National Institute of Child Health and Human Development Neonatal Research Network. *J Pediatr* 129: 63–71.

Stuart SM and Lane AT (1992) Candida and Malassezia as nursery pathogens. *Semin Dermatol* 11: 19–23.

Taira CL, Okay TS, Delgado AF, Ceccon ME, de Almeida MT and Del Negro GM (2014) A multiplex nested PCR for the detection and identification of Candida species in blood samples of critically ill paediatric patients. *BMC Infect Dis* 14: 406.

Tieu KD, Satter EK, Zaleski L and Koehler M (2012) Congenital cutaneous candidiasis in two full-term infants. *Pediatr Dermatol* 29: 507–10.

Visser D, Monnens L, Feitz W and Semmekrot B (1998) Fungal bezoars as a cause of renal insufficiency in neonates and infants—recommended treatment strategy. *Clin Nephrol* 49: 198–201.

Wade KC, Benjamin DK Jr, Kaufman DA, et al. (2009) Fluconazole dosing for the prevention or treatment of invasive candidiasis in young infants. *Pediatr Infect Dis J* 28: 717–23.

Wade KC, Wu D, Kaufman DA, et al. (2008) Population pharmacokinetics of fluconazole in young infants. *Antimicrob Agents Chemother* 52: 4043–9.

Warris A, Semmekrot BA and Voss A (2001) Candidal and bacterial bloodstream infections in premature neonates: a case-control study. *Med Mycol* 39: 75–9.

Wurthwein G, Groll AH, Hempel G, Adler-Shohet FC, Lieberman JM and Walsh TJ (2005) Population pharmacokinetics of amphotericin B lipid complex in neonates. *Antimicrob Agents Chemother* 49: 5092–8.

Wynn JL, Tan S, Gantz MG, et al. (2012) Outcomes following candiduria in extremely low birth weight infants. *Clin Infect Dis* 54: 331–9.

Xia H, Wu H, Xia S, et al. (2014) Invasive Candidiasis in preterm neonates in China: a retrospective study from 11 NICUS during 2009-2011. *Pediatr Infect Dis J* 33: 106–9.

Zaoutis TE, Argon J, Chu J, Berlin JA, Walsh TJ and Feudtner C (2005) The epidemiology and attributable outcomes of candidemia in adults and children hospitalized in the United States: a propensity analysis. *Clin Infect Dis* 41: 1232–9.

Zaoutis TE, Heydon K, Localio R, Walsh TJ and Feudtner C (2007) Outcomes attributable to neonatal candidiasis. *Clin Infect Dis* 44: 1187–93.

CHAPTER 36

Fungal infections in intensive therapy units

Rosemary A. Barnes and Matthijs Backx

Introduction to fungal infections in the intensive care unit

Advances in the delivery of healthcare have facilitated the survival of critically unwell and severely immunocompromised patients for extended periods of time. The at-risk population is not only limited to severely immunocompromised hosts but also patients on surgical and medical intensive care units (ICUs), burns units, and neonatal units. These patients may not be classically immunocompromised but have acquired risk factors and degrees of immunoparesis associated with critical illness (Kox et al. 2000; Vandewoude et al. 2004). Epidemiological surveys suggest that invasive fungal disease (IFD) represents one of the most rapidly growing infectious complications in the intensive care unit.

The majority of IFDs in Western Europe involve opportunistic pathogens such as *Candida* spp., *Aspergillus* spp., *Cryptococcus neoformans*, and *Pneumocystis jirovecii*. This is in contrast to areas of North America and the developing world, where the endemic mycoses may cause community-acquired infections and contribute to the burden of IFD.

The relative risk of infection and the distribution of fungal pathogens depend on the geographic location, patient mix, referral patterns, illness-severity, and policies regarding antifungal therapy and prophylaxis within institutions. However, in all geographic areas, IFDs on the ICU are predominantly nosocomial and, in the majority of cases, caused by *Candida* species.

Epidemiology

Obtaining exact data regarding the epidemiology of IFDs is challenging as these are not notifiable diseases. The majority of large studies evaluating IFD epidemiology have been performed in North America. These have demonstrated that since the 1980s, opportunistic IFDs have become increasingly prevalent (Beck-Sague and Jarvis 1993; Pfaller 1994; Nicolle et al. 1998). Surveillance of epidemiological trends in Europe has been less comprehensive. Data derived from individual institutions, single countries, or specific high-risk population groups cannot be applied to the intensive care population as a whole. Differences in study design, case mix, diagnostic pathways, and therapeutic strategies often hinder comparison and make it difficult to establish epidemiological trends. There is no doubt, however, that fungi are a significant nosocomial pathogen in critically ill patients (Vincent et al. 1995; Spencer 1996; Tortorano et al. 2002; Kibbler et al. 2003; Harrison et al. 2013).

Candidiasis

Of the IFDs, epidemiological data pertaining to invasive candidiasis are likely to be most robust owing to the relative ease of microbiological diagnosis, which is predominantly, but not exclusively, established via culture of the pathogen from blood. A five-fold increase was observed between 1980 and 1990 in the United States (Wey et al. 1988; Banerjee et al. 1991; Beck-Sague and Jarvis 1993; Fisher-Hoch and Hutwagner 1995). This period coincided with rapid advances in medicine, including dramatic changes within critical care and an increase in the number of transplantation procedures. Subsequent data have shown that the incidence of *Candida* bloodstream infections has stabilized and may be declining both in the United States and other geographic areas (Banerjee et al. 1991; Kao et al. 1999; Gradel et al. 2014; Cleveland et al. 2015). It has been postulated that the introduction of azole drugs at the end of the 1980s and improvements in hygiene and disease management in the 1990s have resulted in this stabilization—and in some cases decreasing rates—of disease. However, *Candida* species remain the most common cause of IFD on the ICU, accounting for over 90% of reported cases (Eubanks et al. 1993; Voss et al. 1997).

A large prospective multi-centre study of critical care admissions in the UK between 2009 and 2011 found an incidence of *Candida* bloodstream infections of 3.3 per 1,000 ICU admissions (Harrison et al. 2013), which was comparable to that found in other studies within the UK and Europe (Nolla-Salas et al. 1997; Blot et al. 2002; Leleu et al. 2002). Marked changes in the distribution of *Candida* species have been observed over time, with a significant decrease in the proportion of *C. albicans* infections (Price et al. 1994). The widespread use of azoles has been implicated for this shift in species distribution as it coincided with the introduction of fluconazole in the 1980s (Wingard et al. 1991; Wingard et al. 1993; Odds 1996). *C. albicans* now accounts for less than 50% of cases of candidaemia in the UK, according to Public Health England data (PHE 2015). This overall trend appears to be driven by changes observed in haematology and transplant patients in whom azole prophylaxis use is high, and has not been observed on the ICUs where *C. albicans* still predominates, accounting for over 69% of isolates (Leleu et al. 2002; Kibbler et al. 2003; Kett et al. 2011; Harrison et al. 2013).

Aspergillosis

Although the incidence of invasive aspergillosis (IA) is low compared with that of invasive candidiasis, it is increasingly being recognized as an important cause of morbidity and mortality on the ICU, both within the classic at-risk group and in those with chronic respiratory and liver disease. Patients may develop IA whilst on the ICU but IA is more commonly acquired elsewhere, and patients are transferred onto the ICU for respiratory support (Humphreys et al. 1991; Janssen et al. 1996). Incidences rates of up to 5.8% have been reported on ICUs, but vary greatly depending on the case mix and access to diagnostic tools (Meersseman et al. 2004; Garnacho-Montero et al. 2005; Vandewoude et al. 2006).

Cryptococcosis and *Pneumocystis jirovecii* pneumonia

Candidiasis and IA constitute the vast majority of IFDs on the ICU. Patients with cryptococcosis and *Pneumocystis jirovecii* pneumonia (PCP) are most often diagnosed and treated outside the ICU setting, although some are transferred to the ICU for organ support.

The incidence of invasive cryptococcosis on the ICU has not been described but is likely to be low compared with that of candidiasis. The incidence of PCP on the ICU has also not been characterized, but is likely to be low.

Emerging fungal infections

A variety of emerging pathogens have been reported as causes of infections on the ICU, including non-*Candida* yeasts such as *Rhodotorula rubra, Malassezia furfur, Trichosporon beigelii*, and *Pichia anomala,* which have been implicated in line-associated infections (Gueho et al. 1998). Moulds such as *Fusarium and Scedosporium* spp. and the Mucorales can cause syndromes similar to IA. Additionally, *Scedosporium* infection has been associated with near-drowning incidents (Kowacs et al. 2004), and a variety of fungi have been reported to cause wound infection, particularly following trauma sustained as a result of military conflict or natural disasters (Benedict and Park 2014).

Risk factors for IFD in the ICU

Candidiasis

Several systematic reviews have identified risk factors for the development of candidiasis in the non-neutropenic critically unwell patient: surgery, total parenteral nutrition, fungal colonization, renal replacement therapy, infection and sepsis, mechanical ventilation, diabetes, and APACHE (Acute Physiology and Chronic Health Evaluation) II or APACHE III scores (Pittet et al. 1994; Paphitou et al. 2005; Leon et al. 2006; Ostrosky-Zeichner et al. 2007; Chow et al. 2008). Cardiopulmonary bypass time, acute renal failure, broad-spectrum antibiotics, red blood cell transfusion, antifungal medication, central venous catheters, diarrhoea, and peripheral catheter use were also found to be statistically significant, but each in single studies only. Many of these risk factors are common to hospitalized patients, especially those in an ICU. Prediction rules and scoring systems have been proposed to identify subpopulations of ICU patients who would benefit from prophylaxis. These rules identify different percentages of patients—up to 85% in some centres. Few are practical and none have proven robustness across all ICU populations. Further work is needed to develop risk models that would allow targeted prophylaxis of high-risk groups, thereby avoiding indiscriminate use of antifungals with their associated cost, side-effects, and potential for the development of antifungal resistance (Muskett et al. 2011).

Aspergillosis

Risk factors for IA in this population include chronic obstructive pulmonary disease treated with steroids, liver cirrhosis, and influenza infection (Fischer and Walker 1979; Bulpa et al. 2007; Meersseman et al. 2007).

Clinical presentation

Candidiasis

The clinical presentation and management of *Candida* infection on the ICU is challenging. Unlike classically immunosuppressed patients, who usually have a clearly defined immunological insult with a known attributable morbidity and mortality, critically unwell patients represent a heterogeneous population with multiple underlying clinical problems, non-specific immune paresis, and extensive physiological derangement where the assessment of likelihood of fungal infection is difficult and the presentation of fungal disease is varied and non-specific.

The classification of candidiasis depends to what degree candidaemia and focal organ involvement dominate the clinical picture. It can be classified into candidaemia, acute disseminated candidiasis, chronic disseminated candidiasis, and deep organ candidiasis (Dean and Burchard 1996). Chronic disseminated candidiasis is found almost exclusively in patients with haematological malignancies who are recovering from a period of prolonged neutropenia (Rex et al. 1998).

The mean length of stay on the ICU prior to the diagnosis of candidaemia is 14–30 days, and patients frequently have multiple risk factors including central venous catheters, fungal colonization, and prior exposure to broad-spectrum antibiotics (Wey et al. 1988; Fraser et al. 1992; Eubanks et al. 1993; Nolla-Salas et al. 1997; Voss et al. 1997; Borzotta and Beardsley 1999). Candidaemia is usually associated with a non-specific systemic inflammatory response (Matson et al. 1991; Young et al. 1991; Vincent et al. 1998). Positive blood cultures should prompt the immediate initiation of therapy and the search for metastatic foci (Pappas et al. 2009; Cuenca-Estrella et al. 2012).

Candida peritonitis following abdominal surgery is one of the most common forms of candidiasis on the adult ICU (BSAC 1994). *Candida* species are part of the normal bowel flora and are frequently isolated from abdominal drain fluid in patients with perforation of the gastrointestinal tract or post-surgical anastomotic dehiscence (Solomkin 1993; BSAC 1994; Vincent et al. 1998). In a clinically stable patient this is of doubtful clinical significance and may not be predictive of subsequent candidiasis (Rutledge et al. 1986; Calandra et al. 1989). Intra-abdominal candidiasis is often poly-microbial, primarily associated with acute necrotizing pancreatitis and persistent gastrointestinal perforation or anastomotic breakdown, and manifests as peritonitis or intra-abdominal abscess formation with fever, abdominal pain, distension, or paralytic ileus (Calandra et al. 1989; Keiser and Keay 1992; Hoerauf et al. 1998; Grewe et al. 1999; Sandven et al. 2002). Infection may remain localized or result in acute disseminated candidiasis (Eggimann et al. 1999; Rex and Sobel 1999).

Candiduria is common in hospitalized patients, especially in those that are catheterized, those receiving broad-spectrum antibiotics, and diabetics (Kauffman et al. 2000; Alvarez-Lerma et al. 2003; Sobel et al. 2011). The true incidence of renal tract candidiasis on ICUs is difficult to quantify owing to the difficulty of distinguishing between urinary catheter colonization and urinary tract infection. Ascending infection usually occurs in the setting of urinary tract abnormalities (Irby et al. 1990). Candiduria as a source of candidaemia usually occurs in the setting of either urinary tract obstruction and/or secondary to urinary tract surgery or instrumentation (Ang et al. 1993; Gross et al. 1998). Candidaemia as a consequence of candiduria in the absence of obstruction or surgery is uncommon in hospitalized patients, including those on the ICU (Kauffman et al. 2000; Bougnoux et al. 2008). The kidneys are the most commonly involved organ in disseminated candidiasis, and candiduria can occur as a consequence (Lehner 1964). Patients may present with abdominal and/or flank tenderness with preservation of renal function, although this is difficult to assess in the unconscious patient. Ascending infection may result in the formation of a fungal ball or a perinephric abscess. Flank pain developing over a period of days to weeks may be present, but systemic signs including fever are usually absent.

Candida is frequently isolated from deep respiratory specimens obtained from critically ill patients. In nearly all instances this represents contamination with oropharyngeal flora, and *Candida* pneumonia is rare. Quantitative cultures from bronchoalveolar lavage fluids or protected specimen brushes have little diagnostic value and lung biopsy is needed for confirmation.

Endogenous ocular candidiasis occurs as a result of haematogenous spread to the eye with the subsequent development of chorioidoretinitis and progression to endophthalmitis. Intravenous drug abuse, particularly with heroin, is a specific risk factor (Connell et al. 2010). The reported incidence of ocular candidiasis in hospitalized patients with candidiasis varies widely from 0% to 45% (McDonnell et al. 1985; Brooks 1989; Fraser et al. 1992; Donahue et al. 1994; Petri et al. 1997). The exact incidence on the ICU is not known as serial ophthalmic examination is not normally performed, even though it is recommended in those with suspected or proven candidiasis. In conscious patients, ocular candidiasis presents with a decrease in visual acuity in one or both eyes, which may be painful. Cases present within days to weeks of the onset of candidaemia, and if untreated, this infection may result in permanent vision loss (Solomkin 1993; Donahue et al. 1994).

Aspergillosis

The features of IA are discussed in Chapters 10, 30, and 37.

Diagnosis

In 2002, the European Organisation for Research and Treatment of Cancer/Invasive Fungal Infections Cooperative Group and the National Institute of Allergy and Infectious Diseases Mycoses Study Group (EORTC/MSG) published standard definitions for invasive fungal infections. These were developed to facilitate the identification of a homogenous group of patients for clinical and epidemiological research (Ascioglu et al. 2002) and focused largely on those with haematological malignancy and undergoing transplantation. Critically ill patients in the ICU were not included. Although these definitions (revised in 2008—see De Pauw et al. (2008)—and currently under further revision) provide some guidance, it should be borne in mind that some patients may have IFD and yet not fulfil these diagnostic criteria. It should also be noted that the required EORTC/MSG host criteria may preclude this framework from being used in the critical care setting where non-immunocompromised patients are nonetheless at risk of developing invasive fungal disease. In fact, the critical care population account for approximately 45% of reported candidaemias (Kibbler et al. 2003).

The diagnosis of IFD in the ICU setting is similar to that in other patient populations and is discussed in Section 5.

Treatment strategies

Candidiasis

Untreated candidaemia has a 60% mortality rate, which is reduced to 30–40% with appropriate therapy (Fraser et al. 1992; Andes et al. 2012; Clancy and Nguyen 2012). Delays in treatment result in an increase in mortality (Blot et al. 2002; Morrell et al. 2005; Garey et al. 2006). Current validated diagnostics have a relatively long turnaround time and it is for this reason that there is interest in antifungal prophylaxis and pre-emptive treatment.

Several meta-analyses have been performed which have examined the impact of azole prophylaxis in the critically unwell non-neutropenic patient (Cruciani et al. 2005; Ho et al. 2005; Shorr et al. 2005; Playford et al. 2006a, 2006b; Vardakas et al. 2006). Although there was heterogeneity of the individual studies with regard to patient groups, they demonstrated a homogenous effect of antifungal prophylaxis with a reduction in the risk of IFD as well as a possible reduction in all-cause mortality (Playford et al. 2006b).

On the ICU, fluconazole prophylaxis may be considered where there is a breach of the gastrointestinal tract through oesophageal rupture, recurrent abdominal perforation, or anastomotic breakdown (Calandra et al. 1989; Eggimann et al. 1999; Bauer et al. 1996). However, studies evaluating the impact of antifungal prophylaxis on more heterogeneous ICU populations failed to show an impact primarily due to low incidences of invasive candidiasis (Ostrosky-Zeichner et al. 2014; Knitsch et al. 2015).

Many of the risk factors for the development of invasive candidiasis identified in studies of non-neutropenic critically unwell individuals are common to hospitalized patients, especially those on the ICU. It is clear that methods need to be developed to identify those individuals that would benefit most from prophylaxis whilst minimizing the indiscriminate use of antifungals with their associated costs, toxicity, and risk of promoting resistance (Brion et al. 2007). A multi-centre study was undertaken in patients admitted to UK NHS adult general care units in order to generate and internally validate risk models for the identification of patients who would benefit from antifungal prophylaxis (Table 36.1)(Harrison et al. 2013). Overall, the incidence of IFD was found to be low at 0.6%, with the vast majority caused by *Candida* species. At low incidence levels the effectiveness of prediction rules diminish, even if these have relatively high specificity. This was reflected by the analysis, which showed that adoption of the generated risk models would likely reduce mean hospital costs if prophylaxis were to be introduced when the risk of developing IFD exceeded 1–2%. However, this would require 5–12% of the ICU population to receive prophylaxis. With a lower threshold risk for invasive candidiasis infection of 0.5%, the most cost-effective prophylaxis strategy would require around 30% of eligible patients to receive antifungal prophylactic, which raises concerns about cost, toxicity, and resistance.

In all risk groups, *Candida* colonization is an independent risk factor for infection and precedes infection in most cases. This is supported by the evidence that colonization and infection are often caused by the same strain (Pittet et al. 1991). In addition, heavy

Table 36.1 A comparison of models for the prediction of invasive candidiasis on the intensive care unit

				Performance				
Study	**Design**	**Incidence IFD (%)**	**Model/rules**	**Proportion of ICU patients at risk (%)**	**Sensitivity (%)**	**Specificity (%)**	**PPV (%)**	**NPV (%)**
Harrison et al. 2013	Multicentre, prospective, 60,778 patients	0.6	Risk prediction at the end of day 3 following admission to the critical care unit: pancreatitis; number of CVCs (day 1–3); number of drains (day 1–3); highest heart rate (day 1); number of samples positive for fungal colonization (day 1–3)	27.1* (risk threshold 0.5%) 15.7* (risk threshold 1%) 6.4* (risk threshold 2%)	54.1 40.5 24.3	73.0 84.5 93.6	0.87 1.13 1.65	99.7 99.7 99.6
Leon et al. 2006	Multicentre, prospective, 1,699 patients	5.7	Bedside score ≥3: severe sepsis (2) and one of TPN (1), surgery (1), or multifocal *Candida* colonization (1) *or* all three risk factors	NR	81	74	NR	NR
Ostrosky-Zeichner et al. 2007	Multicentre, retrospective, 2,890 patients	3	Any antibiotics (day 1–3) *or* CVC (day 1–3) *and* at least two of: any surgery (day –7 – 0); immunosuppressive use (day –7 – 0); pancreatitis (day –7 – 0); TPN (day 1–3), dialysis (day 1 – 3); steroid use (day –7 – 3)	10.6	34	90	9	97
Paphitou et al. 2005	Single centre, retrospective, 327 patients	11	At least one of diabetes mellitus; TPN (day –7 – 0); new onset haemodialysis (day –7 – 0); broad-spectrum antibiotics (day –7 – 3)	52	78–83	NR	11–17	NR
Pittet et al. 1994	Multicentre, prospective, 29 patients	38	*Candida* colonization index ≥0.5 *Candida*-corrected colonization index ≥0.4	NR NR	100 100	69 100	66 100	100 100

* Performance of clinical decision rules at the end of the third calendar day following admission to the ICU in the full validation sample (n=8488).

CVC = central venous catheter; ICU = intensive care unit: IFD = invasive fungal disease; NPV = negative predictive value; NR = not recorded; PPV = positive predictive value; TPN total parenteral nutrition

growth, colonization at multiple sites, and isolation of *C. tropicalis* are additional risk factors for infection (Neumann and Rakower 1978; Pittet et al. 1994; Sheridan et al. 1995). The definitive diagnosis of candidiasis is difficult and is often made at a late stage. For this reason treatment is often initiated at an earlier stage in septic high-risk patients who are colonized with *Candida* at multiple sites and are not responding to broad-spectrum antibiotics. It has been suggested that a rational approach to the management of candidiasis on the ICU should involve screening potential sites of colonization in high-risk patients through an active surveillance programme. Identification and sensitivity testing of the isolated organism would not only help delineate the epidemiology of *Candida* species on individual ICUs but would also inform the antifungal agent of choice for therapy. Although early presumptive treatment with source control was associated with reduced mortality in patients with invasive candidiasis in retrospective analyses, this strategy has not been validated in prospective studies (Garey et al. 2006; Leon et al. 2009; Andes et al. 2012; Kollef et al. 2012; Puig-Asensio et al. 2014).

For established infection, fluconazole, echinocandin, and amphotericin-based therapies are effective for invasive candidiasis in non-neutropenic patients. Numerous guidelines exist, although the evidence base supporting them is generally of low quality (Pappas et al. 2009; Ullmann et al. 2012). There is general consensus that in septic patients who may be hyper-catabolic, have large volumes of distribution, and may or may not be on haemofiltration for renal support, there is a risk of under-dosing with azoles, so echinocandins are preferred. Similarly, patients who have received azoles previously—either as treatment or as prophylaxis—are more likely to develop infection with azole-resistant yeasts and should be treated empirically with echinocandins. Once patients are stabilized and susceptibility profiles are available, patients may be switched to azole therapies if appropriate. Amphotericin B in the form of lipid preparation is of value in neonates and in patients with severe hepatic dysfunction or intolerance of other drugs. Duration of treatment is generally 10–14 days but is dependent on adequate source control.

All candidaemic patients should have ophthalmic evaluation looking for intraocular candidiasis. In addition, central venous catheters should be removed or changed, unless the patient is to receive palliative care only, as they are often the source of the infection. Clearance of fungaemia occurs more quickly when lines are removed, and higher rates of mortality have been reported with retention of central venous catheters (Soutter and Todd 1986; Nguyen et al. 1995; Rex et al. 1995; Stamos and Rowley 1995; Asmundsdottir et al. 2005; Labelle et al. 2008; Andes et al. 2012; Fernandez-Ruiz et al. 2014). This approach has been generally accepted, although the evidence for it is not robust (Walsh and Rex 2002; Mermel et al. 2009; Pappas et al. 2009; Brass and Edwards 2010).

Aspergillosis

Prophylaxis with mould-active drugs can prevent invasive aspergillosis. Which specific patients will benefit from prophylactic strategies remains ill-defined and is partly dependent upon patient characteristics and the epidemiology of invasive fungal infections at individual institutions. Trials suggest that primary prophylaxis with mould-active therapy is beneficial if the incidence of IA is at least 6% (Cornely et al. 2007; Ullmann et al. 2007). At this prevalence there is no role for prophylaxis in the ICU outside of high-risk patients with haematological malignancy or following transplantation.

Empiric antifungal treatment after a defined duration of persistent fever refractory to antibacterial agents is of no benefit to ICU patients. Screening using combination galactomannan and polymerase chain reaction testing has been successfully used as part of a pre-emptive approach in high-risk haematology patients, but has not been studied in other settings such as the ICU (Barnes et al. 2009; Morrissey et al. 2013; Rogers et al. 2013).

Voriconazole is an effective treatment but side-effects and drug interactions may compromise use in the ICU. Liposomal amphotericin B is also appropriate. Posaconazole is increasingly used, and echinocandins are considered second line for aspergillosis.

Prevention

Candidiasis

In the ICU environment, the risk of cross-infection is a present but preventable hazard. Up to 75% of nursing staff carry *Candida* on their hands and it is recognised that horizontal transmission of yeast can occur from patient to patient and via the hands of health care workers resulting in outbreaks, particularly on the neonatal unit (Romano et al. 1994; Strausbaugh et al. 1994). Hand hygiene and attention to aseptic techniques can reduce transmission of yeasts (Pfaller 1994).

Reduction of the endogenous fungal carriage may reduce the colonisation load of the skin and gastrointestinal tract and thereby prevent infection via these sites (Lingnau et al. 1998). Despite its modest effect on ICU mortality and bacteraemia rates, selective decontamination of the oropharyngeal and digestive tracts using antimicrobials has been advocated in many liver transplant and neonatal units (Damjanovic et al. 1993; Arnow et al. 1996; de Smet et al. 2009; Price et al. 2014). Uncertainty regarding long-term effects on emerging antimicrobial resistance has however inhibited more widespread uptake of this practice.

Infection control and antimicrobial stewardship should be central to any preventative strategy. Intravenous longlines and urinary catheters provide a potential portal of entry for infection and may serve as a persistent focus. Care bundles should be introduced for the insertion and maintenance of longlines and catheters.

Aspergillosis

Aspergillus species are ubiquitous in the environment and disease occurs primarily through inhalation of airborne conidia. Hospital building works and renovation may result in aerosolisation of conidia and has been associated with outbreaks of IA, including on the ICU (Harvey et al. 1988; Humphreys et al. 1991; Pittet et al. 1996; Manuel and Kibbler 1998; Fitzpatrick et al. 1999). Awareness of the problem is crucial and high-risk patients should be nursed away from areas where the potential for dust contamination exists.

References

Alvarez-Lerma F, Nolla-Salas J, Leon C, et al. (2003) Candiduria in critically ill patients admitted to intensive care medical units. *Intensive Care Med* 29: 1069–76.

Andes DR, Safdar N, Baddley JW, et al. (2012) Impact of treatment strategy on outcomes in patients with candidemia and other forms of invasive candidiasis: a patient-level quantitative review of randomized trials. *Clin Infect Dis* 54: 1110–22.

Ang BS, Telenti A, King B, Steckelberg JM and Wilson WR (1993) Candidemia from a urinary tract source: microbiological aspects and clinical significance. *Clin Infect Dis* 17: 662–6.

Arnow PM, Carandang GC, Zabner R and Irwin ME (1996) Randomized controlled trial of selective bowel decontamination for prevention of infections following liver transplantation. *Clin Infect Dis* 22: 997–1003.

Ascioglu S, Rex JH, De Pauw B, et al. (2002) Defining opportunistic invasive fungal infections in immunocompromised patients with cancer and hematopoietic stem cell transplants: an international consensus. *Clin Infect Dis* 34: 7–14.

Asmundsdottir LR, Erlendsdottir H and Gottfredsson M (2005) Improving survival of patients with candidaemia: analysis of prognostic factors from a long-term, nationwide study in Iceland. *Scand J Infect Dis* 37: 111–20.

Banerjee SN, Emori TG, Culver DH, et al. (1991) Secular trends in nosocomial primary bloodstream infections in the United States, 1980–9. National Nosocomial Infections Surveillance System. *Am J Med* 91: 86S–89S.

Barnes RA, White PL, Bygrave C, Evans N, Healy B and Kell J (2009) Clinical impact of enhanced diagnosis of invasive fungal disease in high-risk haematology and stem cell transplant patients. *J Clin Pathol* 62: 64–9.

Bauer TM, Dupont V and Zimmerli W (1996) Invasive candidiasis complicating spontaneous esophageal perforation (Boerhaave syndrome). *Am J Gastroenterol* 91: 1248–50.

Beck-Sague C and Jarvis WR (1993) Secular trends in the epidemiology of nosocomial fungal infections in the United States, 1980-1990. National Nosocomial Infections Surveillance System. *J Infect Dis* 167: 1247–51.

Benedict K and Park BJ (2014) Invasive fungal infections after natural disasters. *Emerg Infect Dis* 20: 349–55.
Blot SI, Vandewoude KH, Hoste EA and Colardyn FA (2002) Effects of nosocomial candidemia on outcomes of critically ill patients. *Am J Med* 113: 480–5.
Borzotta AP and Beardsley K (1999) Candida infections in critically ill trauma patients: a retrospective case-control study. *Arch Surg* 134: 657–64; discussion 664–5.
Bougnoux ME, Kac G, Aegerter P, D'enfert C and Fagon JY (2008) Candidemia and candiduria in critically ill patients admitted to intensive care units in France: incidence, molecular diversity, management and outcome. *Intensive Care Med* 34: 292–9.
Brass EP and Edwards JE (2010) Should the guidelines for management of central venous catheters in patients with candidemia be changed now? *Clin Infect Dis* 51: 304–6.
Brion LP, Uko SE and Goldman DL (2007) Risk of resistance associated with fluconazole prophylaxis: systematic review. *J Infect* 54: 521–9.
Brooks RG (1989) Prospective study of Candida endophthalmitis in hospitalized patients with candidemia. *Arch Intern Med* 149: 2226–8.
BSAC (1994) Management of deep Candida infection in surgical and intensive care unit patients. British Society for Antimicrobial Chemotherapy Working Party. *Intensive Care Med* 20: 522–8.
Bulpa P, Dive A and Sibille Y (2007) Invasive pulmonary aspergillosis in patients with chronic obstructive pulmonary disease. *Eur Respir J* 30: 782–800.
Calandra T, Bille J, Schneider R, Mosimann F and Francioli P (1989) Clinical significance of Candida isolated from peritoneum in surgical patients. *Lancet* 2: 1437–40.
Chow JK, Golan Y, Ruthazer R, et al. (2008) Risk factors for albicans and non-albicans candidemia in the intensive care unit. *Crit Care Med* 36: 1993–8.
Clancy CJ and Nguyen MH (2012) The end of an era in defining the optimal treatment of invasive candidiasis. *Clin Infect Dis* 54: 1123–5.
Cleveland AA, Harrison LH, Farley MM, et al. (2015) Declining incidence of candidemia and the shifting epidemiology of Candida resistance in two US metropolitan areas, 2008-2013: results from population-based surveillance. *PLoS One* 10: e0120452.
Connell PP, O'neill EC, Amirul Islam FM, et al. (2010) Endogenous endophthalmitis associated with intravenous drug abuse: seven-year experience at a tertiary referral center. *Retina* 30: 1721–5.
Cornely OA, Maertens J, Winston DJ, et al. (2007) Posaconazole vs. fluconazole or itraconazole prophylaxis in patients with neutropenia. *N Engl J Med* 356: 348–59.
Cruciani M, De Lalla F and Mengoli C (2005) Prophylaxis of Candida infections in adult trauma and surgical intensive care patients: a systematic review and meta-analysis. *Intensive Care Med* 31: 1479–87.
Cuenca-Estrella M, Verweij PE, Arendrup MC, et al. (2012) ESCMID* guideline for the diagnosis and management of Candida diseases 2012: diagnostic procedures. *Clin Microbiol Infect* 18 (Suppl. 7): 9–18.
Damjanovic V, Connolly CM, Van Saene HK, et al. (1993) Selective decontamination with nystatin for control of a Candida outbreak in a neonatal intensive care unit. *J Hosp Infect* 24: 245–59.
Dean DA and Burchard KW (1996) Fungal infection in surgical patients. *Am J Surg* 171: 374–82.
De Pauw B, Walsh TJ, Donnelly JP, et al. (2008) Revised definitions of invasive fungal disease from the European Organization for Research and Treatment of Cancer/Invasive Fungal Infections Cooperative Group and the National Institute of Allergy and Infectious Diseases Mycoses Study Group (EORTC/MSG) Consensus Group. *Clin Infect Dis* 46: 1813–21.
De Smet AM, Kluytmans JA, Cooper BS, et al. (2009) Decontamination of the digestive tract and oropharynx in ICU patients. *N Engl J Med* 360: 20–31.
Donahue SP, Greven CM, Zuravleff JJ, et al. (1994) Intraocular candidiasis in patients with candidemia. Clinical implications derived from a prospective multicenter study. *Ophthalmology* 101: 1302–9.
Eggimann P, Francioli P, Bille J, et al. (1999) Fluconazole prophylaxis prevents intra-abdominal candidiasis in high-risk surgical patients. *Crit Care Med* 27: 1066–72.
Eubanks PJ, De Virgilio C, Klein S and Bongard F (1993) Candida sepsis in surgical patients. *Am J Surg* 166: 617–19; discussion 619–20.
Fernandez-Ruiz, M., Aguado, J. M., Almirante, B., et al. (2014) Initial use of echinocandins does not negatively influence outcome in Candida parapsilosis bloodstream infection: a propensity score analysis. *Clin Infect Dis* 58: 1413–21.
Fischer JJ and Walker DH (1979) Invasive pulmonary aspergillosis associated with influenza. *JAMA* 241: 1493–4.
Fisher-Hoch SP and Hutwagner L (1995) Opportunistic candidiasis: an epidemic of the 1980s. *Clin Infect Dis* 21: 897–904.
Fitzpatrick F, Prout S, Gilleece A, Fenelon LE and Murphy OM (1999) Nosocomial aspergillosis during building work—a multidisciplinary approach. *J Hosp Infect* 42: 170–1.
Fraser VJ, Jones M, Dunkel J, Storfer S, Medoff G and Dunagan WC (1992) Candidemia in a tertiary care hospital: epidemiology, risk factors, and predictors of mortality. *Clin Infect Dis* 15: 414–21.
Garey KW, Rege M, Pai MP, et al. (2006) Time to initiation of fluconazole therapy impacts mortality in patients with candidemia: a multi-institutional study. *Clin Infect Dis* 43: 25–31.
Garnacho-Montero J, Amaya-Villar R, Ortiz-Leyba C, et al. (2005) Isolation of Aspergillus spp. from the respiratory tract in critically ill patients: risk factors, clinical presentation and outcome. *Crit Care* 9: R191–9.
Gradel KO, Schonheyder HC, Arpi M, Knudsen JD, Ostergaard C and Sogaard M (2014) The Danish Collaborative Bacteraemia Network (DACOBAN) database. *Clin Epidemiol* 6: 301–8.
Grewe M, Tsiotos GG, Luque De-Leon E and Sarr MG (1999) Fungal infection in acute necrotizing pancreatitis. *J Am Coll Surg* 188: 408–14.
Gross M, Winkler H, Pitlik S and Weinberger M (1998) Unexpected candidemia complicating ureteroscopy and urinary stenting. *Eur J Clin Microbiol Infect Dis* 17: 583–6.
Gueho E, Boekhout T, Ashbee HR, Guillot J, Van Belkum A and Faergemann J (1998) The role of Malassezia species in the ecology of human skin and as pathogens. *Med Mycol* 36 (Suppl. 1): 220–9.
Harrison D, Muskett H, Harvey S, et al. (2013) Development and validation of a risk model for identification of non-neutropenic, critically ill adult patients at high risk of invasive Candida infection: the Fungal Infection Risk Evaluation (FIRE) Study. *Health Technol Assess* 17: 1–156.
Harvey IM, Leadbeatter S, Peters TJ, Mullins J, Philpot CM and Salaman JR (1988) An outbreak of disseminated aspergillosis associated with an intensive care unit. *Community Med* 10: 306–13.
Ho KM, Lipman J, Dobb GJ and Webb SA (2005) The use of prophylactic fluconazole in immunocompetent high-risk surgical patients: a meta-analysis. *Crit Care* 9: R710–17.
Hoerauf A, Hammer S, Muller-Myhsok B and Rupprecht H (1998) Intra-abdominal Candida infection during acute necrotizing pancreatitis has a high prevalence and is associated with increased mortality. *Crit Care Med* 26: 2010–15.
Humphreys H, Johnson EM, Warnock DW, Willatts SM, Winter RJ and Speller DC (1991) An outbreak of aspergillosis in a general ITU. *J Hosp Infect* 18: 167–77.
Irby PB, Stoller ML and McAninch JW (1990) Fungal bezoars of the upper urinary tract. *J Urol* 143: 447–51.
Janssen JJ, Strack Van Schijndel RJ, Van Der Poest Clement EH, Ossenkoppele GJ, Thijs LG and Huijgens PC (1996) Outcome of ICU treatment in invasive aspergillosis. *Intensive Care Med* 22: 1315–22.
Kao AS, Brandt ME, Pruitt WR, et al. (1999) The epidemiology of candidemia in two United States cities: results of a population-based active surveillance. *Clin Infect Dis* 29: 1164–70.
Kauffman CA, Vazquez JA, Sobel JD, et al. (2000) Prospective multicenter surveillance study of funguria in hospitalized patients. The National Institute for Allergy and Infectious Diseases (NIAID) Mycoses Study Group. *Clin Infect Dis* 30: 14–18.
Keiser P and Keay S (1992) Candidal pancreatic abscesses: report of two cases and review. *Clin Infect Dis* 14: 884–8.
Kett DH, Azoulay E, Echeverria PM and Vincent JL (2011) Candida bloodstream infections in intensive care units: analysis of the extended

prevalence of infection in intensive care unit study. *Crit Care Med* 39: 665–70.

Kibbler CC, Seaton S, Barnes RA, et al. (2003) Management and outcome of bloodstream infections due to Candida species in England and Wales. *J Hosp Infect* 54: 18–24.

Knitsch W, Vincent JL, Utzolino S, et al. (2015) A randomized, placebo-controlled trial of preemptive antifungal therapy for the prevention of invasive candidiasis following gastrointestinal surgery for intra-abdominal infections. *Clin Infect Dis* 61: 1671–8.

Kollef M, Micek S, Hampton N, Doherty JA and Kumar A (2012) Septic shock attributed to Candida infection: importance of empiric therapy and source control. *Clin Infect Dis* 54: 1739–46.

Kowacs PA, Soares Silvado CE, Monteiro DE Almeida S, et al. (2004) Infection of the CNS by Scedosporium apiospermum after near drowning. Report of a fatal case and analysis of its confounding factors. *J Clin Pathol* 57: 205–7.

Kox WJ, Volk T, Kox SN and Volk HD (2000) Immunomodulatory therapies in sepsis. *Intensive Care Med* 26 (Suppl. 1): S124–8.

Labelle AJ, Micek ST, Roubinian N and Kollef MH (2008) Treatment-related risk factors for hospital mortality in Candida bloodstream infections. *Crit Care Med* 36: 2967–72.

Lehner T (1964) Systemic candidiasis and renal involvement. *Lancet* 2: 1414–16.

Leleu G, Aegerter P and Guidet B (2002) Systemic candidiasis in intensive care units: a multicenter, matched-cohort study. *J Crit Care* 17: 168–75.

Leon C, Ruiz-Santana S, Saavedra P, et al. (2006) A bedside scoring system ('Candida score') for early antifungal treatment in nonneutropenic critically ill patients with Candida colonization. *Crit Care Med* 34: 730–7.

Leon C, Ruiz-Santana S, Saavedra P, et al. (2009) Usefulness of the 'Candida score' for discriminating between Candida colonization and invasive candidiasis in non-neutropenic critically ill patients: a prospective multicenter study. *Crit Care Med* 37: 1624–33.

Lingnau W, Berger J, Javorsky F, Fille M, Allerberger F and Benzer H (1998) Changing bacterial ecology during a five-year period of selective intestinal decontamination. *J Hosp Infect* 39: 195–206.

Mcdonnell PJ, Mcdonnell JM, Brown RH and Green WR (1985) Ocular involvement in patients with fungal infections. *Ophthalmology* 92: 706–9.

Manuel RJ and Kibbler CC (1998) The epidemiology and prevention of invasive aspergillosis. *J Hosp Infect* 39: 95–109.

Matson A, Soni N and Sheldon J (1991) C-reactive protein as a diagnostic test of sepsis in the critically ill. *Anaesth Intensive Care* 19: 182–6.

Meersseman W, Lagrou K, Maertens J and Van Wijngaerden E (2007) Invasive aspergillosis in the intensive care unit. *Clin Infect Dis* 45: 205–16.

Meersseman W, Vandecasteele SJ, Wilmer A, Verbeken E, Peetermans WE and Van Wijngaerden E (2004) Invasive aspergillosis in critically ill patients without malignancy. *Am J Respir Crit Care Med* 170: 621–5.

Mermel LA, Allon M, Bouza E, et al. (2009) Clinical practice guidelines for the diagnosis and management of intravascular catheter-related infection: 2009 update by the Infectious Diseases Society of America. *Clin Infect Dis* 49: 1–45.

Morrell M, Fraser VJ and Kollef MH (2005) Delaying the empiric treatment of candida bloodstream infection until positive blood culture results are obtained: a potential risk factor for hospital mortality. *Antimicrob Agents Chemother* 49: 3640–5.

Morrissey CO, Chen SC, Sorrell TC, et al. (2013) Galactomannan and PCR versus culture and histology for directing use of antifungal treatment for invasive aspergillosis in high-risk haematology patients: a randomised controlled trial. *Lancet Infect Dis* 13: 519–28.

Muskett H, Shahin J, Eyres G, Harvey S, Rowan K and Harrison D (2011) Risk factors for invasive fungal disease in critically ill adult patients: a systematic review. *Crit Care* 15: R287.

Neumann PR and Rakower SR (1978) The risk of positive cultures for Candida in the critically ill patient. *Crit Care Med* 6: 73–6.

Nguyen MH, Peacock JE Jr, Tanner DC, et al. (1995) Therapeutic approaches in patients with candidemia. Evaluation in a multicenter, prospective, observational study. *Arch Intern Med* 155: 2429–35.

Nicolle L, Rotstein C, Bourgault A, St-Germain G and Garber G (1998) Invasive fungal infections in Canada from 1992 to 1994. *Can J Infect Dis* 9: 347–52.

Nolla-Salas J, Sitges-Serra A, Leon-Gil C, et al. (1997) Candidemia in non-neutropenic critically ill patients: analysis of prognostic factors and assessment of systemic antifungal therapy. Study Group of Fungal Infection in the ICU. *Intensive Care Med* 23: 23–30.

Odds FC (1996) Epidemiological shifts in opportunistic and nosocomial Candida infections: mycological aspects. *Int J Antimicrob Agents* 6: 141–4.

Ostrosky-Zeichner L, Sable C, Sobel J, et al. (2007) Multicenter retrospective development and validation of a clinical prediction rule for nosocomial invasive candidiasis in the intensive care setting. *Eur J Clin Microbiol Infect Dis* 26: 271–6.

Ostrosky-Zeichner L, Shoham S, Vazquez J, et al. (2014) MSG-01: A randomized, double-blind, placebo-controlled trial of caspofungin prophylaxis followed by preemptive therapy for invasive candidiasis in high-risk adults in the critical care setting. *Clin Infect Dis* 58: 1219–26.

Paphitou NI, Ostrosky-Zeichner L and Rex JH (2005) Rules for identifying patients at increased risk for candidal infections in the surgical intensive care unit: approach to developing practical criteria for systematic use in antifungal prophylaxis trials. *Med Mycol* 43: 235–43.

Pappas PG, Kauffman CA, Andes D, et al. (2009) Clinical practice guidelines for the management of candidiasis: 2009 update by the Infectious Diseases Society of America. *Clin Infect Dis* 48: 503–35.

Petri MG, Konig J, Moecke HP, et al. (1997) Epidemiology of invasive mycosis in ICU patients: a prospective multicenter study in 435 non-neutropenic patients. Paul-Ehrlich Society for Chemotherapy, Divisions of Mycology and Pneumonia Research. *Intensive Care Med* 23: 317–25.

Pfaller MA (1994) Epidemiology and control of fungal infections. *Clin Infect Dis* 19 (Suppl. 1): S8–13.

Phe (Public Health England) (2015) *Surveillance of Candidaemia in England, Wales and Northern Ireland, 2014* (Health Protection Report, Volume 9, Number 33), https://www.gov.uk/government/uploads/system/uploads/attachment_data/file/462010/hpr3315_cnddm14.pdf, accessed 30 May 2017.

Pittet D, Huguenin T, Dharan S, et al. (1996) Unusual cause of lethal pulmonary aspergillosis in patients with chronic obstructive pulmonary disease. *Am J Respir Crit Care Med* 154: 541–4.

Pittet D, Monod M, Filthuth I, Frenk E, Suter PM and Auckenthaler R (1991) Contour-clamped homogeneous electric field gel electrophoresis as a powerful epidemiologic tool in yeast infections. *Am J Med* 91: 256S–263S.

Pittet D, Monod M, Suter PM, Frenk E and Auckenthaler R (1994) Candida colonization and subsequent infections in critically ill surgical patients. *Ann Surg* 220: 751–8.

Playford EG, Webster AC, Sorrell TC and Craig JC (2006a) Antifungal agents for preventing fungal infections in non-neutropenic critically ill and surgical patients: systematic review and meta-analysis of randomized clinical trials. *J Antimicrob Chemother* 57: 628–38.

Playford EG, Webster AC, Sorrell TC and Craig JC (2006b) Antifungal agents for preventing fungal infections in non-neutropenic critically ill patients. *Cochrane Database Syst Rev*, CD004920. doi: 10.1002/14651858.CD004920.pub3

Price MF, Larocco MT and Gentry LO (1994) Fluconazole susceptibilities of Candida species and distribution of species recovered from blood cultures over a 5-year period. *Antimicrob Agents Chemother* 38: 1422–4.

Price R, Maclennang and Glen J (2014) Selective digestive or oropharyngeal decontamination and topical oropharyngeal chlorhexidine for prevention of death in general intensive care: systematic review and network meta-analysis. *BMJ* 348: g2197.

Puig-Asensio M, Peman J, Zaragoza R, et al. (2014) Impact of therapeutic strategies on the prognosis of candidemia in the ICU. *Crit Care Med* 42: 1423–32.

Rex JH, Bennett JE, Sugar AM, et al. (1995) Intravascular catheter exchange and duration of candidemia. NIAID Mycoses Study Group and the Candidemia Study Group. *Clin Infect Dis* 21: 994–6.

Rex JH and Sobel JD (1999) Preventing intra-abdominal candidiasis in surgical patients. *Crit Care Med* 27: 1033–4.

Rex JH, Walsh TJ and Anaissie EJ (1998) Fungal infections in iatrogenically compromised hosts. *Adv Intern Med* 43: 321–71.

Rogers TR, Morton CO, Springer J, et al. (2013) Combined real-time PCR and galactomannan surveillance improves diagnosis of invasive aspergillosis in high risk patients with haematological malignancies. *Br J Haematol* 161: 517–24.

Romano F, Ribera G and Giuliano M (1994) A study of a hospital cluster of systemic candidosis using DNA typing methods. *Epidemiol Infect* 112: 393–8.

Rutledge R, Mandel SR and Wild RE (1986) Candida species. Insignificant contaminant or pathogenic species. *Am Surg* 52: 299–302.

Sandven P, Qvist H, Skovlund E and Giercksky KE (2002) Significance of Candida recovered from intraoperative specimens in patients with intra-abdominal perforations. *Crit Care Med* 30: 541–7.

Sheridan RL, Weber JM, Budkevich LG and Tompkins RG (1995) Candidemia in the pediatric patient with burns. *J Burn Care Rehabil* 16: 440–3.

Shorr AF, Chung K, Jackson WL, Waterman PE and Kollef MH (2005) Fluconazole prophylaxis in critically ill surgical patients: a meta-analysis. *Crit Care Med* 33: 1928–35; quiz 1936.

Sobel JD, Fisher JF, Kauffman CA and Newman CA (2011) Candida urinary tract infections—epidemiology. *Clin Infect Dis* 52 (Suppl. 6): S433–6.

Solomkin JS (1993) Pathogenesis and management of Candida infection syndromes in non-neutropenic patients. *New Horiz* 1: 202–13.

Soutter DI and Todd TR (1986) Systemic candidiasis in a surgical intensive care unit. *Can J Surg* 29: 197–9.

Spencer RC (1996) Predominant pathogens found in the European Prevalence of Infection in Intensive Care Study. *Eur J Clin Microbiol Infect Dis* 15: 281–5.

Stamos JK and Rowley AH (1995) Candidemia in a pediatric population. *Clin Infect Dis* 20: 571–5.

Strausbaugh LJ, Sewell DL, Ward TT, Pfaller MA, Heitzman T and Tjoelker R (1994) High frequency of yeast carriage on hands of hospital personnel. *J Clin Microbiol* 32: 2299–300.

Tortorano AM, Biraghi E, Astolfi A, et al. (2002) European Confederation of Medical Mycology (ECMM) prospective survey of candidaemia: report from one Italian region. *J Hosp Infect* 51: 297–304.

Ullmann AJ, Akova M, Herbrecht R, et al. (2012) ESCMID* guideline for the diagnosis and management of Candida diseases 2012: adults with haematological malignancies and after haematopoietic stem cell transplantation (HCT). *Clin Microbiol Infect* 18 (Suppl. 7): 53–67.

Ullmann AJ, Lipton JH, Vesole DH, et al. (2007) Posaconazole or fluconazole for prophylaxis in severe graft-versus-host disease. *N Engl J Med* 356: 335–47.

Vandewoude KH, Blot SI, Benoit D, Colardyn F and Vogelaers D (2004) Invasive aspergillosis in critically ill patients: attributable mortality and excesses in length of ICU stay and ventilator dependence. *J Hosp Infect* 56: 269–76.

Vandewoude KH, Blot SI, Depuydt P, et al. (2006) Clinical relevance of Aspergillus isolation from respiratory tract samples in critically ill patients. *Crit Care* 10: R31.

Vardakas KZ, Samonis G, Michalopoulos A, Soteriades ES and Falagas ME (2006) Antifungal prophylaxis with azoles in high-risk, surgical intensive care unit patients: a meta-analysis of randomized, placebo-controlled trials. *Crit Care Med* 34: 1216–24.

Vincent JL, Anaissie E, Bruining H, et al. (1998) Epidemiology, diagnosis and treatment of systemic Candida infection in surgical patients under intensive care. *Intensive Care Med* 24: 206–16.

Vincent JL, Bihari DJ, Suter PM, et al. (1995) The prevalence of nosocomial infection in intensive care units in Europe. Results of the European Prevalence of Infection in Intensive Care (EPIC) Study. EPIC International Advisory Committee. *JAMA* 274: 639–44.

Voss A, Le Noble JL, Verduyn Lunel FM, Foudraine NA and Meis JF (1997) Candidemia in intensive care unit patients: risk factors for mortality. *Infection* 25: 8–11.

Walsh TJ and Rex JH (2002) All catheter-related candidemia is not the same: assessment of the balance between the risks and benefits of removal of vascular catheters. *Clin Infect Dis* 34: 600–2.

Wey SB, Mori M, Pfaller MA, Woolson RF and Wenzel RP (1988) Hospital-acquired candidemia. The attributable mortality and excess length of stay. *Arch Intern Med* 148: 2642–5.

Wingard JR, Merz WG, Rinaldi MG, Johnson TR, Karp JE and Saral R (1991) Increase in Candida krusei infection among patients with bone marrow transplantation and neutropenia treated prophylactically with fluconazole. *N Engl J Med* 325: 1274–7.

Wingard JR, Merz WG, Rinaldi MG, Miller CB, Karp JE and Saral R (1993) Association of Torulopsis glabrata infections with fluconazole prophylaxis in neutropenic bone marrow transplant patients. *Antimicrob Agents Chemother* 37: 1847–9.

Young B, Gleeson M and Cripps AW (1991) C-reactive protein: a critical review. *Pathology* 23: 118–24.

CHAPTER 37

Fungal disease in cystic fibrosis and chronic respiratory disorders

Chris Kosmidis, David W. Denning, and Eavan G. Muldoon

Introduction to fungal infection in chronic respiratory disease

Chronic respiratory diseases such as asthma, chronic bronchitis, emphysema, bronchiectasis, or sarcoidosis have not been previously thought of as predisposing to fungal diseases. However, in recent years, there has been accumulating evidence on the susceptibility of these patients to aspergillosis and other fungal diseases, as well as on the role of fungi in asthma pathogenesis and exacerbation.

Most published data on fungal diseases in patients with chronic lung disease pertain to aspergillosis, with only rare case reports implicating other fungi. The main clinical syndromes include invasive pulmonary aspergillosis (IPA), chronic pulmonary aspergillosis (CPA) and allergic bronchopulmonary aspergillosis or mycosis (ABPA or ABPM). The diagnosis of fungal disease in these patients requires a high index of suspicion. Symptoms are non-specific, low-grade, and may resemble those of the underlying disease or other infectious aetiologies. As a result, the recognition and treatment of fungal disease may be delayed. The mainstay of treatment is oral triazole antifungals, often administered for prolonged periods, resulting in issues regarding side effects, toxicity, and cost.

In this section, we discuss fungal infection in patients with chronic lung disease other than cystic fibrosis (CF). Because of its unique features, CF is discussed separately in 'Introduction to fungal infection in cystic fibrosis'.

Epidemiology

The epidemiology of IPA has been extensively studied and reviewed in immunocompromised patients (see Chapters 10, 30, and 32). In recent years, however, it has been recognized in other patient groups such as those with chronic obstructive pulmonary disease (COPD) (Bulpa et al. 2007; Guinea et al. 2010) The setting is mostly intensive care unit (ICU) admissions. In one study, around 7% of consecutive medical admissions to ICU had *Aspergillus* isolated in respiratory samples; the majority did not have a haematological malignancy, and half of those with proven or probable IPA had COPD (Meersseman et al. 2004) In a prospective study of ICU admissions, 13 out of 55 consecutive COPD patients were diagnosed with IPA (He et al. 2011). However, the incidence of IPA in COPD patients is difficult to assess because of the lack of a standardized definition and the challenges in distinguishing colonization from infection.

The use of corticosteroids has been highlighted as the most important predictive factor in the development of IPA in COPD patients. In a retrospective study of COPD patients with *Aspergillus* isolation, IPA was associated with ICU admission, accumulated dose of corticosteroids before and after admission, antibiotic use, and heart failure (Guinea et al. 2010). Patients with more severe COPD, defined as the Global Initiative for Chronic Obstructive Pulmonary Disease (GOLD) score III or IV, are more likely to have IPA.

CPA has only recently been recognized as an important global health problem and its incidence appreciated (Denning et al. 2011). As CPA develops in lungs with a pre-existing cavity or other structural abnormality, previous tuberculosis (TB) is the most common underlying condition worldwide. Co-infection with non-tuberculous mycobacteria is also commonly diagnosed, and may be as common as previous TB in low-prevalence areas. In a CPA referral centre in Manchester, UK, 33.3% of referred patients diagnosed with CPA also had COPD, although COPD was thought to be the primary underlying condition in less than 10% of patients, indicating that usually there are multiple predisposing factors for CPA (Smith and Denning 2011). Pneumothorax with presence of bullae was seen in 16.7% of patients, previous chest surgery in 14.3%, previous treatment for lung cancer in 10.3%, and sarcoidosis in 7.1%. In addition, 14.3% of patients had previously been diagnosed with ABPA.

Exposure to fungi affects symptom severity in large numbers of people with asthma. The prevalence of mould-induced asthma appears to be increasing, and fungi may have become the most important trigger agent (Piipari and Keskinen 2005). In children, outdoor fungal spore counts were linked to asthma exacerbations, although this was not observed in adults (Atkinson et al. 2006). *Aspergillus* is implicated in asthma exacerbation, and increased *Aspergillus* spore concentrations were detected in indoor air sampled from the homes of patients with worsening symptoms of asthma (Chen et al. 2014; Zubairi et al. 2014). In addition, patients admitted to ICUs with life-threatening asthma were more likely to have evidence of sensitization to fungi such as *Alternaria,*

Cladosporium, Helminthosporium, or *Epicoccum* (Black et al. 2000). '*Trichophyton* asthma' is a recognized entity in several countries; one Japanese study showed that a high *Trichophyton*-specific IgE (immunoglobulin E) is more common with increasing asthma severity (Matsuoka et al. 2009).

The prevalence of ABPA in asthma varies from 0.7% to 3.5% in studies from various countries, allowing the estimation that there are up to 4.8 million adults with ABPA complicating asthma (Denning et al. 2013). The prevalence of severe asthma with fungal sensitization may be even higher (Denning et al. 2014). Other less commonly implicated fungi are *Candida, Bipolaris, Schizophyllum*, and *Curvularia*.

Immunosuppression

Invasive fungal disease (IFD) typically occurs in the neutropenic patient. However, fungal diseases are being increasingly recognized in non-neutropenic patients, including patients with chronic lung diseases.

The use of steroids is predisposing to IPA; their multiple effects on the immune system—including inhibition of monocyte-mediated damage to fungal hyphae, neutrophil function, and lymphocyte action—accounts for this association (Diamond 1983). In addition, corticosteroids promote the *in vitro* growth of *Aspergillus* (Ng et al. 1994). In a prospective study of COPD patients admitted to ICUs, an accumulated dose of steroids (>350 mg of prednisolone) before ICU admission was an independent risk factor for IPA (He et al. 2011). Other studies implicated higher daily steroid doses (Rello et al. 1998; Bulpa et al. 2001). Once IPA is diagnosed, limiting subsequent steroid use, if possible, does lead to better outcomes.

Although aspergillosis can rarely occur in the normal host, particularly after massive exposure to spores after activities such as cleaning mouldy houses, some form of immune defect, usually subtle, is thought to contribute to the pathogenesis of fungal disease in patients with chronic lung disease. Interferon-gamma deficiency has been linked to CPA, and interferon-gamma treatment may be beneficial to patients not responding to antifungals (Smith and Denning 2014). In addition, genetic susceptibility to CPA and ABPA has been attributed to alterations in mannose-binding lectin and surfactant A2 (Crosdale et al. 2001; Kaur et al. 2006; Vaid et al. 2007; Harrison et al. 2012; Moss 2014).

Clinical presentation

IPA in COPD patients presents with non-specific findings, and only a minority of patients will have fever. Features include wheezing, increasing sputum or thick secretions, and respiratory failure that may progress rapidly. In the ICU setting, the clinical presentation may closely resemble other infections and therefore IPA may not be suspected unless *Aspergillus* grows from respiratory samples. Imaging is also non-specific; bronchoscopy may reveal pseudomembranes (He et al. 2011).

CPA usually has an indolent presentation, with symptoms present for months or years before it is recognized. Symptoms are initially attributed to progression of the underlying disease (e.g. COPD, bronchiectasis, or sarcoidosis). Patients are usually middle-aged and most often male. The main symptoms are worsening breathlessness, chest pain, cough with or without haemoptysis, sweats, fever, malaise, and weight loss. Haemoptysis usually indicates presence of an aspergilloma. If not recognized and treated, CPA can result in profound deterioration and poor functional status.

The natural course of CPA is variable; some patients may remain stable for years, whereas others may deteriorate rapidly. Faster progression may be seen in patients with some form of immunosuppression (diabetes, steroid treatment, AIDS, alcoholism), which may be reflected by worsening findings on imaging such as enlarging cavities, consolidation, or necrosis. This pattern is termed 'subacute invasive pulmonary aspergillosis' (or 'chronic necrotizing pulmonary aspergillosis'). CPA in sarcoidosis may have a worse prognosis, possibly because of the ongoing need for steroids. The majority of patients have a more indolent presentation, termed 'chronic cavitary pulmonary aspergillosis' (CCPA), characterized by slowly evolving single or multiple lung cavities. A small number of patients may go on to develop extensive fibrosis, involving the entire lung (chronic fibrosing pulmonary aspergillosis) (Denning et al. 2003).

The *Aspergillus* nodule is a distinct presentation of fungal disease. It may be an incidental finding, and prompt investigations for malignancy. CT-guided or excisional biopsy confirms the diagnosis. *Aspergillus* bronchitis in the immunocompetent individual is a recently described clinical entity, especially in the setting of bronchiectasis or CF. It may account for a subset of immunocompetent patients with evidence of *Aspergillus* (either microbiological or serological) but without pulmonary parenchymal disease. These patients usually have a history of recurrent chest infections unsuccessfully managed with antibiotics (Chrdle et al. 2012).

ABPM should be suspected in any patient with poorly controlled asthma. Typically, exacerbations are treated with several steroid and antibiotic courses before the diagnosis is considered. Other symptoms are haemoptysis, fever, malaise, and expectoration of mucus plugs. If the condition is not recognized and treated, it results in further lung damage in the form of bronchiectasis or secondary CPA.

Fungi other than *Aspergillus* have been reported to cause clinical syndromes in chronic lung disease patients, although reports are rare. *Candida* species are considered to be colonizers of the respiratory tract rather than pathogens, but have been reported to occasionally cause tracheobronchitis or chronic bronchitis (Karnak et al. 2007; Johnson 2012). *Scedosporium apiospermum* has been reported as a cause of fungus ball in sarcoidosis (Belitsos et al. 1974). *Pneumocystis jirovecii* colonization is more common in COPD patients and may be associated with enhanced inflammation, although the clinical significance is not clear (Calderon et al. 2004; Fitzpatrick et al. 2014).

Diagnosis

A high index of suspicion is required for the diagnosis of fungal disease in patients with chronic lung disease as the symptoms are non-specific and the sensitivity of respiratory sample cultures for fungi is poor. Respiratory samples (sputum or bronchoalveolar lavage [BAL]) should be cultured on fungal media in order to improve sensitivity. Fungal stains should be used to identify the presence of hyphae in the sample. Because of the poor sensitivity of culture, multiple samples should be sent. *Aspergillus* PCR (polymerase chain reaction) and galactomannan (GM) have a role in diagnosis as their sensitivity is better than culture. Among critically ill patients with COPD, BAL GM at a cut-off of 0.8 was found to be more sensitive than fungal culture or serum GM for the diagnosis of IPA (He et al. 2012). Serum galactomannan is rarely positive in the non-neutropenic patient with chronic lung disease. Real-time *Aspergillus* PCR also showed good sensitivity in BAL and sputum in COPD patients (Guinea et al. 2013). A combination of culture,

GM, and PCR may improve sensitivity without compromising specificity (Aquino et al. 2012).

CPA requires the detection of *Aspergillus* in sputum or BAL by culture, PCR, or GM and/or serological evidence of *Aspergillus* infection by precipitins or IgG ELISA (enzyme-linked immunosorbent assay), accompanied by compatible findings on imaging. Recently, diagnostic and classification criteria for ABPA were reviewed by the ABPA Complicating Asthma Working Group of the International Society for Human and Animal Mycology (Figure 37.1) *Aspergillus*-specific IgE is used as a screening test; a total IgE >1,000 IU/mL is then used as a diagnostic criterion for ABPA in asthma (Agarwal et al. 2013).

Imaging plays a key role in diagnosing fungal disease in patients with chronic lung conditions. Chest X-ray may reveal the presence of cavities or fibrosis but is often non-specific, unless an aspergilloma is seen. A computed tomography (CT) scan is more useful and should be performed when there is a suspicion of aspergillosis or other fungal disease. IPA in COPD patients may present as infiltrates, nodules, or cavities on CT scan, but the characteristic findings seen in neutropenic patients, such as the halo sign, are rarely seen. CPA may present as thick-walled cavities usually in the upper lobes with or without intracavitary material or aspergilloma; multiple cavities are often present. Infiltrates, lung nodules, or fibrosis with volume loss may also be seen. Figure 37.2 shows CT scans of various forms of aspergillosis. Radiologically, the main differential diagnosis includes mycobacterial infection and malignancy. Serial imaging over time is important in order to define the rate of progression and response to treatment (Figure 37.3). ABPA presents as transient infiltrates, and in later stages with bronchiectasis, which is typically central (Figure 37.4).

Treatment strategies

COPD patients with IPA should be managed along the same principles as other patients with IPA, according to established guidelines. Voriconazole is the preferred antifungal as it has been associated with survival advantage. As these patients are often on steroids, rapid tapering should be pursued where possible. Prognosis of IPA in this population is poor, as these are usually patients with multiple comorbidities, ongoing need for steroids, and advanced or end-stage COPD.

Management of CPA in patients with respiratory conditions is challenging and requires a multidisciplinary approach (Box 37.1). Azoles are the initial choice for therapy; itraconazole is usually the first choice because of cost, followed by voriconazole and posaconazole. Response is variable: 35% of patients on itraconazole for six months reported an improvement, 41% remained stable, and 23% deteriorated. Unfortunately, six months after treatment was stopped, 30% of patients relapsed (Agarwal et al. 2013). However, if treatment is continued beyond six months, continued improvement can be seen, as documented using the St George's

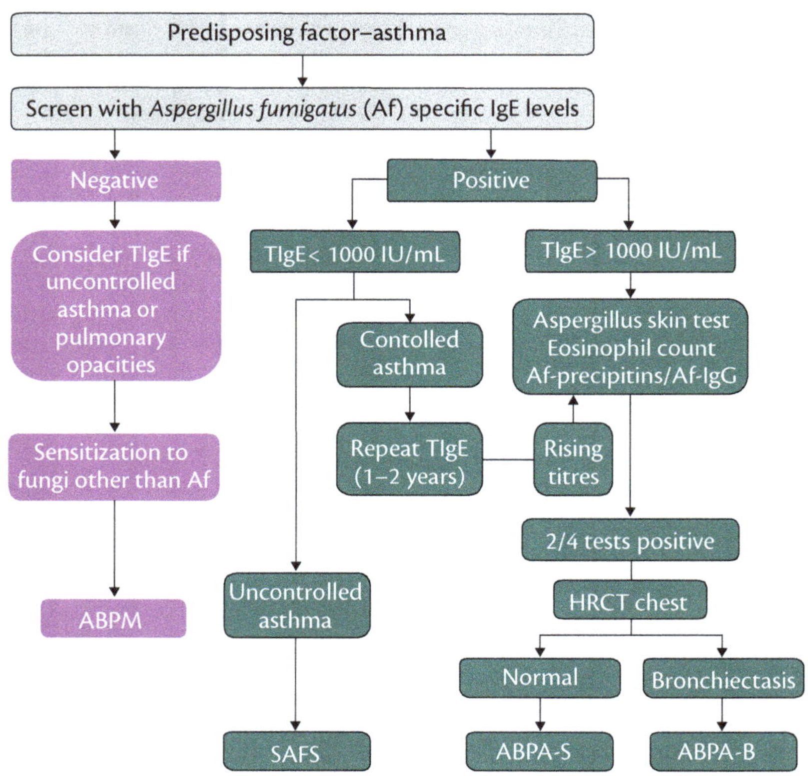

Figure 37.1 Classification of allergic fungal disease in asthma.

ABPA-B = ABPA-bronchiectasis; ABPA-S = ABPA-seropositive; ABPM = allergic bronchopulmonary mycosis; HRCT = high-resolution computed tomography; SAFS = severe asthma with fungal sensitization; TIgE = total IgE

Reproduced with permission from Agarwal R., Chakrabarti A., Shah A., Gupta D., Meis J. F., Guleria R., Moss R., & Denning D. W., 'Allergic bronchopulmonary aspergillosis: review of literature and proposal of new diagnostic and classification criteria', *Clinical and Experimental Allergy*, Volume 43, Issue 8, pp. 850–73, Copyright © 2013 John Wiley & Sons Ltd. DOI: 10.1111/cea.12141.

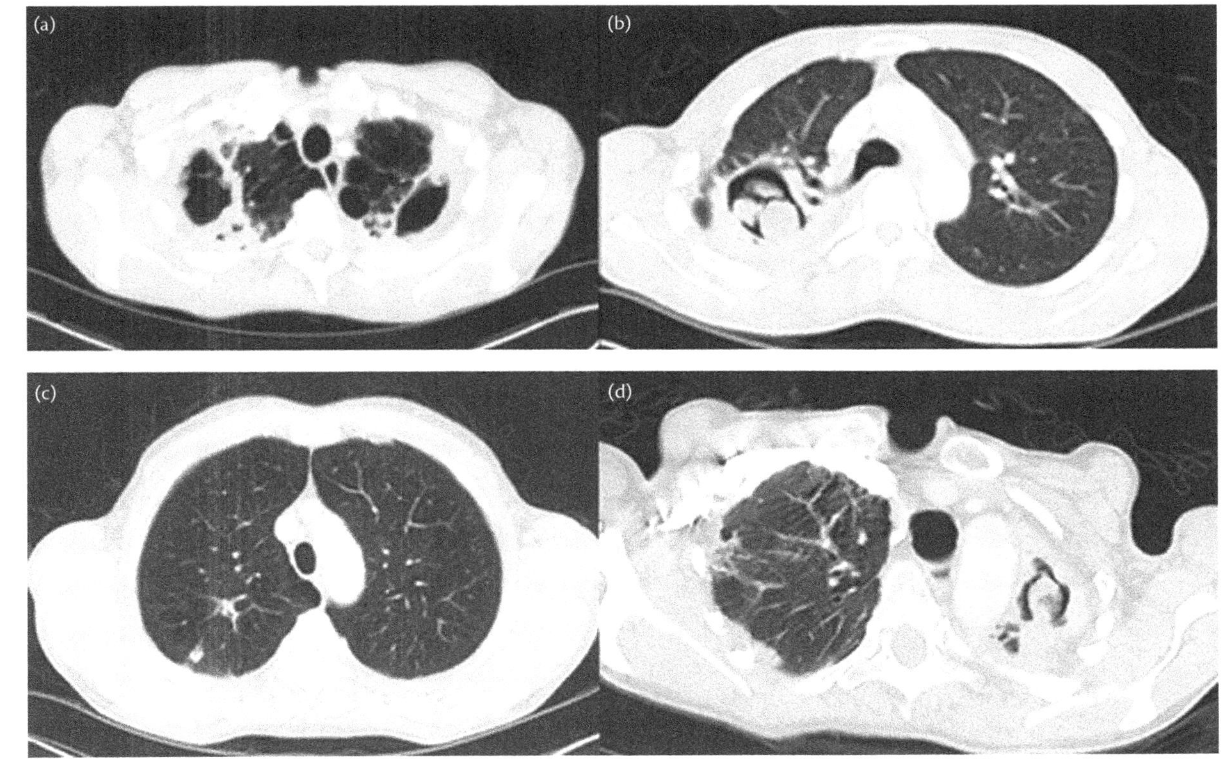

Figure 37.2 High-resolution computed tomography images from patients with various forms of chronic pulmonary aspergillosis.
a,b Chronic cavitary pulmonary aspergillosis; **c** *Aspergillus* nodule; **d** Chronic fibrosing pulmonary aspergillosis.

Respiratory questionnaire (Al-Shair et al. 2013). Therefore, these patients usually remain on prolonged courses of antifungals, often limited by cost, side-effects, and resistance. Intravenous antifungals may be used in cases of intolerance, lack of response, or resistance to oral azoles.

Surgical treatment has a role in patients with limited disease or recurrent or life-threatening haemoptysis and otherwise preserved lung function, and can be curative. Surgical resection is also often undertaken in cases of diagnostic uncertainty—that is, in pulmonary nodules subsequently found to be *Aspergillus* nodules. Procedures may include lobectomy, pneumonectomy, or segmental resection (Farid et al. 2013). Outcomes are better with simple aspergilloma than with CCPA; complications may arise from spillage of fungal material into the pleural cavity, while recurrence is a concern in CCPA, estimated at 25%. Bronchial artery embolization can achieve temporary control of bleeding until surgery is planned or if surgery is contraindicated.

Acute exacerbations of ABPA are managed with systemic corticosteroid therapy, although there are no established guidelines on the dose, and a dose of 0.5 mg/kg of prednisolone for a few weeks is

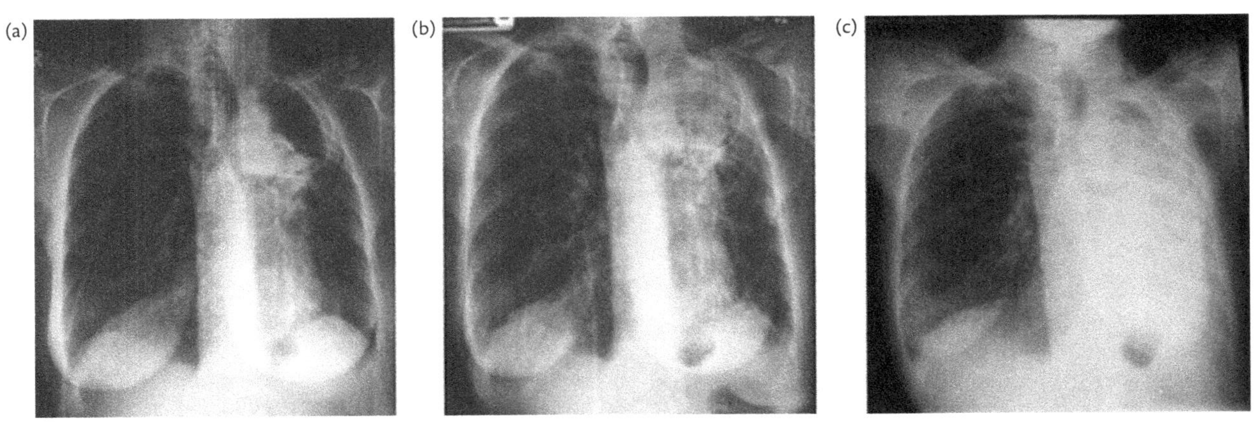

Figure 37.3 Serial chest radiographs of patient with chronic cavitating pulmonary aspergillosis.
a At baseline; **b** Two years later; **c** Four years later.

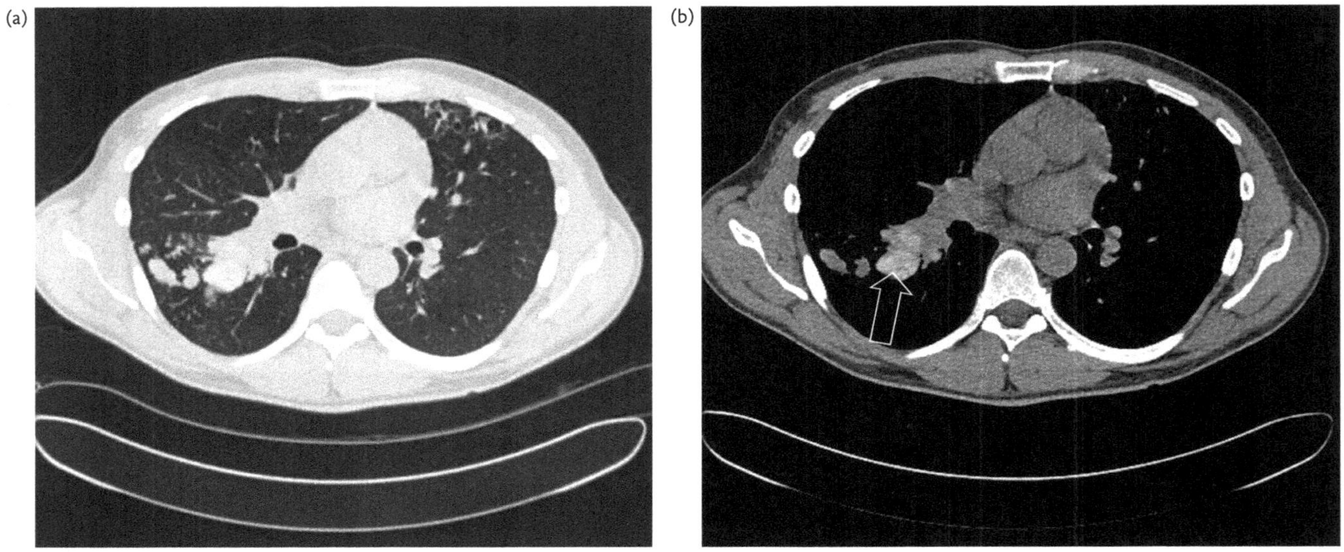

Figure 37.4 High-resolution computed tomography images of patient with allergic bronchopulmonary aspergillosis.
a Lung window; **b** Mediastinal window showing hyperlucent high-density mucus plugging (arrow).

usually used. Patients with significant symptoms or frequent exacerbations may benefit from antifungals, which reduce the fungal burden and help control symptoms, thereby exhibiting a steroid-sparing effect. Inhaled amphotericin B may also have a role in cases of itraconazole intolerance (Box 37.1).

Azole resistance occurs and may be acquired from inhalation of a resistant isolate present in the environment (probably a consequence of azole fungicide use on crops) or may occur during therapy. It is recommended that all isolates of *A. fumigatus* cultured from patients on therapy, or in whom antifungal therapy is to be given, are susceptibility tested.

Prevention

Patients with asthma and COPD may benefit from avoiding exposure to fungi, for example mouldy or damp areas at home, or handling compost or bark chippings. Face masks should be used when doing activities leading to exposure to large numbers of fungal spores. Rooms should be well aerated and drying clothes indoors after washing should be avoided if possible.

IPA in COPD patients could potentially be prevented by limiting unnecessary use of steroids or tapering their use as soon as possible. There are no defined strategies for prevention of CPA. Efforts should focus on rapid detection, mainly by maintaining a high index of suspicion for fungal disease in patients with pre-existing cavities, such as patients with previously treated TB or patients being treated for non-tuberculous mycobacteria. Patients with TB should have an end-of-treatment X-ray as a baseline.

Box 37.1 Chronic fungal diseases and their management

ABPA:

Corticosteroids are used in acute exacerbations.
Itraconazole is used as a steroid-sparing agent.
Inhaled amphotericin B has a role in itraconazole failure or intolerance.

CPA:

Triazoles for prolonged periods are the mainstay of treatment (itraconazole, voriconazole, posaconazole).
Intravenous agents (echinocandins, amphotericin B) are used in azole-resistant aspergillosis or after triazole failure.
Surgery can have a role in limited disease.

Introduction to fungal infection in cystic fibrosis

Cystic fibrosis (CF) patients are commonly colonized with bacterial and fungal species, and it is recognized that such colonization impacts upon patient outcomes. However, whilst fungi are frequently isolated from the respiratory tract in CF patients (Pihet et al. 2009), their role in the progression of disease has been less clear, and the significance of fungal isolates in this patient group is still being investigated. It would seem that we are only just beginning to understand the fungal diversity of the CF lung microbiome (Paganin et al. 2015).

Epidemiology

In CF, risk factors which have been associated with the isolation of *Aspergillus* species from the respiratory tract include increasing age, steroid use, and antibiotic exposure (Pihet et al. 2009). *Aspergillus fumigatus* colonization has also been associated with *Pseudomonas* spp. colonization in CF patients (Amin et al. 2010). The numbers of CF patients colonized with *Aspergillus* species appear to be increasing, having doubled in the United States between 1995 and 2005, and up to one-third of patients may have filamentous fungi isolated from respiratory secretions over the course of a year (Nielsen et al. 2014). Differentiating between colonization and infection in CF patients remains challenging (Baxter et al. 2013). It is estimated that 6–15% of patients with CF will develop ABPA, starting in childhood (Armstead et al. 2014). In ABPA patients without CF, 13% have been reported to be carriers of a CFTR gene mutation (Eaton et al. 2002).

While *Aspergillus* species are the most commonly isolated moulds in CF patients, *Scedosporium* species have also been reported, and pose difficult therapeutic challenges due to their patterns of antifungal resistance, and its relevance post lung transplantation (Blyth et al. 2010a, 2010b; Nielsen et al. 2014). Isolation of *Scedoporium* species is associated with the presence of mucoid *Pseudomonas* species and the prior use of flucloxacillin therapy to treat *S. aureus* colonization and/or infection (Blyth et al. 2010)

Candida species are commonly isolated from the respiratory secretions of CF patients and have long been thought of as contaminants from the oropharynx. Recently however, the isolation of *Candida* species from CF patients has been associated with a decline in lung function, while the absence of any fungi was not (Chotirmall et al. 2010; Nagano et al. 2010; Paganin et al. 2015). Some studies have found *Candida* species isolated from respiratory secretions in up to 97% of CF patients (Nagano et al. 2010).

Other fungi which have been identified in the respiratory secretions of CF patients are *Malassezia* spp., *Rhodotorula* spp., *Saccharomyces cerevisiae, Trichosporon* spp., *Exophiala* spp., *Penicillium* spp., *Aureobasidium* spp., *Fusocoporia* spp., *Fusarium* spp., *Acremonium* spp., *Cladosporium* spp., and *Thanatephorus* spp. (Nagano et al. 2010). However, the clinical relevance of these fungi remains unclear. *Exophiala* species may be isolated from the respiratory secretions of up to 20% of CF patients. Their presence is associated with pancreatic insufficiency, non-tuberculous mycobacteria, *Pseudomonas* spp. colonization, and increased use of intravenous antibiotics (Kondori et al. 2011, 2014). Additionally, patients have been found to have higher levels of inflammation (i.e. high white cell counts and inflammatory markers) and positive IgG response to *Exophiala* species (Kondori et al. 2014). Domestic dishwashers have been implicated as a habitat for such black moulds (Zalar et al. 2011).

Immunosuppression

Cystic fibrosis is the most common genetic condition among Caucasian populations. It is an autosomal recessive disease and occurs because of mutations in the cystic fibrosis transmembrane regulator (CFTR) gene on chromosome 7. It is estimated that in European Union countries, one in every 2,000–3,000 newborns will have CF. While patients with CF are not classically immunocompromised, they are at risk of respiratory infection owing to thick viscous respiratory secretions, impaired mucociliary clearance, and the development of bronchiectasis. Additionally, they often receive either inhaled or oral corticosteroids, particularly if they also have asthma.

As a result, CF patients fail to remove *Aspergillus* or other fungal conidia, which are inhaled, and the conidia may then germinate. The conidia of *A. fumigatus* have been shown to be immunologically inert, as they have a rodlet/hydrophobin layer which is removed by germination (Aimanianda et al. 2009). Additionally, CFTR-deficient cells are less efficient at ingesting and eliminating conidia than CFTR-competent cells (Chaudhary et al. 2012). This colonization of the airway by fungi in CF patients may stimulate T helper (Th) type 2 cell based responses, triggering the development of ABPM (Romani 1997), which may account, in part, for the high prevalence of ABPM in the CF population.

Clinical presentation

In cystic fibrosis, the patterns of *Aspergillus* disease mirror those of the non-CF population, and can be categorized into the following (Felton and Simmonds 2014): 1) colonization, 2) sensitization, 3) ABPA, 4) *Aspergillus* bronchitis, and 5) aspergilloma.

In children with CF, ABPA is associated with the most severe progression of decline in lung function, compared with *Aspergillus* colonization or chronic *Pseudomonas* infection. Additionally, sensitization to *Aspergillus* is almost always preceded by chronic *Pseudomonas* colonization (Kraemer et al. 2006). While *Aspergillus* is the most common cause of allergic fungal disease in CF patients, it should be noted that ABPM can occur with other fungi, such as *Scedosporium* species or *Candida* species.

Children chronically colonized with *Aspergillus* species appear to have significantly worse lung function than those who have never had *Aspergillus* isolated from respiratory secretions, and have a higher frequency of pulmonary exacerbations requiring hospitalization (Amin et al. 2010). Similarly, in adults, the severity of bronchiectasis—as determined by computed tomography—is significantly worse in patients colonized with *Aspergillus* species (McMahon et al. 2012). However, the data are conflicting, and the association between *Aspergillus* colonization and progression in lung function decline has not been borne out in longitudinal analysis (De Vrankrijker et al. 2011), although it is not clear that *Aspergillus* bronchitis was separated from true colonization. There is a paucity of data in this area, and the role of *Aspergillus* colonization in the progression of CF disease remains uncertain (Speirs et al. 2012).

While *Scedosporium* species are the second most frequently isolated moulds in CF patients, few studies have examined the impact of infection and/or colonization on the progression of CF disease. In small studies, no significant differences in disease severity parameters have been identified (Blyth et al. 2010).

Candida species have traditionally been considered contaminants from the oropharynx, and of no clinical significance in CF. Risk factors for colonization with *Candida* species are pancreatic insufficiency, osteopenia, and colonization with *Pseudomonas* species and *Aspergillus* species (Chotirmall et al. 2010). Colonization with *Candida* species has been shown to affect both body mass index and lung function in CF patients (Chotirmall et al. 2010; Paganin et al. 2015).

The absence of fungi in the respiratory secretions of patients with CF has been shown to have a protective effect with regard to lung function when the lung microbiota is analyzed (Paganin et al. 2015).

Aspergilloma is a rare but recognized presentation of *Aspergillus* disease in CF patients and is often intra-bronchial.

Diagnosis

Fungi are commonly found in respiratory secretions of CF patients and may or may not reflect disease. However, there is a lack of standardization of how respiratory samples should be processed to maximize the isolation and identification of fungi (Liu et al. 2013). This leads to complexity when comparing diagnostic criteria, and the epidemiology and incidence of fungal disease, in the published literature. Additionally, there may be overgrowth of bacterial species such as *Burkholderia* species or *Pseudomonas* species, making it difficult to identify fungi. Molecular techniques or the use of selective media may increase the identification of fungi from the respiratory secretions of CF patients (Blyth et al. 2010; Nagano et al. 2010). The use of PCR techniques has been shown to increase the identification of fungal species by 60% in a CF population (Nagano et al. 2010). Microbiota studies have also identified fungi in respiratory secretions of CF patients, further increasing our understanding of the diversity of the lung microbiota in CF (Delhaes et al. 2012; Paganin et al. 2015).

Diagnostic criteria for the diagnosis of ABPA in patients with CF have traditionally been based on clinical condition, serum total IgE, *Aspergillus*-specific IgE or cutaneous reactivity, *Aspergillus*-specific IgG, and chest radiography abnormalities. Minimal diagnostic criteria were a variation of these features, with lower cut-off values for serology applied (Stevens et al. 2003). However, these criteria are somewhat outdated, and do not recognize *Aspergillus* sensitization or *Aspergillus* bronchitis, which are now well recognized within the CF population. Additionally, the use of steroids (either inhaled or oral) can make the serological markers more difficult to interpret. The increased use of molecular techniques, such as PCR and the use of biomarkers such as galactomannan in sputum, has led to the proposal of new diagnostic criteria (Baxter et al. 2013), recognizing the variants of *Aspergillus* sensitization and *Aspergillus* bronchitis which were absent from the previous criteria. *Aspergillus* sensitization is easily distinguished from ABPA by the lack of a serum *Aspergillus* IgG antibody and negative galactomannan antigen in respiratory secretions (Baxter et al. 2013). *Aspergillus* bronchitis is defined by high sputum galactomannan antigen, high DNA levels by PCR, and positive *Aspergillus* IgG antibody in serum.

Diagnosis of aspergilloma in the CF population is the same as for non-CF patients.

Treatment strategies

There is a distinct paucity of evidence on how best to treat fungal diseases in CF patients. The mainstay of therapy in ABPM remains corticosteroids. The use of the triazole antifungals in ABPA/ABPM in CF has not been evaluated; however, azole resistance in *A. fumigatus* has been found in approximately 4% of CF isolates in Europe in 2015.

One randomized controlled trial failed to show any benefit from the use of itraconazole for *Aspergillus* colonization, but only 43% of study participants achieved therapeutic itraconazole levels (Aaron et al. 2012). In contrast, a single-centre, open-label study has suggested a benefit with itraconazole (Coughlan et al. 2012). Alternative triazole antifungal drugs such as voriconazole and posaconazole may also have a role to play in the management of ABPA/ABPM in CF patients, but have not been prospectively evaluated.

It is interesting to note that intermittent antibacterial therapy has been associated with a decrease in *Aspergillus* signal, using both PCR and galactomannan antigen in respiratory secretions (Baxter et al. 2013).

Prevention

Prevention strategies in the CF population are not well defined. Precautions should be taken to protect from potential *Aspergillus* and other fungal exposures during inpatient stays (Schaffer 2015). To our knowledge, no studies to date have evaluated the use of masks to prevent fungal infection and/or colonization, although this approach has not been successful in preventing invasive aspergillosis in an oncology setting (Maschmeyer et al. 2009).

References

Aaron SD, Vandemheen KL, Freitag A, et al. (2012) Treatment of Aspergillus fumigatus in patients with cystic fibrosis: a randomized, placebo-controlled pilot study. *PLoS One* 7: e36077.

Agarwal R, Chakrabarti A, Shah A, et al. (2013) Allergic bronchopulmonary aspergillosis: review of literature and proposal of new diagnostic and classification criteria. *Clin Exp Allergy* 43: 850–73.

Agarwal R, Vishwanath G, Aggarwal AN, Garg M, Gupta D and Chakrabarti A (2013) Itraconazole in chronic cavitary pulmonary aspergillosis: a randomised controlled trial and systematic review of literature. *Mycoses* 56: 559–70.

Aimanianda V, Bayry J, Bozza S, et al. (2009) Surface hydrophobin prevents immune recognition of airborne fungal spores. *Nature* 460: 1117–21.

Al-Shair K, Atherton GT, Harris C, Ratcliffe L, Newton PJ and Denning DW (2013) Long-term antifungal treatment improves health status in patients with chronic pulmonary aspergillosis: a longitudinal analysis. *Clin Infect Dis* 57: 828–35.

Amin R, Dupuis A, Aaron SD and Ratjen F (2010) The effect of chronic infection with Aspergillus fumigatus on lung function and hospitalization in patients with cystic fibrosis. *Chest* 137: 171–6.

Aquino VR, Nagel F, Andreolla HF, et al. (2012) The performance of real-time PCR, galactomannan, and fungal culture in the diagnosis of invasive aspergillosis in ventilated patients with chronic obstructive pulmonary disease (COPD). *Mycopathologia* 174: 163–9.

Armstead J, Morris J and Denning DW (2014) Multi-country estimate of different manifestations of aspergillosis in cystic fibrosis. *PLoS One* 9: e98502.

Atkinson RW, Strachan DP, Anderson HR, Hajat S and Emberlin J (2006) Temporal associations between daily counts of fungal spores and asthma exacerbations. *Occup Environ Med* 63: 580–90.

Baxter CG, Dunn G, Jones AM, et al. (2013) Novel immunologic classification of aspergillosis in adult cystic fibrosis. *J Allergy Clin Immunol* 132: 560–6.e10.

Baxter CG, Rautemaa R, Jones AM, et al. (2013) Intravenous antibiotics reduce the presence of Aspergillus in adult cystic fibrosis sputum. *Thorax* 68: 652–7.

Belitsos NJ, Merz WG, Bowersox DW and Hutchins GM (1974) Allescheria boydii mycetoma complicating pulmonary sarcoid. *Johns Hopkins Med J* 135: 259–67.

Black PN, Udy AA and Brodie SM (2000) Sensitivity to fungal allergens is a risk factor for life-threatening asthma. *Allergy* 55: 501–4.

Blyth CC, Harun A, Middleton PG, et al. (2010) Detection of occult Scedosporium species in respiratory tract specimens from patients with cystic fibrosis by use of selective media. *J Clin Microbiol* 48: 314–16.

Blyth CC, Middleton PG, Harun A, Sorrell TC, Meyer W and Chen SC (2010) Clinical associations and prevalence of Scedosporium spp. in Australian cystic fibrosis patients: identification of novel risk factors? *Med Mycol* 48 (Suppl. 1): S37–44.

Bulpa P, Dive A and Sibille Y (2007) Invasive pulmonary aspergillosis in patients with chronic obstructive pulmonary disease. *Eur Respir J* 30: 782–800.

Bulpa PA, Dive AM, Garrino MG, et al. (2001) Chronic obstructive pulmonary disease patients with invasive pulmonary aspergillosis: benefits of intensive care? *Intensive Care Med* 27: 59–67.

Calderon E, de la Horra C, Medrano FJ, et al. (2004) Pneumocystis jirovecii isolates with dihydropteroate synthase mutations in patients with chronic bronchitis. *Eur J Clin Microbiol Infect Dis* 23: 545–9.

Chaudhary N, Datta K, Askin FB, Staab JF and Marr KA (2012) Cystic fibrosis transmembrane conductance regulator regulates epithelial cell response to Aspergillus and resultant pulmonary inflammation. *Am J Respir Crit Care Med* 185: 301–10.

Chen CH, Chao HJ, Chan CC, Chen BY and Guo YL (2014) Current asthma in schoolchildren is related to fungal spores in classrooms. *Chest* 146: 123–34.

Chotirmall SH, O'Donoghue E, Bennett K, Gunaratnam C, O'Neill SJ and McElvaney NG (2010) Sputum Candida albicans presages FEV(1) decline and hospital-treated exacerbations in cystic fibrosis. *Chest* 138: 1186–95.

Chrdle A, Mustakim S, Bright-Thomas RJ, Baxter CG, Felton T and Denning DW (2012) Aspergillus bronchitis without significant immunocompromise. *Ann N Y Acad Sci* 1272: 73–85.

Coughlan CA, Chotirmall SH, Renwick J, et al. (2012) The effect of Aspergillus fumigatus infection on vitamin D receptor expression in cystic fibrosis. *Am J Respir Crit Care Med* 186: 999–1007.

Crosdale DJ, Poulton KV, Ollier WE, Thomson W and Denning DW (2001) Mannose-binding lectin gene polymorphisms as a susceptibility factor for chronic necrotizing pulmonary aspergillosis. *J Infect Dis* 184: 653–6.

Delhaes L, Monchy S, Frealle E, et al. (2012) The airway microbiota in cystic fibrosis: a complex fungal and bacterial community—implications for therapeutic management. *PLoS One* 7: e36313.

Denning DW, Pashley C, Hartl D, et al. (2014) Fungal allergy in asthma-state of the art and research needs. *Clin Transl Allergy* 4: 14.

Denning DW, Pleuvry A and Cole DC (2011) Global burden of chronic pulmonary aspergillosis as a sequel to pulmonary tuberculosis. *Bull World Health Organ* 89: 864–72.

Denning DW, Pleuvry A and Cole DC (2013) Global burden of allergic bronchopulmonary aspergillosis with asthma and its complication chronic pulmonary aspergillosis in adults. *Med Mycol* 51: 361–70.

Denning DW, Riniotis K, Dobrashian R and Sambatakou H (2003) Chronic cavitary and fibrosing pulmonary and pleural aspergillosis: case series, proposed nomenclature change, and review. *Clin Infect Dis* 37 (Suppl. 3): S265–80.

de Vrankrijker AM, van der Ent CK, van Berkhout FT, et al. (2011) Aspergillus fumigatus colonization in cystic fibrosis: implications for lung function? *Clin Microbiol Infect* 17: 1381–6.

Diamond RD (1983) Inhibition of monocyte-mediated damage to fungal hyphae by steroid hormones. *J Infect Dis* 147: 160.

Eaton TE, Weiner Miller P, Garrett JE and Cutting GR (2002) Cystic fibrosis transmembrane conductance regulator gene mutations: do they play a role in the aetiology of allergic bronchopulmonary aspergillosis? *Clin Exp Allergy* 32: 756–61.

Farid S, Mohamed S, Devbhandari M, et al. (2013) Results of surgery for chronic pulmonary Aspergillosis, optimal antifungal therapy and proposed high risk factors for recurrence—a National Centre's experience. *J Cardiothorac Surg* 8: 180.

Felton IC and Simmonds NJ (2014) Aspergillus and cystic fibrosis: old disease—new classifications. *Curr Opin Pulm Med* 20: 632–8.

Fitzpatrick ME, Tedrow JR, Hillenbrand ME, et al. (2014) Pneumocystis jirovecii colonization is associated with enhanced Th1 inflammatory gene expression in lungs of humans with chronic obstructive pulmonary disease. *Microbiol Immunol* 58: 202–11.

Guinea J, Padilla C, Escribano P, et al. (2013) Evaluation of MycAssay Aspergillus for diagnosis of invasive pulmonary aspergillosis in patients without hematological cancer. *PLoS One* 8: e61545.

Guinea J, Torres-Narbona M, Gijon P, et al. (2010) Pulmonary aspergillosis in patients with chronic obstructive pulmonary disease: incidence, risk factors, and outcome. *Clin Microbiol Infect* 16: 870–7.

Harrison E, Singh A, Morris J, et al. (2012) Mannose-binding lectin genotype and serum levels in patients with chronic and allergic pulmonary aspergillosis. *Int J Immunogenet* 39: 224–32.

He H, Ding L, Li F and Zhan Q (2011) Clinical features of invasive bronchial-pulmonary aspergillosis in critically ill patients with chronic obstructive respiratory diseases: a prospective study. *Crit Care* 15: R5.

He H, Ding L, Sun B, Li F and Zhan Q (2012) Role of galactomannan determinations in bronchoalveolar lavage fluid samples from critically ill patients with chronic obstructive pulmonary disease for the diagnosis of invasive pulmonary aspergillosis: a prospective study. *Crit Care* 16: R138.

Johnson DC (2012) Chronic candidal bronchitis: a consecutive series. *Open Respir Med J* 6: 145–9.

Karnak D, Avery RK, Gildea TR, Sahoo D and Mehta AC (2007) Endobronchial fungal disease: an under-recognized entity. *Respiration* 74: 88–104.

Kaur S, Gupta VK, Shah A, Thiel S, Sarma PU and Madan T (2006) Elevated levels of mannan-binding lectin [corrected] (MBL) and eosinophilia in patients of bronchial asthma with allergic rhinitis and allergic bronchopulmonary aspergillosis associate with a novel intronic polymorphism in MBL. *Clin Exp Immunol* 143: 414–19.

Kondori N, Gilljam M, Lindblad A, Jonsson B, Moore ER and Wenneras C (2011) High rate of Exophiala dermatitidis recovery in the airways of patients with cystic fibrosis is associated with pancreatic insufficiency. *J Clin Microbiol* 49: 1004–9.

Kondori N, Lindblad A, Welinder-Olsson C, Wenneras C and Gilljam M (2014) Development of IgG antibodies to Exophiala dermatitidis is associated with inflammatory responses in patients with cystic fibrosis. *J Cyst Fibros* 13: 391–9.

Kraemer R, Delosea N, Ballinari P, Gallati S and Crameri R (2006) Effect of allergic bronchopulmonary aspergillosis on lung function in children with cystic fibrosis. *Am J Respir Crit Care Med* 174: 1211–20.

Liu JC, Modha DE and Gaillard EA (2013) What is the clinical significance of filamentous fungi positive sputum cultures in patients with cystic fibrosis? *J Cyst Fibros* 12: 187–93.

McMahon MA, Chotirmall SH, McCullagh B, Branagan P, McElvaney NG and Logan PM (2012) Radiological abnormalities associated with Aspergillus colonization in a cystic fibrosis population. *Eur J Radiol* 81: e197–202.

Maschmeyer G, Neuburger S, Fritz L, et al. (2009) A prospective, randomised study on the use of well-fitting masks for prevention of invasive aspergillosis in high-risk patients. *Ann Oncol* 20: 1560–4.

Matsuoka H, Niimi A, Matsumoto H, et al. (2009) Specific IgE response to trichophyton and asthma severity. *Chest* 135: 898–903.

Meersseman W, Vandecasteele SJ, Wilmer A, Verbeken E, Peetermans WE and Van Wijngaerden E (2004) Invasive aspergillosis in critically ill patients without malignancy. *Am J Respir Crit Care Med* 170: 621–5.

Moss RB (2014) Treatment options in severe fungal asthma and allergic bronchopulmonary aspergillosis. *Eur Respir J* 43: 1487–500.

Nagano Y, Elborn JS, Millar BC, et al. (2010) Comparison of techniques to examine the diversity of fungi in adult patients with cystic fibrosis. *Med Mycol* 48: 166–76.e1.

Ng TT, Robson GD and Denning DW (1994) Hydrocortisone-enhanced growth of Aspergillus spp.: implications for pathogenesis. *Microbiology* 140 (Pt 9): 2475–9.

Nielsen SM, Kristensen L, Sondergaard A, Handberg KJ, Stenderup J and Norskov-Lauritsen N (2014) Increased prevalence and altered species composition of filamentous fungi in respiratory specimens from cystic fibrosis patients. *APMIS* 122: 1007–12.

Paganin P, Fiscarelli EV, Tuccio V, et al. (2015) Changes in cystic fibrosis airway microbial community associated with a severe decline in lung function. *PLoS One* 10: e0124348.

Pihet M, Carrere J, Cimon B, et al. (2009) Occurrence and relevance of filamentous fungi in respiratory secretions of patients with cystic fibrosis—a review. *Med Mycol* 47: 387–97.

Piipari R and Keskinen H (2005) Agents causing occupational asthma in Finland in 1986-2002: cow epithelium bypassed by moulds from moisture-damaged buildings. *Clin Exp Allergy* 35: 1632–7.

Rello J, Esandi ME, Mariscal D, Gallego M, Domingo C and Valles J (1998) Invasive pulmonary aspergillosis in patients with chronic obstructive pulmonary disease: report of eight cases and review. *Clin Infect Dis* 26: 1473–5.

Romani L (1997) The T cell response against fungal infections. *Curr Opin Immunol* 9: 484–90.

Schaffer K (2015) Epidemiology of infection and current guidelines for infection prevention in cystic fibrosis patients. *J Hosp Infect* 89: 309–13.

Smith NL and Denning DW (2011) Underlying conditions in chronic pulmonary aspergillosis including simple aspergilloma. *Eur Respir J* 37: 865–72.

Smith NL and Denning DW (2014) Clinical implications of interferon-gamma genetic and epigenetic variants. *Immunology* 143: 499–511.

Speirs JJ, van der Ent CK and Beekman JM (2012) Effects of Aspergillus fumigatus colonization on lung function in cystic fibrosis. *Curr Opin Pulm Med* 18: 632–8.

Stevens DA, Moss RB, Kurup VP, et al. (2003) Allergic bronchopulmonary aspergillosis in cystic fibrosis—state of the art: Cystic Fibrosis Foundation Consensus Conference. *Clin Infect Dis* 37 (Suppl. 3): S225–64.

Vaid M, Kaur S, Sambatakou H, Madan T, Denning DW and Sarma PU (2007) Distinct alleles of mannose-binding lectin (MBL) and surfactant proteins A (SP-A) in patients with chronic cavitary pulmonary aspergillosis and allergic bronchopulmonary aspergillosis. *Clin Chem Lab Med* 45: 183–6.

Zalar P, Novak M, de Hoog GS and Gunde-Cimerman N (2011) Dishwashers—a man-made ecological niche accommodating human opportunistic fungal pathogens. *Fungal Biol* 115: 997–1007.

Zubairi AB, Azam I, Awan S, Zafar A, Imam AA (2014): Association of airborne Aspergillus with asthma exacerbation in Southern Pakistan. *Asia Pac Allergy*, 4(2):91–8.

SECTION 5

Diagnosis

CHAPTER 38

Biosafety and quality assurance in the mycology laboratory

Michael D. Palmer and Shila Seaton

Biosafety aspects of medical mycology

Laboratory-acquired infections

When considering the biosafety aspects of a medical mycology laboratory, it is important to avoid focusing on fungi and the potential infections that they can cause alone, but to take a wider look at biosafety with respect to other microorganisms which may be present in samples sent for mycological investigation.

Evidence in the literature has shown that laboratory-acquired infections (LAIs) with viral or bacterial agents far outweigh the reported cases of LAI with fungi (Table 38.1).

LAI has been recognized since before the 1940s. However, there is no real formal mechanism available to collect data pertaining to LAIs. Instead, researchers have had to rely on information obtained from voluntary questionnaires and personal communications. It is therefore likely that the number of LAIs has been under-reported in these and similar surveys, not only due to laboratories not wishing to admit to particular incidents, but also to the fact that some LAIs may be subclinical or have an uncharacteristic presentation due to atypical infection routes (Pike 1979). Furthermore, some LAIs may be missed if they cannot be related to defined laboratory incidents. However, these data highlight documented infections, and therefore, the importance of biosafety as a prime consideration for the clinical laboratory.

Biosafety regulation

Although it is difficult to ascertain the actual rate of LAIs, by comparing the available data it has been suggested that the incidences are decreasing (Biosafety in Microbiological and Biomedical Laboratories 2007/2009, Singh 2009). This is thought to be due in part to improvements in laboratory design, protective equipment, and training, but the introduction of formal guidelines and legislation has also been of importance.

The primary legislation pertaining to occupational health and safety in the UK is the Health and Safety at Work Act 1974, among others. Other UK legislation of major importance to clinical laboratories in terms of biological agents are: Management of Health and Safety at Work Regulations 1999, Control of Substances Hazardous to Health (COSHH) regulations 2002, and Genetically Modified Organisms (Contained Use) Regulations 2000. In Europe, the key legislation is the directive on the protection of workers exposed to biological agents at work (last revised February 28, 2006) (European Economic Community [2000] Directive 2000/54/EC and Directive 90/679/EEC).

In the USA, advisory documents include *Biosafety in Microbiological and Biomedical Laboratories (BMBL)* (5th edn, 2007; revised 2009) and the *National Institutes of Health* (US) *Guidelines for Research Involving Recombinant DNA Molecules* (2002).

Globally, the World Health Organization's *Laboratory Biosafety Manual* (3rd edn, 2004) is an important source of safety information. It is important that individuals are familiar with the regulations in force in their particular country before commencing work with a biological agent.

Risk assessment for biological agents

A risk assessment is a process to identify risks in the workplace so that suitable control measures may be put in place to mitigate harmful occurrences. The process of a biological agent risk assessment can be applied to various areas—for instance, general risk assessments, manual handling, and equipment—and should be an integral part of all health & safety legislation and approved codes of practice or guidance. In the UK, biological risk assessment is required under the Control of Substances Hazardous to Health Regulations 2002 (COSHH). In general, the risk assessment process must consider the following (Health and Safety Executive 2014):

- What hazards are present?
- Who is at risk and how harm can arise?
- What is the likelihood that harm will arise?
- What control measures can be put in place and how can findings be recorded?
- How can the assessment be reviewed and revised?

Information, instruction, and training must be provided for all aspects of the processes, reagents, and biological agents involved.

Classification of biological agents into hazard/risk groups

Microorganisms can be grouped into four hazard or risk groups as determined by US, European, and World Health Organization (WHO) policies (Table 38.2). The containment level that a particular biological agent must be handled at is generally associated with

Table 38.1 Summary of eight surveys undertaken to assess the incidence of laboratory-acquired infections

	Sulkin & Pike 1951 (USA 1930–1950)	Sulkin et al. 1965 (worldwide 1950–1963)	*Wedum & Kruse 1969	*Pike 1976 (USA & rest of world top ten organisms)	Sewell 1995 (UK 1980–1989)	Walker & Campbell 1999 (UK 1994–1995)	Harding & Byers 2006 (USA 1979–2004)	Baron and Miller 2008 (2002–2004)
Total no. reported cases/labs surveyed	1,342	641	2,912	3,921	95	9/397	2,156	41/88
Bacterial	775	191	1,087	1,351	69	7	658	39
Viral	265	250	244	375	19	2	1,038	
Fungal	63	58	273	325	0	0	6	2
Parasites	39	35		116	0		53	
Rickettsia	200	107	82	124	0		401	
Coxiella			184	278	0			
Chlamydia psittaci			70	116	0			

* Cumulative survey

its hazard/risk group; the containment level generally increases in terms of safety requirements and controls as the hazard/risk group of the biological agent increases (Health and Safety Executive 2001), though this is not the case with all agents. Biological agents might be handled at different containment levels in different parts of the world and it is also possible that, after a thorough risk assessment, some biological agents can be assigned to either a higher or lower containment level than their hazard group suggests. This is because the risk assessment looks at other factors than the hazard or risk group alone. A few examples are: mode of transmission, procedural protocols, exposure

Table 38.2 Classification of biological agents into hazard/risk groups

Risk/Hazard Group	National Institutes of Health (US) Guidelines for Research Involving Recombinant DNA Molecules 2002	European Economic Community (2000) Directive 2000/54/EC and Directive 90/679/EEC. Advisory Committee on Dangerous Pathogens	World Health Organization Laboratory Biosafety Manual 3rd edn, 2004
1	Agents not associated with disease in healthy adult humans	A biological agent that is unlikely to cause human disease	(No or low individual and community risk) A microorganism unlikely to cause human or animal disease
2	Agents associated with human disease that is rarely serious and for which preventive or therapeutic interventions are often available	A biological agent that can cause human disease and might be a hazard to workers; it is unlikely to spread to the community; there is usually effective prophylaxis or treatment available.	(Moderate individual risk; low community risk) A pathogen that can cause human or animal disease but is unlikely to be a serious hazard to laboratory workers, the community, livestock, or the environment. Laboratory exposures may cause serious infection, but effective treatment and preventive measures are available and the risk of spread of infection is limited.
3	Agents associated with serious or lethal human disease for which preventive or therapeutic interventions may be available (high individual risk but low community risk)	A biological agent that can cause severe human disease and present a serious hazard to workers; it may present a risk of spreading to the community, but there is usually effective prophylaxis or treatment available.	(High individual risk; low community risk) A pathogen that usually causes serious human or animal disease but does not ordinarily spread from one infected individual to another. Effective treatment and preventive measures are available.
4	Agents likely to cause serious or lethal human disease for which preventive or therapeutic interventions are not usually available (high individual risk and high community risk)	A biological agent that causes severe human disease and is a serious hazard to workers; it may present a high risk of spreading to the community; there is usually no effective prophylaxis or treatment available	(High individual and community risk) A pathogen that usually causes serious human or animal disease and can be readily transmitted from one individual to another, directly or indirectly. Effective treatment and preventive measures are not usually available.

Source: data from National Institutes of Health 2002; European Economic Community 2000; Advisory Committee on Dangerous Pathogens 2004.

control measures, and the experience of staff and their immune status. These latter issues are of great importance for laboratory staff handling fungi.

The containment levels of most interest that are related directly to the isolation and culturing of fungi are containment/biosafety level 2 (CL2) and containment/biosafety level 3 (CL3).

Hazard/Risk Group 3 fungi

Whilst most clinically important fungi are in Hazard/Risk Group 2 (HG2), there are a number of fungi classified within Hazard Risk Group 3 (HG3). These can be divided into the thermally dimorphic HG3 fungi, namely: *Blastomyces dermatitidis and B. gilchristii, Coccidioides immitis and C. posadasii, Histoplasma capsulatum* and *H. duboisii, Paracoccidioides brasiliensis* and *P. lutzii*, and *Talaromyces marneffei* (formerly *Penicillium marneffei*). It has recently been suggested that *Emmonsia* species should also be considered within HG3 (Kenyon et al. 2013). A smaller group of HG3 fungi are dematiaceous, namely: *Cladophialophora bantiana* and *Rhinocladiella mackenziei* (formerly *Ramichloridium mackenziei*). It has been proposed that *Cladophialophora devriesii* and *C. arxii* should also be considered within HG3 (Howard et al. 2006).

Fungi and laboratory safety

Hanel and Kruse (1967) produced the first detailed review on laboratory-acquired mycoses, describing more than 288 cases, including 108 cases of coccidioidomycosis, 81of histoplasmosis, 7 of sporotrichosis, and 84 cases of dermatophytosis. Apart from the dermatophyte LAIs, the majority (87%) were a result of aerosol inhalation. The reported incidences of laboratory-acquired mycoses, in particular coccidioidomycosis, have reduced considerably since the Hanel and Kruse review and have dropped from the top ten common organisms causing LAIs (Table 38.3).

Despite this, the infection risk to laboratory workers remains. The dermatophytes are HG2 fungi, which pose little risk to the laboratory worker even though they are highly adapted to invading the tissue of humans with normal immunity and are contagious. However, they are restricted to keratin-containing tissues and rarely invade deep tissue. The majority of LAIs with dermatophytes are a result of inoculation injuries during work with animals. The other HG2 fungi, although capable of causing serious infections and fatalities, are generally opportunistic, relying on the impaired immunity of the host. Reports of LAIs with these saprophytic fungi are rare and usually a result of inoculation incidents.

The HG3 fungi are endemic species, being prevalent in various locations in the world, highlighting the importance of travel history to the triage of samples to determine processing at CL3. Most HG3 fungi are soil and vegetation saprophytes that have adapted to infect mammalian tissue with the capacity to cause non-contagious, life-threatening, and fatal disease in people with apparently normal immune function. The route of infection with the neurotropic dematiaceous HG3 fungi is poorly understood, whereas the major risk of LAI with the dimorphic species is by inhalation of their conidia from cultures grown at <30°C. The infectious dose has been estimated to be only ten conidia for *Coccidioides* species (Converse et al. 1962). For this reason the use of a microbiological safety cabinet at CL3 is mandatory when handling cultures or samples suspected of containing these fungi.

In a busy clinical laboratory it is not usually practical to culture all deep-site samples at CL3, so a triage system should be implemented to separate samples that are likely to contain HG3 fungi as well as other HG3 biological agents.

The following mycology samples should be handled at CL3:

- All specimens from deep sites (e.g. biopsies, fluids)—besides fungi, these may contain other HG3 biological agents
- Moulds isolated from samples taken from a deep site (including BAL & sputum), until they are shown not to be a HG3 fungus
- Yeasts isolated from blood cultures or deep sites if a dimorphic pathogen is suspected, or there is relevant travel history

HG3 moulds should only be sub-cultured onto slopes or flasks, not plates, to reduce the risk of LAI due to inhalation.

The role of external quality assessment (EQA) in mycology laboratory quality assurance

For the provision of precise and accurate analyses in cases of known or suspected fungal infection and in order to support optimal patient care, full commitment to quality assurance (QA) is essential in clinical diagnostic laboratories (Snell et al. 1999). QA is the total process whereby the quality of laboratory results, from specimen collection, to analysis of tests and reporting of results, can be guaranteed and enable mycological diagnosis and effective treatment. Components of QA include: good laboratory practice, internal quality control, audit, validation, internal quality assessment, accreditation, evaluation, education, and external quality assessment. In the mycology laboratory the need for comparability of results requires good QA practices, and the complementary discipline of EQA is thus very important. The majority of clinical laboratories employ three complementary quality control or assurance activities:

1 Internal quality control (IQC)

IQC is carried out continually within the laboratory to ensure that the systems are performing to pre-defined specifications. IQC

Table 38.3 The ten most common reported organisms causing laboratory-acquired infections

1930–1978	*Brucella* spp., *Coxiella burnetii*, hepatitis B virus (HBV), *Salmonella typhi*, *Francisella tularensis*, *Mycobacterium tuberculosis*, *Blastomyces dermatitidis*, Venezuelan equine encephalitis virus, *Chlamydia psittaci*, and *Coccidioides immitis*
1979–1998	*Mycobacterium tuberculosis*, *Coxiella burnetii*, hantavirus, arboviruses, HBV, *Brucella* spp., *Salmonella* spp., *Shigella* spp., hepatitis C virus, and *Cryptosporidium* spp.

Source: data from U.S. Department of Health and Human Services (2007), *Biosafety in Microbiological and Biomedical Laboratories*, Fifth Edition, Revised December 2009, Copyright © 2007 Centers for Disease Control and Prevention, National Institute of Health.

assesses and monitors test performance in real time to ensure consistent performance and reproducible results. This process monitors or measures reproducibility, but not necessarily the accuracy. The majority of IQC procedures involve the analysis of the control material or international standards where available, and compares this to the accepted levels predetermined at the validation stage of the test procedure. For example, fungal antigen tests such as the galactomannan test include several control samples that must yield results within a certain range to validate the assay.

2 Internal quality assessment (IQA)

IQA is a system in which clinical specimens are anonymously re-introduced back through the diagnostic laboratory process. This ensures that the processes are operating at an acceptable level and monitors performance of staff and test procedures, ensuring they are consistent. Within the mycology laboratory this is usually straight forward, although there may be occasional problems. For example, some sample types, such as nails where the presence of the fungus is often heterogeneous, may result in different microscopy and culture results between original testing and IQA repeats which are difficult to interpret.

3 External quality assessment (EQA)

The terms EQA or proficiency testing are used to describe a method that allows comparison of a laboratory's competence in testing, to an external source. This process can be defined as a system for objectively checking the laboratory's performance using an external provider. The main objectives of an EQA are to provide inter-laboratory comparability and standardization of diagnostic testing, and to act fundamentally as an educational tool. In a specialist field such as mycology, the educational aspect of EQA can be very important for non-specialist personnel.

Types of EQA

Two EQA methods or processes are commonly used:

1 An EQA provider distributes undisclosed samples for testing to registered participating laboratories (UK NEQAS Microbiology, 2016). The results from all the laboratories are collated, analyzed, and compared. These results are reported back to each individual laboratory (Figure 38.1). The samples can include isolates of fungi for identification and antifungal susceptibility testing, patient samples of serum for fungal antibody studies, and serum samples spiked with antifungals to assess quality in antifungal drug level testing.

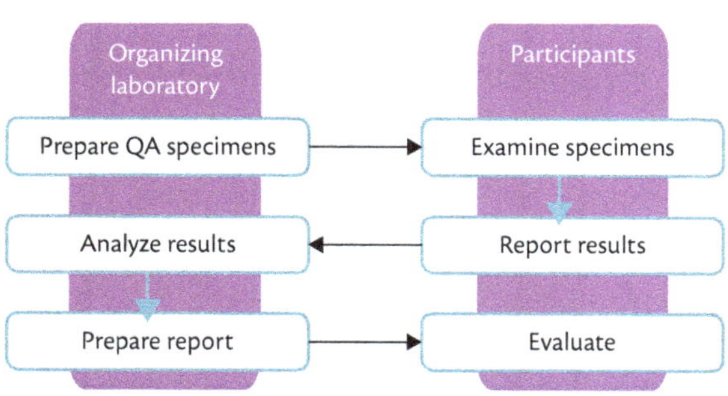

Figure 38.1 Basic external assessment.
Reproduced courtesy of Shila Seaton.

2 Inter-laboratory comparison is the exchange of samples among two or more laboratories (often referred to as 'round-robin testing') for when no proficiency testing is available. At present there is no EQA for the detection of galactomannan in serum samples and a laboratory may analyze a clinical specimen and circulate the remaining specimen to other interested laboratories. Results are collated and analyzed by consensus. This approach is often the only one available for some of the rarer tests in mycology, but discrepancies between laboratories may be difficult to resolve.

Benefits of EQA

Participation in an external quality assessment programme provides valuable data and information. A laboratory participating in EQA for identification allows it to assess its own performance with the specimens distributed for examination in comparison with the intended results, and with the performance of the other test sites. It can highlight issues, at an early stage, involving systematic problems or inadequacies associated with kits or operations. An example is the now widespread use of MALDI-TOF MS (matrix-assisted laser desorption/ionization–time-of-flight mass spectrometry), for the identification of yeasts, superseding conventional testing. *Candida haemulonii* is not identifiable to species level with conventional testing alone (Cendejas-Bueno et al. 2012) but can only be identified by MALDI-TOF MS or molecular methods; distribution of species in this way for identification in an EQA sample may trigger re-evaluation of a laboratory's methodology.

EQA can provide objective evidence and efficacy of testing pathways, help monitor the efficacy of IQC procedures, provide an educational stimulus for improvement, and help identify as well as support staff training needs. Using collections of EQA fungal isolates will enable laboratory staff to improve identification skills on species they might rarely see in practice and for example, train new employees.

The role of ISO standards in quality management

ISO 17025 is the internationally recognized standard that specifies the competence and quality management system requirements for laboratories that provide testing and/or calibration services. ISO 15189:2012 can be used by medical mycology laboratories in developing their quality management systems and assessing their own competence. It can also be used to confirm or recognize the competence of medical laboratories by laboratory customers, regulating authorities, and accreditation bodies.

Factors affecting EQA performance assessment

The EQA performance of a mycology laboratory can provide management with an insight into the quality of the routine work of their laboratories. The qualifying factor required is that EQA results will only provide an effective insight into routine results if the samples are treated in the same way as routine samples. If EQA samples are treated differently from routine samples, then the results may be excellent but nothing will be learnt about the quality of the routine service. For example, if a sample for the identification of a fungal isolate is processed by more experienced staff than those who examine similar routine patient samples, then the quality of identification for that fungus may be high but the quality of the routine service may still be suspect. Similarly, if a serum sample for fungal antibody or antigen testing is subjected to more thorough checking procedures, such as repeat testing, than is routinely performed, the quality management system will not be properly assessed.

Mycology EQA schemes

Types of programmes available for mycological investigations provided by EQA providers are:

- Isolation and identification of pathogenic/non-pathogenic fungal isolates
- Antifungal susceptibility testing of clinically significant fungal isolates
- Therapeutic drug monitoring assays to determine the concentration of an antifungal agent in patient serum
- The detection of fungal antigens or antibodies in sterile bodily fluids

Many mycology EQA schemes distribute fungal spore suspensions for isolation and identification, and include the most commonly encountered filamentous fungi from superficial and deep-seated infections (Campbell et al. 2013). Correct identification of *Aspergillus terreus* species complex has important clinical implications, as unlike most other *Aspergillus* species, it is often resistant to amphotericin B. More than 86% of participants correctly identified this isolate and 97.5% correctly reported its resistance to amphotericin when recently distributed in a UK EQA scheme. From an educational perspective, rare isolates causing fungal disease may also be distributed. One example of an educational EQA was the distribution in the UK scheme of *Exserohilum rostratum*, a rare fungus causing a human infection. This fungus caused a major outbreak of meningitis in the USA in September 2012 following the use of contaminated methylprednisolone acetate injections to treat back and joint pain in immunocompetent individuals (Casadevall and Pirofski 2013; see Chapters 14 and 22).

This fungal isolate was challenging as it phenotypically and microscopically resembles *Bipolaris* species. Participants had the opportunity to culture and examine microscopically and phenotypically a fungus not usually encountered in their own clinical settings. Encouraging results were obtained from the 384 participating laboratories, with 91.4% attaining the correct genus and 88% the correct species.

Antifungal susceptibility schemes distribute yeast species and common filamentous fungi for identification and antifungal susceptibility testing. Yeasts are a common cause of invasive fungal infections in certain patient populations, for example severely immunocompromised patients. Such schemes provide participating laboratories with the opportunity to assess their performance in identification and antifungal susceptibility testing for a variety of clinically significant yeasts and filamentous fungi. Laboratories also have the opportunity to assess whether the appropriate interpretation of results have been correctly followed. Reports published on the data collated detail the most common methods used by laboratories and the percentage concordance of antifungal susceptibilities of the fungal isolate tested with the intended results. In some cases immunologists provide EQA schemes relevant to mycology—for example, the detection of *Aspergillus* and *Candida* antibodies (precipitins).

EQA providers should be continually developing schemes to meet current or new mycology protocols or assays that have been implemented in laboratories. Following successful results from recent pilot studies, the detection of serum antigen galactomannan, (a diagnostic test in widespread use for the diagnosis of invasive aspergillosis for more than a decade), is now available as an established EQA scheme.

Conclusions

Optimal patient care and the safety of healthcare scientists depend upon the provision of precise and consistent laboratory procedures and assays, which should be performed in a safety-focused environment.

All diagnostic mycology laboratories need to integrate QA procedures as part of maintaining professional standards of service, although requirements may differ according to circumstances and clinical application.

Full and regular participation in appropriate EQA schemes is a necessary and integral part of the rational provision of a reliable mycology laboratory service. EQA should be viewed as educational and utilized as a tool to help drive improvement efforts in the laboratory, and is one of the critical elements of a laboratory quality management system.

Ultimately, EQA specimens must be treated as patient samples, following routine testing methods, and the procedure must involve personnel who routinely perform the testing.

References

Baron JO and Miller JM (2008) Bacterial and fungal infections among diagnostic laboratory workers: evaluating the risks. *Diagn Microbiol Infect Dis* 60: 241–6.

Biological agents: Managing the risks in laboratories and healthcare premises. Published by the Health and Safety Executive 05/05

Biosafety in Microbiological and Biomedical Laboratories. (2007/09) US Department of Health and Human Services, Public Health Service, Centres for Disease Control and Prevention, National Institutes of Health, HHS Publication No. (CDC) 21-1112 Revised December 2009 (BMBL 2009)

Campbell CK, Johnson EM and Warnock DW (2013) *Identification of Pathogenic Fungi* (2nd edn, Oxford: Wiley-Blackwell).

Casadevall A and Pirofski LA (2013) *Exserohilum rostratum* fungal meningitis associated with methylprednisolone injections. *Future Microbiol* 8:135–7.

Cendejas-Bueno E, Kolecka A, Alastruey-Izquierdo A, et al. (2012) Reclassification of the *Candida haemulonii* complex as *Candida haemulonii* (*C. haemulonii* Group I), *C. duobushaemulonii* sp. nov. (*C. haemulonii* Group II), and *C. haemulonii* var. *vulnera* var. nov.: three multiresistant human pathogenic yeasts. *J Clin Microbiol* 50: 3641–51.

Converse JL, Castleberry MW, Besemer AR and Snyder EM (1962) Immunization of mice against coccidioidomycosis Journal of bacteriology. *J Bacteriol* 84: 46–52.

Hanel, E. Jr., Kruse, R. H. (1967). Laboratory- Acquired Mycoses, Misc. Pub!. 28. Industrial Health and Safety Office.Ft. Detrick, Md: Dept. Army. 55 pp.

Harding AL and Byers KB (2006) Epidemiology of laboratory-associated infections, *in* DO Flemming and DL Hunt (eds), *Biological Safety: Principles and Practices* (4th edn, Washington, DC: ASM Press), 53–77.

Health and Safety Executive (2001). The management, design and operation of microbiological containment laboratories. Advisory Committee on Dangerous Pathogens

Health and Safety Executive. (2014) Risk assessment: A brief guide to controlling risks in the workplace. Leaflet INDG163(rev4)

Howard SJ, Walker SM, Borman AM, Johnson EM and Denning DW (2006) Sub-cutaneous phaeohyphomycosis caused by Cladophialophora devriesii in a United Kingdom resident. *Med Mycol* 44: 553–6.

Kenyon C, Bonorchis K, Corcoran C, et al. (2013) A dimorphic fungus causing disseminated infection in South Africa. *N Engl J Med* 369: 1416–24.

Pike RM (1976) Laboratory-associated infections. Summary and analysis of 3921 cases. *Health Lab Sci* 13: 105–14.

Pike RM (1979) Laboratory associated infections: incidence, fatalities, causes, and prevention. *Annu Rev Microbiol* 33: 41–66.

Sewell DL (1995) Laboratory-associated infections and biosafety. *Clin Microbiol Rev* 8: 389–405.

Singh K (2009) Laboratory-acquired Infections. *Clin Infect Dis* 49: 142–7.

Snell JJS, Brown DFJ and Roberts C (eds) (1999) *Quality Assurance: Principles and practice in the microbiology laboratory* (London: Public Health Laboratory Service).

Sulkin SE and Pike RM (1951) Survey of laboratory-acquired infections. *Am J Public Health Nations Health* 41: 769–81.

Sulkin SE, Pike RM and Schulze ML (1965) Continuing importance of laboratory acquired infections. *Am J Public Health Nations Health* 55: 190–9.

UK NEQAS Microbiology 2016 http://www.ukneqasmicro.org.uk/

Walker D and Campbell D (1999) A survey of infections in United Kingdom laboratories, 1994–1995. *J Clin Pathol* 52: 415–18.

Wedum AG and Kruse RH (1969) Assessment of risk of human infection in the microbiological laboratory, *in*: Publication No. 30 (2nd edn, Department of the Army, Fort Detrick MD, USA).

CHAPTER 39

Microscopy and culture of fungal disease

Gillian S. Shankland

Microscopy

Introduction

Often, seeing fungal elements in a sample is the first encounter with the fungus and may be the first indication that a fungal infection is involved in the pathology of the disease. Therefore, microscopy is an important part of the repertoire of diagnostic tests and often one that can be performed rapidly so a presumptive diagnosis can sometimes be made. This may be on a wet direct mount from keratinous material, tissue, or body fluid, or a histological slide.

Although fungi are significantly larger than bacteria, they may be present in a specimen in smaller numbers or be more localized; therefore several parts of the preparation need to be examined. It should be borne in mind that microscopy is not as sensitive a technique as culture, as by the nature of the method the quantity of sample examined is less and there is no amplification of the original numbers of organisms. The exceptions to this are nails, where seeing a fungus may be more likely than growing a dermatophyte, as viability is lost in older, slow-growing nails or material from samples from individuals on antifungal therapy when the fungus may no longer be viable (Bonifaz et al. 2013). Microscopy may also help with determining the significance of an isolate cultured from bronchoalveolar lavage or sputum samples as a positive microscopic examination excludes the cultured organism as being merely a contaminant.

The success of visualization of fungi relies on the expertise and diligence of the observer, in addition to careful preparation of the sample. In some instances, it is important to concentrate the sample by centrifugation or filtration. Urgent samples such as cerebrospinal fluid (CSF) should be reported by telephone or electronically, ensuring a very rapid turnaround for results (Schelenz et al. 2015).

Superficial samples

These samples should be collected in folded coloured paper. The use of paper facilitates the capture of the skin, nail, and hair fragments, as they can be scraped directly onto the surface and therefore reduces specimen loss. There are several customized packaging systems commercially available. They have many advantages as they allow safe transport of the samples through the postal system, are compact for storage within the laboratory, are convenient platforms on which to prepare the sample for microscopy and culture, and help reduce bacterial contamination while allowing for the survival of fungi. The use of plastic containers should be avoided (see Chapter 23).

The visibility of fungal elements in skin, nail, and hair is enhanced with the use of potassium hydroxide (KOH) or a potassium hydroxide/dimethyl sulphoxide (KOH/DMSO) mixture. A range of concentrations is employed by mycologists for preparation of wet mounts, from 10–30% KOH, to digest keratin and clear the specimen. This author's preference is for 20% KOH. However, KOH is corrosive and requires careful handling to prevent damage to the microscope or digestion of the handler's own skin. KOH clears the keratin, and although heating can speed up the process, it may cause crystallization of the KOH and obscure the sample. It is sometimes useful, especially with thick dystrophic nails, for preparations to be incubated in a humidity chamber—either at 37°C for a couple of hours, or overnight at room temperature. The lighting used on the microscope is critical and may require stopping-down of the iris diaphragm in the condenser to obtain maximum refractive variation between the fungus and the sample. If a fluorescent microscope is available, these KOH preparations can include fluorescent brighteners to enhance the natural fluorescence of the fungi (Bonifaz et al. 2013). The fluorophore Calcofluor White (CFW), which binds to cell wall chitin, is the most commonly used, with the fungi fluorescing blue/white or green (Figure 39.1a). The inclusion of a fluorescent brightener may help to differentiate fungi. However, the user must be aware of the optimal conditions for the product they are using and the most efficient wavelength for the excitation and emission filters. Other mycologists prefer phase contrast (Milne 1989). Parker, Quink, or some such premier quality ink may be added to help with the visualization of fungi in wet KOH preparations, particularly with *Malassezia* species (Clayton and Midgley 1985).

The keratinous material to be examined is chopped using a scalpel while being held by forceps or a mounted needle, and selected small fragments from all areas of the specimen are lifted onto a droplet of KOH on a microscope slide, usually with a mounted needle. A coverslip is placed gently on top and the preparation kept until ready to be examined. This may be within an hour or longer depending on the thickness of the specimen. Before examination the mount should be gently squashed—a monolayer of cells is the ideal.

On brightfield microscopy, dermatophyte hyphae appear as slightly greenish and refractive. They are sinuous and sparingly branched and can be seen to grow through the skin and nail cells.

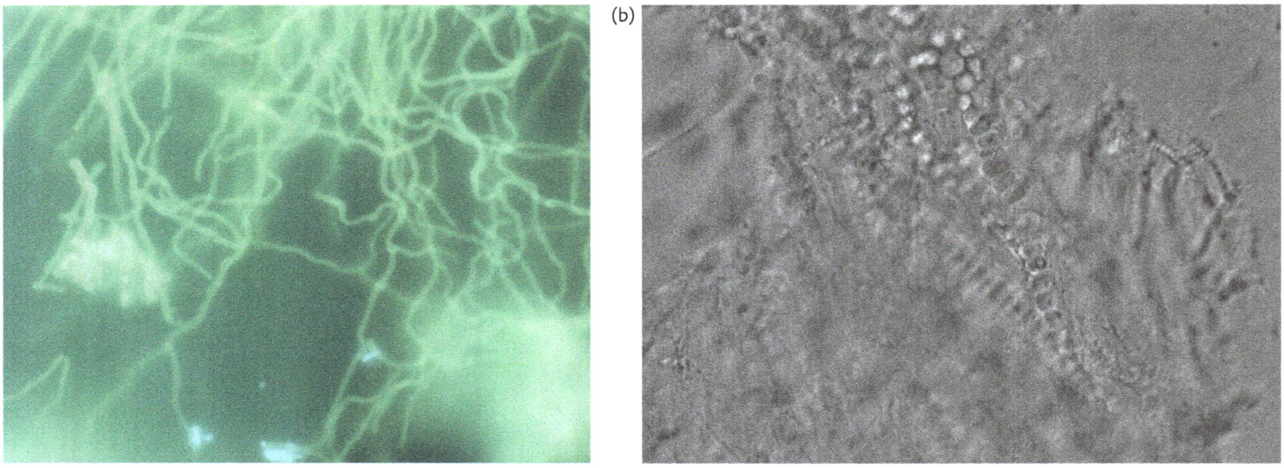

Figure 39.1 **a** Potassium hydroxide—Calcoflour mount of skin showing classic hyphae of a dermatophyte infection.
b Potassium hydroxide mount of skin showing arthroconidia—light microscopy.

Dermatophytes often lay down crosswalls to produce simple brick-like spores termed arthroconidia (Figure 39.1b). There is a great variation in the appearance of fungi on KOH preparations; the fungi are not evenly distributed in the material and may be sparse in one area and dense in another. It is not possible to identify which genus or species of dermatophyte is causing an infection based on the appearance on direct examination.

The presence of artefacts is common, and filaments from socks or other items of clothing may be misidentified as fungus as cotton and linen fibres will also fluoresce with brighteners. Another common artefact is the presence of irregular, discrete branching threads which follow the contours of the epithelial cells; this was named 'mosaic fungus' by Weidman in 1927. Unlike true fungal hyphae this can be seen to trace the outline of the host's cells and has variable diameter; it is likely caused by the presence of a high level of cholesterol. Davidson and Gregory (1935) reported it to consist of piled masses of the flat rhombic crystals of cholesterol. Getz et al. (1955) confirmed it to be an artefact as it did not stain as true fungi. They reported that cultures were not positive in any of the cases where 'mosaic fungus' alone was found in skin scrapings, and 'mosaic fungi' were found in 90% of 'normal' persons in specimens taken from the thick skin on the sole of the foot. They hypothesized that it was a product of oxidation of fats in the epidermis and appeared on the feet because of the well-developed horny layer, creating the time and necessary conditions for the oxidation to take place.

The optimal hair sample includes the hair root and the first half-centimetre. Twenty minutes at room temperature is sufficient time in KOH prior to examination (Public Health England 2015a). In hair samples there are three modalities of hair invasion that can be determined by microscopy: endothrix, ectothrix, and favus. Hyphae may be sparse, but if arthroconidia are present, they are often in abundance and round off, from the brick-like structures formed from partitioning of hyphae, to become spherical. Different specialized dermatophyte species invade hair differently, and the putative causal agent may be identified by observation of the type of hair invasion and epidemiological details from the patient (Table 39.1).

Moulds such as *Aspergillus, Fusarium, Scopulariopsis*, and *Neoscytalidium* can cause nail diseases that may be identified as non-dermatophyte infections on microscopic examination. Their appearance may be that of hyphae that are indistinguishable from dermatophytes or they may demonstrate thickening and fronding, allowing a diagnosis of non-dermatophyte fungus to be made and the relevance of the presence of a saprophyte on culture to be realized. *Scopulariopsis brevicaulis* may produce spores in nail samples that are similar to those produced in culture, with the presence of a characteristic truncate base; this is an infection that can be diagnosed by microscopy, but in practice culture is also undertaken in case there is a concomitant dermatophyte infection.

Examination of superficial samples may indicate the presence of yeast cells. *Candida* species may be demonstrated by the presence of blastoconidia in addition to true hyphae and pseudohyphae. *Malassezia* infections can often be diagnosed solely on microscopic evidence. The characteristic appearance of this lipophylic yeast with

Table 39.1 Hair invasion—presentation

Small-spored ectothrix	Large-spored ectothrix	Endothrix	Favus
Microsporum audouinii	*T. verrucosum*	*T. tonsurans*	*T. schoenleinii*
Microsporum canis		*T. violaceum*	
Trichophyton mentagrophytes		*T. soudanense*	
Trichophyton erinacei			

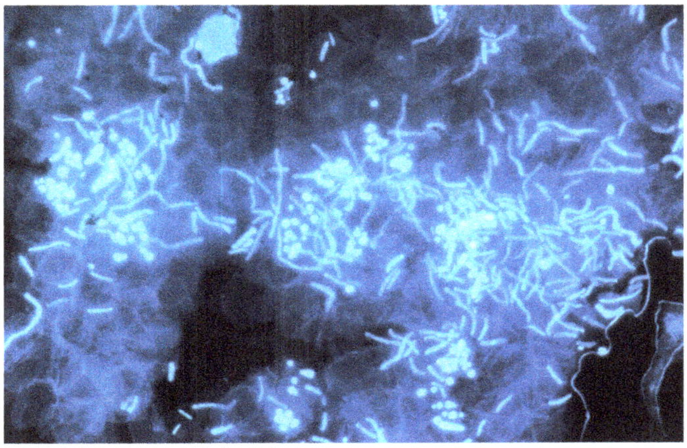

Figure 39.2 PV using potassium hydroxide with Calcofluor White showing characteristic 'spaghetti and meatball' appearance.

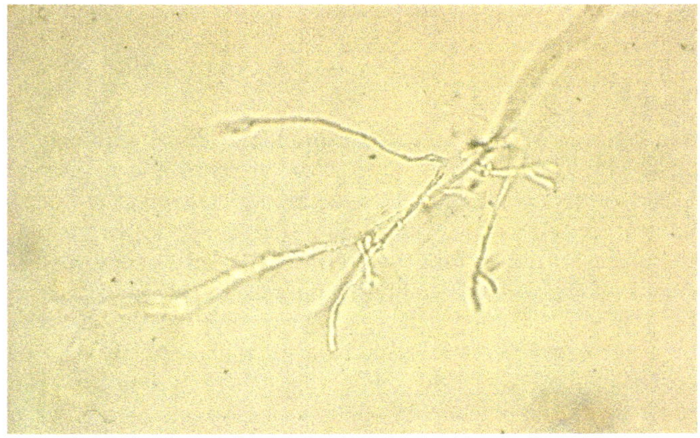

Figure 39.3 *Aspergillus* hyphae in a bronchoalveolar lavage sample from an immunocompromised individual. Note the dichotomous branching.

its short hyphae, which has been described as resembling 'spaghetti & meat balls' or 'grapes & bananas', is sufficient to make a diagnosis (Figure 39.2) (Ashbee 2007).

Corneal scrapings and vitrectomy samples

The preparation of corneal scraping mounts is as described for other superficial infections. The sensitivity and specificity of detecting fungal keratitis by microscopic examination have been reported by Sharma et al. (2002) to be 61.1% and 99.0%, respectively, in the early stages of infection using KOH + CFW, and as 87.7% and 83.7%, respectively, in advanced keratitis. They concluded that predictive values were high for microscopic diagnosis of fungal infection, and decisions could reliably be based on KOH+CFW-stained corneal scrapings for initiation of antifungal therapy in mycotic keratitis (see Chapter 28).

Vitrectomy samples should be centrifuged prior to being examined, and a positive result will lead to a rapid diagnosis of conditions such *Candida* endophthalmitis.

Body fluids

The use of UK containment level 2 (or equivalent) is recommended for handling samples of body fluids, unless a Hazard Group 3 organism is suspected. However, all manipulations which could result in infectious aerosols must be conducted in a microbiological safety cabinet. Centrifugation must be performed in sealed buckets which are opened in a microbiological safety cabinet (see Chapter 38).

Respiratory tract specimens

Sputum, bronchoalveolar lavage (BAL) fluid, and bronchial aspirates are the specimens that are most often encountered by the laboratory. The viscosity of some sputum samples makes them difficult to manipulate and they may be digested prior to processing, although this increases the possibility of contamination. The paucity of fungal fragments in sputum samples makes them less favourable than BALs for visualizing fungi. As BALs are more fluid, digestion is not necessary, but they should be concentrated by centrifugation prior to examination. However prepared, the sample should be mixed with an equivalent volume of KOH. Ensuring there are no air bubbles, it is recommended that a large 22 mm × 40 mm coverslip is placed prior to examination. If four aliquots are spun, then three can be used for culture and the pellet from one used for microscopy. Given the lack of sensitivity of the method, a negative result is not conclusive. Yeast cells and pseudohyphae may be visible, and if there is any delay in the sample reaching the laboratory, *Candida* species will readily grow while in transit, increasing their numbers. The significance of *Candida* yeasts in such samples is dubious as it may well reflect colonization in the mouth or oesophagus and they are rarely a cause of true infection of the lung. The presence of endemic fungi is, however, significant; therefore, the patients' details and clinical and travel history are important (see Chapters 30 and 37).

Throughout the world *Aspergillus* is the major cause of opportunistic lung disease, although a range of other saprophytes such as the Mucorales, *Scedosporium, Fusarium*, and dematiaceous moulds may be implicated. In the absence of yeast the presence of true hyphae is significant and the definitive diagnosis of fungal infection can be made. However, the identification of the causal organism may not be possible from the wet mount as sporing heads are a very rare phenomenon. Nevertheless, the structure, size, and branching pattern will give a strong indication as to the causative organism. Mucorales are coenocytic, infrequently producing crosswalls and having large irregular hyphae that branch at 90°, whereas when causing invasive disease *Aspergillus* has septate dichotomously branched hyphae with parallel sides (Figure 39.3).

Cerebrospinal fluid

The time between collection of the cerebrospinal fluid (CSF) and processing should be kept to a minimum, and the sample should be refrigerated at 4°C if there is any delay. As the capsulate yeast, *Cryptococcus* is the most frequently encountered fungal pathogen in the CSF; an India ink preparation is useful for demonstrating the presence of capsule formation (Public Health England 2015b). The specimen should first be centrifuged to sediment yeast cells, then the pellet emulsified with some India ink and examined under brightfield microscopy. A capsule is identifiable by the presence of a clear halo surrounding the yeast cell; budding cells may also be seen. Preparations from a culture of *Candida* and a known *Cryptococcus* species are useful for comparative purposes, particularly for the inexperienced. The addition of detergent to the India ink helps the carbon particles remain evenly dispersed and prevents them clustering (see Chapter 22).

Tissue

The accuracy of biopsies has improved and can be attributed to advances in imaging methods that are able to act as a guide to locate the area of concern. It is paramount that sufficient material is processed for histopathological diagnosis prior to attempting a wet preparation on a tissue sample. Handlers should also be cognizant of possible infectious agents and whether the technique being used is suitable for the specimen. A drop of KOH is placed on a microscope slide followed by a small piece of tissue plus a coverslip. These are left for ten minutes and then squashed prior to viewing under the microscope.

Culture

Introduction

Few fungal diseases can be diagnosed clinically, so clinicians are reliant on laboratory-based colleagues to recover the infecting organism and give it an identity so that appropriate therapy can be initiated. Primary isolation of fungi from clinical material and interpretation of its significance rely on the optimal collection and transportation of the sample to ensure the viability of the fungus and diminish the possibility of contamination. Good communication with the laboratory is fundamental to guarantee that the correct type of sample is taken for the patient's history with the minimal chance of contamination, to ensure the subsequently cultured fungi are clinically significant. The selection of media is based on the fungi most likely to be isolated from that particular site from patients with that specific clinical condition.

Fungi have a longer generation time than bacteria and consequently the majority take longer to grow. Most opportunistic fungi that infect humans are not fastidious organisms and many will thrive on standard bacteriological media. However, the selection of primary isolation media is crucial as it must sustain growth of the potential pathogen while inhibiting or restricting the growth of competitors such as bacteria and insignificant fungi. As the appearance of some fungi can change with the constituents of the media, it is beneficial to subculture any isolates sent to the laboratory onto a medium familiar to the mycologist, and preferably one that promotes the production of spores or characteristic growth. For general isolation, Sabouraud's dextrose agar or malt extract agar (with 2% or 4% malt extract) may be used, while for certain samples requiring a high degree of selectivity, specialist media such as brain heart infusion, and Sabouraud's agar with cycloheximide to suppress the growth of non-dermatophyte fungi, may be used. Petri dishes, with their large surface area for selection of single colonies and adequate aeration, are preferable except if a Hazard Group 3 fungus is suspected, when slopes should be used.

Many factors can influence the laboratory's ability to obtain the maximum yield of significant fungal organisms as various samples require different methods of processing to obtain the most commonly isolated fungi from each site. The presence of a specific group of fungi depends upon a patient's immune status, site sampled, animal contact, travel history, and any therapy; furthermore, the laboratory should be informed of all of these factors. All deep sites should be sterile and devoid of fungi, so their isolation from such samples should always be investigated. The challenge is to determine whether the isolated fungus is significant and not a contaminant introduced to the specimen during or after collection. Before identification of any fungus is possible within the general microbiology laboratory, or prior to an isolate being referred to a specialist expert laboratory, it must be a pure monoculture.

Superficial samples

As fungi are presumed to be randomly distributed within samples from superficial sites, it is essential to culture sufficient material to ensure the best chance of growing the causative agent, especially if it is a fastidious fungus such as a dermatophyte (Weitzman and Summerbell 1995). The ideal method is to chop the material into as small fragments as is possible, select pieces from all areas of the specimen, and plant them onto the plates, ensuring good contact with the culture media (20 plants per plate is recommended). Alternatively, the sample can be scattered on the surface of the agar. It is preferable to deep-fill the agar plates in order for the sample to endure an incubation period of up to three weeks. Plates with 4% malt containing chloramphenicol and cycloheximide for skin, and the inclusion of an additional Sabouraud plate for nails to allow the growth of non-dermatophyte moulds inhibited by cycloheximide, is an optimal strategy. The majority of the plates should be incubated at 28°C. Exceptions to this are specimens from patients with suspected *Trichophyton verrucosum*, these should additionally be inoculated onto nutrient agar and incubated at 37°C.

There are 11 currently recognized species of *Malassezia* and no single medium can reliably recover them all. Many of them have a requirement for lipids, and selective media have been formulated such as Dixon's medium (containing Tween 40 and glycerol mono-oleate) and Leeming and Notman agar (containing Tween 60, glycerol, and full-fat cow's milk) (Ashbee 2007). Recovery of *Malassezia* can take 5–14 days, depending on the species, and some have optimal growth at 35°C. If an adhesive strip has been used to collect the sample, this can be laid straight onto the agar surface and removed after a few days' incubation.

Corneal scrapings

The best method is to inoculate the scrape directly into the agar in the clinic. In the experience of this author, 2% malt extract agar will give a better isolation yield than other mycological media.

Respiratory tract specimens

Sputum and BAL samples may contain Hazard Group 3 organisms and consequently should be processed in a biological safety cabinet within containment level 3 facilities. Mycological media is preferable to bacteriological media for the isolation of fungi, especially *Aspergillus*. 4% Malt will slightly inhibit the growth of commensal yeasts, allowing for a greater yield of *Aspergillus* species. Sputum can be spread directly onto the media without prior treatment, although in some cases digestion may be preferred. However, this does increase the risk of sample contamination (Schelenz et al. 2015). In addition, contamination from the oral cavity or the environment is likely in such samples. Respiratory specimens such as BAL or bronchial aspirates are obtained by more invasive techniques but with less risk of upper airway contamination, so the growth of *Aspergillus* from such samples is considered more significant. These specimens should be centrifuged in sealed buckets as four aliquots, where sufficient. One pellet can be used for microscopy and the other three for culture. It is useful to spot the concentrated sample on the media with one aliquot in each quadrant and one in the centre (as colonies at the edge of the plate may be contaminants).

For all respiratory tract specimens, three incubation temperatures can be used. First, 28°C will give an indication of how 'clean' the specimen is, as any saprophytic yeasts and moulds will grow at this temperature and if the sample appears full of contaminants, then any *Aspergillus* isolated at other temperatures may not necessarily be significant.

Second, 35°C is the optimal temperature for growth of pathogenic fungi, and any yeasts or moulds isolated are potential pathogens.

Third, 45°C deters the growth of yeast contaminants while supporting the growth of *Aspergillus fumigatus* and some *Mucorales.* Hence, this temperature allows the growth of clinically significant fungi which may otherwise be swamped by competing organisms. Should there only be sufficient material for two temperatures, choose 35°C and 45°C, and if only sufficient for one temperature, choose 35°C.

If there are several samples to be incubated together, then the inclusion of uninoculated plates between each sample will reduce the chance of cross-contamination and highlight any contamination within the incubator. The use of sterile incubation tins ensures that any *Aspergillus* spores from samples are contained and maintains the cleanliness of the incubator.

The recovery of dimorphic fungi can be enhanced using the enriched brain heart infusion agar in addition to Sabouraud's agar and 4% malt extract agar. Growth of *Histoplasma capsulatum* is inhibited by growth of *Candida* species (Richardson and Evans 1989). The inoculation of primary material in a biological safety cabinet in containment level 3 and the use of agar on slopes or cell culture flasks, as opposed to Petri dishes, are important.

Blood

Blood culture methods have seen a drive to improve the recovery of fungi from blood. Positive blood cultures are common in opportunistic infections such as those caused by yeasts for example *Candida, Trichosporon, Cryptococcus,* and *Malassezia* species. Fungaemia is also seen in *Fusarium, Scedosporium,* and more rarely from unusual mould infections. *Aspergillus* species, including *A. terreus,* are isolated only in exceptional cases (Alexander and Pfaller 2006).

Candida and other yeasts can be detected with a high degree of sensitivity (i.e. from very low numbers of circulating organisms) using automated blood culture systems including: BACTEC (Becton Dickinson) and BacT/Alert (BioMerieux). The introduction of specialized broths and constant agitation have improved the isolation of yeasts, and some studies have shown comparable results with lysis centrifugation methods (Geha and Roberts 1994). However, other reports have revealed that recovery of *H. capsulatum, M. furfur,* and *Fusarium* may be better with lysis centrifugation methods (Magadia and Weinstein 2001). Nevertheless, despite the advances in technique, blood cultures are frequently negative even in the presence of disseminated disease (Clancy and Nguyen 2013).

Cerebrospinal fluid

CSF requires concentration for recovery of the optimal number of fungi. The sediment should be cultured on Sabouraud's agar at 35–37°C (Public Health England 2015b) although if *Cryptococcus* is suspected, a better yield and optimal capsule formation are achieved on 4% malt extract agar at 28°C (personal observation). The detection of mucopolysaccaride antigen is a more sensitive method than microscopy or culture (Saldanha et al. 2009).

Vulvovaginal samples

Some guidelines recommend that vaginal swabs should only be cultured if the patient is under 16 years or over 55 years and from women of reproductive age under the following circumstances; recurrent symptoms, treatment failure, postpartum or post gynaecological instrumentation or when microscopy is inconclusive. Once streaked on a plate, preferably containing chromogenic media for the identification of mixed cultures of *Candida,* the plates should be incubated for 48 hours at 35⁰C. The interpretation can be challenging as one or two colonies may not represent a true infection but it is well established that microscopy lacks sensitivity (Sobel 1997).

Microscopic examination and culture are still the corner-stones of mycological diagnosis although the newer automated techniques may one day render them obsolete. However, that day has not yet arrived.

References

Alexander BD and Pfaller MA (2006) Contemporary tools for the diagnosis and management of invasive mycoses. *Infect Dis* 43 (Suppl. 1): S15–27. doi: 10.1086/504491

Ashbee HR (2007) Update on the genus Malassezia. *Medical Mycology* 45: 287–303.

Bonifaz A, Rios-Yuil JM, Arenas R, et al. (2013) Comparison of direct microscopy, culture and calcofluor white for the diagnosis of onychomycosis. *Rev Iberoam Micol* 30:109–11.

Clancy CJ and Nguyen MH (2013) Finding the "missing 50%" of invasive candidiasis: how nonculture diagnostics will improve understanding of disease spectrum and transform patient care. *Clin Infect Dis* 56: 1284–92.

Clayton YM and Midgley G (1985) *Medical Mycology*, Pocket Picture Guides to Clinical Medicine (London: Gower Medical).

Davidson AM and Gregory FH (1935) The so-called mosaic fungus as an intercellular deposit of cholesterol crystals. *JAMA* 105: 1262–3.

Geha DJ and Roberts GD (1994) Laboratory detection of fungemia. *Clin Lab Med* 14: 83–97.

Getz K, Skillern SD and Ulrich JA (1955) Studies on "mosaic fungus". *J Invest Dermatol* 25: 29–32.

Magadia R and Weinstein MP (2001) Laboratory diagnosis of bacteremia and fungemia. *Infect Dis Clin North Am* 15: 1009–24.

Milne LJR (1989) Direct microscopy, *in*: EGV Evans and M Richardson (eds) *Medical Mycology: A practical approach* (Oxford: Oxford University Press), 17–45.

Public Health England (2015a) Investigation of dermatological specimens for superficial mycoses, UK Standards for Microbiology Investigations B 39 i3, www.gov.uk/government/uploads/system/uploads/attachment_data/file/453489/B_39i3.pdf, accessed 30 May 2017.

Public Health England (2015b) Investigation of cerebrospinal fluid shunts. UK Standards for Microbiology Investigation B27i6, https://www.gov.uk/government/uploads/system/uploads/attachment_data/file/434627/B_22i6.1.pdf, accessed 30 May 2017.

Richardson MD and Evans EGV (1989) Culture and isolation of fungi, *in*: EGV Evans and M Richardson (eds) *Medical Mycology: A practical approach* (Oxford: Oxford University Press).

Saldanha Dominic RM, Prashanth HV, Shenoy S and Baliga S (2009) Diagnostic value of latex agglutination in cryptococcal meningitis. *J Lab Physicians* 1: 67–8.

Schelenz S, Barnes RA, Barton RC, et al. (2015) British Society for Medical Mycology best practice recommendations for the diagnosis of serious fungal diseases *Lancet Infect Dis* 15: 461–74.

Sharma S, Kunimoto DY, Gopinathan U, Athmanathan S, Garg P and Rao GN (2002) Evaluation of corneal scraping smear examination methods in the diagnosis of bacterial and fungal keratitis. A survey of eight years of laboratory experience. *Cornea* 21: 643–7.

Sobel JD (1997) Vaginitis. *N Engl J Med* 337: 1896–903.

Weidman F (1927) Laboratory aspects of epidermatophytosis. *Arch Dermat & Syph* 15: 415.

Weitzman I and Summerbell RC (1995) The dermatophytes. *Clin Microbiol Rev* 8: 240–59.

CHAPTER 40

Histopathology of fungal disease

Sebastian B. Lucas

Introduction to the role of histopathology in the diagnosis of mycotic infections

Histopathology involves the examination of 4–5μ-thick sections of tissue on glass slides. The tissues are either fresh and unfixed or, more usually, fixed in formalin solutions and processed through to, and embedded in, paraffin (FFPE). To render objects visible under the microscope, the sections can be stained with general or specific dyes, with labelled antibodies against target epitopes, or (as in *in-situ* hybridization) with labelled target gene-sequences. These methods apply to both biopsy- and autopsy-derived material.

Histopathology has a special place in mycological diagnosis for two reasons, in addition to its speed relative to standard culture methods when an experienced pathologist views the slides:

1 The diagnostic sample is often fixed in its entirety, so that culture is not possible.

2 By observing the infection and its context (e.g. location and pattern of cellular reaction), not only can the fungus be identified, but its significance can be assessed—that is, whether it is a true pathogen or merely a contaminant (i.e. evincing no host reaction or causing no pathology).

The sensitivity of histopathology in identifying fungi is generally high, but its specificity depends on the type of fungus and the experience of the observer (Schelenz et al. 2009). Moreover, numerous microscopic objects can mimic fungi in appearance ('pseudo-fungi'), and other infectious agents such as bacteria and algae can resemble fungi whilst causing rather similar lesions.

The standard histological diagnostic process for fungal infections starts with the general haematoxylin & eosin (H&E) stain, and the most useful 'special stains' for fungi are the Grocott methenamine silver stain (GMS) and periodic acid-Schiff (PAS) stain. Fungus cell walls are rich in polysaccharide which can be converted by oxidation to aldehydes, and thus detected by Schiff's reagent and hexamine silver solution.

If the diagnosis is still uncertain, then FFPE material can be used in the polymerase chain reaction (PCR) technique for molecular diagnostics (Paterson et al. 2003; Hay and Morris Jones 2010; Ruangritchankul et al. 2015). Few laboratories have panels of specific antibodies to fungi, and immunohistochemistry has, for most genera, been supplanted by PCR (Guarner and Brandt 2011; Rickerts et al. 2011); the exception is *Pneumocystis*, as immunocytochemistry is used to increase the sensitivity of bronchial secretion rapid analysis, and the antibodies work well on FFPE tissues (Radio et al. 1990). Similarly, *in-situ* hybridization is no longer widely used. Hereon, only H&E and special stain diagnostics will be discussed and illustrated, along with other special stains such as Gram (most fungi are Gram-positive) and Ziehl-Neelsen (ZN) stains, which are helpful in identifying infections that look like fungal infections.

Every organ in the body can be affected by fungi of many types (Bennett et al. 2010). But clinico-pathologically, there are more limited sets of patterns that arise from the interaction of the four critical pathogenetic variables depicted in Figure 40.1.

Histomorphological features of certain fungal infections

Among the thousands of genera and species of fungi, there are a small number that represent the bulk of infections that present to histopathologists, and cause problems in differential diagnosis. Table 40.1 presents the main groups and genera with their morphological features and key differential diagnoses.

The common histopathological reactions to fungal infections

Fungi induce very varied reactions in host tissues, in immunocompetent as well as immunocompromised hosts. Nonetheless there are general clues here to fungal infections (their presence and sometimes the type) which can be identified (Guarner and Brandt 2011):

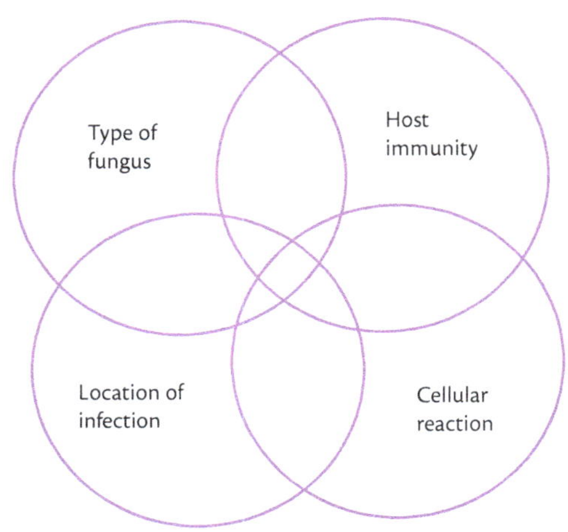

Figure 40.1 The four sets of variables that determine the clinical pathology of fungal infections.

Reproduced courtesy of Sebastian B. Lucas.

- mixed granulomatous reaction (i.e. purulent centres within granulomas)—both yeast and filamentous fungi can induce these;
- granulomas with caseation necrosis, mimicking mycobacterial infections—several yeasts characteristically induce this reaction, including *Histoplasma* and *Coccidioides* species;
- vascular invasion and secondary thrombosis with infarction and haemorrhage—Mucorales moulds and *Aspergillus* species are typical causes of this pattern of organ damage;
- in skin, epithelial hyperplasia, mixed inflammation, and abscesses within the epidermis—characteristic of cutaneous mycoses;
- in the subcutis, mixed inflammation and surrounding fibrosis—characteristic of mycetomas;
- no host cell reaction at all—in immunocompromised patients, pulmonary *Pneumocystis* and disseminated *Cryptococcus* infections often induce no reaction at all.

Host immunity and mycotic infections

Whilst no one is immune to fungal infections of any organ, people with certain types of abnormal host immunity are significantly more likely to develop mycoses—both invasive and localized (Health Protection Agency 2006; Antachopoulos 2010) (see Box 40.1 and Section 4 for more details).

The pathological effect of these conditions is, in general:

- to enable the fungus to multiply more so the visible infection density is greater

Table 40.1 Histomorphological features of fungi important in presumptive identification

Fungus	Size (diameter)	Other features	Key histological differential diagnosis
Yeast or yeast-like appearance			
Blastomyces dermatitidis	5–15μ	Broad-based budding, refractile thick cell wall	*Cryptococcus* spp., *Paracoccidioides brasiliensis*, lobomycosis
Candida glabrata	3–15μ	No pseudohyphae, yeasts only	*H. capsulatum*, *Candida albicans*
Chromoblastomycosis*	5–15μ	Brown-pigmented yeasts that split rather than bud; often a Hoeppli-Splendore reaction, and pseudo-epitheliomatous reaction	Sporotrichosis
Coccidioides immitis / *C. posadasii*	15–100μ	Large yeast-like structures containing endospores	Tuberculosis; protothecosis
Cryptococcus neoformans	5–15μ	Clear mucoid capsule surrounding yeast cells	*Histoplasma capsulatum*
Emmonsia and *Chrysosporium* spp. (adiaspiromycosis)	15–500μ	Thick walled yeasts in early stage of infection, not distinctive; but when enlarged to 500μ, they are pathognomonic	*Blastomyces*, *Coccidioides* spp.
Histoplasma capsulatum	3–5μ	Intracellular; often birefringent	*Leishmania*, *Talaromyces marneffei*, *C. neoformans*
Paracoccidioides brasiliensis	3–15μ	Multiple buds off a single yeast, resembling a ship steering wheel	*Blastomyces*, *Cryptococcus*
Pneumocystis jirovecii	3–5μ	Fine honeycomb	Fibrin exudates, alveolar proteinosis
Sporothrix schenckii	3–15μ	Yeast may be scanty; induces pseudo-epitheliomatous hyperplasia; Hoeppli-Splendore reaction around yeasts	Mycobacterial infection, chromoblastomycosis
Talaromyces (*Penicillium*) *marneffei*	3–15μ	Yeasts divide by splitting rather than budding	*H. capsulatum*, *Leishmania*
Hyphae only			
Aspergillus spp.	5–15μ	Septate; branching at 45 degree	Less common hyphae eg *Fusarium*, *Alternaria* and *Scedosporium* spp. (hyaline), *Rhinocladiella* spp. (pigmented)
Moulds of the order Mucorales *	15–100μ	Usually non-septate; hyphal folding can mimic septation; irregular diameter hyphae, bizarre morphologies	*Aspergillus* spp.
Mycetoma*	5–15μ	Colonies or grains; pigmented or pale (hyaline); expanded chlamydospores at periphery of colonies; Hoeppli-Splendore reaction around the grain; much host fibrosis	Bacterial colonies of *Actinomyces* and *Nocardia* spp.
Subcutaneous phaeo-hyphomycosis*	5–15μ	Usually brown pigmented (as seen in H&E stained sections)	Mycobacterial infection
Dermatophyte infection*	5–15μ	Usually hyphae, but may be dimorphic and exhibit arthroconidia; typically seen in the epidermis, keratin, and within hair shafts	Staphylococcal folliculitis
Mixed hyphae and yeasts (dimorphism)			
Candida albicans and related spp.	3–15μ	Usually hypha-like structures (pseudohyphae) and yeasts seen	Aspergillosis, *Cryptococcus* spp.
Malassezia spp.	5–15μ	Mainly hyphae with some yeasts	Other dermatophyte fungi

* Many genera and species of fungi.

Adapted from *The Lancet Infectious Diseases*, Volume 15, Issue 4, Schelenz S. et al., 'British Society for Medical Mycology best practice recommendations for the diagnosis of serious fungal diseases', pp. 461–474, http://www.sciencedirect.com/science/article/pii/S147330991570006X

Box 40.1 Congenital and acquired immunodeficiency syndromes, and other disease states, that predispose to mycotic infections

1 HIV-related impairment of cell-mediated immunity (CMI)
2 Congenital immune disorders:
  a chronic granulomatous disease
  b hyper-IgE syndrome
  c severe combined immunodeficiency
  d X-linked hyper-IgM syndrome
  e Wiskott–Aldrich syndrome
  f DiGeorge syndrome
  g common variable immunodeficiency
  h defects in the interferon-γ-interleukin-12 axis
  i myeloperoxidase deficiency
3 Burns
4 Diabetes mellitus
5 Cystic fibrosis
6 Chronic renal failure and dialysis
7 Iatrogenic damage to the immune system
  a malignancies per se (eg leukaemia)
  b cancer chemotherapy treatments
  c transplantation and anti-rejection regimes
    i solid organ
    ii bone marrow allograft
  d specific immunosuppressive therapy (e.g. anti-TNF)
  e steroid therapy
  f intensive care organ support systems (including vascular catheter lines as the means of ingress of infection)
8 Old age, with resultant impaired CMI

- to reduce the effective host cellular reaction against the fungus
- to reduce the granulomatous response to certain fungi
- to permit more generalized organ dissemination of infection, via bloodstream and lymphatics

Organ patterns of mycotic infections

Since fungi are widespread in nature and we are constantly exposed, mycotic infections can broadly be categorized into those arising acutely from a new infection, and those emerging from a previous clinical or subclinical latent infection. This section indicates the main fungi causing disease in the major organs.

Cutaneous infections

The skin surface commonly bears fungi in the keratin and superficial hair shafts, and the host reaction varies from nothing, to hyperkeratosis, to dermal inflammation, to folliculitis and subsequent ulceration ('ringworm'). There are three main genera of dermatophyte fungi (*Epidermophyton, Trichophyton, Microsporum*). They all are seen as hyphae in keratin, hair shafts, and dermis. Molecular diagnostics are now available to identify the species (Hay and Morris Jones 2010). If a yeast plus hyphal fungal infection (i.e. dimorphic) is seen in superficial skin biopsies, then it will be either a *Malassezia* species (the cause of pityriasis versicolor) or a *Candida* species.

Deeper dermal infections are notably commoner in immunosuppressed persons, the infections arriving by bloodstream from a primary lesion (usually in the lung). The agents include *Blastomyces, Paracoccidioides, Histoplasma capsulatum*, and *Cryptococcus* spp.

Subepithelial infections such as those due to *Sporothrix schenckii* and *Paracoccidioides,* when located in skin or mouth, can cause a pseudo-epitheliomatous epidermal hyperplasia that mimics squamous carcinoma. Lobomycosis (*Lacazia loboi*) is a rare cause of skin granulomatous lesions.

Cutaneous mucormycosis can follow implantation of Mucorales fungi by penetrating trauma during unusual environmental events such as tornadoes (Neblett Fanfair et al. 2012). One such epidemic caused severe morbidity and some mortality. Histopathology found gangrenous tissue damage caused by infection and thrombotic occlusion of limb arteries. The agent—*Apophysomyces trapeziformis*—was identified by molecular diagnostics on both unfixed and FFPE material.

Finally, people with mental health problems have been known to inject themselves with baker's yeast to create inflammatory lesions.

Subcutaneous and bone infections

These lesions are due to fungi implanted from nature, and they cause chronic inflammatory lesions that include four major clinicopathological categories:

Phaeohyphomycosis. This is a subcutaneous cystic chronic abscess caused mainly by pigmented hyphal infections (including *Exophiala, Bipolaris*, and *Curvularia* spp.). The border is fairly well defined with a granulomatous and fibrotic capsule (thus aiding surgical excision), and the fungi are seen at the inside edge of the semi-liquid cystic cavity along with acute inflammation. Being pigmented, the fungi stain brown with H&E stains. Rarely, hyaline fungi (e.g. some strains of *Alternaria*) can cause this syndrome. It must be distinguished from other forms of eumycetoma which are more fibrosing, and have different treatment.

Chromoblastomycosis. This is caused by pigmented yeast genera (*Fonsecaea* and *Cladophialophora*) these chronic lesions characteristically induce a mixed acute and granulomatous inflammatory reaction. The fungal cells are characteristic in dividing by splitting in two, then four, daughter cells (so-called sclerotic bodies or muriform cells).

Subcutaneous phycomycosis. Implanted Mucorales fungi of the Entomophthoromycotina subphylum, typically *Basidiobolus ranarum*, cause these chronic expanding fibrotic lesions. They can invade vessels and cause local necrosis. The clinical differential diagnosis includes tumoural calcinosis, onchocercoma, and soft tissue tumour.

Mycetoma. This classical infection is a deep implanted infection arising from the presence of pigmented and pale (hyaline) fungal hyphae. The agents include *Madurella mycetomatis* (the commonest pigmented genus), *Acremonium, Scedosporium*, and *Fusarium* spp. (non-pigmented). The infection produces dense colonies visible as grains to the naked eye and compact on histology. At the periphery, chlamydospore expansions are characteristic. The surrounding inflammation causes tissue destruction and dense fibrosis, and progressively involves local bone (Zijlstra et al. 2016). Specific diagnosis requires culture or molecular diagnostics.

The critical differential diagnosis is between a true fungal mycetoma (eumycetoma) and clinically similar bacterial lesions caused by *Actinomadura* and *Nocardia* spp.

For further discussion, please refer to Chapters 20 and 23.

Ophthalmic infections

The most important part of the eye to be infected with fungi is the surface—conjunctiva and cornea—a particular risk factor being the wearing of contact lenses. *Fusarium* species cause this fungal keratitis. Histologically there is necrosis of the conjunctiva and cornea, acute and chronic inflammation, and hyaline hyphae.

Internal vitreous and choroid mycosis may be part of disseminated infection in immunosuppressed individuals (e.g. candidiasis, cryptococcosis, and paracoccidioidomycosis). Aspergillosis and Mucorales fungi may involve the eye as part of orbital invasion.

Facial and sinonasal infections

Aspergillus and Mucorales infections are the major agents of these lesions. Aspergillosis causes a chronic fibrosing granulomatous inflammatory mass, as does the entomophthoromycosis caused by *Conidiobolus coronatus*. However, in diabetic patients who acquire mucormycosis of the sinuses and orbit (typically from *Rhizopus* and *Mucor* spp.), the infection is virulent, necrotizing, destructive, and invasive. On biopsy, it must be distinguished from non-Mucorales hyphal infections promptly.

Intracranial infections

The clinico-pathological patterns of CNS mycotic infections are varied and include (Lucas 2015):

- diffuse encephalitis
- meningitis
- intracranial and intra-spinal mycetoma of the meninges
- space-occupying lesions in CNS parenchyma—granulomas and abscesses
- infarction from vascular invasion and thrombosis, causing stroke
- haemorrhage from mycotic aneurysm and rupture

The commonest agents include meningoencephalitis from *Cryptococcus neoformans* and *C. gattii*, necrotic lesions caused by *Aspergillus* species, and diffuse encephalitis or abscesses from a variety of moulds such as *Scedosporium* (hyaline hyphae) and *Rhinocladiella* (pigmented hyphae) species (Jabeen et al. 2011). Recently, an epidemic of *Exserohilum* meningitis occurred in the USA from spinal injection of steroid solutions that were contaminated during manufacture (Ritter et al. 2013) (see Chapters 7 and 22).

Lung infections

Most of the systemic mycoses enter the body via inhalation and cause a primary lung lesion that may be subclinical. Thus, in immunocompetent persons, histoplasmosis, cryptococcosis, paracoccidioidomycosis, coccidioidomycosis, and blastomycosis cause acute pneumonic lung lesions that are initially a mixed acute and granulomatous inflammation with variable necrosis—and they may persist there for decades. These lung lesions are frequently removed as suspicious of lung cancer. Whether systemic spread develops depends on host immunity.

Pneumocystis jirovecii is different: although most people have antibodies indicating infection in childhood, there is no primary lung lesion. Immunosuppression—particularly from HIV (human immunovirus) infection and malnutrition in childhood—permit the development of pneumonia. Occasionally it spreads to hilar lymph nodes, or further to gut, spleen, and other organs.

Aspergillosis has a predilection to cause various forms of disease in those with chronic lung disease, and disseminated necrotizing lung disease in patients who are immunosuppressed (e.g. advanced HIV disease and after transplantation). Additionally, there is a risk in ITU settings when patients are ventilated for prolonged periods—and especially with extracorporeal membrane oxygenation support.

A wide range of unusual fungi can also cause pneumonia in susceptible subjects, for example the small yeast *Arxula adeninivorans* in cystic fibrosis (Roehmel et al. 2015); histopathology alone will not be able to specify such infections. However, the rare pulmonary adiaspiromycosis (*Emmonsia parva* and *E. crescens*), typically inhaled from pet animal exhalations, is the largest yeast infection of all (diameter up to 500μ), and so is diagnosable on histology (Anstead et al. 2012).

Gut infections

The main fungi encountered in the gastrointestinal tract are:

- *Candida albicans* in the oropharynx and oesophagus
- *Histoplasma capsulatum* in small and large bowel, in the lamina propria macrophages as part of systemic haematogenous spread in immunocompromised persons
- Mucorales fungi as agents of necrotizing enterocolitis in infants and other groups with severe immunosuppression

Systemic multi-organ infections

Haematogenous spread of yeast and hyphal fungal infections is a feature of severe immunosuppression, and all organs can be involved. The yeasts involved are usually those which are phagocytosed by monocytes/macrophages, and are found throughout the lymphoreticular system (lymph nodes, spleen, bone marrow, lung macrophages, liver Kupffer cells, gut macrophages). They include *H. capsulatum*, *Talaromyces marneffei*, and *C. neoformans*. Bone marrow biopsy is a sensitive diagnostic tool, and often the yeasts are visible in Giemsa-stained blood smear monocytes.

Aspergillus, *Candida*, and *Rhizopus* infections can disseminate rapidly by the blood stream to all organs in immunocompromised patients, with high mortality from tissue destruction.

Histopathological features of specific common infections

Aspergillus

Aspergillus spp. infections, along with *Candida*, are the fungi that histopathologists encounter most often, at least in Europe. Generally, as shown in Table 40.1, the hyphae are pale (hyaline), septate, and branch regularly at 45° (Figure 40.2a). In immunosuppressed patients (e.g. those with advanced HIV disease, and those with low blood neutrophil counts), the infection disseminates via the bloodstream to form dense colonies which resemble starbursts,

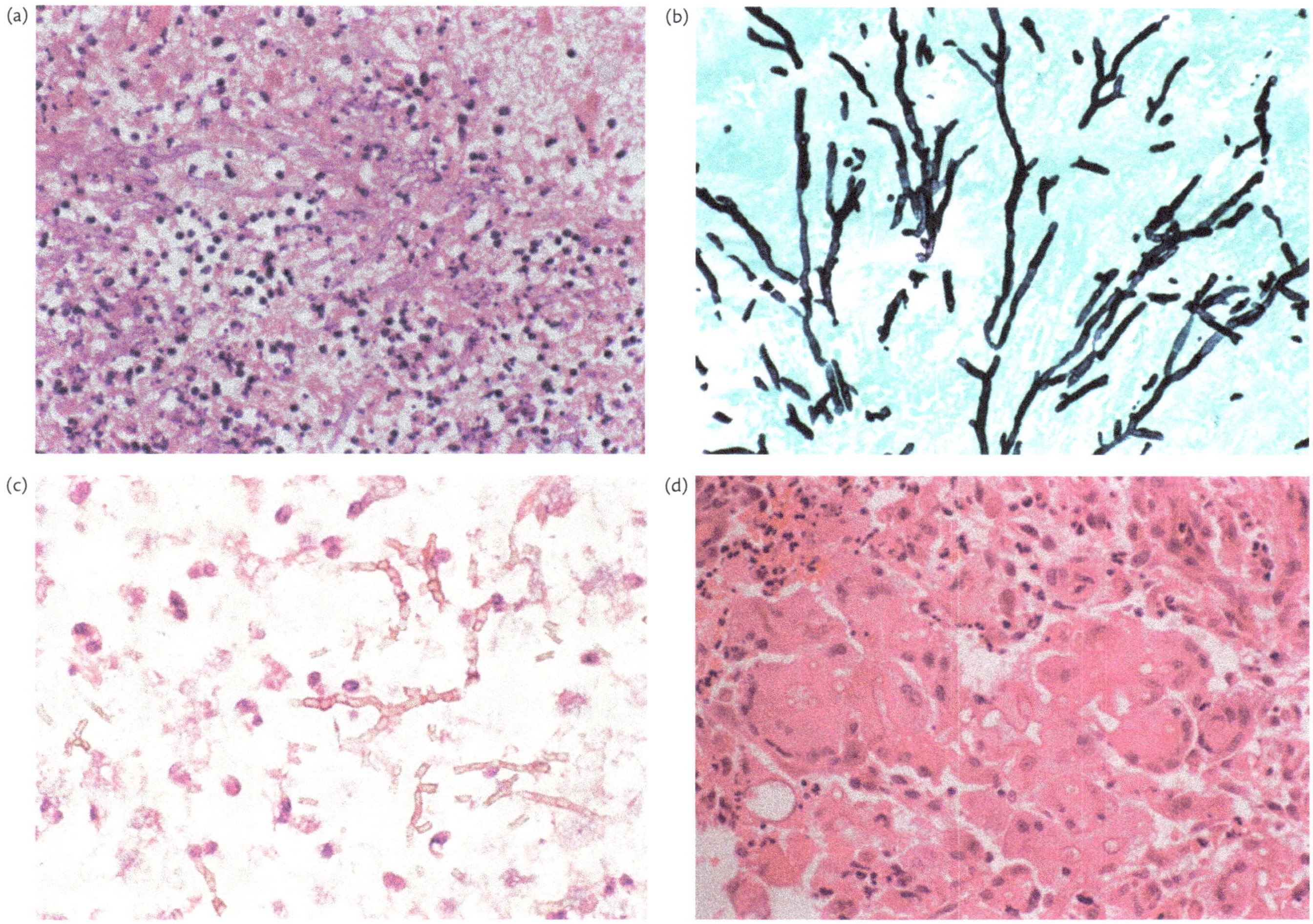

Figure 40.2 Hyphae.

a *Aspergillus* species in brain. Pale haematoxyphilic hyphae, branching and with septa, amidst necrosis and inflammation. Haematoxylin & eosin (H&E) stain.

b *Fusarium* species in the eye. Hyphae similar in shape and size to *Aspergillus*. Methenamine silver stain.

c Chromomycosis (*Rhinocladiella* species) in brain. There are more septa than in *Aspergillus*; the hyphae are bulbous, and are discernibly coloured brown. H&E stain.

d Mucorales infection of the orbit (*Rhizopus* species). The bizarre irregular hyphae, with thin walls and appearing empty, are seen in the macrophage reaction. H&E stain.

Reproduced courtesy of Sebastian B. Lucas.

and obstructs and causes thrombosis in vessels, which in turn causes infarction and haemorrhage. Typically, the lungs, brain, and heart show this pattern.

But other clinico-pathological patterns occur, best exemplified in the respiratory tract (Table 40.2).

The differential diagnosis of aspergillosis is important. Modern chemotherapy for mycotic infections is increasingly sophisticated and dependent on knowing the genus of the infection. But most histopathologists do not know of any pale hyphal fungi beyond *Aspergillus*, and so label them all as that (Ruangritchankul et al. 2015). Whilst the following genera do not branch as acutely as *Aspergillus*, they look similar microscopically: *Alternaria, Fusarium* (Figure 40.2b), and *Scedosporium* species. Thus it is wise to term these lesions as '*Aspergillus*-like' if there is doubt. *Fusarium* hyphae may contain vacuoles and chlamydoconidia as distinctive features. If the hyphae are brown, then the lesion is a phaeohyphomycosis with a completely different set of possible fungal genera, for example *Exophiala* species and *Rhinocladiella mackenziei* (Figure 40.2c).

Mucorales moulds

These moulds, in human tissues, have distinctive morphology (Table 40.1): non-septate, irregularly and bizarrely shaped, thin-walled hyphae that are much wider than those of *Aspergillus* and similar genera (Dhaliwal et al. 2015) (Figure 40.2d). They tend to be angio-invasive and can cause necrosis by ischaemia. Some are relatively non-virulent, such as the agents causing entomophthoromycosis, while others, such as *Rhizopus* species, are very tissue-destructive and have high mortality, particularly when involving the nasal sinuses and gut wall.

Candida species

Candida species are ubiquitous in the oropharynx, lower genital tract, and intestinal tract, colonizing the surface. *C. albicans* is *dimorphic* in histomorphology, having both a yeast and a hyphal form (Figure 40.3a). Locally invasive candidiasis, such as in the oesophagus, retains the dimorphic (and diagnostic) picture. In

Table 40.2 Respiratory tract aspergillosis syndromes

Pattern of respiratory tract aspergillosis	Pathological features
Paranasal granulomatous aspergillosis	Sinus and subcutaneous swelling from non-necrotizing granulomatous reaction to hyphae; these are usually seen as single fragments without much branching; much fibrosis.
Allergic aspergillus sinusitis	Single hyphae in a fibrin- and eosinophil-rich exudate; abundant Charcot–Leyden crystals.
Allergic bronchopulmonary aspergillosis	Moderate density of hyphae within an eosinophil-rich exudate obstructing bronchial lumens; Charcot–Leyden crystals seen; it may locally invade.
Cavitary aspergillus mycetoma, of which there are three subtypes: 1 simple aspergilloma 2 chronic cavitary pulmonary aspergillosis 3 fibrosing pulmonary aspergillosis	In old tuberculosis cavities and emphysematous spaces; a mycelium of *Aspergillus*, with species-specific fruiting bodies at the periphery (from contact with air). Usually non-invasive (simple aspergilloma), but can show limited invasion with progressive destruction (chronic cavitary form). The fibrosing pattern of dense pericavity fibrosis is a reaction to persistent infection with chronic inflammation, usually non-granulomatous.
Invasive necrotizing aspergillosis	Haematogenous dissemination and florid vascular & tissue invasion; dense starburst clusters of hyphae; thrombosis, necrosis, and haemorrhage

disseminated tissue invasive infections, the fungi may be more variable by being mostly hyphae or yeasts, so raising other possible fungal diagnoses.

C. glabrata is less common than *C. albicans*, but can involve mucosal surfaces and cause systemic disease in immunosuppressed hosts. It is not dimorphic, so only small yeasts are seen (Fidel et al. 1999). Other *Candida* species are difficult to discriminate on histology.

Coccidioides immitis

Many people infected by this fungus (in the Americas) have no symptoms of infection; only a few develop a pneumonia. The asymptomatic cases may present as nodules on chest imaging, suggesting a cancer; the only way to identify the true cause is needle biopsy or nodule resection. The large thick-walled spherules with endospores are characteristic (Figure 40.3b). This infection may reactivate and disseminate as host defences decline (e.g. with age or HIV infection).

Cryptococcus neoformans and *C. gattii*

Both of these *Cryptococcus* species cause disease in immunocompetent and immunocompromised persons, though *C. gattii* is the more virulent in immunocompetent patients and induces more inflammation (Franco-Paredes et al. 2015). In lung and subcutis, there are granulomatous lesions with moderate numbers of yeasts. These are seen budding, within clear polysaccharide capsular spaces. The capsular material can be stained red with a mucicarmine stain (its only use in myco-histology). The amount of mucin is variable, and when the capsule is small, the fungi can resemble other medium-sized yeasts (Table 40.1).

In immunosuppressed patients, typically in those with HIV, there is less host reaction, and the budding encapsulated yeasts proliferate to fill spaces in the meninges, in the Virchow-Robin spaces of the brain, and extend into the neurophil; in the lungs, liver, spleen, and lymph nodes, they often aggregate to form a pool of mucoid fungal mass.

An unusual histological differential diagnosis of cryptococcosis is *Rhodotorula* species, which look very like *Cryptococcus*, minus the capsule (Worth et al. 2012).

Histoplasma capsulatum

Histologically, *H. capsulatum* yeasts look like small fried eggs with a refractile cytoplasm on H&E stains. They are seen within macrophages, often in large numbers. The main fungal differential diagnoses are *Candida glabrata* and *Talaromyces marneffei*. *T. marneffei* cells are of similar size but multiply by splitting, not budding. PAS stains show internal structure, whilst the GMS stain merely indicates a uniform, black, small, oval yeast (Figure 40.3c). *Leishmania donovani* and *L. infantum* amastigotes are of similar size, but the cells contain a DNA haematoxyphilic kinetoplast, and do not stain with PAS or GMS stains. Histoplasmosis can reactivate and disseminate from an occult lung lesion if the person becomes immunosuppressed.

Pneumocystis jirovecii

The typical *Pneumocystis* pneumonia (PCP) shows alveoli packed with an eosinophilic honeycomb of yeast-like cyst forms, which contain a tiny haematoxyphylic nucleus. The GMS stain indicates the partly flattened round discs, and the silver-positive dot on one side of the cell wall (Figure 40.3d). The host reaction is variable: in adult advanced HIV-infection, there is minimal inflammation in and around the alveoli, whilst in children there is more mononuclear infiltration, hence the synonym 'plasma cell pneumonia'. The honeycomb appearance is maintained when the fungus infects other, solid, organs also. Occasionally, the cell induces a granulomatous reaction, mimicking military tuberculosis. This is the only mycosis where specific immunohistochemistry has a diagnostic role.

Effects of antifungal and other therapies

Chemotherapy is effective in systemic mycoses, when it can be delivered to the target infection through the bloodstream. Damaged and killed fungi are phagocytosed by macrophages, which reduces their density in tissues and changes their shape, usually rendering them smaller. This can cause confusion in yeast infections such as *Cryptococcus neoformans*: the capsule can shrink, so removing a diagnostic feature of the infections, and the cell body shrinks or crenates, so that they may resemble smaller yeasts such as *Histoplasma*

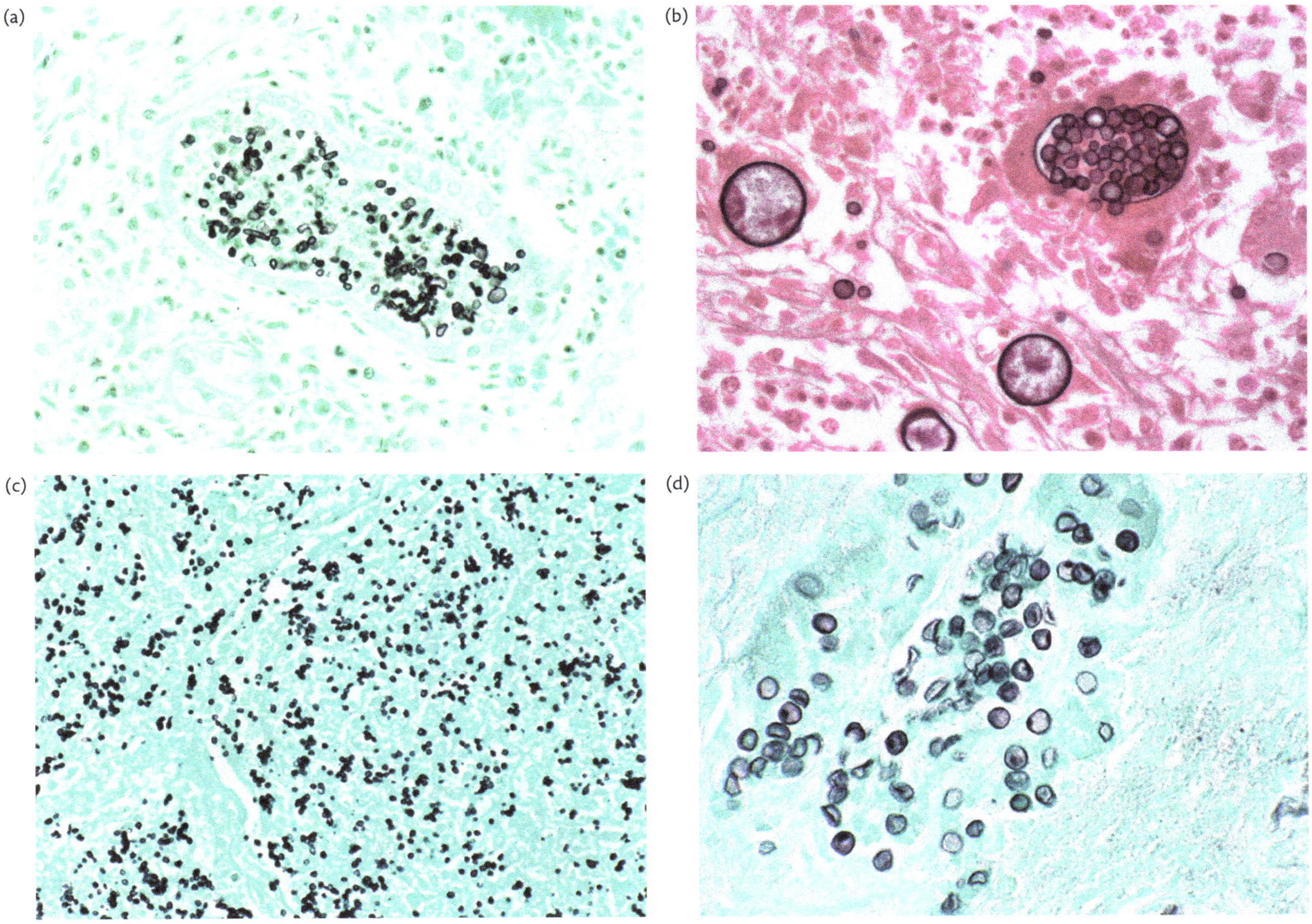

Figure 40.3 Yeasts.

a *Candida albicans* in kidney. The combination of small- to medium-sized yeasts with short hyphae is characteristic of this infection (dimorphism). Methenamine silver stain.

b *Coccidioides immitis* in lymph node. Medium- to large-sized spherules, some collapsing. One contains characteristic small endospores. Methenamine silver stain.

c *Histoplasma capsulatum* in lung. Uniform small yeasts which are budding. Methenamine silver stain.

d *Pneumocystis jirovecii* in lung. Small yeast-like cysts with the pathognomonic 'dot' density on one side of the cell wall. Methenamine silver stain.

Reproduced courtesy of Sebastian B. Lucas.

capsulatum. Treated PCP results in the yeast cells shrinking to a compact granular mass, though still discernible as small discs with the GMS stain.

The hyphae of treated aspergillosis can also become distorted and may resemble a Mucorales.

A related phenomenon is the immune reconstitution inflammatory syndrome (IRIS), when treatments bring depressed host immunity back towards normal. This is most commonly seen in HIV infection following specific antiretroviral therapy, where the host reaction (often previously minimal or absent) becomes granulomatous, or a mixed granulomatous-acute inflammation, with or without necrosis (Lucas and Nelson 2015). Cryptococcosis is particularly susceptible to IRIS reactions, and in the meninges the augmented granulomatous reaction can lead to hydrocephalus and death.

Eumycotic mycetomas are notable for their resistance to antifungal chemotherapy. The grains of the pigmented *Madurella mycetomatis* are coated in a melanin derived from the fungus which inhibits their destruction by macrophages, enzymatic lysis, and oxidants, as well as their killing by drugs (Zijlstra et al. 2016).

Pseudo-fungi and other differential diagnoses

From experience, mycotic infections can be overdiagnosed on histopathology, there being a wide range of fungal look-alikes which include both non-infection and other-infection entities.

Liesegang rings. These are rounded structures that derive from breakdown of cell material and mucins that resemble large yeasts, and so cause confusion with *Coccidioides* and parasite eggs. The lack of consistent structure, internal cell structure, and staining with GMS and PAS indicate they are not fungi.

'Pseudo-fungi' is a term sometime applied to free and intracellular structures that resemble hyphae, even apparently septate and branching, but they are degenerate host collagen material that has become encrusted in iron and/or calcium, and so appear brown or blue on H&E stains (Lyapichev et al. 2016). The fungal special stains are negative.

Myospherulosis. In chronic tissue lesions with haemorrhage (often with previous antibiotic treatment), the red cells may die but remain visible as spheres, and around clusters there forms an encircling eosinophilic membrane (Figure 40.4a). Thus, this can resemble *Coccidioides* with its endosphere, or a parasitic infection. Again, GMS and PAS stains are negative.

Fibrin strands. Within vessels, fixation and tissue processing can make fibrin polymerize into strands that look like fungal hyphae. PAS and GMS stains are negative, and the pseudohyphae lack internal structure.

Lysosomal junk. PAS and GMS stains inevitably incur visible 'noise', such as granules within macrophages that might resemble small yeasts. These are large lysosomes with phagocytosed debris; the lack of internal structure and their irregular morphology indicate that they are not yeast cells.

Pulmonary alveolar proteinosis (PAP). The proteinaceous eosinophilic material in PAP can resemble pneumocystosis, but it lacks the internal nuclei of the yeast, and does not stain with PAS and GMS.

There are also several genuine infections that histologically resemble yeasts and hyphae:

Algal infection and protothecosis. Algal infections are uncommon in man, but, when they occur, look very like yeast infections histologically. Skin infection with *Prototheca* species, following traumatic implantation, results in rounded medium-large cells which are PAS and GMS positively stained (Figure 40.4b). These can also contain two to eight tightly-packed endospores, but the organisms are smaller than *Coccidioides* species. Joint and disseminated infections, including meningitis, are rare (Bennett et al. 2010).

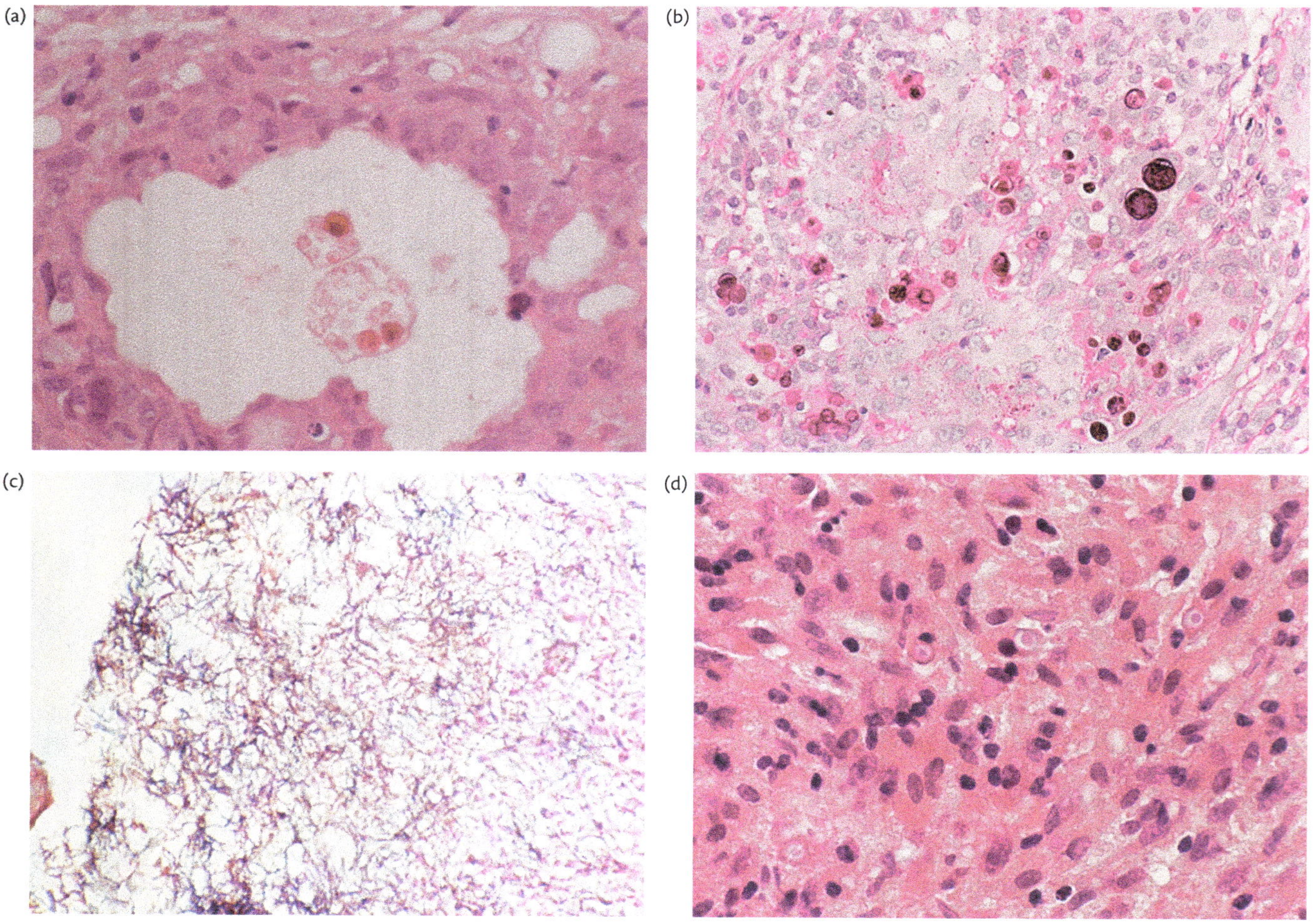

Figure 40.4 Pseudo-fungi.

a Myospherulosis in the subcutis. Chronic inflammation around a cyst-like structure which contains yeast-like bodies—these are denatured red blood cells. Haematoxylin & eosin (H&E) stain.

b Protothecosis in the subcutis. Very irregular yeast-like bodies, some of which contain multiple internal nuclei. Periodic acid-Schiff stain.

c Actinomycosis in the lung. A mass of branching, fragmenting, and beaded thin bacilli; at 1-2 μ thick, they are narrower than fungal hyphae which are >5 μ thick. Gram stain.

d Malakoplakia in the kidney. Several macrophages contain haematoxyphilic intra-cytoplasmic bodies, some of them 'targetoid' in form. H&E stain.

Reproduced courtesy of Sebastian B. Lucas.

Rhinosporidiosis. Rhinosporidium seeberi is a chronic infection of mucus membranes in cattle and man. Most cases occur in the Indian sub-continent. Previously considered to be a fungus, by DNA analysis it is now known to be a protistan parasite. As well as in the nose, polyps form on the conjunctiva, containing large numbers of the infectious agent. The histopathology is pathognomonic, with large sporangia containing numerous endospores.

Bacterial infections—actinomycosis, nocardiosis, streptomycosis, botryomycosis, and malakoplakia

Actinomycosis. Actinomyces israelii is a commensal in the oropharynx, but can cause infection with abscesses in the lungs, liver, appendix, and female genital tract. The bacilli are branching, beaded, and gram/GMS positive, and have a diameter <1 μ (Figure 40.4c).

Nocardiosis. Nocardia species are morphologically similar to *A. israelii* infection when disseminated; also, these species are usually weakly-ZN staining. *Nocardia* and *Actinomadura* species are also common causes of mycetoma, along with *Streptomyces somaliensis*, where the morphology is of small compact colonies. Again, the thin filaments are gram/GMS-positive. Eumycetomas are, in comparison, true hyphal infections with diameters >5 μ.

Botryomycosis refers to dense clumps of bacteria, usually gram-positive *Staphylococcus aureus*, within acute inflammation, in the meninges, lung, and solid tissues; it can look like a small yeast infection, but the cocci are only 1–2 μ.

Finally, *malakoplakia*—a chronic gram-negative bacillus inflammatory process—has characteristic Michaelis-Gutmann intracytoplasmic bodies in macrophages, which can resemble small- to medium-sized yeasts (Figure 40.4d). These are haematoxyphilic blobs, which do not take up silver stains.

Conclusion

Histopathology has a critical role in the diagnosis of fungal infections—both for confirmation and exclusion. In many instances, the only tissue available is fixed and paraffin-embedded (FFPE), so the onus is on the pathologist to identify fungi and to specify them if possible. As a technical advance, molecular diagnostic techniques increasingly work well on FFPE tissue.

In summary, multidisciplinary collaboration—involving clinical, imaging, culture, cytological morphology, histopathology, and molecular methods—is the key to accurate diagnosis and optimum management of patients with fungal infections.

References

Anstead GM, Sutton DA and Graybill JR (2012) Adiaspiromycosis causing respiratory failure and a review of human infections due to *Emmonsia* and *Chrysosporium* spp. *J Clin Microbiol* 50: 1346–54.

Antachopoulos C (2010) Invasive fungal infections in congenital immunodeficiencies. *Clin Microbiol Infect* 16: 1335–42.

Bennett JE et al. (2010) Mycoses, *in*: GL Mandell, JE Bennett and R Dolin, eds, *Principles and Practice of Infectious Diseases* (7th edn, Philadelphia: Churchill Livingstone), 3221–408.

Dhaliwal HS, Singh A, Sinha SK, et al. (2015) Diagnosed only if considered: isolated renal mucormycosis. *Lancet* 385: 2322.

Fidel PL, Vazquez JA and Sobel JD (1999) *Candida glabrata*: review of epidemiology, pathogenesis, and clinical disease with comparison to *C. albicans. Clin Microbiol Rev* 12: 80–96.

Franco-Paredes C, Womack T, Bohlmeyer T, et al. (2015) Management of *Cryptococcus gattii* meningoencephalitis. *Lancet Infect Dis* 15: 348–55.

Guarner J and Brandt ME (2011) Histopathologic diagnosis of fungal infections in the 21st century. *Clin Microbiol Rev* 24: 247–80.

Hay RJ and Morris Jones R (2010) New molecular tools in the diagnosis of superficial fungal infections. *Clin Dermatol* 28: 190–6.

Health Protection Agency (2006) Fungal diseases in the UK—the current provision of support for diagnosis and treatment: assessment and proposed network solution. Report of a working group of the HPA Advisory Committee for Fungal Infection and Superficial Parasites, Health Protection Agency, London.

Jabeen K, Farooqi J, Zafar A, et al. (2011) *Rhinocladiella mackenziei* as an emerging cause of cerebral phaeohyphomycosis in Pakistan: a case series. *Clin Infect Dis* 15: 213–17.

Lucas SB (2015) Fungal infections, *in*: S Love, H Budka, JW Ironside and A Perry, eds, *Greenfield's Neuropathology*, Vol. II (9th edn, Boca Raton, FL: CRC Press), 1281–96.

Lucas S and Nelson AM (2015) HIV and the spectrum of human disease. *J Pathol* 235: 229–41.

Lyapichev KA, Agarwal A, Rosenberg AE and Chapman JR (2016) Pseudofungi: a diagnostic pifall. *Int J Surg Pathol* 24: 528–31.

Neblett Fanfair R, Benedict K, Bos J, et al. (2012) Necrotizing cutaneous mucormycosis after a tornado in Joplin, Missouri, in 2011. *N Engl J Med* 167: 2214–25.

Paterson PJ, Seaton S, McLaughlin J and Kibbler CC (2003) Development of molecular methods for the identification of aspergillus and emerging moulds in paraffin wax embedded tissue sections. *Mol Pathol* 56: 368–70.

Radio SJ, Hansen S, Goldsmith J and Linder J (1990) Immunohistochemistry of Pneumocystis carinii infection. *Mol Pathol* 3: 462–9.

Rickerts V, Mousset S, Lambrecht E, et al. (2011) Comparison of quantitative real time PCR with sequencing and ribosomal RNA-FISH for the identification of fungi in formalin fixed, paraffin-embedded tissue specimens. *BMC Infect Dis* 11: 202. doi: 10.1186/1471-2334-11-202

Ritter JM, Muehlenbachs A, Blau DM, Paddock CD, and the *Exserohilum* Infections Working Group (2013) *Exserohilum* infections associated with contaminated steroid injections: a clinicopathologic review of 40 cases. *Am J Pathol* 183: 881–92.

Roehmel JF, Tintelnot K, Bernhardt A, Siebold M, Staab D and Schwartz C (2015) *Arxula adeninivorans* causing invasive pulmonary mycosis and fungaemia in cystic fibrosis. Lancet 385: 1476.

Ruangritchankul K, Chindamporn A, Worasilchai N, Poumsuk U, Keelawat S and Bychkov A (2015) Invasive fungal disease in university hospital: a PCR-based study of autopsy cases. *Int J Clin Exp Pathol* 8: 14840–52.

Schelenz S, Barnes RA, Barton RC, et al. (2015) British Society for Medical Mycology best practice recommendations for the diagnosis of serious fungal infections. *Lancet Infect Dis* 15: 461–74.

Schelenz S, Barnes RA, Kibbler CC, Jones BL and Denning DW (2009) Standards of care for patients with invasive fungal infections within the UK: a national audit. *J Infect* 58: 145–53.

Worth F and Goldani LZ (Review Article: Epidemiology of *Rhodotorula*: an emerging pathogen. *Interdiscip Perspect Infect Dis* 2012, Article ID 465717. doi: 10.1155/2012/465717

Zijlstra EE, van de Sande WWJ, Welsh O, Mahgoub ES, Goodfellow M and Fahal AH (2016) Mycetoma: a unique neglected tropical disease. *Lancet Infect Dis* 16: 100–12.

CHAPTER 41

The imaging of fungal disease

Joanne Cleverley

Introduction to the imaging of fungal infection

Imaging is routinely used to diagnose and assess the extent of fungal infection. There are several imaging modalities available which can be used to aid in the diagnosis of fungal infection, these are: the plain radiograph, computed tomography (CT), magnetic resonance imaging (MRI), ultrasound and nuclear medicine isotope imaging such as CT–positron emission tomography (CT-PET). Deciding on the most appropriate imaging modality to use depends upon which is the most appropriate to answer the clinical question, the organ or organs to be imaged, and the patient's state of health.

Plain radiography, CT, and CT-PET use ionizing radiation to obtain an image, whereas ultrasound and MRI use non-ionizing radiation.

CT imaging is used to image the thorax, sinuses, head, and abdomen. When describing how CT imaging has been obtained, different terms have been used over time, including high-resolution CT (HRCT), spiral or helical CT, and latterly multi-detector CT (MDCT). HRCT is a traditional axial CT examination of the thorax to assess lung parenchyma in fine detail and was used to diagnose pulmonary fungal infection. Only one image 1–3 mm thick was obtained for each rotation of the X-ray tube at 10 mm intervals; consequently, only a portion of the thorax was imaged. With developments in CT technology, initially spiral CT was developed where the X-ray tube and a single row of opposite detectors rotated whilst the patient moved through the CT scanner. This enabled contiguous images to be obtained in a single breath hold in contrast to the required breath holds in traditional axial CT. MDCT is an advancement over spiral CT as multiple detectors—often 128 or 256—are used to obtain the images, enabling higher acquisition speed, greater coverage of the patient, and improved resolution with a volumetric data set. Images can then be reconstructed in the axial, coronal, and sagittal planes (Sundaram et al. 2010). Intravenous iodinated contrast can be used to show blood vessels and organ enhancement, though its use is contraindicated with allergy to iodine and decreased renal function (The Royal College of Radiologists 2015). Imaging can be obtained in the arterial phase approximately 30 seconds after injection of contrast—and/or in the venous phase, approximately 60–70 seconds after injection. Imaging in the arterial phase highlights arteries and any mass with an arterial blood supply, whereas imaging in the portal phase shows the organs such as the pleura of the lung, liver, and kidneys in more detail and any lesions within them. CT can also be used for biopsy of suspected fungal lesions to obtain a tissue diagnosis.

MRI is used to image the sinuses, brain, and abdomen. In a similar way to CT, images can be obtained in the axial, coronal, and sagittal planes. The examination lasts longer than a CT examination, is more claustrophobic, and very unwell patients often cannot be safely monitored. The advantage of MRI over CT is the extent of soft tissue detail and its ability to detect lesions which are not apparent on CT. MRI uses different pulse imaging sequences of proton relaxation times to show abnormality. The commonest used sequences are T1-weighted and T2-weighted, where T1 represents longitudinal relaxation time and T2 represents transverse relaxation time. T1-weighted images are used to differentiate anatomical structures where fat appears bright and water is black; T2-weighted images are used to demonstrate pathology as the majority of lesions contain a high water content, which appear bright. Fungal infection on MR images appears bright on T2-weighted images, but as fungal infection often causes haemorrhage, the signal may be reduced or the image may appear black owing to the paramagnetic effect of haemoglobin and paramagnetic particles (iron and manganese) often found in some fungi. Correspondingly, on T1-weighted images some fungal lesions are bright. These signal changes should raise the suspicion of possible fungal infection. T1-weighted images with intravenous gadolinium can also be used to show fungal abscess more clearly and—similar to CT images—can be obtained in the arterial and venous phase. Gadolinium is potentially contraindicated in renal disease with a low estimated glomerular filtration rate (<30 mL/min) because of the risk of developing nephrogenic systemic fibrosis (The Royal College of Radiologists 2015). Other imaging sequences such as FLAIR (fluid-attenuated inversion recovery), which is a heavily T2-weighted sequence, diffusion-weighted images, and apparent diffusion coefficients, which image how quickly protons can diffuse, can be used to show subtle lesions more clearly, helping to confirm the diagnosis (Luthra et al. 2007).

Ultrasonography has the advantage over CT and MRI in that it is portable and can be used by the bedside. It used in the imaging and management of pleural effusion, imaging the abdomen, neck, and brain of the neonate via the fontanelle. Ultrasonography can also be used to biopsy suspected fungal lesions and drain fluid collections such as a pleural effusion.

CT-PET, which is hybrid imaging where the radio-isotope image is merged with the CT image to pin-point areas of abnormal increased metabolic activity, may have a role in quantifying the extent of fungal disease and the organs involved. However, the findings can be non-specific and similar to those found with disseminated malignancy and other infections (Sharma et al. 2014).

Imaging of thoracic fungal infection

The lungs are the commonest site of fungal infection owing to inhalation of fungus and fungal spores. Chest radiography, MDCT imaging, and ultrasonography are the imaging modalities routinely used to investigate fungal disease in the thorax. The chest radiograph is the initial investigation of choice for assessment and follow-up of fungal infection. Although it does have limitations—it can appear normal despite the patient being symptomatic—there is a lag time before abnormality is detected compared with CT, which provides more accurate information as to the extent and location of fungal infection. The CT appearances can be diagnostic and may lead to a change in managing infections (Barloon et al. 1991; Heussel et al. 1996; Gruden et al. 1997). Using MDCT, contiguous 1 mm sections are obtained in a similar way to traditional HRCT except that all of the thorax is imaged in one breath hold and the images are then reconstructed in the axial, coronal, and sagittal planes (Sundaram et al. 2010). Post-processing of MDCT images using multi-intensity projection allows small lesions to be identified more clearly (Gruden et al. 2002). Intravenous iodinated contrast media is used to assess for mediastinal, pleural, and vascular disease. Ultrasonography is used to assess for pleural disease and effusion with a view to potential drainage.

Many radiographic abnormalities—identified by a chest radiograph and CT examination, which can be seen in fungal infection. The Fleischner Society has described and defined these abnormalities in its glossary of terms; these are outlined in Table 41.1 (Hansell et al. 2008).

Pulmonary aspergillosis

There is a wide spectrum of pulmonary disease caused by *Aspergillus* species, usually *A fumigatus,* that often overlaps and is related to the immune status of the host (Franquet et al. 2001; Kousha et al. 2011) (see Chapters 30 and 37). It is recognized that pulmonary aspergillosis can be divided radiographically into five categories (Franquet et al. 2001; Desai et al. 2015): saprophytic, hypersensitivity (such as allergic bronchopulmonary aspergillosis, ABPA), chronic pulmonary, airway-invasive, and angio-invasive.

Saprophytic aspergillosis or simple aspergilloma (fungus ball) is due to colonization, but not tissue invasion, of pre-existing lung cavities, cysts, or bronchiectatic airways by aspergillosis infection (Franquet et al. 2001). Colonization occurs commonly in cavities due to previous tuberculosis and sarcoidosis. The radiographic findings are of single or multiple upper lobe cavities containing an aspergilloma (Figure 41.1a). The aspergilloma is separated from the wall by an airspace called an 'air crescent and, classically, the aspergilloma changes in position in relation to the position of the patient (Franquet et al. 2001). CT is of value as the size and wall thickness of the cavity and fungus ball can be assessed, and not all aspergillomas are apparent on the chest radiograph (Figure 41.1b) (Kousha et al. 2011).

ABPA is a hypersensitivity response to aspergillosis and is commonly seen in patients with a long history of asthma or cystic fibrosis. The condition is characterized by the formation of bronchial mucoid plugs containing aspergillosis infection and eosinophils. The radiographic findings are tubular opacities extending towards the lung periphery—commonly in the upper lobes—which have the appearance of 'a finger in a glove' on the chest radiograph due to the impacted bronchial mucoid plugs (Franquet et al. 2001). Bronchiectasis develops over time and CT is more sensitive at defining the bronchiectasis and the extent of involvement (Figure 41.1c) (Franquet et al. 2001).

Chronic pulmonary aspergillosis (CPA) is a term used to cover the spectrum, often with overlap of the different types of chronic pulmonary aspergillosis infection, which include chronic cavitary pulmonary aspergillosis (CCPA), pulmonary chronic fibrosing pulmonary aspergillosis, and subacute invasive aspergillosis (Denning et al. 2016). When suggesting a diagnosis of CPA, reviews of

Table 41.1 Description of radiographic and CT abnormalities seen in fungal chest infection adapted from the Fleischner Society: glossary of terms

Abnormality	Description
Air bronchogram	Air filled bronchus on a background of opaque airless lung
Air crescent	Crescentic shape of air seen between a wall of a cavity and aspergilloma
Airspace	A gas-containing part of the lung. The term is often used to describe consolidation, increased opacification and nodules.
Bronchiectasis	Irreversible bronchial dilatation
Cavity	A gas-filled space seen within consolidation, mass, or nodule
Centrilobular	The site of the centre of the secondary pulmonary nodule where the respiratory bronchiole and intralobular pulmonary artery are situated
Consolidation	Homogenous increase in lung density obscuring the margins of vessels and bronchi
Cyst	An airspace surrounded by a wall of variable thickness
Ground-glass opacity	Increased area of hazy opacification; less dense than consolidation on the radiograph and CT scan. On CT, there is preservation of bronchial and vascular margins.
Halo sign	Ground glass opacification surrounding a nodule or mass
Mass and nodule	Mass is an opacity seen on radiographs or CT scans >3 cm in diameter. A nodule is an opacity <3 cm in size.
Reverse halo sign	A round area of ground-glass opacity surrounded by a ring of consolidation

Source: data from Hansell D. M. et al., 'Fleischner Society: glossary of terms for thoracic imaging', *Radiology*, Volume 246, Issue 3, pp. 697–722. Copyright © 2008 Radiological Society of North America. DOI: 10.1148/radiol.2462070712.

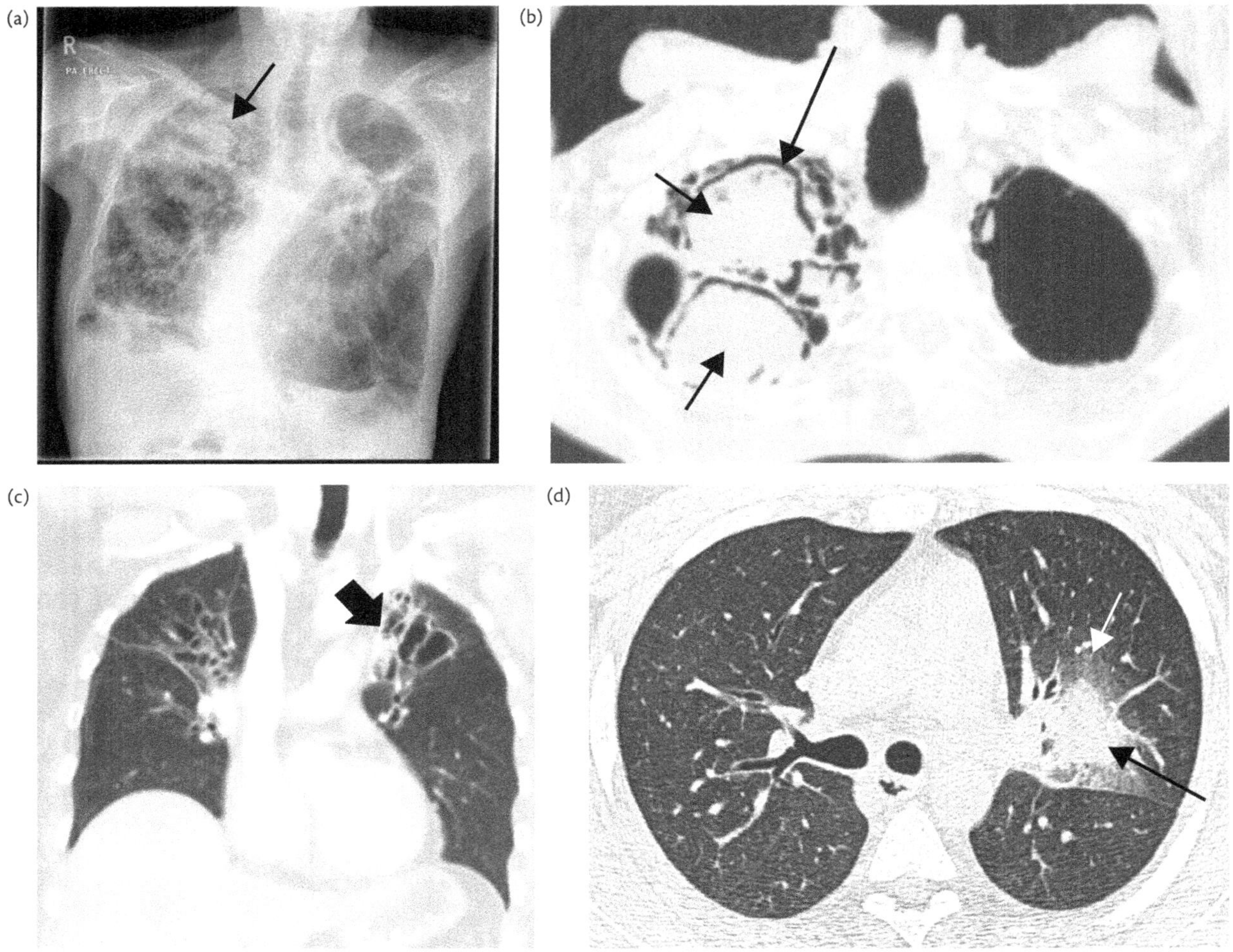

Figure 41.1 **a** Aspergilloma: chest radiograph of a 72-year-old male with a past history of tuberculosis. The chest radiograph shows fibrotic cavitary disease in both apices. In the right apex there is a mass surrounded by a crescent of air (arrow). In the left apex there is a large cavity.

b Aspergilloma: computed tomography (CT) image of the same patient at the lung apices on lung windows shows two right upper lobe aspergillomas (short arrows) with one only clearly identified on the chest radiograph surrounded by an air crescent (long arrow). There is a large left apical cavity containing air.

c Allergic bronchopulmonary aspergillosis (ABPA): coronal CT image at the level of the superior vena cava on lung windows of a 74-year-old female with known ABPA and bronchiectasis. The CT examination shows multiple proximal severely dilated upper lobe bronchi (arrow).

d Angio-invasive aspergillosis, halo sign: axial CT image of a 28-year-old male with relapsed acute myeloid leukaemia with neutropenic sepsis and previous proven fungal infection. CT scan shows a left upper nodule (black arrow) surrounded by a halo of ground-glass opacification (white arrow).

Reproduced courtesy of Joanne Cleverley.

serial chest radiographs are probably the most important diagnostic tool as they are used to assess serial change (Desai et al. 2015). The radiographic findings are those of persistent consolidation often involving a whole lobe of lung, leading to single or multiple cavities which may contain material with an upper zone predilection and pleural thickening (Desai et al. 2015). Without treatment, consolidation can progress to complete opacification of the lung and volume loss; this appearance is termed 'chronic fibrosing pulmonary aspergillosis' (Denning et al. 2016). CT findings are similar to those of the chest radiograph, though they provide more accurate detail as to the extent of cavitation, material seen within cavities, consolidation, and pleural thickening adjacent to areas of consolidation and cavitation, which is characteristic (Desai et al. 2015).

Airway-invasive aspergillosis is defined as invasion of the *Aspergillus* into the basement membrane of the airway (Franquet et al. 2001). Infection occurs in immunocompromised hosts and is more commonly seen in patients with AIDS, in patients post lung transplant, and in chemotherapy-induced neutropenia. The condition causes a tracheobronchitis, bronchiolitis, and bronchopneumonia. The imaging findings are often non-specific and cannot be distinguished from other bronchopneumonias. The CT findings are those of peribronchial consolidation and small airways involvement with centrilobular nodules (Franquet et al. 2001).

Angio-invasive aspergillosis occurs in those patients with profound neutropenia, and is due to invasion of pulmonary arteries by *Aspergillus* species.

The CT features are classically characterized as a soft tissue nodule surrounded by a ground-glass halo—the 'halo sign' (Figure 41.1d)—which, in the clinical setting of neutropenic sepsis, is often considered diagnostic for invasive *Aspergillus* infection

(Caillot et al. 2001, Franquet et al. 2001). The CT appearances correspond to a central area of necrosis with peripheral haemorrhagic ground-glass change, although the 'halo sign' has been described in immunosuppressed patients with *Candida*, cytomegalovirus, mucormycosis, and herpes simplex infection (Caillot et al. 2001; Franquet et al. 2001). With immune reconstitution and antifungal treatment, the halo sign is transitory and the central nodule cavitates with an air crescent identified on chest radiographs and CT scans (Franquet et al. 2001). A less specific CT finding of angio-invasive aspergillosis is of pleural-based wedge-shaped areas of consolidation consistent with haemorrhagic invasion. CT pulmonary angiography using intravenous contrast to opacify the pulmonary arteries may show small vessel occlusion subtending an area of wedge-shaped consolidation, confirming a diagnosis of pulmonary infarction rather than a bacterial pneumonia (Sonnet et al. 2005).

Thoracic candidiasis

Candida infection in the thorax is seen in the immunocompromised host. As it is a normal commensal of the mouth, oesophageal candidiasis is common. Barium studies of the oesophagus show impaired motility, with a narrowing of the oesophageal lumen, a "cobblestone" appearance of the oesphageal wall, and ulceration (Lewicki and Moore 1975). Pulmonary infection is seen less commonly, and the CT findings of *Candida* infection are those primarily of random small nodules and consolidation (Franquet et al. 2005). The halo sign is also a recognized though unusual finding, and the appearances are indistinguishable from angio-invasive aspergillosis (Franquet et al. 2005).

Pneumocystis jirovecii infection

Pneumocystis jirovecii infection is commonly associated with HIV (human immunovirus) infection and a low CD4 count. The radiographic presentation is of a bilateral perihilar or diffuse symmetrical pattern and has a finely granular, reticular, or ground-glass appearance (Boiselle et al. 1999). It is recognized that CT accurately diagnoses *Pneumocystis* pneumonia, particularly when the radiograph is non-diagnostic (Gruden et al. 1997). The CT findings are of extensive ground-glass change (Figure 41.2) in a patchy or geographic distribution (Boiselle et al. 1999). Septal lines and consolidation may be present. Additional findings are of lung cysts or pneumatoceles of variable size and shape (Boiselle et al. 1999).

Pulmonary Mucorales infection

Pulmonary mucormycosis is seen in those patients who are immunocompromised or diabetic, often with other organs involved (McAdams 1997; Chung et al. 2010). The radiographic findings are often non-specific with single or multiple areas of consolidation, nodules, cavitation, and adenopathy (McAdams 1997). It is recognized that nodules with a halo sign can initially be seen on CT examination, which then evolve rapidly and increase in size, changing into a nodule with a reverse halo sign (Figure 41.3). This evolutionary change should be considered potentially diagnostic (Chung et al. 2010).

Endemic and other fungal pulmonary infection

The imaging of pulmonary cryptococcosis and endemic fungal infection due to histoplasmosis, coccidioidomycosis, blastomycosis, and paracoccidioidomycosis, is non-specific, often with a myriad of radiographic findings on the chest radiograph and CT examination, as outlined in Table 41.2, leading to a potential delay in diagnosis. The imaging findings often mimic TB, carcinoma, and lymphoma (Figure 41.4) (Hansell et al. 2005). The reverse halo sign is identified in paracoccidioidomycosis infection, and in the appropriate clinical setting is considered diagnostic (Gasparetto 2005). Pleural effusion occurs rarely.

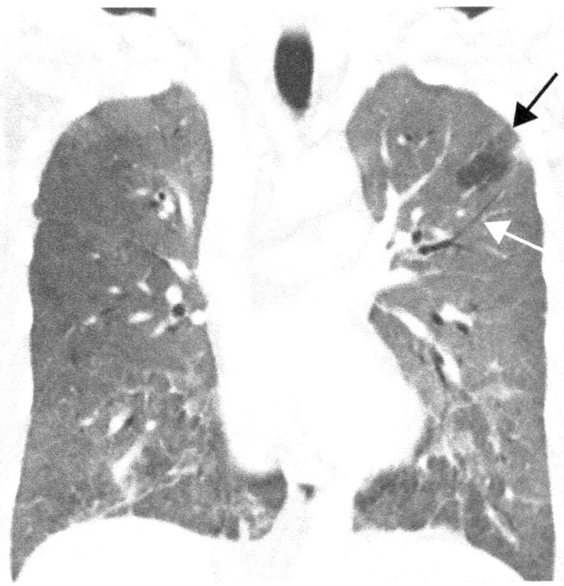

Figure 41.2 *Pneumocystis jirovecii* infection. CT examination with intravenous contrast of a 30-year-old male newly diagnosed with HIV who presented with a history of cough and worsening breathlessness. Coronal image on lung windows at the level of the superior vena cava shows extensive ground-glass change in both lungs, and normal black bronchus (white arrow). There is a small focal area of ground-glass sparing in the left upper lobe (black arrow).
Reproduced courtesy of Joanne Cleverley.

Imaging of sinonasal fungal infection

CT is the initial investigation for suspected sinonasal fungal infection as plain radiographs are insensitive (Lund et al. 2000). Magnetic resonance imaging with intravenous gadolinium enhancement is used to complement the CT examination, assessing for suspected intracranial and orbital extension (Lund et al. 2000).

Aspergillus, *Candida*, and mucoraceous mould species are commonly associated with fungal sinonasal infection, presenting as a chronic sinusitis which has not responded to conventional therapy. Sinonasal fungal infection can be classified into four subcategories, which can have different radiological appearances: fungal ball or mycetoma, allergic fungal rhinosinusitis, acute fulminant invasive sinusitis infection in immunocompromised hosts, and chronic invasive infection in immunocompetent hosts (Lund et al. 2000).

The fungus ball usually involves a single sinus with the maxillary sinus commonly involved; it is non-invasive with no bony destruction (Lund et al. 2000). On CT, the fungus ball is usually polypoid in appearance, though the sinus can be completely opacified (Lund et al. 2000; Madani and Beale 2009). The density of the fungus ball is often higher on CT owing to calcium, manganese, and iron found in fungal hyphae, and because these elements have paramagnetic properties, the fungus ball is hypointense on T1-weighted and T2-weighted

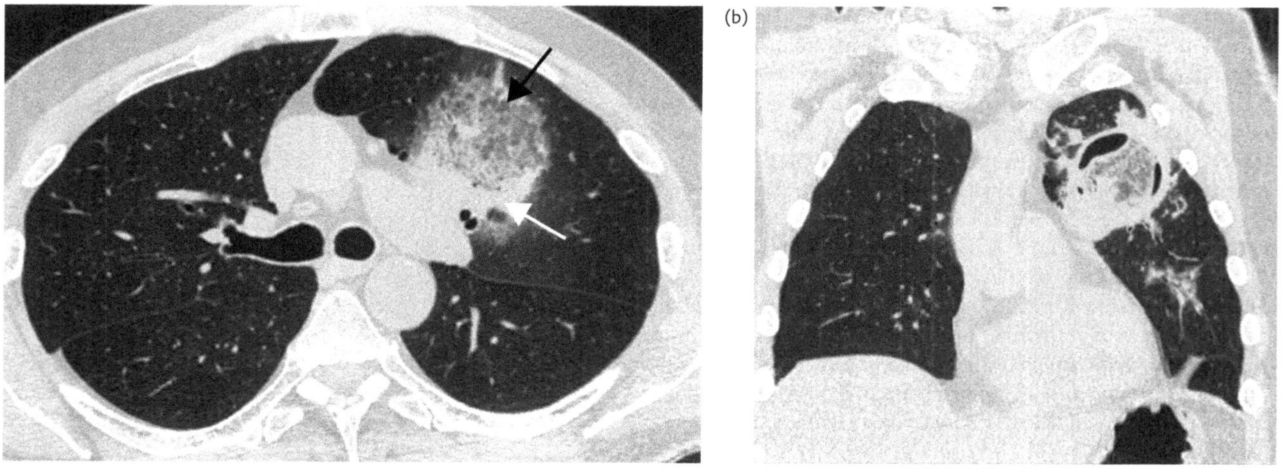

Figure 41.3 **a** Reverse halo sign: computed tomography (CT) image of lung windows of a 64-year-old male with relapsed acute myeloid leukaemia post bone marrow transplant presenting with neutropenic sepsis. The initial axial CT scan shows a left upper lobe mass which is predominantly of ground-glass density (black arrow) with a peripheral posterior curvilinear area of solid density or consolidation (white arrow).

b CT three-week-later coronal image shows that this mass has become more organized with a circumferential ring of solid tissue, with a decrease in size of the central ground-glass density and early cavitation seen as an area of blackness between the outer rim and the ground-glass change. The patient went on to have a left upper lobe lobectomy and the lesion was due to *Aspergillus* infection, which is an unusual but recognized cause of the reverse halo sign.

Reproduced courtesy of Joanne Cleverley.

Table 41.2 Radiographic findings in thoracic endemic fungal infection

Histoplasmosis	***Acute form:*** Single or multifocal consolidation; hilar adenopathy Multiple nodules—often miliary ***Chronic form:*** Fibrocavitary upper lobe disease Histoplasmoma—slow-growing nodule, mimicking carcinoma Mediastinal fibrosis and granuloma formation with compression of mediastinal structures Calcified granuloma in lungs and lymph nodes
Coccidioidomycosis	***Acute form:*** Single or multifocal consolidation Consolidation with cavitation Nodules with cavitation on CT scan Nodules with halo sign on CT mediastinal and hilar adenopathy ***Chronic form:*** Coccidioidomycoma—nodule mimicking carcinoma Cavities with fibroapical disease
Blastomycosis	***Acute form:*** Single or multiple areas Non-segmental consolidation Nodules of variable size; can be large Can mimic lung carcinoma Miliary nodules often seen in disseminated infection Cavities thin or thick walled, single or multiple; can mimic TB and histoplasmosis
Paracoccidioidomycosis	***Chronic form:*** Lung most commonly involved: Nodules Cavities Consolidation Fibrosis CT 'reverse halo sign'
Cryptococcosis	Immunocompetent—multiple nodules of variable size Immunocompromised—consolidation, solid and cavitary nodules

Source: data from Hansell D. M., Armstrong P., Lynch D. A. and McAdams H. P. (2005) *Imaging of Diseases of the Chest*, Fourth Edition, Philadelphia: Elsevier Mosby, Copyright © Mosby 2010

MR images, causing a possible signal void which can mimic air (Lund et al. 2000).

Allergic fungal rhinosinusitis causes extensive, often complete, bilateral sinus opacification with bony expansion (Figure 41.5). The CT findings are those of opacified sinuses containing foci of calcium, which is often central and fine (Madani and Beale 2009). The MR findings are similar to those found in a fungal ball owing to paramagnetic materials contained within the fungal hyphae (Lund et al. 2000).

Acute fulminant invasive sinusitis occurs in the immunocompromised host, generally in those with profound neutropenia or poorly controlled diabetes. The CT and MR findings are those of sinus disease with bony destruction and invasion of adjacent structures: orbits, nasopharynx, skull base, and intracranial extension. MRI demonstrates a greater sensitivity at defining the extent of this

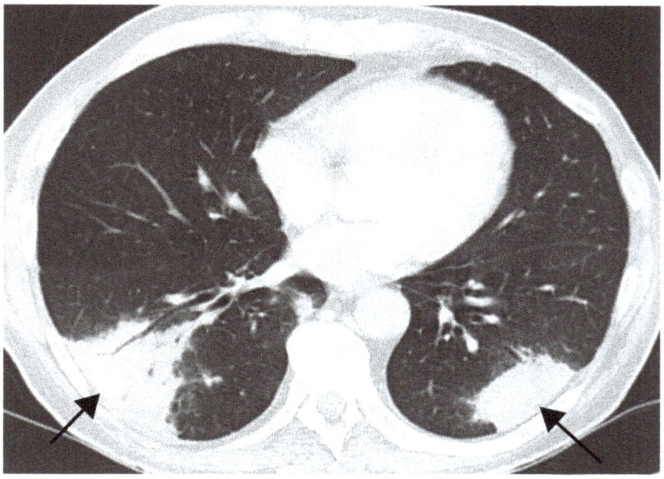

Figure 41.4 A *Cryptococcus* 64-year-old male post liver transplant is non-specifically unwell. Contrast-enhanced computed tomography (CT) examination of the lower lobes on lung windows shows multifocal areas of consolidation (black arrows). The differential diagnosis prior to biopsy was infection, cryptogenic organizing pneumonia, or lymphoma. CT-guided biopsy confirmed *Cryptococcus* infection.
Reproduced courtesy of Joanne Cleverley.

sinus disease (Lund et al. 2000; Madani and Beale 2009). As the infection is acute, high-density fungal material is often absent on CT (Lund et al. 2000).

Chronic invasive rhinosinusitis is more indolent and can be difficult to distinguish from allergic fungal sinusitis (Lund et al. 2000), although, over time, CT and MRI demonstrate invasion of adjacent bone and structures (Lund et al. 2000).

Imaging of fungal infection of the central nervous system

In suspected CNS fungal infection due to *Aspergillus*, *Candida*, and *Cryptococcus* species, CT and/or MRI is used to assess for abnormality and extent. In neonates, ultrasonography is routinely used and can have similar findings to MRI (Huang et al. 1998). CT is often the initial investigation in the acute setting as it is a relatively short examination and readily available.

Aspergillus infection of the central nervous system

CNS *Aspergillus* infection occurs in the immunocompromised host and arises either because of haematogenous spread commonly from lung, or by direct sinonasal invasion. There are three recognized imaging patterns of CNS aspergillosis infection: angio-invasive infarction, ring-enhancing mass lesions, and dural enhancement due to direct invasion (Ashdown et al. 1994).

As aspergillosis is angio-invasive, it causes multiple areas of infarction, which may lead to haemorrhagic infarction. The infarction occurs at the corticomedullary junction, but additionally involves the basal ganglia, corpus callosum, and brainstem owing to involvement of the small perforating arteries, not commonly seen in other infections (Delone et al. 1999). The imaging findings of infarction are of focal areas of low density on CT, and hyperintensity on T2-weighted images, at these sites. If there is associated haemorrhage, these areas are of increased density on CT, and hypointense on T2-weighted MR images (Ashdown et al. 1994).

Ring-enhancing mass lesions may be due to *Aspergillus* abscesses; these are often irregular in outline and thick walled, unlike a pyogenic abscess (Ashdown et al. 1994). CT and MRI show peripheral ring enhancement following intravenous

(a) (b)

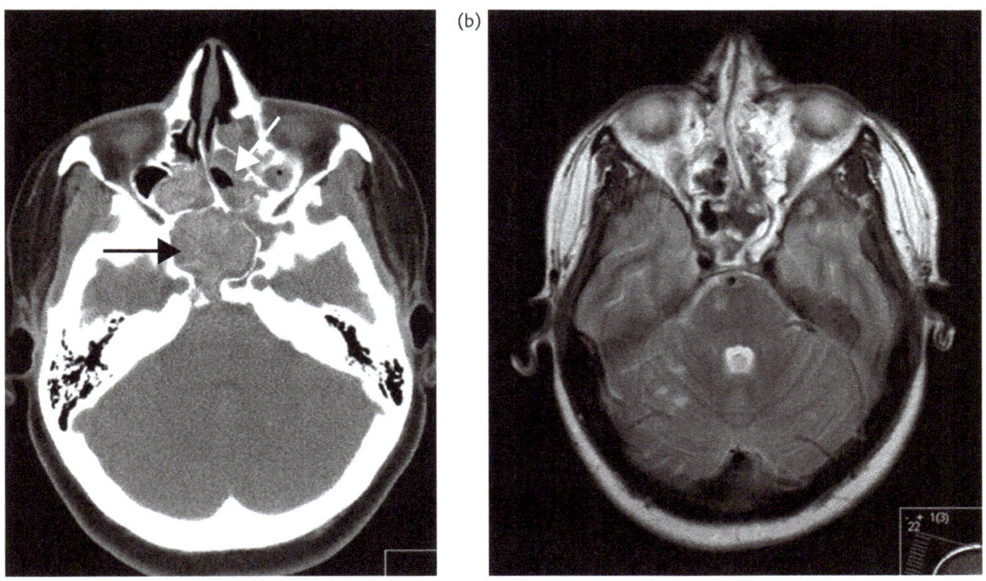

Figure 41.5 **a** Computed tomography (CT) image of chronic allergic fungal sinusitis in a 30-year-old female with headache. Axial CT on soft-tissue windows at the level of the sphenoid sinus showing the extent of bony expansion (black arrow) and the central high fungal density material within the sphenoid and the ethmoid sinuses (white arrow).

b Axial magnetic resonance T2-weighted image at a similar level to Figure 4a showing the signal voids in the sphenoid and ethmoid sinuses.
Reproduced courtesy of Joanne Cleverley.

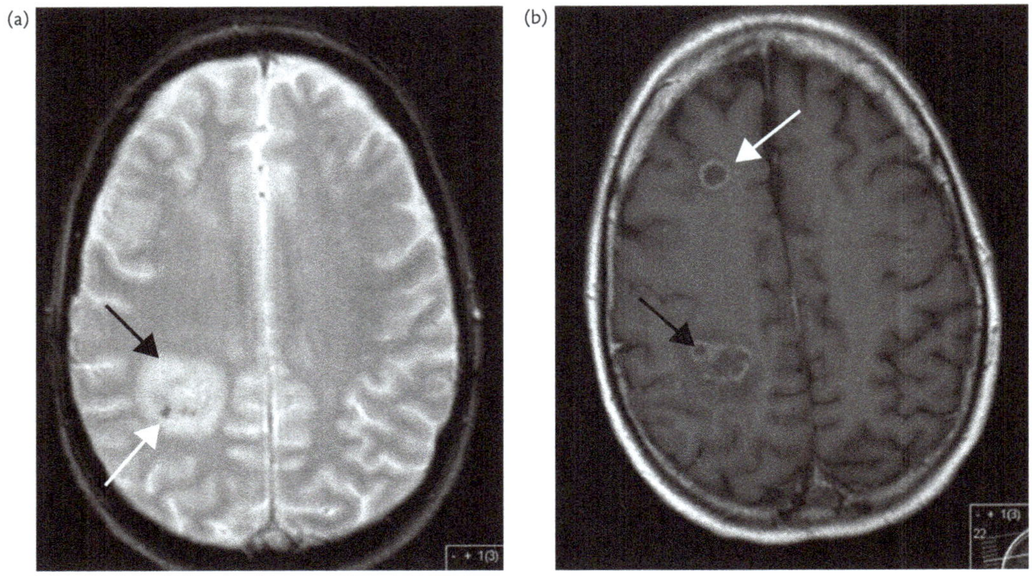

Figure 41.6 **a** Magnetic resonance (MR) scan of cerebral *Aspergillus* abscesses proven on stereotactic brain biospy. A 33-year-old male who has presented with ischaemic bowel with protracted long hospital stay presents with grand mal fits. Computed tomography examination shows ring-enhancing space-occupying lesions. The patient went on to have an MR examination to clarify further. Axial gradient T2-weighted image shows a mass lesion in the right parietal lobe (black arrow) with small foci of low signal within it, suggesting blood products or paramagnetic minerals (white arrow).

b T1-weighted axial post-intravenous gadolinium enhancement at the same level shows that the lesion in the parietal lobe is ring enhancing with an irregular wall, with an additional small satellite ring-enhancing nodule (black arrow). An additional ring-enhancing lesion is seen in the right frontal lobe (white arrow), which is not very visible on the corresponding T2-weighted image.

Reproduced courtesy of Joanne Cleverley.

contrast, though the extent of enhancement is often related to the patient's immune status (Yuh et al. 1994). On MRI examination, the abscess is usually hypointense on unenhanced T1-weighted images, though foci of high signal can be seen owing to either haemorrhage or paramagnetic particles, and on T2-weighted images the wall is hypointense with inner hyperintensity (Figure 41.6) (Ashdown et al. 1994).

Dural involvement, due to local invasion and direct extension from nasosinuses, orbit, or calvarium, is identified on MRI examination as dural thickening with enhancement post intravenous contrast. Further extension can then lead to local cerebral abscess formation and cavernous sinus thrombosis (Ashdown et al. 1994).

Candida infection of the central nervous system

CNS *candida* infection is often related to a central venous line infection, causing meningitis or cerebral abscesses. The abscesses can vary in size, though multiple microabscesses are often seen (Lai et al. 1997). It is a recognized infection in low birth weight premature neonates, with cranial ultrasound examination showing abscesses with an echogenic rim and hydrocephalus (Huang et al. 1998).

Cryptococcus infection of the central nervous system

Cryptococcus infection is commonly seen in patients with HIV infection who often present with meningitis. The imaging in these patients can be diverse with minimal abnormality identified. The recognized imaging findings are of leptomeningeal enhancement, with nodules, hydrocephalus, cysts in the basal ganglia, and intraventricular or parenchymal ring-enhancing cryptococcomas (Smith et al. 2008; Tien et al. 1991). The presence of non-enhancing and rapidly growing cysts or pseudocysts in the basal ganglia, due to dilated Virchow-Robin spaces, which are hyperintense on T2-weighted and hypointense on T1-weighted MR images, are considered diagnostic (Smith et al. 2008).

Imaging of other fungal infections of the central nervous system

The endemic mycotic infections blastomycosis, coccidioidomycosis, and paracoccidioidomycosis can cause CNS infection, although the imaging findings are normal or non-specific, which include ring-enhancing abscesses and/or leptomeningeal disease with thickened dura (Elias et al. 2005; Fang et al. 2007; Lammering et al. 2013).

Mucormycosis infection is either due to haematogenous spread in drug users with non-specific ring-enhancing cerebral abscesses or the consequence of sinonasal infection extending to involve the orbit and the basal portions of the cerebral hemispheres, brainstem, and hypothalamus. This typically appears hyperintense on T2-weighted MR images (Press et al. 1988; Siddiqi and Freedman 1994).

Imaging of fungal infection in the abdomen and pelvis

Ultrasonography, CT, and MRI can all be used to investigate suspected abdominal fungal infection. Ultrasonography is a quick, portable investigation and does not involve radiation, though it is less sensitive than CT or MRI (Moore et al. 2003). Contrast-enhanced CT or MRI have similar sensitivity and specificity for investigation of fungal infection (del Campo et al. 2014), although CT may be preferred in the first instance as it is quick and patients can be more easily monitored.

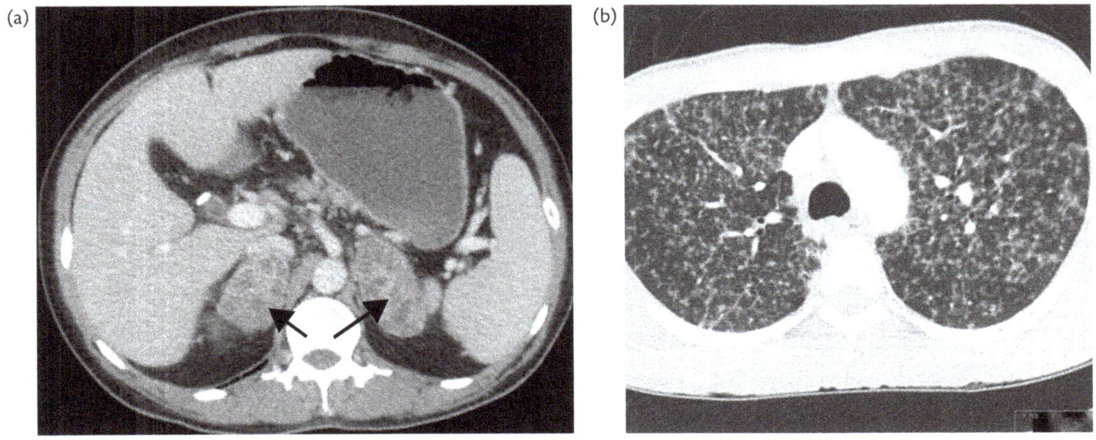

Figure 41.7 **a** Adrenal histoplasmosis. Axial computed tomography (CT) image of the upper abdomen of a 61-year-old male who presented with Addisonian crisis. CT examination of the adrenal glands post intravenous contrast shows symmetrical enlargement of the adrenal glands with heterogeneous enhancement (black arrows). The patient went on to have a CT-guided biopsy which confirmed the diagnosis of histoplasmosis.

b Pulmonary histoplasmosis. Axial CT scan with intravenous contrast of the upper lobes on lung windows of a 40-year-old male recently diagnosed with HIV shows widespread military nodules. Initially this was thought to be tuberculosis, but polymerase chain reaction and bronchoscopy were positive for histoplasmosis.

Reproduced courtesy of Joanne Cleverley.

Abdominal fungal infection in the neutropenic patient

Neutropenic fungal infection in the abdomen is usually due to *Aspergillus* and *Candida* species, often associated with disseminated infection. The liver, spleen, and kidneys are most commonly affected, though gastrointestinal tract involvement can occur, which is also associated with mucormycosis infection.

The imaging findings in the liver, spleen, and kidneys are similar with the development of abscesses and focal areas of infarction (del Campo et al. 2014). The hepatic fungal abscesses are often small and multiple and appear as ring enhancing on CT and MR examinations post intravenous contrast, and on ultrasound examination with an echogenic rim similar to that of a 'bull's eye' (del Campo et al. 2014). CT has similar sensitivity to MRI for detecting hepatic fungal abscesses when images are obtained in the arterial and portal venous phase, as the abscesses are more conspicuous in the arterial phase (del Campo et al. 2014). On MRI, the abscesses appear as focal hyperintense lesions on T2-weighted images, and iso- or hypo-intense on T1-weighted images.

In renal infection, mycetomas (fungal bezoars) can also form in the collecting system of the kidney, identified as irregular filling defects causing urinary obstruction (del Campo et al. 2014) (see Chapter 29).

Fungal gastrointestinal tract involvement is due to haemorrhagic invasion of the blood vessels causing vascular occlusion with haemorrhagic change and infarction seen within the bowel wall. Contrast-enhanced CT shows circumferential bowel wall thickening, which is poorly enhanced due to the infarcted and necrotic bowel (Schmit et al. 2008).

Abdominal endemic fungal infection

Histoplasmosis infection in the abdomen is more commonly associated with disseminated disease, particularly in those patients who are immunosuppressed and HIV positive (Radin 1991). The contrast-enhanced CT findings are those of lymphadenopathy, which often comprise necrosis (similar to TB infection), hepatosplenomegaly—with the spleen having areas of low density within it—and bilateral and symmetrical adrenal gland enlargement (Figure 41.7) (Radin 1991). Foci of calcium are often seen in the liver, spleen, and adrenal glands, indicating previous histoplasmosis infection in the immunocompetent host (Conces 1996).

Acute paracoccidioidomycosis in the acute phase causes hepatosplenomegaly and widespread adenopathy, similar to TB or lymphoma (Pereira et al. 2004). Adrenal gland involvement is a recognized finding in chronic disease where there is unilateral or asymmetrical bilateral adrenal gland enlargement. On contrast-enhanced CT the adrenal glands are irregular in outline and have a peripheral enhancing ring (Faiçal et al. 1996).

In summary, this chapter provides a current overview of the role of different imaging modalities and the radiographic findings in aiding the diagnosis of fungal infection in immunocompetent and immunocompromised hosts. In the future it is envisaged that advances in diagnosing fungal infection are to be made at a molecular level using hybrid imaging with radiolabelled antifungal or antifungal peptides to detect and monitor fungal infection (Gemmel et al. 2009).

Bone and joint fungal infection imaging

The imaging of bone and joint fungal infection is discussed in Chapter 20.

References

Ashdown BC, Tien RD and Felsberg GJ (1994) Aspergillosis of the brain and paranasal sinuses in immunocompromised patients: CT and MR imaging findings. *AJR Am J Roentgenol* 162: 155–9.

Barloon TJ, Galvin JR, Mori M, Stanford W and Cingrich RD (1991) High-resolution ultrafast CT in the clinical management of febrile bone marrow transplant patients with normal or nonspecific chest roentgenograms. *Chest* 99: 928–33.

Barretto MM, Marchiori E, Amorim VB, et al. (2012) Thoracic paracoccidioidomycosis: radiographic and CT findings. *Radiographics* 32: 71–84.

Boiselle PM, Crans CA and Kaplan MA (1999) The changing face of Pneumocystis carinii pneumonia in AIDS patients. *AJR Am J Roengenol* 172: 1301–9.

Caillot D, Couailler J-F, Bernard A, et al. (2001) Increasing volume and changing characteristics of invasive pulmonary aspergillosis on sequential thoracic computed tomography scans in patients with neutropenia. *J Clin Oncol* 19: 253–9.

Chung JH, Godwin JD, Chien JW and Pipavath SJ (2010) Case 160: Pulmonary mucormycosis. *Radiology* 256: 667–70.

Conces DJ Jr (1996) Histoplasmosis. *Semin Roetgenol* 16: 14–27.

del Campo L, León NG, Palacios DC, Lagana C and Tagarro D (2014) Abdominal complications following hematopoietic stem cell transplantation. *Radiographics* 34: 396–412.

DeLone DR, Goldstein RA, Petterman G, et al. (1999) Disseminated aspergillosis involving the brain: distribution and imaging characteristics. *AJNR Am J Neuroradiol* 20: 1597–604.

Denning DW, Cadranel J, Biegelman-Aubry C, et al. (2016) Chronic pulmonary aspergillosis: rational and clinical guidelines for diagnosis and management. *Eur Respir J* 47: 45–68.

Desai SR, Hedayati V, Patel K and Hansell DM (2015) Chronic aspergillosis of the lungs: unraveling the terminology and radiology. *Eur Radiol* 25: 3100–7.

Elias J Jr, dos Santos A, Carlotti CG Jr, et al. (2005) Central nervous system paracoccidioidomycosis: diagnosis and treatment. *Surg Neurol* 63 (Suppl. 1): S13–21.

Faiçal S, Borri ML, Hauache DM and Ajzen S (1996) Addison's disease caused by paracoccidioidomycosis brasiliensis: diagnosis by needle aspiration biopsy of the adrenal gland. *AJR Am J Roentgenol* 166: 461–2.

Fang W, Washington L and Kumar N (2007) Imaging manifestations of blastomycosis: a pulmonary infection with potential dissemination. *Radiographics* 27: 641–55.

Franquet T, Müller NL, Giménez A, Guembe P, de la Torre J and Bagué S (2001) Spectrum of pulmonary aspergillosis: histologic, clinical, and radiologic findings. *Radiographics* 21: 825–37.

Franquet T, Müller NL, Lee KS, Oikonomou A and Flint JD (2005) Pulmonary candidiasis after hematopoietic stem cell transplantation: thin-section CT findings. *Radiology* 236: 332–7.

Gasparetto EL, Escuissato DL, Davaus T, de Cerqueira EM, Souza AS Jr., Marchiori E and Müller NL (2005) Reversed halo sign in pulmonary paracoccidioidomycosis. *AJR Am J Roentgenol* 184: 1932–4.

Gemmel F, Dumary N and Welling M (2009) Future diagnostic agents. *Semin Nucl Med* 39: 11–36.

Gruden JF, Huang L, Turner J, et al. (1997) High-resolution CT in the evaluation of clinically suspected Pneumocystis carinii pneumonia in AIDS patients with normal, equivocal, or nonspecific radiographic findings. *AJR Am J Roentgenol* 169: 967–75.

Gruden JF, Ouanounou S, Tigges S, Norris DS and Klausner TS (2002) Incremental benefit of maximum-intensity-projection images on observer detection of small pulmonary nodules revealed by multidetector CT. *AJR Am J Roentgenol* 179: 149–57.

Hansell DM, Armstrong P, Lynch DA and McAdams HP (2005) *Imaging of Diseases of the Chest* (4th edn, Philadelphia: Elsevier Mosby).

Hansell DM, Bankier AA, MacMahon H, McLoud TC, Müller NL and Remy J (2008) Fleischner Society: glossary of terms for thoracic imaging. *Radiology* 246: 697–722.

Heussel CP, Kauczor H-U, Heussel GE, Fischer B, Mildeberger P and Thelen M (1996) Early detection of pneumonia in febrile neutropenic patients: use of thin section CT. *AJR Am J Roentgenol* 169: 1347–53.

Huang CC, Chen CY, Yang HB, Wang SM, Chang YC and Liu CC (1998) Central nervous system candidiasis in very low-birth-weight premature neonates and infants: ultrasound characteristics and histopathologic and MR imaging correlates in five patients. *Radiology* 209: 49–56.

Kousha M, Tadi R and Soubani AO (2011) Pulmonary aspergillosis: a clinical review. *Eur Respir Rev* 20: 156–74.

Lai PH, Lin SM, Pan HB and Yang CF (1997) Disseminated military cerebral candidiasis. *AJNR Am J Neuroradiol* 18: 1303–6.

Lammering JC, Iv M, Gupta N, Pandit R and Patel MR (2013) Imaging spectrum of CNS coccidioidomycosis: prevalence and significance of concurrent brain and spinal disease. *AJR Am J Roentgenol* 200: 1334–46.

Lewicki AM and Moore JP (1975) Esophageal moniliasis. A review of common and less frequent characteristics. *Am J Roentgenol Radium Ther Nucl Med* 125: 218–25.

Lund VJ, Lloyd G, Savy L and Howard D (2000) Radiology in focus. Fungal rhinosinusitis. *J Laryngol Otol* 114: 76–80. doi: 10.1258/0022215001903762

Luthra G, Parihar A, Nath K, et al. (2007) Comparative evaluation of fungal, tubercular, and pyogenic brain abscesses with conventional and diffusion MR imaging and proton MR spectroscopy. *AJNR Am J Neuroradiol* 28: 1332–8.

Madani G and Beale TJ (2009) Sinonasal inflammatory disease. *Semin Ultrasound CT MR* 30: 17–24.

McAdams HP, Rosado de Christenson M, Strollo DC and Patz EF Jr. (1997) Pulmonary mucormycosis: radiologic findings in 32 cases. *AJR Am J Roentgenol* 168: 1541–8.

Moore NJE, Leef JL and Pang Y (2003) Systemic candidiasis. *Radiographics* 23: 1287–90.

Pereira RM, Bucaretchi F, de Melo Barison E, Hessel G and Tresoldi AT (2004) Paracoccidioidomycosis in children: clinical presentation, follow-up and outcome. *Rev Inst Med Trop Sao Paulo* 46: 127–31.

Press GA, Wiendling SM, Hesselink JR, Ochi JW and Harris JP (1988) Rhinocerebral mucormycosis: MR manifestations. *J Comput Assist Tomogr* 12: 744–9.

Radin DR (1991) Disseminated histoplasmosis: abdominal CT findings in 16 patients. *AJR Am J Roentgenol* 157: 955–8.

Schmit M, Bethge W, Beck R, Faul C, Claussen CD and Horger M (2008) CT of gastrointestinal complications associated with hematopoietic stem cell transplantation. *AJR Am J Roentgenol* 190: 712–19.

Sharma P, Mukherjee A, Karunanithi S, Bal C and Kumar R (2014) Potential role of ^{18}F-FDG PET/CT in patients with fungal infections. *AJR Am J Roentgenol* 203: 180–9.

Siddiqi SU and Freedman JD (1994) Isolated central nervous system mucormycosis. *South Med J* 87: 997–1000.

Smith AB, Smirniotopoulos JG and Rushing EJ (2008) From the archives of the AFIP: central nervous system infections associated with human immunodeficiency virus infection: radiologic-pathologic correlation. *Radiographics* 28: 2033–58.

Sonnet S, Buitrago-Téllez C, Tamm M, Christen S and Steinbrich W (2005) Direct detection of angioinvasive pulmonary aspergillosis in immunosuppressed patients: preliminary results with high-resolution 16-MDCT angiography. *AJR Am J Roentgenol* 185: 746–51.

Sundaram B, Chughtai AR and Kazerooni EA (2010) Multidetector high-resolution computed tomography of the lungs. Protocols and applications. *J Thorac Imaging* 25: 125–41.

The Royal College of Radiologists (2015) Standards for intravascular contrast agent administration to adult patients, 3rd edn, https://www.rcr.ac.uk/sites/default/files/Intravasc_contrast_web.pdf, accessed 1 June 2017.

Tien RD, Chu PK, Hesselink JR, Duberg A and Wiley C (1991) Intracranial cryptococcosis in immunocompromised patients: CT and MR findings in 29 cases. *AJNR Am J Neuroradiol* 12: 283–9.

Yuh WT, Nguyen HD, Gao F, et al. (1994) Brain parenchymal infection in bone marrow transplantation patients: CT and MR findings. *AJR Am J Roentgenol* 162: 425–30.

CHAPTER 42

Serology of fungal disease

Richard Barton

Introduction to serology

The diagnosis of a fungal infection through the examination of serum originally involved the detection of antibodies specific for fungal pathogens and is now over 50 years old (Pepys et al. 1959). The term serodiagnosis within mycology has since broadened to also include direct detection of fungal antigens in serum and also within other body fluids such as cerebrospinal fluid (CSF) and bronchoalveolar lavage (BAL). Serodiagnostic assays may either enable a rapid diagnosis without invasive procedures or, together with culture, radiology, and molecular biology, provide a contribution towards compound approaches to diagnosis that are increasingly common (De Pauw et al. 2008). Serological assays have a variety of diagnostic uses including making use of their negative and positive predictive values and likelihood ratios, or in monitoring the response to treatment.

Methodology

A wide range of serological methods have been, and are being, applied to the serodiagnosis of fungal disease. One of the first approaches to antibody detection was a simple precipitin test. Serum placed in a well cut out of an agarose slab diffusing into antigen that is diffusing from an adjacent well and binding a complementary antigen may precipitate and produce a visible line in the gel, which can also be fixed by drying and staining the gel on a glass slide. The method is very simple and easy to apply and still represents a standard method of analysis for infections such as histoplasmosis (Guimarães et al. 2006) (Figure 42.1) and coccidioidomycosis (Pappagianis and Zimmer 1990). Precipitin tests lack sensitivity and will only detect certain IgG classes. Sensitivity can be increased by concentrating the serum—as is used in detecting antibodies to *Coccidioides*. Applying an electrophoretic step to the precipitation reaction using a running buffer with a pH matching the pH of immunoglobulins—8.2—and making up the agarose gel with half the running buffer strength will cause most antigens to migrate to the anode, while antibodies are carried by endosmosis towards the cathode. In this way the numbers of lines of precipitation and levels of detectable antibody increased (Philpot and MacKenzie 1976). Levels of antibody can be determined semi-quantitatively by titration. However, this method has lost out to more rapid enzyme-linked immunosorbent assay (ELISA) methods that can easily determine a quantitative measure of a specific immunoglobulin class (Sepulveda et al. 1979). Sandwich ELISAs are also effective in antigen detection. Agglutination methods have the advantage of being rapid. Whole-cell agglutination can make use of antibodies binding and agglutinating heat-killed yeast cells, but tends to be insensitive (Kozinn et al. 1978). Haemagglutination works by animal erythrocytes, sensitized with fungal extracts, binding and agglutinating in the presence of antibody to the fungus. Although there are commercial assays available, this approach not been widely adopted. Latex agglutination, where either antigen or monoclonal antibodies are covalently fixed to latex beads, has found use in a range of assays including the very effective cryptococcal latex agglutination test (Bloomfield et al. 1963). A recently launched commercial *Aspergillus* antibody assay makes use of strips of a nitrocellulose-type matrix blotted with *Aspergillus* antigens separated out by gel electrophoresis and incubated with a colorimetric substrate. Any bands on the strip from the patient test can then be compared with those on the control strip to determine both the presence and level of individual antibody reactions (Oliva et al. 2015). Many IgG antibody molecules fix complement, and this can be exploited in complement fixation tests, where patient serum antibody is incubated with a fungal antigen, sheep erythrocytes, complement, and haemolysin, and the presence of specific antibodies is indicated by a clearly visible pellet of intact erythrocytes. Although this approach is lengthy, laborious, hard to control, and prone to variation, it remains part of the gold-standard serodiagnostic approach for histoplasmosis and coccidioidomycosis. Finally, there has been recent interest in rapid lateral flow assays for antigen detection, where a sample is absorbed onto a membrane and flows through a conjugate antibody. Antigen binding the conjugate and moving by lateral flow to a test line and binding to immobilized antibody there will result in the development of a coloured line. This method has the advantages of speed, simplicity, and sensitivity. A cryptococcal antigen assay is now in widespread use (Jarvis et al. 2011) and an *Aspergillus* antigen assay has also been licensed (Thornton 2012).

In general, fungal serology tests are moving towards the detection of well-defined antigens, or antibodies to well-defined antigens which may improve the specificity of assays. In a recent study Tanimoto et al. (2015) determined that by using IgE responses to two cloned *Aspergillus fumigatus* antigens—Asp f1 and f2—allergic bronchopulmonary aspergillosis could be differentiated from *Aspergillus*-sensitized asthma.

Cryptococcosis

Cryptococcus neoformans and *C. gattii* cause serious infections in immunocompromised patients, typically presenting as meningitis. Whilst culture of CSF and blood plays an important role in diagnosis, a capsule antigen—glucuronoxylomannan—is shed in

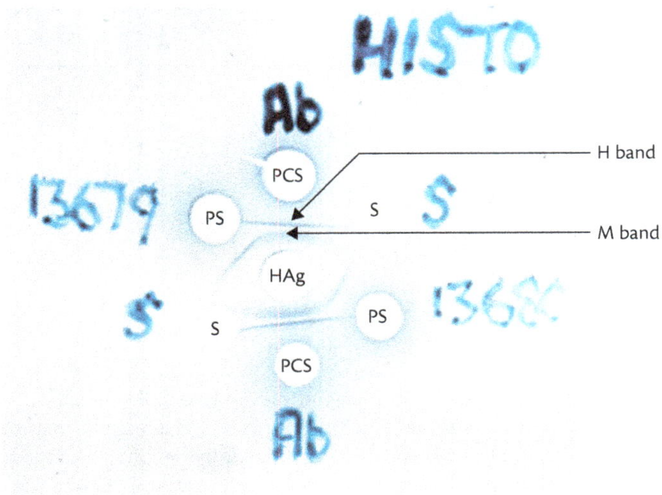

Figure 42.1 Histoplasma double-diffusion test result. An agarose gel with holes cut out is filled with *Histoplasma* antigen (HAg), patient sera (PS), positive control sera (PCS), and saline (S). Two bands—the H band and M band—can be seen with the control sera, and a positive M band with both patients' sera.

significant quantities in both the CSF and blood, and detection of this antigen has been a success story for the serological diagnosis of cryptococcosis. Early studies have shown that cryptococcal antigen could be detected in CSF by a latex agglutination (LA) test (Goodman et al. 1971). Further studies, particularly in HIV-positive patients, demonstrated the very high sensitivity of the LA test when serum is treated with pronase (a protease mixture originally introduced to remove rheumatoid factor from false positives). Dilution of serum and CSF can also overcome the false negatives resulting from the prozone effect seen in samples with extremely high levels of antigen (Hamilton et al. 1991). ELISA versions of the LA test are available and have a lower limit of detection (i.e. are more sensitive) than the original LA test (Scott et al. 1980), but later studies revealed that both tests performed equivalently (Tanner et al. 1994) and the convenience of the LA together with the often high antigen load in many patient samples has made this a popular diagnostic format for this test. While it is often difficult to determine whether cryptococcal antigen tests are more sensitive than culture, most studies suggest they are at least as sensitive (Tanner et al. 1994) and are much more rapid. An important development in recent years has been the lateral flow assay (Jarvis et al. 2011), which has at least as good a sensitivity as the LA test—possibly slightly better (Binnicker et al. 2012)—and has the advantage of being a rapid point-of-care test.

Attempts to detect antibodies to *Cryptococcus* in order to effect a diagnosis have typically been affected by low specificity (Qureshi et al. 2012), possibly reflecting a high level of exposure to cryptococcal antigen in many people.

Aspergillosis

Aspergillosis, typically caused by *A. fumigatus*, can take many forms, and is usually a function of the host's susceptibility, from allergic responses to *Aspergillus* through fungal balls and chronic pulmonary disease to invasive aspergillosis (IA). Anti-*Aspergillus* antibody or *Aspergillus* antigen detection, depending on the host's immune status, can play an important role in diagnosing these diseases (see Chapters 10, 30, and 37).

In the recently described condition severe asthma with fungal sensitization (SAFS), elevated specific IgE antibody to *Aspergillus* and some other fungi is the key biomarker for identifying the disease in patients with severe asthma (Denning et al. 2009). Positive total IgE to *Aspergillus* is also found in allergic bronchopulmonary aspergillosis (ABPA) along with raised total IgE. These two criteria, combined with either elevated *Aspergillus* IgG, raised eosinophil count, or chest radiographic changes, are the recently proposed markers for ABPA (Agarwal et al. 2013). The precise cut-off defining ABPA for total IgE has been problematic, resulting from a confusion over units of measurement (IU/mL or ng/mL). Some authorities have proposed a reference (i.e. normal) level of <417 IU/mL, but Agarwal et al. (2013) have proposed the more widely used <1,000 IU/mL, and this is likely to become standard. There are few studies looking at cutoffs for specific *Aspergillus* IgE, though Baxter et al. (2013) found that >3.7 kUA/L separated ABPA from *Aspergillus* bronchitis in cystic fibrosis (CF). Generally, 'elevated' levels of *Aspergillus* IgE are used in many diagnostic criteria. There is more work on *Aspergillus* IgG levels in ABPA, with reference ranges defined as <35 mg/L (Van Hoeyveld et al. 2006), but in patients with CF where higher levels of colonization lead to higher background levels of antibody, <90 mg/L (Barton et al. 2008) and <75 mg/L (Baxter et al. 2013) have been proposed. High levels of IgG to *Aspergillus* have long been known to be useful for confirming a radiological diagnosis of an *Aspergillus* fungal ball or aspergilloma (Longbottom and Pepys 1964). Generally, positive precipitating antibodies, or more recently IgG levels, are an important finding for the diagnosis of chronic pulmonary aspergillosis, and reference ranges for a number of different test manufacturers have been proposed (Page et al. 2016). In early studies, antibody tests in patients with IA were generally found to be very limited owing to the damaged immune systems of the kinds of immunocompromised patients who are at risk of this form of aspergillosis (Young and Bennett 1971). However, with the development of more sensitive tests, others have found that *Aspergillus* IgG responses in patients prior to immunosuppressive treatments may be useful for predicting subsequent invasive disease when such patients become immunocompromised (Du et al. 2012).

Since *Aspergillus* is rarely grown in blood culture, considerable efforts have been expended to find an effective non-culture blood-based diagnostic for IA. Galactomannan (GM) is an antigen found in the cell walls and other cellular components of *Aspergillus* species and in some other moulds, notably *Fusarium*, *Histoplasma*, and *Talaromyces (Penicillium) marneffei*, though not *Candida*. GM consists of galactofuranose side chains of α-linked mannan chains, and a sensitive commercial ELISA has been developed to detect levels as low as 1 ng/mL GM in serum and BAL samples for the diagnosis of IA, and in the case of BAL, detection of invasive pulmonary aspergillosis and other forms of pulmonary aspergillosis (Mennink Kersten 2004). The best cutoff for GM in serum to define IA took some time to establish, but is now confirmed as an optical density index (ODI) >0.5 (equivalent to approximately 0.5 ng/mL). There is a greater background of GM in BAL samples and the best cut-off has not been universally agreed, though meta-analyses of many studies suggest it should be >1.0 (Zou et al. 2012). Meta-analysis suggests that the sensitivity and specificity of GM in serum are reasonable at 82% and 81%, respectively (Leeflang et al. 2015). When using a cut-off of >0.5 for BAL, the sensitivity is good, though the specificity is worse than for serum (Zou et al. 2012), hence the proposal for a higher cut-off. GM testing is sufficiently robust and useful to have been incorporated in the European Organisation for Research and Treatment of Cancer/Mycoses Study Group criteria for defining fungal infections (De Pauw et al. 2008).

False positives in the GM assay have been found when testing neonates (Siemann et al. 1998), which may relate to a cross-reactive antigen in *Bifidobacterium* found in the guts of neonates (Mennink Kersten et al. 2005), and also to the use of piperacillin/tazobactam (Aubry et al. 2006). Several reports have noted the failure of a proportion of positive GM results to repeat test positive (Oren et al. 2011), though in general these repeat test fail samples correlate with patients who are unlikely to have aspergillosis (Kimpton et al. 2014) and this may reflect a problem with laboratory contamination.

Candidiasis

The development of antibody tests against *Candida* species for the diagnosis of candidiasis, specifically for systemic candidiasis, never met with the early success seen with antibodies to *Aspergillus*. The major problem was with a lack of specificity. This may have reflected the complications of antibodies to *Candida* present in patients with superficial infections. In addition, compared with *Aspergillus* disease, levels of antibodies are generally lower, and this may reflect the fact that *Candida*, particularly *C. albicans*, is a commensal organism for many, possibly most, people and humans have developed a tolerance to *Candida* which may result in relatively low levels of antibody production. During the 1980s and 1990s considerable effort was expended to develop assays to detect antibodies to *Candida*, by counterimmunoelectrophoresis, by fluorescence microscopy, by ELISA, and by immunoblot analysis (Mitsutake et al. 1994). This was developed further by Pemán et al. (2011), who examined antibodies to *C. albicans* germ tubes, and though such assays have claimed respectable clinical utility for the diagnosis of systemic candidiasis, they have never been widely implemented. Some more recent studies have used antigens from individual cloned genes in order to target detection of antibody more specifically. Clancy et al. (2008) found that combining four single *C. albicans* gene product antigens provided a high level of sensitivity and specificity for an IgG ELISA compared with blood culture, and interestingly this was independent of the species of infecting *Candida* species, and of whether the patients were immunocompetent or immunocompromised. While some early studies suggested that antibodies to the *Candida* cell wall carbohydrate antigen, mannan, were very non-specific, and were likely to be found in people with commensal *Candida* (Lehman and Reiss 1980), ironically it has been an anti-mannan antibody which has been commercialized and found to be of most use clinically (Sendid et al. 1999). However, unlike with aspergillosis, Sendid et al. (1999) found that in both immunocompetent and immunocompromised patients, antibody (anti-mannan) and antigen (mannan) could be detected at different times during the course of infection, and indeed a commercial ELISA mannan detection kit is available for use alongside the anti-mannan detection assay. Several studies analyzing the sensitivity and specificity of combined anti-mannan and mannan detection in a variety of patients have been examined in a meta-analysis by Mikulska et al. (2010), and in combination these assays provide a sensitivity of 83% and specificity of 86%.

Endemic mycoses

Culture of the dimorphic fungus *Histoplasma* plays an important role in the diagnosis of histoplasmosis, but it takes a comparatively long time and requires containment level 3 laboratory facilities for safety. Thus, a quick, safe approach to diagnosis is the examination of serum for the presence of antibody or antigen. Two serological assays developed in the 1950s have remained the gold standard of histoplasmosis antibody serodiagnosis: the double diffusion (DD) test and the complement fixation test (CFT) (DiSalvo 1986; Guimarães et al. 2006). The DD test is usually carried out using histoplasmin, an antigen derived from the mould form of *Histoplasma capsulatum*, whilst the CFT makes use of antigens derived from both yeast and mould forms of the fungus. The DD test for antibodies—presumed to be IgG antibodies to *Histoplasma*—classically generates two lines of precipitation (the M and H bands) with a control antibody sample and patient serum placed in wells adjacent to the control antibody. These react with the antigen in a similar way, and the bands in the patient sample are identified as significant if they line up with the control bands (lines of identity) (Figure 42.1). M bands are seen in 80% of patients with histoplasmosis and will last for some time after the resolution of the infection. H bands are seen in about 10–20% of histoplasmosis patients and only during active disease. The CFT again measures IgG response to *Histoplasma*, although it is more sensitive (and unsurprisingly less specific) than the DD test. It is positive in >90% of histoplasmosis cases, with positive reactions to the yeast antigen being more common than with the mycelial antigen. It has been shown that patients with aspergillosis, tuberculosis, and legionellosis may produce false positives with the histoplasma yeast CFT (Wheat et al. 1986). More recently, ELISA tests have been developed to detect antibodies to *Histoplasma*, but these are not widely available (Guimarães et al. 2010). Immunocompromised patients tend to make fewer antibodies to *Histoplasma*, and a *Histoplasma* antigen test detecting a polysaccharide antigen has been developed and been shown to be highly sensitive for diagnosing histoplasmosis in HIV patients. This was initially a polyclonal antibody-based assay, but more recently, monoclonal assays have become available. Interestingly, sensitivity is highest with urine, while the test has reasonable sensitivity for acute pulmonary histoplasmosis but not with chronic disease (Kauffman 2007). Combining antibody and antigen tests may improve the diagnosis further in patients with acute pulmonary histoplasmosis (Richer et al. 2016).

Coccidioidomycosis caused by *Coccidioides immitis* and *C. posadasii* can also be diagnosed serologically. One of the earliest tests to detect antibodies to *Coccidioides* was a tube precipitin (TP) test, detecting IgG which becomes detectable about a month following exposure. Like histoplasmosis, a combination of a DD test and CFT is standard for *Coccidioides* serology. The DD test detects an IgM response which occurs within about two weeks of exposure and then declines rapidly, whilst the CFT detects the slightly later IgG response to the TP-antigen, which may last for years (Pappagianis and Zimmer 1990). An antigen test for coccidioidomycosis has been developed and has found use in both serum (Durkin et al. 2008) and CSF (Bamberger et al. 2015). The assay has high sensitivity and can be useful to complement antibody testing, particularly in the more severe cases of this disease.

Blastomycosis is a disease which is largely confined to North America and is declining in incidence. While DD and CF tests using antigen from *Blastomyces dermatitidis* have been developed and used to diagnose this infection, they have often been found to be insensitive. More recent ELISA assays based on the *B. dermatitidis* surface protein BAD-1 provide improved sensitivity (Richer et al. 2014). Paracoccidioidomycosis, caused by the slow-growing *Paracoccidioides brasiliensis,* is widespread in South America and can be diagnosed by simple, rapid DD tests (de Camargo 2008). Considerable effort has been put into identifying immunodominant antigens such as gp43 which might be useful in antibody and antigen ELISA tests, but such tests have been hampered by the lack of cross-reactivity with the recently identified *P. lutzii* (da Silva et al. 2015).

Sporotrichosis caused by the dimorphic fungus *Sporothrix schenckii* is a subcutaneous fungal infection which is typically diagnosed by culture (see Chapter 23). However, infected patients often have antibodies to the cell wall carbohydrate antigen peptide-rhamnomannan, and commercial assays in the latex agglutination format have been developed and are useful in endemic areas. However, improved diagnostic approaches using detection of antibodies to antigens from the mycelial phase have proved to be both specific and sensitive (Almeida-Paes et al. 2007).

Eumycetoma, following the subcutaneous inoculation of a fungus and its growth in the form of tightly packed hyphal masses called grains, has also been the target of serological tests. It is important to distinguish between eumycetoma caused by fungi and actinomycetoma caused by actinomycetes, which respond well to antibacterial therapy. If grains are not produced, the two are difficult to distinguish, and in this case serology may obviate the need for invasive biopsy. However, eumycetoma may be caused by a wide range of fungi, including mycetoma 'specialists' such as *Madurella grisea* and *M. mycetomatis*, and 'generalist agents' such as *Fusarium, Scedosporium, Aspergillus*, and *Curvularia*. Thus, although precipitin-based antibody tests, using both fungal and actinomycete antigens, have been applied to mycetoma diagnosis, knowing which fungus or actinomycete to target is difficult and this approach to diagnosis has not become widespread (van de Sande et al. 2014).

(1→3) β-D-glucan detection

Some fungal antigens are found in a wide range of fungi; a good example of this is (1→3) β-D-glucan (BDG). BDG is found in the cell wall of *Aspergillus, Candida, Fusarium*, and *Pneumocystis*, though not, or at very low levels, in *Cryptococcus* species and the mucoraceous moulds. A test to develop BDG was developed making use of the fact that part of the *Limulus* amoebocyte clotting cascade is triggered by glucan. The assay can be used to specifically detect glucan using an isothermal colorimetric reaction available in several commercial assays (Figure 42.2) (Odabasi et al. 2004). Technically, the assay is more demanding than an ELISA or precipitin test, and prone to contamination. Despite some early concerns about false positives in patients with Gram-positive bacteraemia, the assay has been shown to provide an accurate diagnosis of several fungal infections. The test can play a role where the negative predictive value is used to guide empiric antifungal therapy if cryptococcal infection and infection due to mucoraceous moulds can either be excluded or determined to be very unlikely. Meta-analysis of the performance of the assay has shown that sensitivities and specificities are generally good (Karageorgopoulos et al. 2011). For *Pneumocystis* pneumonia (PCP), the sensitivity was found to be extremely high, and negative results extremely useful for excluding PCP in HIV patients, though not necessarily in non-HIV patients (Li et al. 2015).

The main drawback of BDG testing is that a positive result cannot necessarily be attributed to a specific fungus, though clinical signs may indicate a likely cause, and further testing is usually required to determine the aetiological agent beyond diagnosis.

The primary role of serology testing is to diagnose an infection. However, it has been realized that the same tests may be useful in monitoring response to treatment, particularly where clinical response may be difficult to discern. Furthermore, there is increasing interest in using diagnostic tests to predict outcome, though this role is necessarily complicated by the diversity of treatment options.

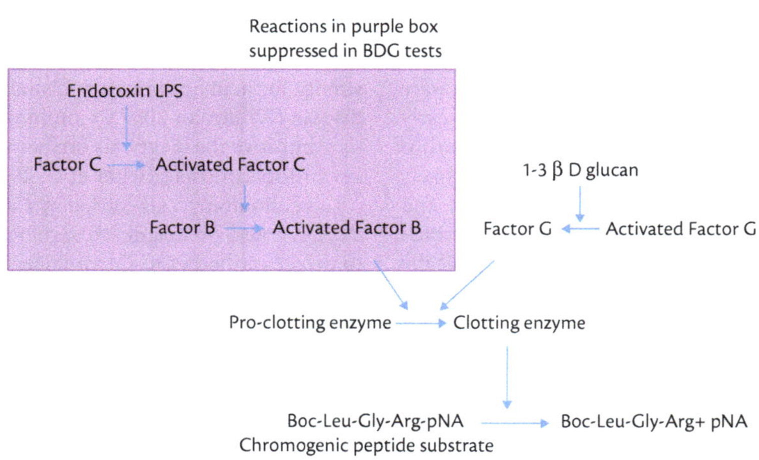

Figure 42.2 Beta-D-glucan reaction pathway. The lipopolysaccharide (LPS) section is suppressed, enabling the reaction to only detect (1→3) β-D-glucan. The cleaving of the substrate generates a product—p-nitroaniline (pNA)—detectable by a spectrophotometer.

Probably the oldest predictive serological marker is the *Coccidioides* CFT assay, where the titre is useful for assessing the extent of disease: using standard methods for CFT, patients with titres of >1/16 are likely to have, or to develop, disseminated disease (Pappagianis and Zimmer 1990). *Aspergillus* antibody levels decline in patients responding to effective treatment (Felton et al. 2010), and this can be useful in supporting a diagnosis where high antibody levels may not necessarily have indicated aspergillosis in complex patients with chronic respiratory disease, where multiple aetiologies are possible. Anecdotal evidence has long suggested that high galactomannan levels in patients with invasive aspergillosis are associated with worse outcomes, and now several studies have corroborated this view. Koo et al. (2010) looked at initial GM levels in patients with IA, and found that for each increase in units of GM ODI, the risk of six-week mortality increased by 25%.

Beyond Diagnosis

It is generally recognized that, for cryptococcal meningitis, a declining antigen level is a poor marker for response to treatment in the short to medium term (Antinori et al. 2005). However, Lortholary et al. (2006) demonstrated that cryptococcal antigen titres >1:512 are a risk factor for increased likelihood of relapse in HIV patients treated for cryptococcal meningitis. Furthermore, Cachay et al. (2010) suggest that high-baseline CSF cryptococcal titres may be a useful indicator for patients likely to develop complicated cryptococcal meningitis with much worse outcomes. BDG levels in patients with PCP have been found to persist for weeks or months, and levels do not correlate well with clinical outcomes (Koga et al. 2011), limiting the role for this assay in monitoring response to treatment.

References

Agarwal RA, Chakrabarti A, Shah D, et al. (2013) Allergic bronchopulmonary aspergillosis: review of literature and proposal of new diagnostic and classification criteria *Clin Exp Allergy* 43: 850–73.

Almeida-Paes R, Pimenta MA, Pizzini CV, et al. (2007) Use of mycelial-phase Sporothrix schenckii exoantigens in an enzyme-linked immunosorbent assay for diagnosis of sporotrichosis by antibody detection. *Clin Vaccine Immunol* 14: 244–9.

Antinori S, Radice A, Galimberti L, Magni C, Fasan M and Parravicini C (2005) The role of cryptococcal antigen assay in diagnosis and monitoring of cryptococcal meningitis. *J Clin Microbiol* 43: 5828–9.

Aubry A, Porcher R, Bottero J, et al. (2006) Occurrence and kinetics of false positive Aspergillus galactomannan test results following treatment with beta-lactam antibiotics in patients with hematological disorders. *J Clin Microbiol* 44: 389–94.

Bamberger DM, Pepito BS, Proia LA, et al. (2015) Cerebrospinal fluid Coccidioides antigen testing in the diagnosis and management of central nervous system coccidioidomycosis. *Mycoses* 58: 598–602.

Barton RC, Hobson RP, Denton M, et al. (2008) Serologic diagnosis of allergic bronchopulmonary aspergillosis in patients with cystic fibrosis through the detection of immunoglobulin G to Aspergillus fumigatus. *Diagn Microbiol Infect Dis* 62: 287–91.

Baxter CG, Dunn G, Jones AM, et al. (2013) Novel immunologic classification of aspergillosis in adult cystic fibrosis. *J Allergy Clin Immunol* 132: 560–6.

Binnicker MJ, Jesperson DJ, Bestrom JE and Rollins LO (2012) Comparison of four assays for the detection of cryptococcal antigen. *Clin Vaccine Immunol* 19: 1988–90.

Bloomfield LB, Gordon MA and Elmendorf DF (1963) Detection of Cryptococcus neoformans antigen in body fluids by latex particle agglutination *Proc Soc Exp Biol Med* 114: 64–7.

Cachay ER, Caperna J, Sitapati AM, Jafari H, Kandel S and Mathews WC (2010) Utility of clinical assessment, imaging, and cryptococcal antigen titer to predict AIDS-related complicated forms of cryptococcal meningitis. *AIDS Res Ther* 7: 29. doi: 10.1186/1742-6405-7-29

Clancy CJ, Nguyen ML, Cheng S, et al. (2008) Immunoglobulin G responses to a panel of Candida albicans antigens as accurate and early markers for the presence of systemic candidiasis. *J Clin Microbiol* 46: 1647–54.

da Silva Jde F, de Oliveira HC, Marcos CM, Assato PA, Fusco-Almeida AM and Mendes-Giannini MJ (2015) Advances and challenges in paracoccidioidomycosis serology caused by Paracoccidioides species complex: an update. *Diagn Microbiol Infect Dis* 84: 87–94.

De Camargo ZL (2008) Serology of paracoccidioidomycosis. *Mycopathologia* 165: 289–302.

Denning DW, O'Driscoll BR, Powell G, et al. (2009) Randomized controlled trial of oral antifungal treatment for severe asthma with fungal sensitization: The Fungal Asthma Sensitization Trial (FAST) study. *Am J Respir Crit Care Med* 179: 11–18.

De Pauw B, Walsh TJ, Donnelly JP, et al. (2008) Revised definitions of invasive fungal disease from the European Organization for Research and Treatment of Cancer/Invasive Fungal Infections Cooperative Group and the National Institute of Allergy and Infectious Diseases Mycoses Study Group (EORTC/MSG) Consensus Group. *Clin Infect Dis* 46: 1813–21.

DiSalvo AF (1986) *Histoplasma capsulatum* serology. *J Clin Microbiol* 24: 905.

Du C, Wingard JR, Chen S, Nguyen MH and Clancy CJ (2012) Serum IgG responses against Aspergillus proteins before hematopoietic stem cell transplantation or chemotherapy identify patients who develop invasive aspergillosis. *Biol Blood Marrow Transplant* 18: 1927–34

Durkin M, Connolly P, Kuberski T, et al. (2008) Diagnosis of coccidioidomycosis with use of the Coccidioides antigen enzyme immunoassay. *Clin Infect Dis* 47: e69–73.

Felton TW, Baxter C, Moore CB, Roberts SA, Hope WW and Denning DW (2010) Efficacy and safety of posaconazole for chronic pulmonary aspergillosis. *Clin Infect Dis* 51: 1383–91.

Goodman JS, Kaufman L and Koenig MG (1971) Diagnosis of cryptococcal meningitis. Value of immunologic detection of Cryptococcal antigen. *N Engl J Med* 285: 434–6.

Guimarães AJ, Nosanchuk JD and Zancopé-Oliveira RM (2006) Diagnosis of histoplasmosis. *Braz J Microbiol* 37: 1–13.

Guimarães AJ, Pizzini CV, De Abreu Almeida M, Peralta JM, Nosanchuk JD and Zancopé-Oliveira RM (2010) Evaluation of an enzyme-linked immunosorbent assay using purified, deglycosylated histoplasmin for different clinical manifestations of histoplasmosis *Microbiol Res (Pavia)* 2: 10.4081.

Hamilton JR, Noble A, Denning DW and Stevens DA (1991) Performance of cryptococcal antigen latex agglutination kits on serum and cerebrospinal fluid specimens of AIDS patients before and after pronase treatment. *J Clin Microbiol* 29: 333–9.

Jarvis JN, Percival A, Bauman S, et al. (2011) Evaluation of a novel point-of-care cryptococcal antigen test on serum, plasma, and urine from patients with HIV-associated cryptococcal meningitis. *Clin Infect Dis* 53: 1019–23.

Karageorgopoulos DE, Vouloumanou EK, Ntziora F, Michalopoulos A, Rafailidis PI and Falagas ME (2011) β-D-glucan assay for the diagnosis of invasive fungal infections: a meta-analysis. *Clin Infect Dis* 52: 750–70.

Kauffman CA (2007) Histoplasmosis: a clinical and laboratory update. *Clin Microbiol Rev* 20: 115–32.

Kimpton G, White PL and Barnes RA (2014) The effect of sample storage on the performance and reproducibility of the galactomannan EIA test. *Med Mycol* 52: 618–26.

Koga M, Koibuchi T, Kikuchi T, et al. (2011) Kinetics of serum β-D-glucan after Pneumocystis pneumonia treatment in patients with AIDS. *Intern Med* 50: 1397–401.

Koo S, Bryar JM, Baden LR and Marty FM (2010) Prognostic features of galactomannan antigenemia in galactomannan-positive invasive aspergillosis. *J Clin Microbiol* 48: 1255–60.

Kozinn PJ, Taschdjian CL, Goldberg PK, et al. (1978) Efficiency of serologic tests in the diagnosis of systemic candidiasis. *Am J Clin Pathol* 70: 893–8.

Leeflang MM, Debets-Ossenkopp YJ, Wang J, et al. (2015) Galactomannan detection for invasive aspergillosis in immunocompromised patients. *Cochrane Database Syst Rev* 2015 Dec 30(12): CD007394. doi: 10.1002/14651858.CD007394.pub2.

Lehman PF and Reiss E (1980) Comparison by ELISA of serum anti-Candida albicans mannan IgG levels of a normal population and in diseased patients. *Mycopathologia* 70: 89–93.

Li WJ, Guo YL, Liu TJ, Wang J and Kong JL (2015) Diagnosis of pneumocystis pneumonia using serum (1-3)-β-D-glucan: a bivariate meta-analysis and systematic review. *J Thorac Dis* 7: 2214–25.

Longbottom JL and Pepys J (1964) Pulmonary aspergillosis: diagnostic and immunological significance of antigens and c-substance in Aspergillus fumigatus. *J Pathol Bacteriol* 88: 141–51.

Lortholary O, Poizat G, Zeller V, et al. (2006) Long-term outcome of AIDS-associated cryptococcosis in the era of combination antiretroviral therapy. *AIDS* 20: 2183–91.

Mennink-Kersten MA, Ruegebrink D, Klont RR, et al. (2005) Bifidobacterial lipoglycan as a new cause for false-positive platelia Aspergillus enzyme-linked immunosorbent assay reactivity. *J Clin Microbiol* 43: 3925–31.

Mikulska M, Calandra T, Sanguinetti M, Poulain D and Viscoli C (2010) The use of mannan antigen and anti-mannan antibodies in the diagnosis of invasive candidiasis: recommendations from the Third European Conference on Infections in Leukemia. *Crit Care* 2010; 14(6): R222. doi: 10.1186/cc9365

Mitsutake K, Kohno S, Miyazaki T, Miyazaki H, Maesaki S and Koga H (1994) Detection of Candida enolase antibody in patients with candidiasis. *J Clin Lab Anal* 8: 207–10.

Odabasi Z, Mattiuzzi G, Estey E, et al. (2004) Beta-D-glucan as a diagnostic adjunct for invasive fungal infections: validation, cutoff development, and performance in patients with acute myelogenous leukemia and myelodysplastic syndrome. *Clin Infect Dis* 39: 199–205.

Oliva A, Flori P, Hennequin C, et al. (2015) Evaluation of the *Aspergillus* Western blot IgG kit for diagnosis of chronic aspergillosis. *J Clin Microbiol* 53: 248–54.

Oren I, Avidor I and Sprecher H (2011) Lack of intra-laboratory reproducibility in using Platelia Aspergillus enzyme immunoassay test for detection of Aspergillus galactomannan antigen. *Transpl Infect Dis* 14: 107–9.

Page ID, Richardson MD and Denning DW (2016) Comparison of six Aspergillus-specific IgG assays for the diagnosis of chronic pulmonary aspergillosis (CPA). *J Infect* 72: 240–9.

Pappagianis D and Zimmer BL (1990) Serology of coccidioidomycosis. *Clin Microbiol Rev* 3: 247–68.

Pemán J, Zaragoza R, Quindós G, et al. (2011) Clinical factors associated with a Candida albicans Germ Tube Antibody positive test in Intensive Care Unit patients. *BMC Infect Dis* Mar 9;11:60. doi: 10.1186/1471-2334-11-60

Pepys J, Riddell RW, Citron KM, Clayton YM and Short EI (1959) Clinical and immunologic significance of *Aspergillus fumigatus* in the sputum. *Am Rev Respir Dis* 80: 167–80.

Philpot M and Mackenzie DW (1976) A comparison of Aspergillus fumigatus antigens by counterimmunoelectrophoresis. *Mycopathologia* 58: 19–20.

Qureshi A, Wray D, Rhome R, Barry W and Del Poeta M (2012) Detection of antibody against fungal glucosylceramide in immunocompromised patients: a potential new diagnostic approach for cryptococcosis. *Mycopathologia* 173: 5–6

Richer SM, Smedema ML, Durkin MM, et al. (2014) Development of a highly sensitive and specific blastomycosis antibody enzyme immunoassay using Blastomyces dermatitidis surface protein BAD-1. *Clin Vaccine Immunol* 21: 143–6.

Richer SM, Smedema ML, Durkin MM, et al. (2016) Improved diagnosis of acute pulmonary histoplasmosis by combining antigen and antibody detection. *Clin Infect Dis* 62: 896–902.

Scott EN, Muchmore HG and Felton FG (1980) Comparison of enzyme immunoassay and latex agglutination methods for the detection of Cryptococcus neoformans antigen. *Am J Clin Pathol* 73: 790–4.

Sendid B, Tabouret M, Poirot JL, Mathieu D, Fruit J and Poulain D (1999) New enzyme immunoassays for sensitive detection of circulating Candida albicans mannan and antimannan antibodies: useful combined test for diagnosis of systemic candidiasis. *J Clin Microbiol* 37: 1510–17.

Sepulveda R, Longbottom J and Pepys J (1979) Enzyme linked immunosorbent assay (ELISA) for IgG and IgE antibodies to protein and polysaccharide antigens of *Aspergillus fumigatus*. *Clin Allergy* 9: 359–71.

Siemann M, Koch-Dorfler M and Gaude M (1998) False-positive results in premature infants with the Platelia *Aspergillus* sandwich enzyme-linked immunosorbent assay. *Mycoses* 41: 373–7.

Tanimoto H, Fukutomi Y, Yasueda H, et al. (2015) Molecular-based allergy diagnosis of allergic bronchopulmonary aspergillosis in Aspergillus fumigatus-sensitized Japanese patients. *Clin Exp Allergy* 45: 1790–800.

Tanner DC, Weinstein MP, Fedorciw B, Joho KL, Thorpe JJ and Reller L (1994) Comparison of commercial kits for detection of cryptococcal antigen. *J Clin Microbiol* 32: 1680–4.

Thornton C, Johnson G and Agrawal S (2012) Detection of invasive pulmonary aspergillosis in haematological malignancy patients by using lateral-flow technology. *J Vis Exp* Mar 22(61). doi: 10.3791/3721

van de Sande WW, Fahal AH, Goodfellow M, Mahgoub el S, Welsh O and Zijlstra EE (2014) Merits and pitfalls of currently used diagnostic tools in mycetoma. *PLoS Negl Trop Dis* 8: e2918.

Van Hoeyveld E, Dupont L and Bossuyt X (2006) Quantification of IgG antibodies to Aspergillus fumigatus and pigeon antigens by ImmunoCAP technology: an alternative to the precipitation technique? *Clin Chem* 52: 1785–93.

Wheat J, French ML, Kamel S and Tewari RP (1986) Evaluation of cross-reactions in *Histoplasma capsulatum* serologic tests. *J Clin Microbiol* 23: 493–9.

Young RC and Bennett JE (1971) Invasive aspergillosis. Absence of detectable antibody response. *Am Rev Respir Dis* 104: 710–16.

Zou M1, Tang L, Zhao S, et al. (2012) Systematic review and meta-analysis of detecting galactomannan in bronchoalveolar lavage fluid for diagnosing invasive aspergillosis. *PLoS One* 7: e43347.

CHAPTER 43

Molecular diagnosis of fungal disease

P. Lewis White and Rosemary A. Barnes

The need for molecular diagnosis in mycology

Delayed treatment of invasive fungal disease (IFD) results in increasing mortality (Von Eiff et al. 1995). A lack of confidence in classical mycology has led to reliance on the often unnecessary overuse of empirical therapy, associated with great expense, frequent patient toxicity, and adverse events (Donnelly and Maertens 2013). Empirical therapy was introduced over 40 years ago when diagnostic tests were unreliable (Donnelly and Maertens 2013). Attempts to overcome the diagnostic limitations have resulted in the development of a range of alternative non-culture techniques, including the detection of fungal nucleic acid in clinical specimens. These have the potential to provide an earlier diagnosis and a reduction in fungal-associated mortality, but more importantly, can also exclude IFD (Barnes et al. 2013; Morrissey et al. 2013; Aguado et al. 2014). Whilst there are a number of ways of demonstrating the presence of fungi in clinical samples, this chapter will concentrate on PCR (polymerase chain reaction) assays.

Disease can be caused by a range of fungal pathogens, and while certain fungi usually present with typical clinical features (e.g. *Pneumocystis* pneumonia or cryptococcal meningitis), others (e.g. *Aspergillus* or *Candida*) cause a wide range of manifestations. Different disease presentations may require different specimen types for optimal diagnosis, which in turn impact on the preferred method of nucleic acid extraction protocol. With extraction identified as the rate-limiting step, this initial process is paramount to success (White et al. 2010).

It is important to understand how best to utilize tests by understanding pre-test probability of disease (determined largely by prevalence), and how different testing strategies can be used to confirm or rule out a diagnosis.

General considerations

Disease manifestation, sample type, and nucleic acid extraction principles

Before taking and testing samples by molecular methods, it is essential to understand a number of principles; the pathogenesis and progression of the disease process; typical manifestation; the aim of the test; and the factors which affect specimen selection. The choice of specimen is the first experimental variable, and if inappropriately taken or stored incorrectly, this can have a detrimental effect and complicate clinical interpretation (Bustin et al. 2009). The sample type will determine the preferred nucleic acid extraction process, but the optimal sample will be governed by the disease manifestation (Figure 43.1) or testing strategy employed.

Blood-based testing

For fungi capable of causing bloodstream infection (yeasts, *Fusarium* spp., *Scedosporium prolificans, Histoplasma* spp., and *Talaromyces marneffei*), the obvious choice of specimen is whole blood (WB). However, for other fungal diseases where blood cultures rarely recover an organism, the use of WB may seem illogical. Yet many fungi invade tissues, often demonstrating angio-invasion (e.g. Mucorales and *Aspergillus*), and cause disseminated disease via the circulation without being recoverable in blood culture. Consequently all IFD provides potential, albeit temporal, targets within the circulation (Figure 43.2). Serum/plasma, WB, and the blood clot have been successfully used for fungal PCR (Tables 43.1–43.3). It can be argued that if the organism is recovered by blood culture, then whole blood should be used and the organism itself targeted. Fractionation required to obtain serum/plasma could theoretically remove fungal elements along with human blood cells, particularly if fungi are intracellular or cell associated. Recommendations for processing whole blood with respect to invasive aspergillosis (IA)-PCR have been published by the European *Aspergillus* PCR Initiative (EAPCRI), and are summarized in Figure 43.1 (White et al. 2010). Critical stages include bead beating and white cell lysis, even though they add to the processing time and complexity of testing. Although it is not clear whether these recommendations will apply to other fungal pathogens, the principles of enhancing performance to detect low fungal burdens in blood are generally applicable to most fungal diseases.

An alternative target in blood is free-circulating DNA (DNAaemia) released by the effects of the host's immune system or antifungal therapy. Targeting DNAaemia permits the testing of serum or plasma and the use of commercially available, frequently automated nucleic acid (NA) extraction platforms, negating the need for additional processes required for WB, which actually remove free DNA (White et al. 2010, 2011, 2015a; Loeffler et al.

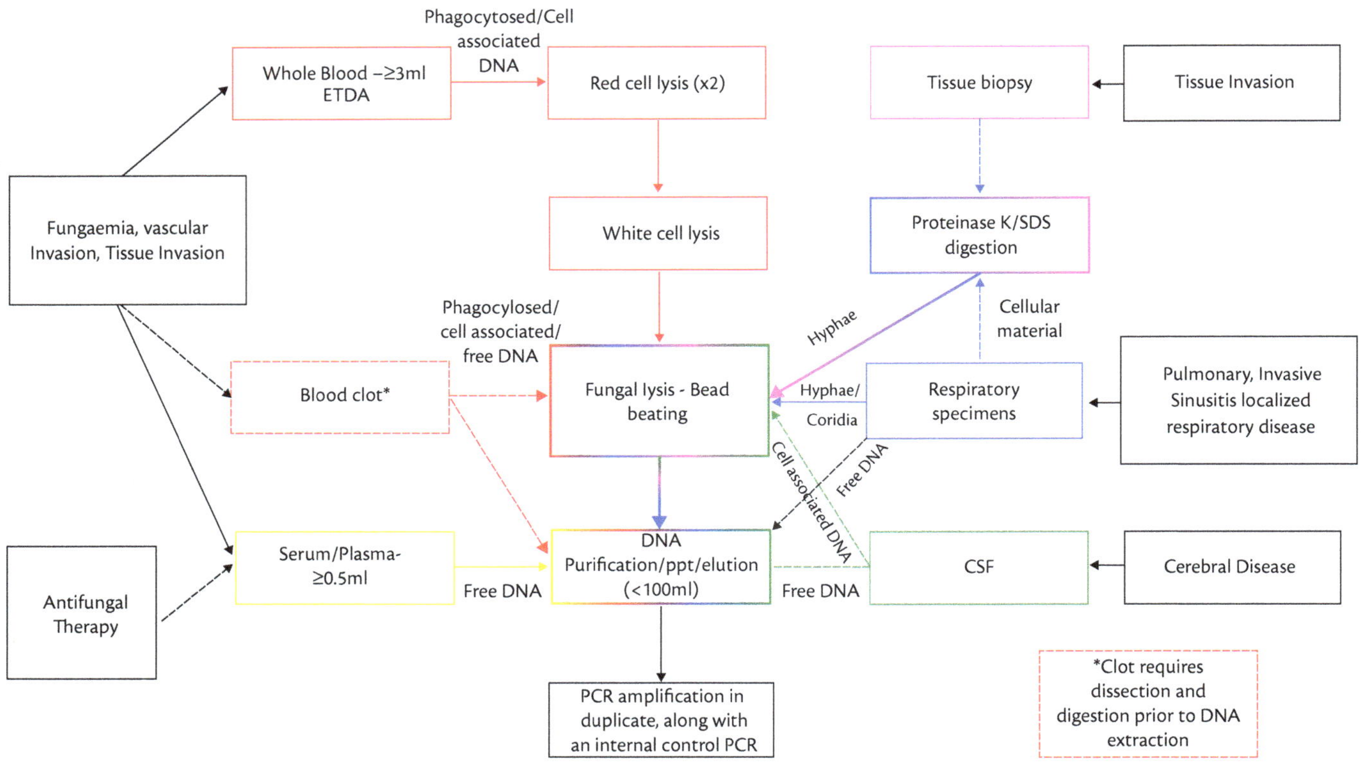

Figure 43.1 An overview of fungal disease manifestations, potential sample types, and resultant molecular processes.

Adapted with permission from White P. L., Perry, M. D., Barnes, R. A., 'Polymerase chain reaction diagnosis of fungal disease: Finally coming of age', *Current Fungal Infection Reports*, Volume 3, Issue 207, Copyright © 2009, Springer Science+Business Media, LLC. DOI: 10.1007/s12281-009-0029-3.

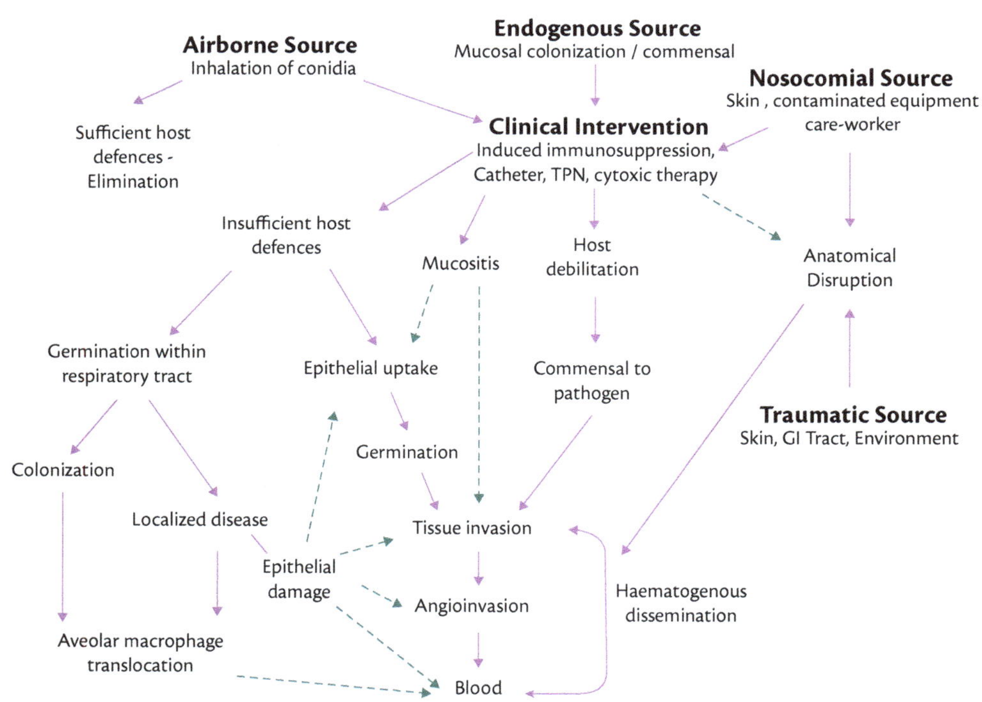

Figure 43.2 Invasive fungal disease and possible routes to the circulation.

Adapted with permission from White P. L., Perry M. D., Barnes R. A., 'Candida', *Molecular Detection of Human Fungal Pathogens*, Copyright © 2011 CRC Press. Published by Taylor and Francis Group.

2015). By removing plasma prior to red-cell lysis and re-introducing it post bead-beating, both cell-associated DNA and DNAaemia can be targeted (Springer et al. 2012). Recommendations specific for *Aspergillus* PCR testing of serum and plasma have been published by the EAPCRI and are summarized in Figure 43.1 (White et al. 2011, 2015a; Loeffler et al. 2015).

One interesting approach involves testing clot material in blood taken for serum samples. In an animal model of IA, the blood clot trapped significantly more fungal DNA than both serum and WB (McCulloch et al. 2009). Unfortunately, to process human clotted blood is technically difficult, and by testing plasma the difficulty of manipulating the clot and the associated losses can be avoided (White et al. 2015a).

Respiratory sample testing

With the origin of most filamentous fungal disease being the inhalation of airborne spores, testing a respiratory specimen seems the obvious choice for a successful approach. Testing respiratory specimens permits detection of any fungi capable of causing pulmonary or sinus disease, including *Aspergillus* spp., the Mucorales, endemic fungi, *Pneumocystis jirovecii, Scedosporium* spp., and *Fusarium* spp. *Candida* species may also be present, but generally represent commensal organisms within the upper respiratory tract and are rare causes of respiratory disease.

The frequency of testing required will limit the application of any test. For deep respiratory samples such as bronchoalveolar lavage fluid (BAL)—usually only taken when there is clinical suspicion of disease—a low frequency of sampling is expected. This largely excludes the use of BAL in pre-emptive or screening strategies. Also, regular exposure to conidia increases the possibility of airway contamination and/or colonization, potentially compromising the specificity and positive predictive value of PCR for invasive disease. However, meta-analyses of *Aspergillus* PCR performed on respiratory samples showed that clinical specificity was not overly compromised (Table 43.1, Tuon 2007; Sun et al. 2011; Avni et al. 2012). Accurate sampling from known areas of infection should generate significantly greater fungal burdens indicative of disease (Kawazu et al. 2003). Through the actions of the immune system or antifungal therapy, free DNA may be released from the fungal cell and be present in the sample. BAL sample volumes vary considerably but no optimal volume has been determined, and striking a balance to attain sufficient sensitivity whilst maintaining specificity and minimizing inhibition is paramount. When targeting fungal cells, both enzymatic (e.g. lyticase) and mechanical disruption (e.g. bead beating) have been successfully applied (Tables 43.1 and 43.3), although the latter is cheaper, quicker, and more efficient for hyphal disruption (Van Burik et al. 1998b). After lysing fungal cells, commercial DNA extraction platforms can be

Table 43.1 Selected *Aspergillus* PCR methods with good clinical performance

Specimen	Year	Basis of extraction	PCR assay	Sensitivity	Specificity	Reference
BAL	2015	Pellet – Bead beating Supernatant – bioMérieux NucliSENS®	PathoNostics AsperGenius®	88.9	89.3	Chong et al. 2015
	2014	GenElute kit	Nest RT, 18S rRNA	78	79	Heng et al. 2014
	2014	Lyticase	Nest, 18S rRNA	70	100	Hoenigl et al. 2014
	2013	MycXtra®	MycAssay™ Aspergillus	87	88	Guinea et al. 2013
	2012	Lyticase	Nest, 18S rRNA	59	87	Reinwald et al. 2012
	2012	MycXtra®	MycAssay™ Aspergillus	100	100	Orsi et al. 2012
	2012	EZ1 DNA tissue	Nest, 18S/5.8S rRNA	26	70	Buess et al. 2012
	2011	Bead beating	RT, 18S rRNA	100	88	Luong et al. 2011
			RT, ITS1 *A. fumigatus*	85	96	
	2011	MycXtra®	MycAssay™ Aspergillus	94.1	98.6	Torelli et al. 2011
	2011	Qiagen kit	RT, 18S rRNA PCR-ELISA	64 71	96 96	Hadrich et al. 2011
	2009	Qiagen kit	RT, MtDNA	64	100	Fréalle et al. 2009
	2008	Bead beating	RT, 18S rRNA	77	88	Khot et al. 2008
	2007	Lyticase	RT, ITS2	100	100	Schabereiter-Gurtner et al. 2007
	2007	Lyticase	RT, MtCB	100	100	Spiess et al. 2007
	2003	Qiagen kit	RT, 18S rRNA	90	100	Sanguinetti et al. 2003
	2001	Lyticase	Nest, 18S rRNA	100	90	Buchheidt et al. 2001
	2001	Proteinase K	Nest, AlkP	100	96	Hayette et al. 2001

(continued)

Table 43.1 (Continued)

Specimen	Year	Basis of extraction	PCR assay	Sensitivity	Specificity	Reference
	1998	Proteinase K	EIA, MtDNA	100	100	Jones et al. 1998
	1994	Bead beating	RSB, 18S rRNA	100	95	Melchers et al. 1994
	2011	Meta-analysis	N/A	79.6	94.1	Sun et al. 2011
	2011	Meta-analysis	N/A	76.8	94.5	Avni et al. 2011
	2007	Meta-analysis	N/A	78.4	93.7	Tuon et al. 2007
Serum/ plasma	2015	Qiagen EZ1 kit	PathoNostics AsperGenius®	78.6	100	White et al. 2015a
	2014	Qiagen kits	MycAssay™ Aspergillus	43.8	63.2	Danylo et al. 2014
	2013	Qiagen/Roche kits	RT, ITS1 and 28S rRNA	79	84	Springer et al. 2013
	2013	Proteinase K	RT, MtDNA	73	45	Schwarzinger et al. 2013
	2012	Proteinase K	Nest, 18S rRNA	80	96	Badiee et al. 2012
	2011	MagNA Pure LC	RT, MtDNA/18S rRNA	65	94	Millon et al. 2011
	2011	Roche High Pure Template DNA	MycAssay™ Aspergillus	70	90.5	White et al. 2011b
	2010	Proteinase K	Con, 18S rRNA	75	92	Lopes da Silva et al. 2010
	2006	Proteinase K	Con 18s rRNA	75	92	El-Mahallawy et al. 2006
	2003	Guanidine thiocyanate	RT, 5.8S rRNA	73	100	Pham et al. 2003
	2002	MagNA Pure LC	RT, MtDNA	70	100	Costa et al. 2002
	2001	Qiagen kit	RT, 18S rRNA	79	92	Kami et al. 2001
	1999	Proteinase K	Nest, 18S rRNA	89	100	Kawamura et al. 1999
Whole blood	2013	Bead beating	Nest, 28S rRNA,	69-87	36-63	Rogers et al. 2013
			RT, ITS1	55-80	57-84	
	2013	Bead beating	RT, 28S rRNA	95	73	White et al. 2013
	2013	Bead beating	RT, ITS1 and 28S rRNA	85	65	Springer et al. 2013
	2013	Biospin Fungus kit	RT, 28S rRNA and ITS 2	90.9	73.4	Li et al. 2013
	2010	Lyticase	RT, 18S rRNA	87	82	Badiee et al. 2010
	2009	Bead beating	RT, 18S rRNA	40	100	Ramirez et al. 2009
	2009	Bead beating	Nest RT, 28S rRNA	88	98	Barnes et al. 2009
	2006	Bead beating	Nest RT, 28S rRNA	92	95	White et al. 2006b
	2006	Lyticase	Nest, 18S rRNA	100	75	Halliday et al. 2006
	2000	Lyticase	RT, 18S, rRNA	100	100	Loeffler et al. 2000
	1998	Lyticase	SB, 18S rRNA	100	100	Van Burik et al. 1998a
	1997	Zymolase	SB, 18S rRNA	100	98	Einsele et al. 1997
Blood-combined	2014	Bead beating/Qiagen EZ1 kit	Renishaw Diagnostics Fungiplex	85.7	87.5	White et al. 2014
	2014	Meta-analysis		84	76	Arvanitis et al. 2014
	2009	Meta-analysis		88	75	Mengoli et al. 2009

AlkP = alkaline phosphatase; EIA = PCR-ELISA; ITS = internal transcribed spacer; MtDNA = mitochondrial DNA; MtDNA = mitochondrial DNA; Nest = nested PCR; RT = real time; RSB = reverse transcriptase-PCR and Southern blot; SB = PCR and Southern blot

Source: data from White P. L., Barnes R., Donnelly P., 'Developments in the molecular diagnosis of invasive fungal disease', *Invasive fungal infections in cancer patients*, Copyright © 2015 Turkish Febrile Neutropenia Society.

Table 43.2 Selected *Candida* PCR methods with clinical evaluation

Specimen	Year	Basis of extraction	PCR assay	Sensitivity	Specificity	Reference
Whole blood	2015	Bead beating	T2MR	71*	98**	Mylonakis 2015
	2014	Bead beating	Renishaw Fungiplex	83	88	White et al. 2014
	2013	Bead beating	Abbott PlexID	73	100	Laffler et al. 2013
	2010	Lyticase	ITS 2 RT	100	97	Badiee et al. 2010
	2009	Enzymatic digestion and Puregene yeast and Gram-positive bacteria kit	ITS 2 RT	100	92	Skovbjerg et al. 2009
	2009	Molysis kit	18S rRNA RT	88	93	Wellinghausen et al. 2009
	2005	Lyticase	18s rRNA Nested RT	95	97	White et al. 2005
	2003	Lyticase	ITS 2 Region RT	100	97	Maaroufi et al. 2003
	2001	Zymolase***	Cytochrome P450 lanesterol demethylase Nested PCR	89	50	Khan and Mustafa 2001
	1999	Yeast lytic enzyme	P450 LDMG RFLP	93	69	Morace et al. 1999
	1999	Zymolase***	18s rRNA SB	100	98	Einsele et al. 1997
Serum/Plasma	2013	QIAamp DNA mini kit	18s rRNA and ITS RT	91	100	Metzgar et al. 2013
	2012	Qiagen Tissue/DNAeasy kits	ITS1/2 RT	80	70	Nguyen et al. 2012
	2008	Qiagen kits with micro-concentration of eluate	ITS 1/2 Nested RT	70	100	McMullan et al. 2008
	2007	QIAamp DNA mini kit	ITS 2 S-nest	93	100	Alam et al. 2007
	2004	QIAamp Blood Kit	ITS Region RT	100	69	Maaroufi et al. 2004
	2002	Guanidine thiocyanate and boiling	ITS 2 S-nest	100	100	Ahmad et al. 2002
	1997	SDS/proteinase K and guanidine thiocyanate	ITS 3-4 PCR-EIA	100	100	Burnie et al. 1997
Tissue	2012	Tissue homogenization and Fast-DNA Spin Kit	Chipron GmbH Fungi 2.1	73	100	Fleischhacker et al. 2012
Blood	2013	Meta-analysis	Roche Septifast	61	99	Chang et al. 2013
Blood-combined	2011	Meta-analysis		95	92	Avni et al. 2011

* Based on detection of five of the seven proven cases (six blood culture and one proven intra-abdominal candidiasis case).

** Based on prospective and contrived arms of the study as published.

*** To avoid potential fungal contamination, zymolase should be replaced with recombinant lyticase.

ITS = internal transcribed spacer; P450 LDMG = cytochrome P450 lanosterol demethylase gene; PCR EIA = PCR enzyme immunoassay; RT = real time; S-nest = semi-nested PCR

Source: data from White, P. L., Barnes, R., Donnelly, P., 'Developments in the molecular diagnosis of invasive fungal disease', *Invasive Fungal Infections in Cancer Patients*, Copyright Turkish Febrile Neutropenia Society.

Table 43.3 Selected real-time or commercial PCR assays with a clinical evaluation for the diagnosis of fungal diseases other than invasive aspergillosis and invasive candidiasis

Detection range	Specimen	Year	Basis of extraction	PCR assay	Sensitivity	Specificity	Reference
Rhizopus spp., *Rhizomucor pusillus*, *Lichtheimia corymbifera*, and *Mucor* spp.	BAL	2014	Bead beating and Zymo Research fungal/bacterial kit	RT-HRM 18S rRNA	100	93	Lengerova et al. 2014
Lichtheimia corymbifera; Mucor amphiborum/circinelloides/ hiemalis/ indicus/mucedo/racemosus/ ramosissimus; Rhizopus azygosporus/ homothalicus/microsporus/ oligosporus/oryzae; Rhizomucor miehei/pusillus/variabilis	Serum	2013	MagNA Pure LC Total NA Large volume	RT 18S rRNA	90	100	Millon et al. 2013
Rhizopus spp., *Rhizomucor* pusillus, *Lichtheimia corymbifera*, and *Mucor* spp.	Fresh and formalin-fixed tissue	2010	Bead beating and Zymo Research fungal/bacterial kit	RT-HRM 18S rRNA	100	100	Hrncirova et al. 2010
Lichtheimia, Mucor, Rhizopus, Cunninghamella, Apophysomyces, and *Saksenaea*	Fresh and formalin- and PE-fixed tissue	2008	SDS/Proteinase K digestion	RT Cytochrome *b* gene	58	100	Hata et al. 2008
Pneumocystis jirovecii	BAL	2012	MycXtra® Fungal DNA kit	MycAssay™ *Pneumocystis*	100	100	McTaggart et al. 2012
	BAL	2012	MycXtra® Fungal DNA kit	MycAssay™ *Pneumocystis*	100	100	Orsi et al. 2012
Other than *Aspergillus* and *Candida* spp: *Pneumocystis, Cryptococcus* spp, *Mucor* spp. and *Rhizopus* spp	BAL	2014	Proteinase K, zirconium beads and ESI-MS DNA preparation kit	Abbott's PLEX-ID	78	64	Lovari et al. 2014
Other than *Aspergillus* and *Candida* ɒ: *Mucor spp., Rhizomucor pusillus,* ·*omucor oryzae/Rhizomucor* ·*us,Rhizomucor azygosporus/* ·*ucor microspores, Rhizomucor* ·*r, Cryptococcus neoformans,* ·*ces variotii, Scedosporium* ·*nd Lichtheimia (Absidia)*	Tissue	2012	Tissue Homogenization and Fast-DNA Spin Kit	Chipron GmbH Fungi 2.1	73[a]	100*	Fleischhacker et al. 2012
	Tissues, BAL other respiratory fluids	2011	Yeast lysis buffer, bead-beating	Luminex xTAG fungal analyte-specific	79	84	Babady et al. 2011
	Blood, CSF and tissue	2011	Lyticase	RT 28S rRNA	96	77	Landlinger et al. 2010
	BAL and other respiratory samples	2009	Lyticase	Luminex – in house assay ITS2	100	ND	Landlinger et al. 2009
	Blood	2005	Lyticase	RT 18S rRNA	75	70	Jordanides et al. 2005

f chronic disseminated candidiasis.

'ysis; ITS = internal transcribed spacer; RT = real time

› 2015

used to complete the DNA clean-up (Figure 43.1). An alternative approach described in Figure 43.1 targets the free DNA and only requires the use of commercially available standard technology.

As respiratory samples can be prone to inhibit PCR, performing an internal control PCR is essential.

While PCR testing of BAL fluid and tissue biopsies may be limited to a single occasion, when presented with a patient with evidence of overt disease, testing samples from the focus of infection is preferable to testing a 'one-off' blood-based sample, potentially with lower sample positivity rates (Verweij 2005).

Alternative sample types

While the testing of specimens targeted to a known focus of disease provides diagnostic confirmation, the invasive procedures necessary to obtain such samples may limit their availability. When testing tissue specimens, efficient digestion is essential so that invading fungal hyphae can be accessed for DNA extraction (Figure 43.1). Fresh, rather than paraffin-embedded/formalin-fixed, specimens are preferable, as the extraction protocol is less complicated, although if microscopic fungal elements have been seen, retrospective molecular identification, using the fixed specimen, may be useful, particularly if no fresh specimen is available. A pan-fungal approach may be required, particularly if non-*Aspergillus* species are suspected. Several studies have explored PCR on fungal DNA extracted from tissue sections (Tables 43.1–43.3). CSF specimens can be used to enhance the diagnosis of fungal meningitis or encephalitis (Verweij et al. 1999). In the recent outbreak of *Exserohilum rostratum* meningitis in the United States, PCR played an important diagnostic role, and specific real-time PCR assays were developed in a time frame that serological diagnostics could not match—essential in responding to outbreaks with emerging pathogens (Zhao et al. 2013a). In CSF, both free and cell-associated DNA sources are possible targets (Figure 43.1).

Testing strategies

For most patient groups the incidence of IFD is relatively low, even in high-risk populations such as patients with acute leukaemia or those undergoing allogeneic stem cell transplantation (incidence 5–10%). Consequently, the pre-test probability of disease is small, compared with the pre-test probability of not having disease (<10% *vs* >90%). In most instances, patient management does not reflect this low probability of IFD, and prophylactic or empirical antifungal therapy is used widely in many patient groups, with little or no evidence of benefit (Harrison et al. 2013; Morrissey et al. 2013).

In this situation, assays are better suited to excluding disease through a high sensitivity and negative predictive value. Regular testing, regardless of signs and symptoms, can be incorporated into a screening strategy of high-risk patients. In other groups (such as most solid organ transplant patients and those on effective anti-mould prophylaxis), the incidence of IFD is <5% and screening cannot be recommended and is unlikely to be cost-effective. In these situations, assays should be used to confirm the diagnosis in patients showing non-specific signs or when breakthrough infections are suspected. The different approaches are not mutually exclusive and can be used to complement one other. While repeated positivity during screening may be sufficient for pre-emptive therapy, it may also be used to trigger an intensive diagnostic work-up, including CT scans and BAL. When performing PCR to confirm disease in patients presenting with clinical signs typical of IFD (e.g. nodules or halo sign), focal/invasive samples (e.g. BAL) are better suited and will have a higher diagnostic value owing to the higher pre-test probability of disease evidenced by the radiological abnormalities. Blood samples may provide false negativity, particularly if an isolated sample is tested (Verweij 2005).

In invasive pulmonary aspergillosis, failure to clear inhaled conidia results in germination and hyphal production, leading to infection through tissue invasion. The characteristic angio-invasion (Figure 43.2) releases fungal components directly into the circulation and disseminates disease in susceptible hosts (Zaas and Alexander 2009). Were this the only route available for the release of biomarkers into the circulation, then pre-empting disease through regular testing of blood specimens would be unlikely to be successful.

However, phagocytosed fungal elements can provide an alternative target in blood (Figure 43.2). Translocation of particle-laden alveolar macrophages to extrapulmonary organs, via the circulation, can be clearly demonstrated (Furuyama et al. 2009). In an animal model study, both serum and WB PCR assays were positive one hour after inoculation, prior to invasive disease (White et al. 2016).

Consequently, testing blood samples may detect exposure to *Aspergillus* preceding infection. Patients may clear the inhaled fungi and never develop disease; in doing so, PCR testing will generate false-positive results. However, knowing that a highly susceptible population has been exposed could identify patients who could benefit from targeted prophylaxis.

For *Pneumocystis* pneumonia (PCP) a meta-analysis of PCR-tested BAL samples generated sensitivity and specificity of 99% and 90%, respectively, with the authors concluding that PCP PCR on respiratory specimens was sufficient to confirm or exclude the disease in high-risk patients (Lu et al. 2011). Moreover, for the diagnosis of candidaemia, a meta-analysis of PCR methods generated equally impressive statistics (sensitivity 95% and specificity 92%), confirming both a diagnostic and a screening capacity (Avni et al. 2011).

PCR performance

Aspergillus PCR

PCR was first used to aid the diagnosis of aspergillosis in 1993, in testing BAL samples (Spreadbury et al. 1993). Since then, the number of published articles has increased significantly. Most testing has been applied to blood-based samples, followed by the testing of BAL, with a range of tissue biopsies and other samples (e.g. cerebrospinal fluid, CSF) also tested. This diversity in sampling is the consequence of the range of disease manifestations that represent IA, but has hampered standardization.

A summary of publications describing *Aspergillus* PCR when testing BAL, whole blood, serum/plasma, and other samples is shown in Table 43.1. The performance of PCR, as determined by the various meta-analyses, avoiding individual assay bias, is at least comparable to that for other biomarkers. When testing BAL fluid from proven/probable cases of IA and control patients with no evidence of IFD, the sensitivity and specificity are consistent, ranging from 76.8–79.65 and 93.7–94.5, respectively (Tuon 2007; Sun et al. 2011;

Avni et al. 2012). As the testing of BAL fluids is suited to confirming a diagnosis of IA, assay specificity is paramount. For PCR testing of BAL samples this specificity appears to be optimal, and the positive likelihood ratio generated by the various meta-analyses is always greater than 10 (range 12.4–13.9). When comparing meta-analyses of GM-ELISA (galactomannan enzyme-linked immunosorbent assay) and PCR testing of BAL fluid, the specificity of PCR is significantly greater (P <0.0001–0.0019) (White et al. 2015b).

When using *Aspergillus* PCR to test blood samples from proven/probable cases of IA and control patients with no evidence of IFD, meta-analytical reviews generated sensitivity and specificity values of 84–88% and 75–76%, respectively (Mengoli et al. 2009; Arvanitis et al. 2014). With blood sampling suited to high-frequency screening strategies, sensitivity and negative predictive value are paramount, and when testing blood samples by *Aspergillus* PCR sensitivity needs to be optimal. Compared with antigen testing of blood (GM-ELISA and β-D-glucan [BDG]), meta-analyses show the specificity of both antigen tests to be significantly higher than for PCR (P <0.0001–0.012), while the sensitivity of PCR is significantly higher than for BDG (P: <0.0001-0.0477) (White et al. 2015b).

When serum and WB testing were compared in over 800 samples from 47 cases with proven/probable IA and 31 control patients, there was a trend towards increased sensitivity when testing WB (85% *vs* 79%), with the reverse true for specificity (65% *vs* 84%) (Springer et al. 2013). WB PCR generally provided an earlier time to positivity and potential diagnosis, although serum PCR is technically less complicated, and better suited for use in general molecular biology laboratories. Plasma and serum PCR have also been compared following international methodological recommendations when testing 19 cases and 42 control patients (White et al. 2015a). Plasma PCR provided the optimal sensitivity (95% *vs* 68%, respectively) and was usually the first assay to generate a positive result. The sensitivity of plasma PCR was comparable with that of WB PCR, but with the benefits of using DNA extraction methodology in line with serum testing.

Candida PCR

Candida species are the most common cause of opportunistic fungal infection and this genus is associated with significant mortality/morbidity, particularly if diagnosis is delayed. Although growth in conventional cultures from blood and other specimens is frequently seen in invasive disease, conventional methods are slow and often miss deep-seated disease. Any molecular advancement that improves sensitivity or time to diagnosis is likely to be beneficial (Pfaller and Diekema 2007). Many publications describe the development and application of PCR, and commercial molecular assays with the capacity to detect candidaemia as part of the investigation of sepsis are available (Table 43.2). However, routine clinical use of PCR to aid in the diagnosis of invasive candidiasis (IC) has not gained widespread acceptance and the necessary standardization of methodology and evaluation of clinical validity and utility is lacking. An interesting concept has been proposed by Clancy and Nguyen (2013), who postulate how non-culture diagnostics, including PCR, may be beneficial in detecting the 'missing 30–50% of blood-culture-negative IC cases'. Estimates suggest that many blood specimens taken for routine culture contain less than one colony-forming unit—well below the limit of detection by routine culture methods. Also, invasive infection can occur without fungaemia, or there may be only transient or only sporadic release of yeasts into the bloodstream. While PCR could potentially detect culture negatives, the limited circulating burden in many cases of candidaemia may be too low for reliable detection even by DNA-based methods (Pfeiffer et al. 2011). The optimal specimen for *Candida* PCR testing is still to be determined, with testing of WB, serum, and plasma all reported. As viable *Candida* cells are present during candidaemia, WB testing, theoretically, should be preferable to testing of serum and plasma. In a meta-analysis of *Candida* PCR testing, WB was associated with improved performance over serum (Avni et al. 2011). Sample positivity for *Candida* PCR was lower when testing plasma than when testing whole blood, in one small study (Innings et al. 2007). Conversely, a preliminary study of PCR performance, testing WB and plasma from 21 cases of IC and 27 controls, showed the sensitivity of plasma PCR to be significantly greater than WB PCR (57% *vs* 14%; P = 0 .008), while specificity was comparable (81% *vs* 96%; P = 0.22) (Nguyen et al. 2012). Similar findings have been reported from other studies (Metwally et al. 2008; Lau et al. 2010).

These data suggest that the cell-free fraction is optimal for *Candida* PCR, but may not reflect differences in disease, and for candidaemia, targeting the organism rather than DNA may be preferential. In the study by Nguyen et al. (2012), the performance of PCR for different manifestations of IC using plasma generated a sensitivity of 59% for cases of candidaemia—lower than when testing cases of intra-abdominal/deep-seated candidiasis (89%; P = 0.0033).

A selection of manuscripts describing *Candida* PCR testing and providing clinical performance is shown in Table 43.2. A meta-analysis of *Candida* PCR methods generated an overall pooled sensitivity and specificity for candidaemia of 95% and 92%, respectively, remaining high when investigating cases of proven/probable IC (sensitivity 93%; specificity 95%), and 100% sensitivity was achieved for cases of candidaemia when testing whole blood (Avni et al. 2011). However, performance is variable, with sensitivity and specificity ranging from 0–100% to 20–100%, respectively, representing the variability in methodology and the need for standardization.

The mucoraceous moulds

Cultures are of limited use and there are few serological assays available for infections caused by mucoraceous moulds. Species identification requires considerable expertise, and for these rapidly growing fungi, any delays in the diagnosis of mucormycosis are clinically detrimental. Clinical specimens are often from necrotic tissues and the fungus fails to grow in culture. The gold standard relies on confirming tissue invasion by histopathological evidence of typical broad non-septate hyphae, but cannot provide species identification (Roden et al. 2005; Kasai et al. 2008). Molecular detection of Mucorales species in clinical samples may aid diagnosis and reduce the high mortality.

The optimal sample type has not been determined. The capacity for tissue invasion suggests that tissue biopsies may be preferable. Pulmonary and rhinocerebral disease follow inhalation, and when coupled with the organism's significant invasive capacity, both respiratory and blood samples could be used. Real-time PCR and high-resolution melt curve analysis of BAL samples generated sensitivity and specificity of 100% and 93%, respectively (Lengerova et al. 2014). PCR was also used to detect Mucorales DNAaemia in serum (Millon et al. 2013; Shigemura et al. 2014). In a study of ten cases of histologically proven mucormycosis and 51 controls, a specific real-time PCR testing achieved a sensitivity and specificity of 90% and 100%, respectively (Millon et al. 2013). Table 43.3 presents a selection of published real-time PCR assays for the identification and direct detection of members of the Mucorales family. Given the low prevalence of this disease, the use of this assay as a primary screen is unwarranted. It could be used as part of a staged diagnostic workup after tests to detect more common respiratory fungal opportunist pathogens (*Aspergillus* and *Pneumocystis*) have been found to be negative.

Pneumocystis PCR

The inability to culture *Pneumocystis jirovecii* has led to the development of many *Pneumocystis* PCR assays (Table 43.3). The development of commercial assays provides standardization and quality control that ensures consistency across centres. In two studies evaluating the MycAssay *Pneumocystis* kit when testing BAL fluids, the sensitivity and specificity were both found to be 100% (McTaggart et al. 2012; Orsi et al. 2012). Excellent performance was confirmed by meta-analysis, where the overall sensitivity and specificity generated were 99% and 90% respectively, with an area under the receiver operator characteristic curve of 0.98 (Lu et al. 2011). Consequently, PCP PCR on respiratory specimens showed excellent diagnostic value with the ability to confirm or exclude the disease.

However, different sample types should be utilized in different strategies. BAL fluids are more sensitive than oropharyngeal washes ($P < 0.001$) and better suited to excluding disease. Conversely, oropharyngeal washes have greater specificity ($P < 0.001$), and if positive, confirm a diagnosis (Lu et al. 2011). Interpretation of results is complicated by the need to differentiate respiratory positives resulting from asymptomatic infection or colonization, compared with those resulting from disease. However, real-time PCR can provide a quantitative result, and if the burden is sufficiently high, results are distinguishable from colonization/exposure using a pre-validated threshold (Flori et al. 2004).

More problematic are the low-level positives typically seen in transplant recipients or in patients with haematological malignancies or receiving immuno-modifying drugs. In these non-HIV patients a greater immune response is likely, resulting in symptomatic patients at lower burdens. Different thresholds may be required for different populations. It is also necessary to target human genes in order to determine the quality of sample.

Other fungi

While infection by other fungi, such as *Scedosporium* or *Fusarium* species, can have high mortality due to antifungal resistance, the incidence of such infections and most other invasive fungal diseases is so low as to render individual assays of little benefit (Nucci and Anaissie 2007). The burden of cryptococcal disease associated with HIV disease in sub-Saharan Africa and Asia is enormous, but antigen testing has been available for many years and provides excellent performance. As a consequence, there are few *Cryptococcus*-specific diagnostic PCR assays described and a clinical need is low (Amjad et al. 2004).

Recently, real-time PCR assays for fusariosis and scedosporiosis have been reported (Castelli et al. 2008; Bernal-Martínez et al. 2012; González et al. 2013; Muraosa et al. 2014). PCR has also been used to detect the black yeast *Exophiala dermatitidis* in cystic fibrosis patients (Nagano et al. 2008). Molecular detection of these infrequent pathogens is better performed as part of a pan-fungal approach.

Pan-fungal detection

Pan-fungal PCR provides a syndromic approach where most, if not all, potential pathogens are targeted (Table 43.3). Using a single probe capable of detecting all fungi will inevitably result in false positivity affecting specificity and positive predictive values, but can also be detrimental to sensitivity. In a clinical evaluation of a pan-fungal PCR utilizing a single all-encompassing probe, the positive predictive value was found to be poor (Jordanides et al. 2005). Environmental fungal contamination has been associated with molecular biology reagents and tubes used to draw blood, and would affect pan-fungal PCR performance (Loeffler et al. 1999; Rimek et al. 1999; Jaeger et al. 2000; Harrison et al. 2010; Perry et al. 2014).

However, being able to detect and identify a range of different fungal species/genera in a single reaction is preferable to utilizing multiple individual real-time PCR assays specific for different fungal pathogens, as this is neither cost-effective nor time-efficient. Performing broad-range PCR amplification in combination with a wide range of specific probes permits identification of multiple pathogens (>20) in a single assay.

Using an in-house semi-nested PCR with 75 specific probes, Luminex xMAP technology was utilized to identify *Aspergillus, Candida, Cryptococcus, Fusarium, Trichosporon, Mucor, Rhizopus, Penicillium, Lichtheimia*, and *Acremonium* species in a single reaction, with a good correlation between classical diagnosis and Luminex identification for 19 out of 20 cases of IFD (Landlinger et al. 2009). Luminex xTAG fungal analyte-specific reagents are also available, and provided good performance (sensitivity 79%, specificity 84%) in one clinical evaluation (Babady et al. 2011). Several other commercial assays have been released for the investigation of broad-ranging fungal pathogens, including the Roche Septifast, Chipron GmbH Fungi 2.1, and the Abbott PlexID system (Table 43.3). Currently, extensive validations for all pathogens are limited and the true value of these tests is yet to be determined.

Future perspectives

Antifungal resistance

Antifungal resistance is emerging and may limit the number of treatment options available. This may relate to increases in inherently resistant species such as *Scedosporium prolificans* or *Aspergillus terreus*, or the emergence of azole in resistance in *A. fumigatus*, and molecular techniques have the potential to identify resistance, even without the need for a cultured organism (Van der Linden et al. 2010). This is significant as the vast majority of possible, probable, and even proven IFD have no cultured isolate available. Indeed, many cases reach a probable diagnosis, through radiological evidence supported by galactomannan (GM) or BDG detection. But with GM not providing a species level of identification and cross-reacting with other fungal species, and BDG detecting a broad range of fungi, PCR is the only non-culture-based assay that can be designed to identify to a species level (Swannink et al. 1997; Cummings et al. 2007). In so doing, it provides accurate epidemiological data and identifies species that may prove resistant to antifungal drugs.

With respect to azole resistance in *A. fumigatus*, molecular-based assays have been used to detect specific mutations that confer resistance (Denning et al. 2011; Zhao et al. 2013b; Spiess et al. 2014; Chong et al. 2015). Direct testing of a clinical sample will overcome the limitations of culture while reducing turn-around time. Amplification of CYP51 regions potentially associated with azole resistance has focused mainly on BAL or tissue specimens (Denning et al. 2011; Zhao et al. 2013b; Spiess et al. 2014; Chong et al. 2015). The development of commercially manufactured assays capable of detecting the main mutations associated with this resistance is a major step forward in the standardization of PCR technology. In a recent study, the PathoNostics AsperGenius® species assay—a multiplex real-time PCR assay capable of detecting *A. fumigatus*, *A. terreus*, and *Aspergillus* species—plus an internal control were evaluated testing BAL samples from haematology patients (Chong et al. 2015). It generated a sensitivity and specificity of 88.9% and 89.3%, respectively, but with the added bonus of a second multiplex with the ability to detect the most prevalent mutations conferring azole resistance (TR34/L98H, TR46/Y121F, and TR46/T289A) in the CYP51A gene of *A. fumigatus*. When testing BAL samples from 11 proven/probable cases, eight mutation profiles were determined directly from the clinical sample, highlighting the potential benefits in both the diagnosis and management of patients with IA (Chong et al. 2015).

Successful application of this test to less invasive samples (e.g. blood) could enhance the application of these assays. However, in the study by Spiess et al. (2014) it was not possible to amplify any regions associated with azole resistance despite using DNA extracted from 25 blood samples that were PCR-positive by the generic *Aspergillus* assay (Spiess et al. 2014). Conversely, when the PathoNostics AsperGenius® assay was retrospectively performed on serum samples from 14 patients with proven/probable IA, the sensitivity and specificity of the species assay were 78.6% and 100%, respectively (White et al. 2015a). For seven cases, at least one genetic region potentially associated with azole resistance was successfully amplified, although no resistance markers were detected. This study utilized protocols that strictly followed international recommendations for DNA extraction from serum, highlighting the benefits of standardization (White et al. 2011, 2015a).

Standardization

Standardized methodology provides intra and inter-assay consistency, quality control, and a consistent approach for the molecular diagnosis of IFD. International attempts to attain standardized methodology have focused entirely on *Aspergillus* PCR, although there have been national efforts focused on *Candida* and *Aspergillus* PCR (White et al. 2006a, 2010, 2011, 2015a; Reichard et al. 2012; Loeffler et al. 2015). Other infectious fungi have not been considered. It is important that this is resolved, particularly for diseases such as *Pneumocystis* pneumonia, where PCR has a significant diagnostic role.

Internationally, the European *Aspergillus* PCR Initiative (EAPCRI) identified that DNA extraction, and not PCR amplification, was the critical factor, and provided recommendations for *Aspergillus* DNA extraction from EDTA (ethylenediaminetetraacetic acid) blood, serum, and plasma (White et al. 2010, 2011, 2015a; Loeffler et al. 2015). All papers are open-access and freely available from the EAPCRI website (http://www.eapcri.eu), and are summarized in Figure 43.1. By combining these recommendations with commercially available *Aspergillus* PCR assays (Table 43.1), a fully standardized approach will be achieved. An independent meta-analysis of these recommendations showed that there was a trend towards improved sensitivity and a significant improvement in specificity (Arvanitis et al. 2014).

The development of an international *Aspergillus* DNA calibrator allows different PCR assays to be confidently compared, and potentially could be used to develop an international standard for *Aspergillus* PCR (Lyon et al. 2013).

Combined diagnostic strategies

For IA, evidence that a combination diagnostic strategy is optimal is emerging. A multi-centre randomized controlled trial comparing non-culture diagnostics (GM-EIA[enzyme immunoassay]/PCR) with culture and histology showed that the non-culture arm provided an effective strategy for managing disease, particularly by excluding disease, significantly reducing the use of empirical antifungal therapy (17%, *P*: 0.002), with no significant effect on all-cause and fungal-related mortality (Morrissey et al. 2013). In another randomized controlled trial, combined PCR/GM-EIA surveillance, compared with GM-EIA alone, in addition to reducing unnecessary empirical antifungal therapy, reduced time to diagnosis and cases of proven/probable IA (Aguado et al. 2014).

Outside the clinical trial setting similar observations were seen in routine clinical practice, where over a five-year period a combined PCR/GM-EIA strategy was used to screen 549 haematological patients (Barnes et al. 2013). The strategy had a sensitivity of 98.1%, where consistently negative tests excluded IA, but if both tests were positive on multiple occasions it was highly suggestive of disease.

References

Aguado JM, Vázquez L, Fernández-Ruiz M, et al. (2014) Serum galactomannan versus a combination of galactomannan and PCR-based *Aspergillus* DNA detection for early therapy of invasive aspergillosis in high-risk hematological patients: a randomized controlled trial. *Clin Infect Dis* 60: 405–14.

Ahmad S, Khan Z, Mustafa AS and Khan ZU (2002) Seminested PCR for diagnosis of candidemia: comparison with culture, antigen detection and biochemical methods for species identification. *J Clin Microbiol* 40: 2483–9.

Alam FF, Mustafa AS and Khan ZU (2007) Comparative evaluation of (1,3)-beta-D-glucan, mannan and anti-mannan antibodies, and *Candida* species-specific snPCR in patients with candidemia. *BMC Infect Dis* 7: 103.

Amjad M, Kfoury N, Cha R and Mobarak R (2004) Quantification and assessment of viability of Cryptococcus neoformans by LightCycler amplification of capsule gene mRNA. *J Med Microbiol* 53: 1201–6.

Arvanitis M, Ziakas PD, Zacharioudakis IM, Zervou FN, Caliendo AM and Mylonakis E (2014) PCR in diagnosis of invasive aspergillosis: a meta-analysis of diagnostic performance. *J Clin Microbiol* 52: 3731–42.

Avni T, Leibovici L and Paul M (2011) PCR diagnosis of invasive candidiasis: systematic review and meta-analysis. *J Clin Microbiol* 49: 665–70.

Avni T, Levy I, Sprecher H, Yahav D, Leibovici L and Paul M (2012) Diagnostic accuracy of PCR alone compared to galactomannan in bronchoalveolar lavage fluid for diagnosis of invasive pulmonary aspergillosis: a systematic review. *J Clin Microbiol* 50: 3652–8.

Babady NE, Miranda E and Gilhuley KA (2011) Evaluation of Luminex xTAG fungal analyte-specific reagents for rapid identification of clinically relevant fungi. *J Clin Microbiol* 49: 3777–82.

Badiee P, Alborzi A, Karimi M, et al. (2012) Diagnostic potential of nested PCR, galactomannan EIA, and beta-D-glucan for invasive aspergillosis in pediatric patients. *J Infect Dev Ctries* 6: 352–7.

Badiee P, Alborzi A, Vojdani R, et al. (2010) Early diagnosis of systemic candidiasis in bone marrow transplant recipients. *Exp Clin Transplant* 8: 98–103.

Barnes RA, Stocking K, Bowden S, Poynton MH and White PL (2013) Prevention and diagnosis of invasive fungal disease in high-risk patients within an integrative care pathway. *J Infect* 67: 206–14.

Barnes RA, White PL, Bygrave C, Evans N, Healy B and Kell J (2009) Clinical impact of enhanced diagnosis of invasive fungal disease in high-risk haematology and stem cell transplant patients. *J Clin Pathol* 62: 64–9.

Bernal-Martínez L, Buitrago MJ, Castelli MV, Rodríguez-Tudela JL and Cuenca-Estrella M (2012) Detection of invasive infection caused by Fusarium solani and non-Fusarium solani species using a duplex quantitative PCR-based assay in a murine model of fusariosis. *Med Mycol* 50: 270–5.

Buchheidt D, Baust C, Skladny H, et al. (2001) Detection of Aspergillus species in blood and bronchoalveolar lavage samples from immunocompromised patients by means of 2-step polymerase chain reaction: clinical results. *Clin Infect Dis* 33: 428–35.

Buess M, Cathomas G, Halter J, et al. (2012) Aspergillus-PCR in bronchoalveolar lavage for detection of invasive pulmonary aspergillosis in immunocompromised patients. *BMC Infect Dis* 12: 237.

Burnie JP, Golbang N and Matthews RC (1997) Semiquantitative polymerase chain reaction enzyme immunoassay for diagnosis of disseminated candidiasis. *Eur J Clin Microbiol Infect Dis* 16: 346–50.

Bustin SA, Benes V, Garson JA, et al. (2009) The MIQE guidelines: minimum information for publication of quantitative real-time PCR experiments. *Clin Chem* 55: 611–22.

Castelli MV, Buitrago MJ, Bernal-Martinez L, Gomez-Lopez A, Rodriguez-Tudela JL and Cuenca-Estrella M (2008) Development and validation of a quantitative PCR assay for diagnosis of scedosporiosis. *J Clin Microbiol* 46: 3412–16.

Chang SS, Hsieh WH, Liu TS, et al. (2013) Multiplex PCR system for rapid detection of pathogens in patients with presumed sepsis—a systemic review and meta-analysis. *PLoS One* 8: e62323.

Chong GL, van de Sande WW, Dingemans GJ, et al. (2015) Validation of a new Aspergillus real-time PCR assay for direct detection of Aspergillus and azole resistance of Aspergillus fumigatus on bronchoalveolar lavage fluid. *J Clin Microbiol* 53: 868–74.

Clancy CJ and Nguyen MH (2013) Finding the 'Missing 50%'of invasive candidiasis: how nonculture diagnostics will improve understanding of disease spectrum and transform patient care. *Clin Infect Dis* 56: 1284–92.

Costa C, Costa JM, Desterke C, Botterel F, Cordonnier C and Bretagne S (2002) Real-time PCR coupled with automated DNA extraction and detection of galactomannan antigen in serum by enzyme-linked immunosorbent assay for diagnosis of invasive aspergillosis. *J Clin Microbiol* 40: 2224–7.

Cummings JR, Jamison GR, Boudreaux JW, et al. (2007) Cross reactivity of non-Aspergillus fungal species in the Aspergillus galactomannan enzyme immunoassay. *Diagn Microbiol Infect Dis* 59: 113–15.

Danylo A, Courtemanche C, Pelletier R and Boudreault AA (2014) Performance of MycAssay Aspergillus DNA real-time PCR assay compared with the galactomannan detection assay for the diagnosis of invasive aspergillosis from serum samples. *Med Mycol* 52: 577–83.

Denning DW, Park S, Lass-Florl C, et al. (2011) High-frequency triazole resistance found in nonculturable *Aspergillus fumigatus* from lungs of patients with chronic fungal disease. *Clin Infect Dis* 52: 1123–9.

Donnelly JP and Maertens J (2013) The end of the road for empirical antifungal treatment? *Lancet Infect Dis* 13: 470–2.

Einsele H, Hebart H, Roller G, et al. (1997) Detection and identification of fungal pathogens in blood by using molecular probes. *J Clin Microbiol* 35: 1353–60.

El-Mahallawy HA, Shaker HH, Ali Helmy H, Mostafa T and Razak Abo-Sedah A (2006) Evaluation of pan-fungal PCR assay and Aspergillus antigen detection in the diagnosis of invasive fungal infections in high risk paediatric cancer patients. *Med Mycol* 44: 733–9.

Fleischhacker M, Schulz S, Jöhrens K, et al. (2012) Diagnosis of chronic disseminated candidosis from liver biopsies by a novel PCR in patients with haematological malignancies. *Clin Microbiol Infect* 18: 1010–16.

Flori P, Bellete B, Durand F, et al. (2004) Comparison between real-time PCR, conventional PCR and different staining techniques for diagnosing Pneumocystis jirovecii pneumonia from bronchoalveolar lavage specimens. *J Med Microbiol* 53: 603–7.

Fréalle E, Decrucq K, Botterel F, et al. (2009) Diagnosis of invasive aspergillosis using bronchoalveolar lavage in haematology patients: influence of bronchoalveolar lavage human DNA content on real-time PCR performance. *Eur J Clin Microbiol Infect Dis* 28: 223–32.

Furuyama A, Kanno S, Kobayashi T and Hirano S (2009) Extrapulmonary translocation of intratracheally instilled fine and ultrafine particles via direct and alveolar macrophage-associated routes. *Arch Toxicol* 83: 429–37.

González GM, Márquez J, Treviño-Rangel Rde J, et al. (2013) Murine model of disseminated fusariosis: evaluation of the fungal burden by traditional CFU and quantitative PCR. *Mycopathologia* 176: 219–24.

Guinea J, Padilla C, Escribano P, et al. (2013) Evaluation of MycAssay™ Aspergillus for diagnosis of invasive pulmonary aspergillosis in patients without hematological cancer. *PLoS One* 8: e61545.

Hadrich I, Mary C, Makni F, et al. (2011) Comparison of PCR-ELISA and Real-Time PCR for invasive aspergillosis diagnosis in patients with hematological malignancies. *Med Mycol* 49: 489–94.

Halliday C, Hoile R, Sorrell T, et al. (2006) Role of prospective screening of blood for invasive aspergillosis by polymerase chain reaction in febrile neutropenic recipients of haematopoietic stem cell transplants and patients with acute leukaemia. *Br J Haematol* 132: 478–86.

Harrison D, Muskett H, Harvey S, et al. (2013) Development and validation of a risk model for identification of non-neutropenic, critically ill adult patients at high risk of invasive Candida infection: the Fungal Infection Risk Evaluation (FIRE) Study. *Health Technol Assess* 17: 1–156.

Harrison E, Stalhberger T, Whelan R, et al. (2010) Aspergillus DNA contamination in blood collection tubes. *Diagn Microbiol Infect Dis* 67: 392–4.

Hata DJ, Buckwalter SP, Pritt BS, Roberts GD and Wengenack NL (2008) Real-time PCR method for detection of Zygomycetes. *J Clin Microbiol* 46: 2353–8.

Hayette MP, Vaira D, Susin F, et al. (2001) Detection of Aspergillus species DNA by PCR in bronchoalveolar lavage fluid. *J Clin Microbiol* 39: 2338–40.

Heng SC, Chen SC, Morrissey CO, et al. (2014) Clinical utility of Aspergillus galactomannan and PCR in bronchoalveolar lavage fluid for the diagnosis of invasive pulmonary aspergillosis in patients with haematological malignancies. *Diagn Microbiol Infect Dis* 79: 322–7.

Hoenigl M, Prattes J, Spiess B, et al. (2014) Performance of galactomannan, beta-d-glucan, Aspergillus lateral-flow device, conventional culture, and PCR tests with bronchoalveolar lavage fluid for diagnosis of invasive pulmonary aspergillosis. *J Clin Microbiol* 52: 2039–45

Hrncirova K, Lengerova M, Kocmanova I, et al. (2010) Rapid detection and identification of mucormycetes from culture and tissue samples by use of high-resolution melt analysis. *J Clin Microbiol* 48: 3392–4.

Innings A, Ullberg M, Johansson A, et al. (2007) Multiplex real-time PCR targeting the Rnase P RNA gene for detection and identification of *Candida* species in blood. *J Clin Microbiol* 45: 874–80.

Jaeger EE, Carroll NM, Choudhury S, et al. (2000) Rapid detection and identification of *Candida, Aspergillus*, and *Fusarium* species in ocular samples using nested PCR. *J Clin Microbiol* 38: 2902–8.

Jones ME, Fox AJ, Barnes AJ, et al. (1998) PCR-ELISA for the early diagnosis of invasive pulmonary aspergillus infection in neutropenic patients. *J Clin Pathol* 51: 652–6.

Jordanides NE, Allan EK, McLintock LA, et al. (2005) A prospective study of real-time panfungal PCR for the early diagnosis of invasive fungal infection in haemato-oncology patients. *Bone Marrow Transplant* 35: 389–95.

Kami M, Fukui T, Ogawa S, et al. (2001) Use of real-time PCR on blood samples for diagnosis of invasive aspergillosis. *Clin Infect Dis* 33: 1504–12.

Kasai M, Harrington SM, Francesconi A, et al. (2008) Detection of a molecular biomarker for Zygomycetes by quantitative PCR assays of plasma, bronchoalveolar lavage, and lung tissue in a rabbit model of experimental pulmonary zygomycosis. *J Clin Microbiol* 46: 3690–702.

Kawamura S, Maesaki S, Noda T, et al. (1999) Comparison between PCR and detection of antigen in sera for diagnosis of pulmonary aspergillosis. *J Clin Microbiol* 37: 218–20.

Kawazu M, Kanda Y, Goyama S, et al. (2003) Rapid diagnosis of invasive pulmonary aspergillosis by quantitative polymerase chain reaction using bronchial lavage fluid. *Am J Hematol* 72: 27–30.

Khan ZU and Mustafa AS (2001) Detection of *Candida* species by polymerase chain reaction (PCR) in blood samples of experimentally infected mice and patients with suspected candidemia. *Microbiol Res* 156: 95–102.

Khot PD, Ko DL, Hackman RC and Fredricks DN (2008) Development and optimization of quantitative PCR for the diagnosis of invasive aspergillosis with bronchoalveolar lavage fluid. *BMC Infect Dis* 8: 73.

Laffler TG, Cummins LL, McClain CM, et al. (2013) Enhanced diagnostic yields of bacteremia and candidemia in blood specimens by PCR-electrospray ionization mass spectrometry. *J Clin Microbiol* 51: 3535–41.

Landlinger C, Preuner S, Bašková L, et al. (2010) Diagnosis of invasive fungal infections by a real-time panfungal PCR assay in immunocompromised pediatric patients. *Leukemia* 24: 2032–8.

Landlinger C, Preuner S, Willinger B, et al. (2009) Species-specific identification of a wide range of clinically relevant fungal pathogens by use of Luminex xMAP technology. *J Clin Microbiol* 47: 1063–73.

Lau A, Halliday C, Chen SCA, Playford EG, Stanley K and Sorrell TC (2010) Comparison of whole blood, serum and plasma for early detection of candidemia by multiplex-tandem PCR. *J Clin Microbiol* 48: 811–16.

Lengerova M, Racil Z, Hrncirova K, et al. (2014) Rapid detection and identification of mucormycetes in bronchoalveolar lavage samples from immunocompromised patients with pulmonary infiltrates by use of high-resolution melt analysis. *J Clin Microbiol* 52: 2824–8.

Li Y, Gao L, Ding Y, et al. (2013) Establishment and application of real-time quantitative PCR for diagnosing invasive aspergillosis via the blood in hematological patients: targeting a specific sequence of Aspergillus 28S-ITS2. *BMC Infect Dis* 13: 255.

Loeffler J, Hebart H, Bialek R, et al. (1999) Contaminations occurring in fungal PCR assays. *J Clin Microbiol* 7: 1200–2.

Loeffler J, Henke N, Hebart H, et al. (2000) Quantification of fungal DNA by using fluorescence resonance energy transfer and the light cycler system. *J Clin Microbiol* 38: 586–90.

Loeffler J, Mengoli C, Springer J, et al. (2015) Analytical comparison of in vitro spiked human serum and plasma for the PCR-based detection of Aspergillus fumigatus DNA—a study by the European Aspergillus PCR Initiative. *J Clin Microbiol* 53: 2838–45.

Lopes da Silva R, Ribeiro P, Abreu N, et al. (2010) Early diagnosis of invasive aspergillosis in neutropenic patients. Comparison between serum galactomannan and polymerase chain reaction. *Clin Med Insights Oncol* 4: 81–8.

Lovari R, Metzgar D, Toleno D, et al. (2014) Characterisation of a PCR/ESI-MS assay for detection and identification of diverse fungi in bronchoalveolar lavage samples. Oral Presentation Abstract O219, ECCMID 2014.

Lu Y, Ling G, Qiang C, et al. (2011) PCR diagnosis of Pneumocystis pneumonia: a bivariate meta-analysis. *J Clin Microbiol* 49: 4361–3.

Luong ML, Clancy CJ, Vadnerkar A, et al. (2011) Comparison of an Aspergillus real-time polymerase chain reaction assay with galactomannan testing of bronchoalveolar lavage fluid for the diagnosis of invasive pulmonary aspergillosis in lung transplant recipients. *Clin Infect Dis* 52: 1218–26.

Lyon GM, Abdul-Ali D, Loeffler J, et al. (2013) Development and evaluation of a calibrator material for nucleic acid-based assays for diagnosing aspergillosis. *J Clin Microbiol* 51: 2403–5.

Maaroufi Y, Ahariz N, Husson M and Crokaert F (2004) Comparison of different methods of isolation of DNA of commonly encountered *Candida* species and its quantitation by using a real-time PCR-based assay. *J Clin Microbiol* 42: 3159–63.

Maaroufi Y, Heymans C, De Bruyne JM, et al. (2003) Rapid detection of *Candida albicans* in clinical blood samples by using a TaqMan-based PCR assay. *J Clin Microbiol* 41: 3293–8.

McCulloch E, Ramage G, Jones B, et al. (2009) Don't throw your blood clots away: use of blood clot may improve sensitivity of PCR diagnosis in invasive aspergillosis. *J Clin Pathol* 62: 539–41.

McMullan R, Metwally L, Coyle PV, et al. (2008) A prospective clinical trial of a real-time polymerase chain reaction assay for the diagnosis of candidemia in nonneutropenic, critically ill adults. *Clin Infect Dis* 46: 890–6.

McTaggart LR, Wengenack NL and Richardson SE (2012) Validation of the MycAssay Pneumocystis kit for detection of Pneumocystis jirovecii in bronchoalveolar lavage specimens by comparison to a laboratory standard of direct immunofluorescence microscopy, real-time PCR, or conventional PCR. *J Clin Microbiol* 50: 1856–9.

Melchers WJ, Verweij PE, van den Hurk P, et al. (1994) General primer-mediated PCR for detection of Aspergillus species. *J Clin Microbiol* 32: 1710–17.

Mengoli C, Cruciani M, Barnes RA, Loeffler J and Donnelly JP (2009) Use of PCR for diagnosis of invasive aspergillosis: systematic review of and meta-analysis. *Lancet Infect Dis* 9: 89–96.

Metwally L, Fairley DJ, Coyle PV, et al. (2008) Comparison of serum and whole-blood specimens for the detection of Candida DNA in critically ill, non-neutropenic patients. *J Med Microbiol* 57: 1269–72.

Metzgar D, Frinder M, Lovari R, et al. (2013) Broad-spectrum biosensor capable of detecting and identifying diverse bacterial and Candida species in blood. *J Clin Microbiol* 51: 2670–8.

Millon L, Grenouillet F, Legrand F, et al. (2011) Ribosomal and mitochondrial DNA target for real-time PCR diagnosis of invasive aspergillosis. *J Clin Microbiol* 49: 1058–63.

Millon L, Larosa F, Lepiller Q, et al. (2013) Quantitative polymerase chain reaction detection of circulating DNA in serum for early diagnosis of mucormycosis in immunocompromised patients. *Clin Infect Dis* 56: e95–101.

Morace G, Pagano L, Sanguinetti M, et al. (1999) PCR-restriction enzyme analysis for detection of *Candida* DNA in blood from febrile patients with hematological malignancies. *J Clin Microbiol* 37: 1871–5.

Morrissey CO, Chen SC, Sorrell TC, et al. (2013) Galactomannan and PCR versus culture and histology for directing use of antifungal treatment for invasive aspergillosis in high-risk haematology patients: a randomised controlled trial. *Lancet Infect Dis* 13: 519–28.

Muraosa Y, Schreiber AZ, Trabasso P, et al. (2014) Development of cycling probe-based real-time PCR system to detect Fusarium species and Fusarium solani species complex (FSSC). *Int J Med Microbiol* 304: 505–11.

Mylonakis E, Clancy CJ, Ostrosky-Zeichner L, et al. (2015) T2 magnetic resonance assay for the rapid diagnosis of candidemia in whole blood: a clinical trial. *Clin Infect Dis* 60: 892–9.

Nagano Y, Elborn JS, Millar BC, Goldsmith CE, Rendall J and Moore JE (2008) Development of a novel PCR assay for the identification of the black yeast, Exophiala (Wangiella) dermatitidis from adult patients with cystic fibrosis (CF). *J Cyst Fibros* 7: 576–80.

Nguyen MH, Wissel MC, Shields RK, et al. (2012) Performance of Candida real-time polymerase chain reaction, β-D-glucan assay, and blood cultures in the diagnosis of invasive candidiasis. *Clin Infect Dis* 54: 1240–8.

Nucci M and Anaissie E (2007) *Fusarium* infections in immunocompromised patients. *Clin Microbiol Rev* 20: 695–704.

Orsi CF, Gennari W, Venturelli C, et al. (2012) Performance of 2 commercial real-time polymerase chain reaction assays for the detection of Aspergillus and Pneumocystis DNA in bronchoalveolar lavage fluid samples from critical care patients. *Diagn Microbiol Infect Dis* 73: 138–43.

Perry MD, White PL and Barnes RA (2014) Comparison of four automated nucleic acid extraction platforms for the recovery of DNA from Aspergillus fumigatus. *J Med Microbiol* 63: 1160–6.

Pfaller MA and Diekema DJ (2007) Epidemiology of invasive candidiasis: a persistent public health problem. *Clin Microbiol Rev* 20: 133–63.

Pfeiffer CD, Samsa GP, Schell WA, Reller LB, Perfect JR and Alexander BD (2011) Quantitation of Candida CFU in initial positive blood cultures. *J Clin Microbiol* 49: 2879–83.

Pham AS, Tarrand JJ, May GS, Lee MS, Kontoyiannis DP and Han XY (2003) Diagnosis of invasive mold infection by real-time quantitative PCR. *Am J Clin Pathol* 119: 38–44.

Ramírez M, Castro C, Palomares JC, et al. (2009) Molecular detection and identification of Aspergillus spp. from clinical samples using real-time PCR. *Mycoses* 52: 129–34.

Reichard U, Buchheidt D, Lass-Flörl C, et al. (2012) Interlaboratory comparison of PCR-based identification of Candida and Aspergillus DNA in spiked blood samples. *Mycoses* 55: 426–34.

Reinwald M, Spiess B, Heinz WJ, et al. (2012) Diagnosing pulmonary aspergillosis in patients with hematological malignancies: a multicenter prospective evaluation of an Aspergillus PCR assay and a galactomannan ELISA in bronchoalveolar lavage samples. *Eur J Haematol* 89: 120–7.

Rimek D, Garg AP, Haas WH and Kappe R (1999) Identification of contaminating fungal DNA sequences in Zymolyase. *J Clin Microbiol* 37: 830–1.

Roden MM, Zaoutis TE, Buchanan WL, et al. (2005) Epidemiology and outcome of zygomycosis: a review of 929 reported cases. *Clin Infect Dis* 41: 634–53.

Rogers TR, Morton CO, Springer J, et al. (2013) Combined real-time PCR and galactomannan surveillance improves diagnosis of invasive aspergillosis in high risk patients with haematological malignancies. *Br J Haematol* 161: 517–24.

Sanguinetti M, Posteraro B, Pagano L, et al. (2003) Comparison of real-time PCR, conventional PCR, and galactomannan antigen detection by enzyme-linked immunosorbent assay using bronchoalveolar lavage fluid samples from hematology patients for diagnosis of invasive pulmonary aspergillosis. *J Clin Microbiol* 41: 3922–5.

Schabereiter-Gurtner C, Selitsch B, Rotter ML, Hirschl AM and Willinger B (2007) Development of novel real-time PCR assays for detection and differentiation of eleven medically important Aspergillus and Candida species in clinical specimens. *J Clin Microbiol* 45: 906–14.

Schwarzinger M, Sagaon-Teyssier L, Cabaret O, Bretagne S, Cordonnier C and PREVERT Investigators (2013) Performance of serum biomarkers for the early detection of invasive aspergillosis in febrile, neutropenic patients: a multi-state model. *PLoS One* 8: e65776.

Shigemura T, Nakazawa Y, Matsuda K, et al. (2014) Serial monitoring of Mucorales DNA load in serum samples of a patient with disseminated mucormycosis after allogeneic bone marrow transplantation. *Int J Hematol* 100: 206–9.

Skovbjerg S, Welinder-Olsson C, Kondori N, et al. (2009) Optimization of the detection of microbes in blood from immunocompromised patients with haematological malignancies. *Clin Microbiol Infect* 15: 680–3.

Spiess B, Postina P, Reinwald M, et al. (2014) Incidence of Cyp51 A key mutations in *Aspergillus fumigatus*—a study on primary clinical samples of immuno-compromised patients in the period of 1995–2013. *PLos Pathog* e103–13.

Spiess B, Seifarth W, Hummel M, et al. (2007) DNA microarray-based detection and identification of fungal pathogens in clinical samples from neutropenic patients. *J Clin Microbiol* 45: 3743–53.

Spreadbury C, Holden D, Aufauvre-Brown A, Bainbridge B and Cohen J (1993) Detection of *Aspergillus fumigatus* by polymerase chain reaction. *J Clin Microbiol* 31: 615–21.

Springer J, Morton CO, Perry M, et al. (2013) Multicenter comparison of serum and whole-blood specimens for detection of Aspergillus DNA in high-risk hematological patients. *J Clin Microbiol* 51: 1445–50.

Springer J, Schloßnagel H, Heinz W, et al. (2012) A novel extraction method combining plasma with a whole-blood fraction shows excellent sensitivity and reproducibility for patients at high risk for invasive aspergillosis. *J Clin Microbiol* 50: 2585–91.

Sun W, Wang K, Gao W, et al. (2011) Evaluation of PCR on bronchoalveolar lavage fluid for diagnosis of invasive aspergillosis: a bivariate meta-analysis and systematic review. *Plos One* 6: e28467.

Swannink CMA, Meis JFGM, Rijs AJMM, Donnelly JP and Verweij PE (1997) Specificity of a sandwich enzyme-linked immunosorbent assay for detecting *Aspergillus* galactomannan. *J Clin Microbiol* 35: 257–60.

Torelli R, Sanguinetti M, Moody A, et al. (2011) Diagnosis of invasive aspergillosis by a commercial real-time PCR assay for Aspergillus DNA in bronchoalveolar lavage fluid samples from high-risk patients compared to a galactomannan enzyme immunoassay. *J Clin Microbiol* 49: 4273–8.

Tuon FF (2007) A systematic literature review on the diagnosis of invasive aspergillosis using the polymerase chain reaction (PCR) from bronchoalveolar lavage clinical samples. *Rev Iberoam Micol* 24: 89–94.

Van Burik JA, Myerson D, Schreckhise RW and Bowden RA (1998a) Panfungal PCR assay for detection of fungal infection in human blood specimens. *J Clin Microbiol* 36: 1169–75.

Van Burik JA, Schreckhise RW, White TC, Bowden RA and Myerson D (1998b) Comparison of six extraction techniques for isolation of DNA from filamentous fungi. *Med Mycol* 36: 299–303.

Van der Linden JW, Snelders E, Arends JP, et al. (2010) Rapid diagnosis of azole resistant aspergillosis by direct PCR using tissue specimens. *J Clin Microbiol* 48: 1478–80.

Verweij PE (2005) Advances in diagnostic testing. *Med Mycol* 43: S121–4.

Verweij PE, Brinkman K, Kremer HP, Kullberg BJ and Meis JF (1999) *Aspergillus* meningitis: diagnosis by non-culture-based microbiological methods and management. *J Clin Microbiol* 37: 1186–9.

von Eiff M, Roos N, Schulten R, Hesse M, Zühlsdorf M, van de Loo J (1995) Pulmonary aspergillosis: early diagnosis improves survival. *Respiration* 1995; 62: 341–7.

Wellinghausen N, Siegel D, Winter J and Gebert S (2009) Rapid diagnosis of candidaemia by real-time PCR detection of Candida DNA in blood samples. *J Med Microbiol* 58 (Pt 8): 1106–11.

White PL, Archer A and Barnes RA (2005) Comparison of non-culture based methods for detection of systemic fungal infections, with an emphasis on invasive *Candida* infections. *J Clin Microbiol* 43: 2181–7.

White PL, Barnes RA, Springer J, et al. (2015a) Clinical performance of Aspergillus PCR when testing serum and plasma—a study by the European Aspergillus PCR Initiative. *J Clin Microbiol* 53: 2832–7.

White PL, Barton R, Guiver M, et al. (2006a) A consensus on fungal polymerase chain reaction diagnosis?: a United Kingdom-Ireland evaluation of polymerase chain reaction methods for detection of systemic fungal infections. *J Mol Diagn* 8: 376–84.

White PL, Bretagne S, Klingspor L, et al. (2010) *Aspergillus* PCR: one step closer to standardization. *J Clin Microbiol* 48: 1231–40.

White PL, Hibbitts SJ, Perry MD, et al. (2014) Evaluation of a commercially developed semi-automated PCR-SERS assay for the diagnosis of invasive fungal disease. *J Clin Microbiol* 52: 3536–43.

White PL, Linton CJ, Perry MD, Johnson EM and Barnes RA (2006b) The evolution and evaluation of a whole blood polymerase chain reaction assay for the detection of invasive aspergillosis in hematology patients in a routine clinical setting. *Clin Infect Dis* 42: 479–86.

White PL, Mengoli C, Bretagne S, et al. (2011a) Evaluation of Aspergillus PCR protocols for testing serum specimens. *J Clin Microbiol* 49: 3842–8.
White PL, Parr C, Thornton C and Barnes RA (2013) Evaluation of real-time PCR, galactomannan enzyme-linked immunosorbent assay (ELISA), and a novel lateral-flow device for diagnosis of invasive aspergillosis. *J Clin Microbiol* 51: 1510–16.
White PL, Perry MD and Barnes RA (2009) Polymerase chain reaction diagnosis of fungal disease: finally coming of age. *Curr Fungal Infect Rep* 3: 207–15.
White Pl, Perry MD and Barnes RA (2011b) *Candida*, *in*: D Liu (ed.) *Molecular Detection of Human Fungal Pathogens* (Florida, USA: CRC Press, Taylor and Francis Group), 551–68.
White PL, Perry MD, Moody A, Follett SA, Morgan G and Barnes RA (2011c) Evaluation of analytical and preliminary clinical performance of Myconostica MycAssay Aspergillus when testing serum specimens for diagnosis of invasive aspergillosis. *J Clin Microbiol* 49: 2169–74.
White PL, Posso RB and Barnes RA (2015b) Analytical and clinical evaluation of the PathoNostics AsperGenius® Assay for detection of Invasive Aspergillosis and resistance to azole antifungal drugs during testing of serum samples. *J Clin Microbiol* 53: 2115–21.
White PL, Wiederhold NP, Loeffler J, et al. (2016) Comparison of nonculture blood-based tests for diagnosing invasive aspergillosis in an animal model. *J Clin Microbiol* 54: 960–6.
White PL, Wingard JR, Bretagne S, et al. (2015c) *Aspergillus* PCR: a systematic review of evidence for clinical use in comparison with antigen testing. *Clin Infect Dis* 61: 1293–303.
Zaas AK and Alexander BD (2009) Invasive pulmonary aspergillosis, *in*: J-P Latge and WJ Steinbach, eds, *Aspergillus fumigatus and Aspergillosis* (Washington, DC: ASM Press), 293–300.
Zhao Y, Petraitiene R, Walsh TJ and Perlin DS (2013a) A real-time PCR assay for rapid detection and quantification of Exserohilum rostratum, a causative pathogen of fungal meningitis associated with injection of contaminated methylprednisolone. *J Clin Microbiol* 51: 1034–6.
Zhao Y, Stensvold CR, Perlin DS and Arendrup MC (2013b) Azole resistance in *Aspergillus fumigatus* from bronchoalveolar lavage fluid samples of patients with chronic diseases *J Antimicrob Chemother* 68: 1497–1504.

CHAPTER 44

Guidelines for the diagnosis of fungal disease

Manuel Cuenca-Estrella

Introduction to the diagnosis of fungal disease

Over recent years there has been a notable increase in the publication of guidelines. Scientific societies, study groups, and expert panels have reported recommendations about the detection and the management of fungal diseases. Several proposals have been published for grading the quality of evidence and strength of recommendations for those strategies. However, most experts agree that guideline development should follow the AGREE II method (Appraisal of guidelines research & evaluation II; http://www.agreetrust.org/resource-centre/agree-ii/). AGREE II is an instrument developed to address the issue of variability in guideline quality as well as to assess the methodological rigour and transparency of guidelines. The AGREE II system evaluates 23 items across six different domains: scope and purpose, stakeholder involvement, rigour of the development, clarity of presentation, applicability, and editorial independence.

The recommendations mentioned in this chapter follow the AGREE II instrument. Thus, reported guidelines have been included only when the overall objectives of the guideline are specifically described, the health questions covered by the guideline are clearly assessed, and the population to whom the guideline is meant to apply is also specifically described. The definition of the strength of recommendation and the quality of the published evidence are defined in Table 44.1.

Tables 44.2 to 44.5 exhibit the recommendations for diagnosing fungal diseases, classified by diagnostic procedure and emphasizing specific information for some mycoses. Most recommendations in this chapter are based on the results of uncontrolled experiments, opinions of respected authorities, clinical experience, descriptive case studies, or reports of expert committees. It should be noted that conventional diagnostic procedures are essential investigations, and their performance often depends on the possibility of obtaining samples of deep tissues. However, in some cases, strengths of recommendations about new non-culture-based techniques for detecting fungal components should be considered as comparative clinical studies in terms of their accuracy and performance.

Summary of recommendations

Microscopy and culture are of great help in identifying superficial fungal infections, but in the case of systemic and deep fungal diseases their performance has limitations, such as reduced sensitivity, and with microscopy it is not possible to identify the species causing the infection (Cuenca-Estrella et al. 2011). Microscopic procedures include fresh and stained examination of samples as well as histopathological studies (Table 44.2 and Table 44.3). Both cytology and examination of histological sections help to detect fungal elements. Histological sections can also be used for nucleic acid amplification, subsequent to the extraction of such nucleic acids from the tissue. According to Buitrago et al. (2014), molecular techniques could become the technique of choice for the identification of fungal species present in tissue samples.

Table 44.4 shows the recommendations for the culture and identification of species that cause fungal disease. Clinical specimens should be cultured in suitable media to support fungal growth. Cultures should be incubated at both 30°C and 37°C. Selective

Table 44.1 System for grading strength of recommendation and quality of evidence regarding diagnostic procedures used in most reported guidelines

Strength of recommendation	
Grade of recommendation	**Definition**
Grade A	Strongly supports a recommendation for use
Grade B	Moderately supports a recommendation for use
Grade C	Marginally supports a recommendation for use
Grade D	Supports a recommendation against use
Quality of evidence accepted	
Level of evidence	**Definition**
Level I	Evidence from at least one properly designed, randomized, controlled multi-centre trial
Level II	Evidence from at least one well-designed clinical trial, without randomization; from cohort or case-controlled analytical studies (preferably from more than one centre); from multiple time series; or from dramatic results of uncontrolled experiments
Level III	Evidence from opinions of respected authorities, based on clinical experience, descriptive case studies, or reports of expert committees

Table 44.2 Summary of recommendations for direct microscopical examination of clinical specimens to detect fungal diseases (including grade and quality of evidences)

Disease	Intention	Diagnostic procedure	SoR	QoE	Comments
All fungal infections	To identify fungal elements in fresh clinical specimens	Direct microscopy	A	III	Essential investigation
All fungal infections	To improve the detection of fungal elements in fresh clinical specimens	Direct microscopy and application of dyes or fluorescent dyes	A	II	Dyes such as Gram staining, Calcofluor White, Uvitex 2B, or Blancophor
All pulmonary infections	To identify fungal elements in respiratory specimens	Liquefaction of respiratory samples using a mucolytic agent (KOH) or sonication and dithiothreitol	A	III	Three sputum samples should be obtained for the detection of respiratory fungi
Pulmonary infections in immunocompromised patients	To identify fungal elements in respiratory samples	Examination of bronchoalveolar lavage (BAL) with centrifugation and investigation of the sediment	A	III	Examination of sputum and other respiratory secretions is not very useful in this population
Aspergillosis and candidiasis	To identify *Aspergillus* or *Candida* in clinical specimens	Fluorescent-antibody staining	B	II	Genus-specific monoclonal antibody is commercially available
Cryptococcosis	To diagnose the infection presumptively	India ink staining	A	II	Recommended in addition to Gram staining
Pneumocystis jirovecii infection	To diagnose the infection	Liquefaction of respiratory samples and direct fluorescent-antibody staining	A	II	Liquefaction is especially relevant for detecting this microorganism

KOH – potassium hydroxide; QoR = quality of evidence; SoR = strength of evidence

media are recommended for non-sterile samples. All fungi obtained from sterile sites should be identified to species level. Isolates from non-sterile specimens should be evaluated in terms of whether the patient has risk, and isolation from a repeated specimen enhances significance (Schelenz et al. 2015).

Characterization to species level is strongly recommended for all clinical isolates collected from deep sites, including urine samples, respiratory samples, and samples from intravenous line tips. Superficial isolates should be identified in patients receiving antifungal therapy and in cases of proven infection. Conventional methods

Table 44.3 Summary of recommendations for the use of histopathological procedures to detect fungal diseases (including grade and quality of evidences)

Disease	Intention	Diagnostic procedure	SoR	QoE	Comments
All fungal infections	To identify fungal elements in histological sections	Histological examination of fresh tissue and stain (applicable to frozen sections and paraffin-embedded tissues)	A	II	Recommended stains: haematoxylin and eosin (HE) as standard stain; silver-based stains and periodic acid-Schiff (PAS) can be used to highlight fungi
All fungal infections	To improve the detection of fungal elements in fresh tissues	Direct microscopy and application of fluorescent dyes	A	II	Dyes such as Calcofluor White, Uvitex 2B or Blancophor; no species identification
All fungal infections	To identify genus in histological sections	Immunohistochemistry; *in-situ* hybridization	B	II	Monoclonal antibodies are commercially available for *Aspergillus*, *Candida*, and some other fungal species
Mucormycosis	Histological examination of fresh tissue and stain	Histological examination of tissue and stain	A	II	Does not allow for genus or species differentiation
Phaeohyphomycosis	Histological examination of fresh tissue and stain	Histological examination of tissue and stain	A	II	Sclerotic bodies, or 'copper pennies', are specific for chromoblastomycosis; other mycoses present as non-specific melanized hyphae or yeast
Endemic dimorphic mycosis	Histological examination of fresh tissue and stain	Histological examination of tissue and stain	A	II	Observation of spherules can presumptively identify coccidioidomycosis

QoR = quality of evidence; SoR = strength of evidence

Table 44.4 Summary of recommendations for the culture and identification of species causing fungal diseases (including grade and quality of evidences)

Disease/population	Intention	Diagnostic procedure	SoR	QoE	Comments
All fungal infections	Definitive diagnosis	Culture of specimen at the sources of infection at 30°C and 37°C for 72 h	A	III	Cultures on Sabouraud dextrose agar, brain-heart infusion agar, or other assay media for fungi
All fungal infections	Isolation from non-sterile samples	Culture of specimens on assay media for fungi supplemented with gentamicin and chloramphenicol	A	III	Isolation of several colonies or repeated isolation of the same fungus from consecutive specimens enhances significance
All fungal infections	Isolation from non-sterile samples	Quantitative cultures	D	II	Does not discriminate infection from colonization
Disseminated infections and fungal endocarditis	Definitive diagnosis	Blood cultures	A	III	Sensitivity of blood cultures can be <50% in most disseminated mycoses
Cerebral abscess	Definitive diagnosis	Culture of specimens taken by guided biopsy	A	II	Useful for diagnosing cases by species such as *Cladophialophora bantiana* and *Rhinocladiella mackenziei*—species commonly found in cerebral abscess
Pulmonary infections	Definitive diagnosis	Culture of bronchoalveolar lavage (BAL) specimens, guided biopsy, or open lung biopsy	A	II	BAL is preferable; biopsies undertaken only if less invasive procedures are not achievable
All fungal infections	Species identification	Macroscopic and microscopic examination from positive cultures	A	III	Accurate species assignment is important for guiding clinical management
All fungal infections	Species identification	Subculture on identification media (2% malt extract agar, etc.) at 25–30°C and 37°C	A	III	Observations should be made of colony colour, and of conidium size, colour, shape, and septation
Candidiasis and other yeast infections	Species identification	Phenotypical identification by biochemical profile	C	II	Non-accurate for rare, emerging, and sibling species
All fungal infections	Species identification	Identification by MALDI-TOF	A	II	Now widely used for yeasts but still problematic for moulds and not yet validated for rare species
All fungal infections	Species identification	Identification by DNA target sequences	A	III	In-house procedures, but essential for classification of some species
All fungal infections	To expand knowledge about local species distribution	Periodical epidemiological surveys	A	III	DNA target sequence is essential for establishing the rate of rare and emerging species

BAL = bronchoalveolar lavage; MALDI-TOF = matrix-assisted laser desorption/ionization–time-of-flight (mass spectrometry); QoR = quality of evidence; SoR = strength of evidence

of classification remain the standard, but nucleic acid sequencing techniques are coming closer to routine clinical practice, and are essential for rare, emerging, and sibling species (Arendrup et al. 2014; Chowdhary et al. 2014; Tortorano et al. 2014).

Macroscopic lesions can be analyzed by radiographic examinations. Imaging is very useful for detecting and managing fungal diseases. Chest radiographs can help to localize the infection, but high-resolution computed tomography (CT) scans of the thorax are recommended in onco-haematological patients and some other populations with respiratory symptoms or a positive fungal biomarker. Cranial CT and MRI (magnetic resonance imaging) scans should be performed in immunocompromised patients with neurological features. A CT scan is also useful in invasive fungal sinus and abdominal infections (De Pauw et al. 2008).

The detection of fungal biomarkers should be implemented as procedure for the early detection of fungal diseases in immunocompromised patients, in cases undergoing intensive-care therapies, and in patients with chronic disorders and lung diseases (Table 44.5). The quantification of antigens is already the gold standard for detecting cryptococcosis in the HIV (human immunovirus) population and in some infections caused by endemic dimorphic fungi (Wheat et al. 2007; Perfect et al. 2010; Limper et al. 2011). In addition, the quantification of galactomannan is strongly recommended for the early detection of aspergillosis in onco-haematological patients (Marchetti et al. 2011; EFISG 2015) and for the detection of beta-D-glucan in candidiasis and pneumocystosis (Limper 2011; Cuenca-Estrella et al. 2012). Polymerase chain reaction (PCR)-based methods are very useful for diagnosing the infection in tissues positive for microscopic fungal elements. In other clinical specimens, those molecular methods can help to detect fungal diseases in combination with conventional techniques (Cornely et al. 2013; Aguado et al. 2014).

Table 44.5 Summary of recommendations for diagnosing fungal diseases using non-cultured procedures (direct biomarker detection, molecular testing, and fungal serology in clinical specimens). Table includes grade and quality of evidences.

Disease	Intention	Diagnostic procedure	SoR	QoE	Comments
Aspergillosis					
Invasive aspergillosis	To diagnose the infection	Detection of antibodies to *Aspergillus*	C	III	Detection of specific antibodies to *Aspergillus* by EIA, agar diffusion, or immunohaemagglutination; low performance in immunosuppressant patients
Chronic pulmonary aspergillosis	To diagnose the infection	Detection of *Aspergillus* IgG and *Aspergillus* precipitins	A	II	Useful in cavitary or nodular pulmonary infiltrate in non-immunocompromised patients
Allergic bronchopulmonary aspergillosis	To diagnose the infection	Detection of total IgE and *Aspergillus*-specific IgE	B	II	Useful in the context of asthma or cystic fibrosis
Invasive aspergillosis in neutropenic patients without anti-mould prophylaxis	To exclude invasive aspergillosis-screening	Detection of galactomannan (GM) blood	A	I	Better performance in prolonged neutropenic patients and allogeneic stem cell transplantation recipients; monitored twice weekly
Invasive aspergillosis in neutropenic patients with anti-mould prophylaxis	To diagnose the infection	Detection of GM blood	D	II	Very low prevalence rate and unacceptable positive predictive value
Invasive aspergillosis in haematological non-neutropenic patients	To diagnose the infection	Detection of GM blood	B	II	Less accurate than in neutropenic patients
Aspergillosis in ICU patients	To diagnose the infection	Detection of GM blood	C	II	Low sensitivity
Aspergillosis in solid organ recipients	To diagnose the infection	Detection of GM blood	C	II	Low sensitivity
Pulmonary aspergillosis	To diagnose the infection	Detection of GM bronchoalveolar lavage (BAL)	A	II	Criterion of probable aspergillosis
Cerebral aspergillosis	To diagnose the infection	Detection of GM cerebrospinal fluid (CSF)	B	II	Less experience than with other methods
Invasive aspergillosis	To exclude invasive aspergillosis-screening	Detection of beta-D-glucan blood	B	II	Pan-fungal assay; twice-weekly assay
Invasive aspergillosis	To diagnose the infection	Detection of beta-D-glucan blood	C	II	Evaluated in mixed population: adult ICU, haematological disorders, transplant recipients; requires further tests to diagnose aspergillosis
Invasive aspergillosis	To diagnose the infection	Detection of beta-D-glucan BAL	C	II	False-positive results due to saprophyte flora
Invasive aspergillosis	To exclude invasive aspergillosis-screening	PCR-based techniques in blood	B	II	Standardization in progress; quantitative techniques are preferable
Invasive aspergillosis	To diagnose the infection	PCR-based technique in tissues microscopic hyphal-positive	A	II	Fresh wax- and paraffin-embedded tissues can be analyzed
Invasive aspergillosis	To diagnose the infection	PCR-based technique in tissues microscopic hyphal-negative	C	II	Low sensitivity
Pulmonary aspergillosis	To diagnose the infection	PCR-based techniques in BAL	B	II	Low positive predictive values in other respiratory secretions; commercial kits are available
Cerebral aspergillosis	To diagnose the infection	PCR-based techniques in CSF	B	III	Less experience than with other sample types
Invasive aspergillosis	To diagnose the infection	Combination of techniques; largely GM plus PCR-based procedures	A	II	Two positive tests can confirm the diagnosis of the infection
Invasive aspergillosis	To monitor response to treatment	Serial GM quantification	C	II	GM index >1 in blood may be considered a sign of therapeutic failure in patients undergoing treatment

Table 44.5 (Continued)

Disease	Intention	Diagnostic procedure	SoR	QoE	Comments
Candidiasis					
All candidiasis	To diagnose the infection	Detection of specific antibodies to *Candida*	D	II	Unable to distinguish colonization and infection
Candidaemia	To exclude the infection	Detection of beta-D-glucan blood	B	II	Pan-fungal assay
Candidaemia	To exclude the infection	Detection of combined mannan antigen and anti-mannan antibody	B	II	Not available in most centres
Candidaemia	To diagnose the infection	PCR-based techniques in blood	C	II	In process of standardization
Invasive candidiasis	To exclude the infection	Detection of beta-D-glucan blood	B	II	Useful in ICU settings
Invasive candidiasis	To exclude the infection	Detection of combined mannan antigen and anti-mannan antibody	C	II	Insufficient data
Invasive candidiasis	To diagnose the infection	PCR-based techniques in blood	C	II	In process of standardization; could be useful as a gold standard in combination with detection of other biomarkers
Chronic disseminated candidiasis	To diagnose the infection	Detection of beta-D-glucan blood	B	II	Dramatic results from uncontrolled studies
Chronic disseminated candidiasis	To diagnose the infection	Detection of combined nannan antigen and anti-mannan antibody	B	II	Dramatic results from uncontrolled studies
Chronic disseminated candidiasis	To diagnose the infection	PCR-based techniques in blood	C	II	Insufficient data
Invasive and chronic disseminated candidiasis	To diagnose the infection	PCR-based techniques in tissues microscopic yeast-positive	B	II	Fresh wax- and paraffin-embedded tissues can be analyzed
Cryptococcosis (by *C. neoformans* or *C. gattii*)					
Disseminated or meningeal cryptococcosis in HIV population	To diagnose the infection	Detection of cryptococcal antigen in CSF, serum, or urine	A	I	A lateral flow device is already available
Cryptococcosis in non-HIV population	To diagnose the infection	Detection of cryptococcal antigen in serum or CSF	B	II	Lower sensitivity than in HIV patients
Pulmonary and other local cryptococcosis	To diagnose the infection	Detection of cryptococcal antigen in serum	B	II	Limited uncontrolled studies
Pulmonary cryptococcosis	To diagnose the infection	Detection of cryptococcal antigen in respiratory specimens	A	II	Good performance in BAL specimens
Other cryptococcosis caused by non-*neoformans* and non-*gattii* species	To diagnose the infection	Detection of cryptococcal antigen	C	III	Less sensitivity for those species
All cryptococcosis	To diagnose the infection	PCR-based techniques	C	II	Insufficient data
All cryptococcosis	To diagnose the infection	Detection of beta-D-glucan blood	D	II	It is a pan-fungal test but beta-D-glucan is not part of the cell wall of *Cryptococcus* or other basidiomycetes
Disseminated cryptococcosis	To monitor response to treatment	Cryptococcal antigen quantification in serum	B	II	Very useful in HIV patients in decisions on continuing maintenance therapy

(continued)

Table 44.5 (Continued)

Disease	Intention	Diagnostic procedure	SoR	QoE	Comments
Infections by other yeasts					
Disseminated infections	To diagnose the infection	Detection of beta-D-glucan blood	C	III	Potentially useful in detecting infections caused by members of Ascomycota as it is a pan-fungal biomarker
Deep local infections	To diagnose the infection	Detection of beta-D-glucan blood	D	III	Sensitivity likely to be too low
All infections by other yeasts	To diagnose the infection	Detection of GM	C	III	Cross-reaction in some species, but not sufficiently evaluated and no species identification
All infections by other yeasts	To diagnose the infection	PCR-based techniques	C	III	Useful in some case studies reported, but not validated
Infection by *Trichosporon*	To diagnose the infection	Detection of cryptococcal antigen	B	II	Cross-reaction with cryptococcal polysaccharide
Infection by *Saccharomyces*	To diagnose the infection	Detection of *Candida* mannan	C	III	Cross- reactivity and single cases reported
Infections by dematiaceous (pigmented) fungi					
All deep infections	To diagnose the infection	Detection of beta-D-glucan blood	C	III	Pan-fungal detection but insufficient data
Pulmonary infections	To diagnose the infection	Detection of beta-D-glucan BAL	D	III	False positives from saprophytic flora
All deep infections	To diagnose the infection	Detection of GM	D	III	Cross-reactivity in some cases, but not analyzed
All deep infections	To diagnose the infection	PCR-based techniques in blood or respiratory specimens	C	III	Not validated
All deep infections	To diagnose the infection	PCR-based technique in tissues microscopic hyphal-positive	A	II	Fresh, wax- and paraffin-embedded tissues can be analyzed
Infections by *Fonseca pedrosoi* and *Cladophialophora carrionii*	To diagnose the infection	In-house ELISA techniques to detect antibodies	C	III	Not validated
Endemic dimorphic fungi					
Acute histoplasmosis	To diagnose the infection	Detection of antibody	D	II	Low performance
Disseminated histoplasmosis in HIV patients	To diagnose the infection and follow up	Detection of *Histoplasma* antigen in urine and blood	A	II	Criterion of probable histoplasmosis
Pulmonary histoplasmosis in non-HIV patients	To diagnose the infection	Detection of *Histoplasma* antigen in BAL	A	II	None
Disseminated histoplasmosis in HIV patients	To diagnose the infection	Detection of *Histoplasma* antigen in BAL	B	II	Lower sensitivity than in urine and blood
Pulmonary histoplasmosis in non-HIV patients	To diagnose the infection	Detection of *Histoplasma* antigen in blood and urine	B	II	Lower sensitivity than in BAL
Chronic complications of histoplasmosis in non-HIV patients	To diagnose the complication	Detection of antibody	A	II	Low sensitivity in immunocompromised populations
All histoplasmosis	To diagnose infections	PCR-based techniques	B	II	Poorly evaluated in chronic complications
Blastomycosis	To diagnose the infection	Detection of antibody	D	II	Positive weeks after acute disease
Blastomycosis	To diagnose the infection	Detection of antigen in urine, blood, and respiratory specimens	B	II	Criterion of probable blastomycosis
Blastomycosis	To diagnose the infection	PCR-based techniques	B	III	Lack of controlled studies

Table 44.5 (Continued)

Disease	Intention	Diagnostic procedure	SoR	QoE	Comments
Coccidioidomycosis	To diagnose the infection and follow up	Detection of antibody	A	II	Positive a few days after infection
Coccidioidomycosis	To diagnose the infection	Detection of antigen in urine, blood, and respiratory specimens	B	II	Criterion of probable coccidioidomycosis
Coccidioidomycosis	To diagnose the infection	PCR-based techniques	B	III	Lack of controlled studies
Paracoccidioidomycosis	To diagnose the infection	Detection of antibody	A	II	Better performance combining two serological techniques; Less useful for the follow-up
Paracoccidioidomycosis in immunocompromised hosts	To diagnose the infection	Detection of antibody	D	II	Low sensitivity
Paracoccidioidomycosis	To diagnose the infection and follow up	Detection of antigen in blood	B	II	Criterion of probable infection
Paracoccidioidomycosis	To diagnose the infection	PCR-based techniques	B	III	Lack of controlled studies
Infections by *Talaromyces (Penicillium) marneffei*	To diagnose the infection	Detection of antibody	D	III	Opportunistic infection in immunocompromised populations
Infections by *Talaromyces (Penicillium) marneffei*	To diagnose the infection	Detection of GM in clinical specimens	B	II	Blood and respiratory samples
Infections by *Talaromyces (Penicillium) marneffei*	To diagnose the infection	PCR-based techniques	B	III	Lack of controlled studies
Infections by other hyaline fungi (*Fusarium* and *Scedosporium*)					
All deep infections	To diagnose the infection	Detection of beta-D-glucan	B	III	Pan-fungal biomarker; utility observed in disseminated infections by *Fusarium*
All deep infections	To diagnose the infection	Detection of GM	C	III	Cross-reaction in some species, but not sufficiently evaluated and no species identification
Al deep infections	To diagnose the infection	PCR-based techniques	C	III	In combination with conventional methods
Infections by mucoraceous fungi					
All deep infections	To diagnose the infection	Detection of beta-D-glucan	D	III	Not a reliable marker in detecting mucoraceous moulds
All deep infections	To diagnose the infection	Detection of GM	B	III	Cross-reactivity and positively evaluated in uncontrolled studies
All deep infections	To diagnose the infection	PCR-based techniques	B	II	Fresh, wax- and paraffin embedded tissues can be analyzed
Infections by *Pneumocystis jirovecii*					
All infections	To diagnose the infection	Detection of beta-D-glucan	A	II	High level of this fungal component in blood of patients with pneumocystosis
All infections	To diagnose the infection	Detection of antibody and specific antigen	C	III	Not evaluated
Pulmonary infections in HIV population	To diagnose the infection	PCR-based techniques in respiratory samples	A	II	Reference technique in many clinical laboratories
Pulmonary infections in non-HIV population	To diagnose the infection	PCR-based techniques in respiratory samples	B	II	In combination with stains

BAL = bronchoalveolar lavage; CSF = cerebrospinal fluid; EIA = enzyme immunoassay; ELISA = enzyme-linked immunosorbent assay; GM = galactomannan; ICU = intensive care unit; QoR = quality of evidence; SoR = strength of evidence

References

Aguado JM, Vázquez L, Fernández-Ruiz M, et al. (2014) Serum galactomannan vs. a combination of galactomannan and PCR-based Aspergillus DNA detection for early therapy of invasive aspergillosis in high-risk hematological patients: a randomized controlled trial. *Clin Infect Dis* 60: 405–14.

Arendrup MC, Boekhout T, Akova M, et al. (2014) ESCMID/ECMM joint clinical guidelines for the diagnosis and management of rare invasive yeast infections. *Clin Microbiol Infect* 20 (Suppl. 3): 76–103.

Buitrago MJ, Bernal-Martinez L, Castelli MV, et al. (2014) Analysis of performance of panfungal and specific PCR-based procedures for etiological diagnosis of invasive fungal diseases on tissue biopsies with proven infection: a seven year retrospective analysis from a reference laboratory. *J Clin Microbiol* 52: 1737–40.

Chowdhary A, Meis JF, Guarro J, et al. (2014) ESCMID/ECMM Joint clinical guidelines for the diagnosis and management of systemic phaeohyphomycosis: diseases caused by black fungi. *Clin Microbiol Infect* 20 (Suppl. 3):47–75.

Cornely OA, Arikan-Akdagli S, Dannaoui E, et al. (2013) ESCMID and ECMM joint clinical guidelines for the diagnosis and management of mucormycosis. *Clin Microbiol Infect* 20 (Suppl. 3): 5–26.

Cuenca-Estrella M, Bassetti M, Lass-Floerl C, et al. (2011) Detection and investigation of invasive mould disease. *J Antimicrob Chemother* 66 (Suppl. 1): i15–24.

Cuenca-Estrella M, Verweij PE, Arendrup MC, et al. (2012) ESCMID guidelines for the diagnosis and management of Candida diseases 2012: diagnostic procedures. *Clin Microbiol Infect* 18 (Suppl. 7): 9–18.

De Pauw B, Walsh TJ, Donnelly JP, et al. (2008) Revised definitions of invasive fungal disease from the European Organisation for Research and Treatment of Cancer/Invasive Fungal Infections Cooperative Group and the National Institute of Allergy and Infectious Diseases Mycoses Study Group (EORTC/MSG) Consensus Group. *Clin Infect Dis* 46: 1813–21.

European Fungal Infection Study Group (EFISG) (2015) Guidelines for the diagnosis and management of Aspergillus diseases of the European Society of Clinical Microbiology and Infectious Diseases. *Clin Microbiol Infect* (in press).

Limper AH, Knox KS, Sarosi GA, et al. (2011) An official American Thoracic Society statement: treatment of fungal infections in adult pulmonary and critical care patients. *Am J Respir Crit Care Med* 183: 96–128.

Marchetti O, Lamoth F, Mikulska M et al. (2011) European Conference on Infections in Leukemia (ECIL) Laboratory Working Groups. (2011) ECIL recommendations for the use of biological markers for the diagnosis of invasive fungal diseases in leukemic patients and hematopoietic SCT recipients. *Bone Marrow Transplant* 47: 846–54.

Perfect JR, Dismukes WE, Dromer F, et al. (2010) Clinical practice guidelines for the management of cryptococcal disease: 2010 update by the infectious diseases society of America. *Clin Infect Dis* 50: 291–322.

Schelenz S, Barnes RA, Barton RC, et al. (2015) British Society for Medical Mycology best practice recommendations for the diagnosis of serious fungal diseases. *Lancet Infect Dis* 15: 461–74.

Tortorano AM, Richardson M, Roilides E, et al. (2014) ESCMID & ECMM joint guidelines on diagnosis and management of hyalohyphomycosis: *Fusarium* spp, *Scedosporium* spp, and others. *Clin Microbiol Infect* 20 (Suppl 3): 27–46.

Wheat LJ, Freifeld AG, Kleiman MB, et al. (2007) Clinical practice guidelines for the management of patients with histoplasmosis: 2007 update by the Infectious Diseases Society of America. *Clin Infect Dis* 45: 807–25.

SECTION 6

Antifungal therapy

CHAPTER 45

Principles of antifungal therapy

Russell E. Lewis

Introduction to antifungal agents

Fungal infections are increasing in incidence and mortality. Fortunately, clinicians now have a greater number of treatment options for combating these life-threatening infections (Figure 45.1). In a little over a decade, six new antifungal agents have been introduced that are as effective, or more effective, than conventional amphotericin B-deoxycholate, but with significantly fewer toxicities (Ostrosky-Zeichner et al. 2010). However, all of the current antifungal agents have limitations for treating invasive fungal disease regarding their spectrum of activity, pharmacokinetic/pharmacodynamic properties, dosing, toxicity, potential for serious drug interactions, and cost. Therefore, there is no single ideal antifungal for all patients. Therapeutic decisions and dosing must be tailored to specific treatment scenarios—that is, the most likely pathogen, the patient's comorbidities and medication profile, and, in some centres, the hospital formulary. This chapter examines some of the general principles that impact on the selection of antifungal therapy for life-threatening mycoses. Chapters 46 to 49 present more detailed discussion of individual antifungal agents.

Patient and drug factors that impact upon the success of antifungal therapy

Several risk factors have been consistently shown to predispose patients to treatment failure during the management of invasive fungal disease. The depth and severity of the immunosuppression of the patient are perhaps the most important determinants of long-term treatment success (Romani 2011). Defects in cellular immunity, particularly profound neutropenia (<100 white blood cells/mm^3), or receipt of high-dose corticosteroid therapy or calcineurin inhibitors to prevent organ rejection or control graft-versus-host disease, are independent risk factors for antifungal treatment failure in clinical trials and case series (Upton et al. 2007; Nivoix et al. 2008; Andes et al. 2010; Nucci et al. 2013). Inadequate source control may also impair immune system clearance of fungal pathogens. In the case of invasive candidiasis, an undrained abscess or failure to remove infected catheters with biofilm-embedded *Candida* species predisposes patients to relapse or progression to sepsis during antifungal therapy (Andes et al. 2010; Bassetti et al. 2014; Micek et al. 2014).

A second variable influencing the outcome of antifungal therapy is the timing of treatment after disease onset. Antifungal agents are less effective if started when the fungal burden is high, tissue invasion or damage is extensive, and dissemination to other organs has occurred. Hence, delayed diagnosis of invasive fungal disease directly reduces the probability of treatment success. In observational studies, treatment delays as little as 24 hours after a positive blood culture for *Candida* species were associated with a near doubling of crude mortality rates in patients with invasive candidiasis (Morrell et al. 2005; Garey et al. 2006; Cornely et al. 2015). Similarly, patients with cryptococcal meningitis who present with a higher baseline fungal burden are more likely to develop increased intracranial pressure and mental status changes, both of which are risk factors for mortality (Brouwer et al. 2004; Bicanic et al. 2009). Patients with invasive aspergillosis in whom antifungal therapy was initiated at the time of the 'halo sign'—an early radiographic finding of mould infection on chest computed tomography (CT) that disappears in one-third of patients within 72 hours—have a 20–25% higher clinical response rate and significantly lower mortality than patients without this early CT finding (Caillot et al. 1997; Brodoefel et al. 2006; Greene et al. 2007).

The final two variables influencing response to antifungal therapy are the closely linked concepts of pharmacokinetic (PK) and pharmacodynamic (PD) variability (Figure 45.2). Pharmacokinetics refers to the time course of drug concentrations in the body, which are determined by the degree and rate of drug absorption from the gastrointestinal tract, tissue distribution, metabolism, and the rate of drug elimination. Variability in the time course of drug concentrations from one patient to the next, or within the same patient from one day to the next, is influenced by drug factors (e.g. molecule lipophilicity, molecular weight, plasma, and tissue protein binding), patient-specific factors (e.g. weight, sex, disease state, organ function), site of infection, and how the drug is dosed.

Pharmacodynamics refers to the rate and extent of pathogen killing versus drug exposure. Pharmacodynamic variability arises primarily from the intrinsic or acquired resistance to the pathogen. The most common index used to identify intrinsic or acquired resistance to both antibacterial and antifungal agents is the minimum inhibitory concentration (MIC).

Indexing plasma pharmacokinetic parameters to the pathogen MIC allows pharmacokinetic exposures to be linked to antifungal effects and the probability of clinical cure. However, the specific PK/PD variable associated with antifungal efficacy varies from one class of antifungals to the next, depending on the shape of the dose–response curve *in vivo*, especially at supra-MIC concentrations (i.e. 4, 8, 16× MIC) (Figure 45.3). For antifungals that display patterns of inhibition or killing that maximize as the drug concentrations approach the MIC (e.g. flucytosine [5-fluorocytosine]), the percentage of time plasma drug concentrations exceed the MIC over a 24-hour dosing interval (%T_{MIC}) is the PK/PD variable most closely linked to antifungal efficacy. Alternatively, for antifungals

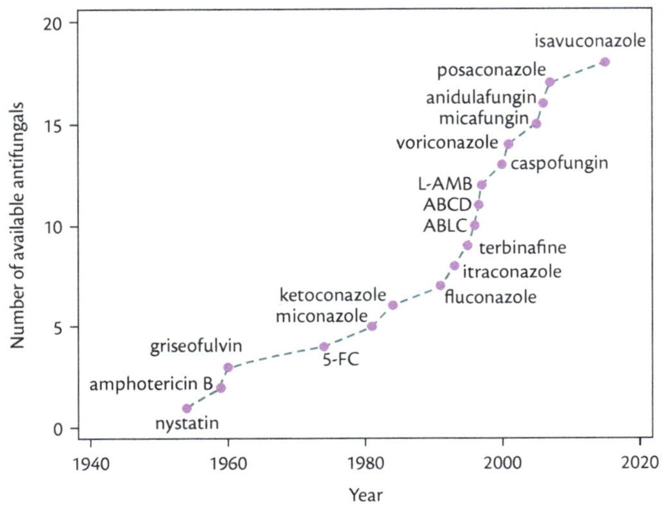

Figure 45.1 Timeline of systemic antifungals.

ABCD = amphotericin B colloidal dispersion; ABLC = amphotericin B lipid complex; L-AMB = liposomal amphotericin B.

that show patterns of increasing rate and extent of antifungal activity with higher multiples above the MIC (i.e. 4–16× MIC), the ratio of peak plasma levels to MIC (C_{max}/MIC) or the 24-hour area under the concentration-time curve ratio (AUC/MIC) are better predictors of efficacy than %T_{MIC}. Antifungals that have mixed time and concentration-dependent pharmacodynamics (triazoles, echinocandins, lipid amphotericin-B formulations) are best described by the AUC/MIC ratio (Sinnollareddy et al. 2012) (Table 45.1).

PK/PD variables are unique because they are controlled by the prescriber—that is, the prescriber controls which antifungal is selected and how it is dosed (Theuretzbacher 2012). Therefore, it is important for clinicians to recognize the drug and patient-related

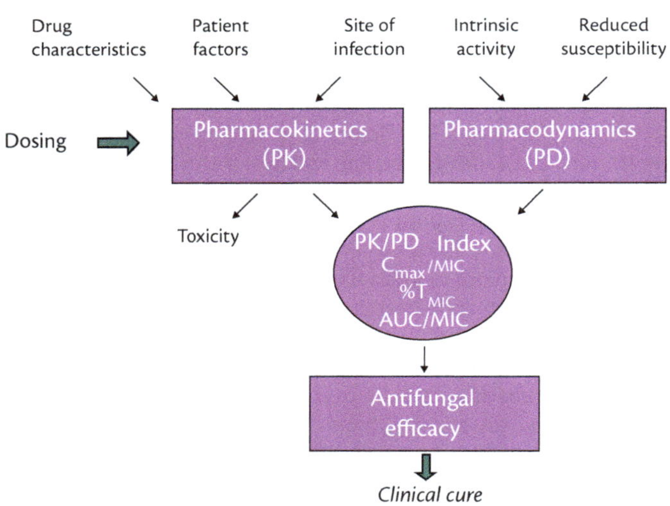

Figure 45.2 Interrelationship between antifungal pharmacokinetics and pharmacodynamics.

Reproduced from Theuretzbacher U, 'Pharmacokinetic and pharmacodynamic issues for antimicrobial therapy in patients with cancer', *Clinical Infectious Diseases*, Volume 54, Issue 12, pp. 1785–92, by permission of Oxford University Press. Copyright © 2012 Oxford University Press. DOI: 10.1093/cid/cis210

variables that can result in PK/PD variability and reduce the probability of clinical cure.

Which factors contribute to the pharmacokinetic variability of antifungals?

Antifungal risk factors

A frequent misconception is that a European Medicine Agency (EMA) or US Food and Drug Administration (FDA) 'approved' dose—as stated on the package labelling—is always appropriate for a specific patient. Doses listed on package labelling are primarily from Phase II/III clinical trials that frequently excluded patients who exhibit significant pharmacokinetic or pharmacodynamic heterogeneity. Indeed, only 10% of non-neutropenic ICU (intensive care unit) patients prospectively evaluated for inclusion in clinical trials of invasive candidiasis are enrolled (Pappas et al. 2003; Rex et al. 2003). Most patients are excluded because of prior antifungal therapy, abnormal laboratory values, age, comorbid conditions, and other considerations. For invasive aspergillosis, fewer than half of patients meet the European Organisation for Research and Treatment of Cancer/Mycoses Study Group (EORTC/MSG) criteria of proven or probable diseases required for trial enrolment, and many patients with poor underlying disease prognosis are not enrolled to limit early deaths that confound analysis of treatment response (Herbrecht et al. 2012). Hence, recommended dosing is derived from patient populations with less pharmacokinetic heterogeneity, and may not be representative of many 'real-life' patients.

Pharmacokinetic variability occurs with all agents, but the degree of variability and its potential impact on outcome varies from one drug to the next. As discussed earlier, the degree of pharmacokinetic variability is linked to the inherent physiochemical properties of the drug (hydrophobic *vs* hydrophilic characteristics, protein binding), oral bioavailability, and the pathways by which the antifungal is metabolized and cleared.

Drug interactions, in particular, are an important source of pharmacokinetic variability for antifungals. Some triazoles are metabolized to varying degrees by human CYP P450 enzymatic pathways (Brüggemann et al. 2009). Consequently, co-administration of triazoles with inducers of CYP P450 accelerates their metabolism and clearance, resulting in sub-therapeutic, if not undetectable, blood levels. As triazoles also act as inhibitors of CYP 3A4, with varying degrees of potency, they have the potential to inhibit the metabolism and clearance of many immunosuppressive and chemotherapy agents, antiviral medications, anaesthetics, and cardiac drugs, resulting in potentially dangerous overdosing. Over 2,000 theoretical drug interactions with triazoles have been predicted based on known pathways of drug metabolism. However, only several hundred of these interactions have been studied, and specific recommendations for using potentially dangerous combinations are frequently unavailable (Brüggemann et al. 2009). Any patient starting or stopping a triazole antifungal therapy should have their medication profile carefully reviewed (including herbal and non-prescription medications) to screen for possibly contraindicated combinations or drugs that require dosing adjustment. This assessment can be aided by point-of-care computerized screening tools and databases, some of which are freely available online or for smartphones

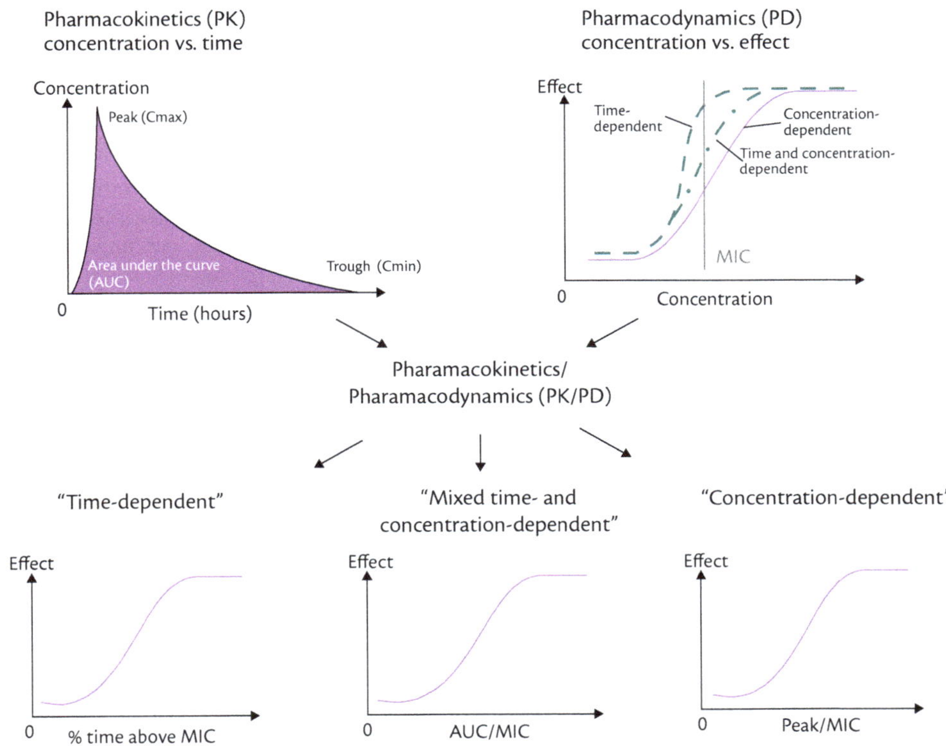

Figure 45.3 Variability and relationship between dosing, pharmacokinetics, pharmacodynamics, and antifungal efficacy that predicts the probability of clinical cure. C_{max}/MIC = peak serum level to MIC ratio; %T_{MIC} = cumulative period of a 24-hour time interval in which the plasma drug exceeds the MIC; AUC/MIC = plasma area under the concentration-time curve over a 24-hour ratio to MIC.

Adapted from Theuretzbacher U, 'Pharmacokinetic and pharmacodynamic issues for antimicrobial therapy in patients with cancer', *Clinical Infectious Diseases*, Volume 54, Issue 12, pp. 1785–92, by permission of Oxford University Press. Copyright © 2012 Oxford University Press. DOI: 10.1093/cid/cis210

Table 45.1 Pharmacokinetic/pharmacodynamic parameters of commonly used systemic antifungal agents.

Antifungal class	PK/PD index	References
Polyenes Amphotericin B	C_{max}/MIC >2.5 (AMB-d) AUC/MIC >13 (AMB-d) AUC/MIC >25 (ABLC) AUC/MIC >150 (L-AMB)	Andes et al. 2001 Al-Nakeeb et al. 2015 Wiederhold et al. 2006
Triazole antifungals Fluconazole Itraconazole Voriconazole Posaconazole Isavuconazole	AUC/MIC Free drug 25–50 Maximal survival, free drug >100	EUCAST 2015 Baddley et al. 2008
Echinocandins Anidulafungin Caspofungin Micafungin	Total drug C_{max}/MIC 3–10 Free drug AUC/MIC_{24} 7–20	Wiederhold et al. 2004 Andes et al. 2010
Flucytosine	%T_{MIC} >50%	Andes and van Ogtrop 2000 Hope et al. 2006

ABLC = amphotericin-B lipid complex; AMB-d = amphotericin B deoxycholate; AUC/MIC = area under the curve/minimum inhibitory concentration; C_{max}/MIC = peak concentration/minimum inhibitory concentration; L-AMB = liposomal amphotericin B; %T_{MIC} = MIC over a 24-hour dosing interval

(e.g. http://www.fungalpharmacology.org and the antifungal interactions PRO program available on Apple iTunes App Store and Google Play App Store).

Patient risk factors

Careful consideration of patient physiological characteristics is important for selecting an antifungal therapy. These characteristics may include weight, renal, and liver function; hypoalbuminaemia, sepsis, or other hyperdynamic conditions associated with altered fluid balance; and the presence of extracorporeal circuits (i.e. renal replacement therapy, extracorporeal membrane oxygenation) (Sinnollareddy et al. 2012; Roberts et al. 2014). Patients with sepsis often exhibit marked alterations in fluid balance owing to capillary leakage into tissue (third spacing) and increased cardiac output. These changes can increase the distribution volume for hydrophilic antifungals, such as fluconazole and flucytosine, resulting in low blood levels with standard doses. Increases in distribution volume during sepsis make the administration of a loading dose for antifungals such as fluconazole critical, as therapeutic levels may not occur for several days with increased volume of distribution (Roberts et al. 2014).

Marked changes in fluid balance are often accompanied by dysfunction of one or more organ systems that could predispose the patient to clinical failure or enhanced toxic effects from the antifungal regimen. For example, use of an amphotericin-B based regimen in a patient with sepsis may not be judicious, even in the absence of markedly elevated serum creatinine, as the risk of acute tubular necrosis is higher in the setting of impaired renal blood flow (Saliba and Dupont 2008).

Although prescribers are frequently aware of the potential for toxicity with antifungals, the problem of under-dosing in critically ill patients may be under-recognized. The multinational Defining Antibiotic Levels in Intensive care unit (DALI) patients point-prevalence pharmacokinetic study examined how frequently ICU patients achieved adequate PK/PD exposures for representative antifungals used in the treatment of invasive candidiasis (fluconazole, anidulafungin, micafungin) (Sinnollareddy et al. 2015). Considerable inter- and intra-individual pharmacokinetic variability was evident for all three antifungals, but was most problematic for fluconazole because a fixed 400 mg dose is frequently administered in patients irrespective of weight or physiological status. One-third of fluconazole-treated patients in the DALI study did not achieve the recommended plasma-free drug (non-protein bound drug) PK/PD target of AUC/MIC >100. This finding was consistent with a retrospective study in 245 invasive candidiasis patients which reported that inadequate initial fluconazole dosing was an independent predictor of mortality (adjusted odds ratio 3.31; 95% CI, range 1.83–6.0; $P = 0.003$), along with receipt of corticosteroids and failure to remove central venous catheters (Labelle et al. 2008). Plasma exposures for anidulafungin and caspofungin in the DALI study were also found to be lower than was previously reported from clinical trials, suggesting that fixed doses of these agents may not be appropriate for all patients, especially in light of increasing echinocandin resistance (Pham et al. 2014).

Some antifungals exhibit substantial pharmacokinetic variability, even in less critically ill agents. Triazoles may display wide inter- and intra-patient pharmacokinetic variability depending on patient age (especially paediatric *vs* adult patients), gastrointestinal function and diet, renal function (fluconazole), hepatic function or disease (itraconazole, voriconazole, posaconazole, isavuconazole), and patient race or pharmacogenomics (voriconazole) (Andes et al. 2009; Ashbee et al. 2014). Up to one-third of patients undergoing haematopoietic stem cell transplantation, for example, may have low or undetectable voriconazole blood levels with the package-insert recommended doses of 200 mg twice daily (Trifilio et al. 2005). Paediatric patients have significantly higher rates of voriconazole clearance, often making it difficult to predict whether the patient has sufficient plasma levels, even with higher weight-based dosing (Neely et al. 2015). However, simply administering higher voriconazole doses to all patients may place them at unacceptable risk for central nervous system toxicities, neuralgias, hepatic toxicity, and other treatment-interrupting adverse effects. In scenarios where inter- and intra-patient pharmacokinetic variability is considerable and jeopardizes the safety and efficacy of standardized doses, direct measurement of plasma drug levels may be the most practical strategy for identifying patients at risk for treatment failure or toxicity (Ashbee et al. 2014). Discussion of the indications and interpretation of therapeutic drug monitoring for antifungals can be found in Chapter 48.

Site of infection

Invasive fungal pathogens frequently disseminate to other organs, including anatomically protected sites such as the eye and central nervous system, where many antifungals poorly penetrate. Published literature on antifungal tissue penetration is often difficult to interpret because data are reported as a ratio of single tissue versus plasma concentration determinations that is highly dependent on when samples are drawn (Felton et al. 2014). Comparison of antifungals from different classes, which have different plasma pharmacokinetics, also results in misleading conclusions when comparing these ratios because of the different denominators (Felton et al. 2014).

Several differences in tissue penetration among antifungals can be assumed based on drug characteristics. Antifungals that have large molecular weights and a high degree of protein binding, such as amphotericin-B formulations and echinocandins, are assumed to have minimal or slow penetration into the eye or cerebrospinal fluid (CSF) because they cannot traverse the tight junctions of the choroid-retinal complex or the blood–brain barrier (Kethireddy and Andes 2007). However, this does not exclude the possibility that these antifungals can achieve therapeutic concentrations in brain parenchyma or meninges. Indeed, brain parenchymal concentrations are often greater than those in the CSF (Kethireddy and Andes 2007). Additionally, CNS inflammation disrupts blood–brain barrier tight junctions, allowing penetration of even larger, less lipophilic molecules into the CSF and brain.

Fluconazole and voriconazole are compounds with intermediate molecular weights and lower degrees of protein binding, and can achieve potentially therapeutic concentrations in anatomically protected sites, especially at higher doses. More lipophilic triazoles with higher molecular weights, such as itraconazole and posaconazole, are less effective than fluconazole or voriconazole in penetrating into the CNS, but may still achieve therapeutic concentrations in brain parenchymal tissue (Kethireddy and Andes 2007). Flucytosine is a low molecular weight compound with limited protein binding that can pass freely into the CSF and aqueous humour. Pharmacokinetically, flucytosine is an ideal adjunctive therapy for infections of the eye and CNS, even though its limited spectrum and the potential for the rapid emergence of resistance requires that it be used in combination with other agents. When administered in combination with amphotericin B for cryptococcal meningitis, flucytosine enhances the rate of fungicidal activity in the CSF and improves patient survival compared with amphotericin-B monotherapy (Brouwer et al. 2004; Day et al. 2013).

Which factors contribute to the pharmacodynamic variability of antifungals?

A fundamental tenet of pharmacodynamics is that as the potency of the drug decreases (or MIC increases), the amount of drug exposure required for microbiological effect correspondingly increases (Drusano 2004). Thus, selection of antifungals with high potency or lower MICs against the probable pathogens, with respect to achievable plasma levels, reduces the probability of treatment failure due to inadequate pharmacokinetic exposures. An accurate assessment of the patient's risk for specific fungal pathogens and knowledge of the local resistance epidemiology is essential for selecting appropriate antifungal therapy. In severely immunocompromised patients, antifungals with fungicidal activity are preferable, although classifications of what constitutes fungistatic versus fungicidal activity *in vivo* are unclear (Lewis and Graybill 2008). In several clinical studies, regimens with greater antifungal potency were associated with improved patient survival, such as amphotericin B plus flucytosine for cryptococcal meningitis (Day et al. 2013), echinocandins for invasive candidiasis (Andes et al. 2010), and a triazole-echinocandin combination regimen for invasive aspergillosis (Marr et al. 2015).

Acquired antifungal resistance in patients—that is, the emergence of resistance in a previously susceptible pathogen—is typically a phenomenon of selective pressure within the host rather than the exogenous acquisition of a resistant strain (Pfaller 2012), although some exceptions to this rule have been noted with environmental azole resistance in *Aspergillus fumigatus* and the recent emergence of multi-drug resistant *Candida auris*. A patient with a history of prior exposure to antifungals, especially for prolonged periods, should, in general, receive empirical therapy with an antifungal from a different class if a breakthrough infection is suspected (Maschmeyer and Patterson 2014). While antifungal susceptibility testing is still not available in many institutions, it remains the most direct indicator for confirming antifungal potency/resistance (Theuretzbacher 2012). Susceptibility testing of isolates recovered from patients with documented infection is also important for defining the local resistance landscape in an institution to help guide empirical therapy. Unfortunately, an understanding of resistance epidemiology among many fungal pathogens is vanishing with the declining number of infections diagnosed by culture and low rates of medical autopsy (Shojania and Burton 2008).

How does antifungal toxicity affect treatment selection?

Unlike previous decades, clinicians now have a greater number of treatment alternatives available if a patient develops intolerance or toxicity to a specific agent. The trade-off of selecting one antifungal over another with respect to spectrum, pharmacokinetic variability, safety, and convenience is weighed differently depending on the treatment phase. Early acute stages of treatment should place greater emphasis on the selection of a broader-spectrum agent (if the pathogen is unknown) with a drug that has predictable pharmacokinetics for the likely site(s) of infection. Once a patient is stable or transitions to a more chronic phase of treatment, greater emphasis should be placed on safety and convenience if an antifungal will be required for several weeks or months (Figure 45.4).

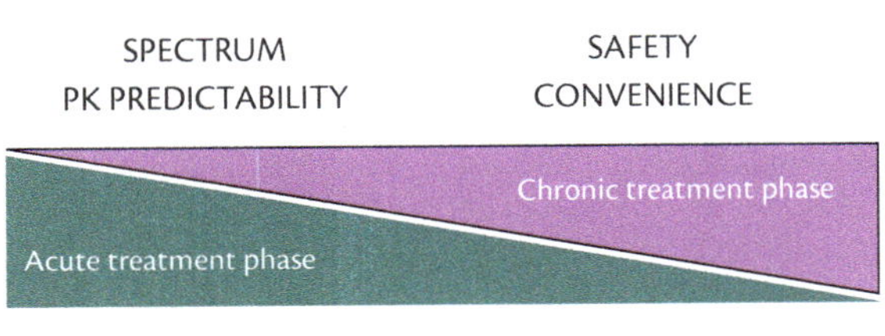

Figure 45.4 How the phase of treatment for invasive fungal disease influences the selection of an antifungal agent.

Summary

Antifungal therapies are life-saving drugs in patients with invasive fungal diseases, but to be used to their full effect clinicians must have knowledge of drug and patient characteristics that lead to pharmacokinetic and pharmacodynamic variability. If assessed carefully, these problems can be accounted for by selecting alternative antifungals or adjusting doses, thereby improving the probability of a favourable outcome.

References

Al-Nakeeb Z, Petraitis V, Goodwin J, Petraitiene R, Walsh TJ and Hope WW (2015) Pharmacodynamics of amphotericin B deoxycholate, amphotericin B lipid complex, and liposomal amphotericin B against *Aspergillus fumigatus*. *Antimicrob Agents Chemother* 59: 2735–45.

Andes D, Diekema DJ, Pfaller MA, Bohrmuller J, Marchillo K and Lepak A (2010) In vivo comparison of the pharmacodynamic targets for echinocandin drugs against *Candida* species. *Antimicrob Agents Chemother* 54: 2497–506.

Andes D, Pascual A and Marchetti O (2009) Antifungal therapeutic drug monitoring: established and emerging indications. *Antimicrob Agents Chemother* 53: 24–34.

Andes DR, Safdar N, Baddley JW, et al. (2012) Impact of treatment strategy on outcomes in patients with candidemia and other forms of invasive candidiasis: a patient-level quantitative review of randomized trials. *Clin Infect Dis* 54: 1110–22.

Andes D, Stamsted T, Conklin R (2001) Pharmacodynamics of amphotericin B in a neutropenic-mouse disseminated-candidiasis model. *Antimicrob Agents Chemother* 45: 922–6.

Andes D and van Ogtrop M (2000) *In vivo* characterization of the pharmacodynamics or flucytosine in a neutropenic murine disseminated candidiasis model. *Antimicrob Agents Chemother* 44: 938–42.

Ashbee HR, Barnes RA, Johnson EM, Richardson MD, Gorton R and Hope WW (2014) Therapeutic drug monitoring (TDM) of antifungal agents: guidelines from the British Society for Medical Mycology. *J Antimicrob Chemother* 69: 1162–76.

Baddley JW, Patel M, Bhavnani SM, Moser SA and Andes DR (2008) Association of fluconazole pharmacodynamics with mortality in patients with candidemia. *Antimicrob Agents Chemother* 52: 3022–8.

Bassetti M, Righi E, Ansaldi F, et al. (2014) A multicenter study of septic shock due to candidemia: outcomes and predictors of mortality. *Intensive Care Med* 40: 839–45.

Bicanic T, Brouwer AE, Meintjes G, et al. (2009) Relationship of cerebrospinal fluid pressure, fungal burden and outcome in patients with cryptococcal meningitis undergoing serial lumbar punctures. *AIDS* 23: 701–6.

Brodoefel H, Vogel M, Hebart H, et al. (2006) Long-term CT follow-up in 40 non-HIV immunocompromised patients with invasive pulmonary aspergillosis: kinetics of CT morphology and correlation with clinical findings and outcome. *Am J Roentgenol* 187: 404–13.

Brouwer AE, Rajanuwong A, Chierakul W, et al. (2004) Combination antifungal therapies for HIV-associated cryptococcal meningitis: a randomised trial. *Lancet* 363: 1764–7.

Brüggemann RJM, Alffenaar JC, Blijlevens NMA, et al. (2009) Clinical relevance of the pharmacokinetic interactions of azole antifungal drugs with other coadministered agents. *Clin Infect Dis* 48: 1441–8.

Caillot D, Casasnovas O, Bernard A, et al. (1997) Improved management of invasive pulmonary aspergillosis in neutropenic patients using early thoracic computed tomographic scan and surgery. *J Clin Oncol* 15: 139–47.

Cornely OA, Gachot B, Akan H, et al. (2015) Epidemiology and outcome of fungemia in a cancer cohort of the Infectious Diseases Group (IDG) of the European Organisation for Research and Treatment of Cancer (EORTC 65031). *Clin Infect Dis* 61: 324–31.

Day JN, Chau TTH, Wolbers M, et al. (2013) Combination antifungal therapy for cryptococcal meningitis. *N Engl J Med* 368: 1291–302.

Drusano G (2004) Antimicrobial pharmacodynamics: critical interactions of 'bug and drug'. *Nat Rev Microbiol* 2: 289–300.

EUCAST (European Committee on Antimicrobial Susceptibility Testing) Antifungal susceptibility testing rationale documents on antifungal agents, http://www.eucast.org/ast_of_fungi/rationale_documents_for_antifungals/, accessed June 1, 2017.

Felton T, Troke PF and Hope WW (2014) Tissue penetration of antifungal agents. *Clin Microbiol Rev* 27: 68–88.

Garey KW, Rege M, Pai MP, et al. (2006) Time to initiation of fluconazole therapy impacts mortality in patients with candidemia: a multi-institutional study. *Clin Infect Dis* 43: 25–31.

Greene RE, Schlamm HT, Oestmann JW, et al. (2007) Imaging findings in acute invasive pulmonary aspergillosis: clinical significance of the halo sign. *Clin Infect Dis* 44: 373–9.

Herbrecht R, Bories P, Moulin JC, Ledoux MP and Letscher-Bru V (2012) Risk stratification for invasive aspergillosis in immunocompromised patients. *Ann NY Acad Sci* 1272: 23–30.

Hope WW, Warn PA, Sharp A, et al. (2006) Derivation of an in vivo drug exposure breakpoint for flucytosine against *Candida albicans* and impact of the MIC, growth rate, and resistance genotype on the antifungal effect. *Antimicrob Agents Chemother* 50: 3680–8.

Kethireddy S and Andes D (2007) CNS pharmacokinetics of antifungal agents. *Expert Opin Drug Metabol Toxicol* 3: 573–81.

Labelle AJ, Micek ST, Roubinian N and Kollef MH (2008) Treatment-related risk factors for hospital mortality in *Candida* bloodstream infections. *Crit Care Med* 36: 2967–72.

Lewis JS and Graybill JR (2008) Fungicidal versus Fungistatic: what's in a word? *Expert Opin Pharmacother* 9: 927–35.

Marr KA, Schlamm HT, Herbrecht R, et al. (2015) Combination antifungal therapy for invasive aspergillosis: a randomized trial. *Ann Intern Med* 162: 81–9.

Maschmeyer G and Patterson TF (2014) Our 2014 approach to breakthrough invasive fungal infections. *Mycoses* 57: 645–51.

Micek ST, Arnold H, Juang P, et al. (2014) Effects of empiric antifungal therapy for septic shock on time to appropriate therapy for *Candida* infection: a pilot study. *Clin Ther* 36: 1226–32.

Morrell M, Fraser VJ and Kollef MH (2005) Delaying the empiric treatment of candida bloodstream infection until positive blood culture results are obtained: a potential risk factor for hospital mortality. *Antimicrob Agents Chemother* 49: 3640–5.

Neely M, Margol A, Fu X, et al. (2015) Achieving target voriconazole concentrations more accurately in children and adolescents. *Antimicrob Agents Chemother* 59: 3090–7.

Nivoix Y, Velten M, Letscher-Bru V, et al. (2008) Factors associated with overall and attributable mortality in invasive aspergillosis. *Clin Infect Dis* 47: 1176–84.

Nucci M, Marr KA, Vehreschild MJ, et al. (2013) Improvement in the outcome of invasive fusariosis in the last decade. *Clin Microbiol Infect* 20: 580–5.

Ostrosky-Zeichner L, Casadevall A, Galgiani JN, Odds FC and Rex JH (2010) An insight into the antifungal pipeline: selected new molecules and beyond. Nat Rev Drug Discov 9: 719–27.

Pappas PG, Rex JH, Lee J, et al. (2003) A prospective observational study of candidemia: epidemiology, therapy, and influences on mortality in hospitalized adult and pediatric patients. *Clin Infect Dis* 37: 634–43.

Pfaller MA (2012) Antifungal drug resistance: mechanisms, epidemiology, and consequences for treatment. Am J Med 125 (Suppl. 1): S3–13.

Pham CD, Iqbal N, Bolden CB, et al. (2014) Role of *FKS* mutations in *Candida glabrata*: MIC values, echinocandin resistance, and multidrug resistance. *Antimicrob Agents Chemother* 58: 4690–6.

Rex JH, Pappas PG, Karchmer AW, et al. (2003) A randomized and blinded multicenter trial of high-dose fluconazole plus placebo versus fluconazole plus amphotericin B as therapy for candidemia and its consequences in nonneutropenic subjects. *Clin Infect Dis* 36: 1221–8.

Roberts JA, Abdul-Aziz MH, Lipman J, et al. (2014) Individualised antibiotic dosing for patients who are critically ill: challenges and potential solutions. *Lancet Infect Dis* 14: 498–509.

Romani L (2011) Immunity to fungal infections. *Nat Rev Immunol* 11: 275–88.

Saliba F and Dupont B (2008) Renal impairment and amphotericin B formulations in patients with invasive fungal infections. *Med Mycol* 46: 97–112.

Shojania KG and Burton EC (2008) The vanishing non-forensic autopsy. *N Engl J Med* 358: 873–5.

Sinnollareddy M, Peake SL, Roberts MS, Lipman J and Roberts JA (2012) Using pharmacokinetics and pharmacodynamics to optimise dosing of antifungal agents in critically ill patients: a systematic review. *Int J Antimicrob Agents* 39: 1–10.

Sinnollareddy MG, Roberts JA, Lipman J, et al. (2015) Pharmacokinetic variability and exposures of fluconazole, anidulafungin, and caspofungin in intensive care unit patients: data from multinational Defining Antibiotic Levels in Intensive care unit (DALI) patients study. *Crit Care* 19: 1–7.

Theuretzbacher U (2012) Pharmacokinetic and pharmacodynamic issues for antimicrobial therapy in patients with cancer. *Clin Infect Dis* 54: 1785–92.

Trifilio S, Ortiz R, Pennick G, et al. (2005) Voriconazole therapeutic drug monitoring in allogeneic stem cell transplant recipients. *Bone Marrow Transplant* 35: 509–13.

Upton A, Kirby KA, Carpenter P, Boeckh M and Marr KA (2007) Invasive aspergillosis following hematopoietic cell transplantation: outcomes and prognostic factors associated with mortality. *Clin Infect Dis* 44: 531–40.

Wiederhold NP, Kontoyiannis DP, Chi J, Prince RA, Tam VH and Lewis RE (2004) Pharmacodynamics of caspofungin in a murine model of invasive pulmonary aspergillosis: evidence of concentration-dependent activity. *J Infect Dis* 190: 1464–71.

Wiederhold NP, Tam VH, Chi J, Prince RA, Kontoyiannis DP and Lewis RE (2006) Pharmacodynamics of amphotericin B deoxycholate is associated with peak plasma concentrations in a neutropenic murine model of invasive pulmonary aspergillosis. *Antimicrob Agents Chemother* 50: 469–73.

CHAPTER 46

Antifungal agents

Donna M. MacCallum

Introduction to antifungal agents

Invasive fungal infections continue to be associated with high mortality and morbidity rates, even with increased choice of antifungal agents. The majority of antifungals target the fungal cell membrane (ergosterol) and wall (beta-glucan). This chapter discusses the current antifungals and their modes of action, formulations, and indications for use.

Amphotericin B

Amphotericin B is a broad-spectrum polyene antifungal agent (Figure 46.1), first extracted from *Streptomyces nodosus* in 1955. It is active against most *Candida* and *Aspergillus* spp., *Cryptococcus neoformans*, and dimorphic fungi (Andes 2013; Pfaller et al. 2015). Amphotericin B binds to ergosterol in the fungal cell membrane, forming pores which allow leakage of ions from the cell (Gray et al. 2012). It also induces oxidative damage through the generation and accumulation of reactive oxygen species (Sokol-Anderson et al. 1986; Mesa-Arango et al. 2014). Amphotericin is cidal, and there is little evidence for the development of antifungal resistance during therapy.

Amphotericin B was originally formulated as amphotericin B deoxycholate, but nephrotoxicity was an issue with prolonged treatment and/or high doses. This was due to amphotericin B interacting with cholesterol in the renal distal tubule membranes, causing tubular damage. Lipid formulations reduce the nephrotoxicity (Hamill 2013). Cholesterol in the formulation binds the drug until it reaches the fungal cell wall. The liposomes in the liposomal formulation then bind to the fungal cell wall, allowing the drug to interact with ergosterol. Various lipid formulations have been produced (Table 46.1), with AmBisome approved by the US Food and Drug Administration (FDA) in 1997. However, not all lipid or liposomal versions are equal in terms of toxicity and clinical effectiveness (Adler-Moore et al. 2016).

Amphotericin B is indicated for the treatment of a wide range of invasive fungal infections (Table 46.1). All versions are administered intravenously, which limits the clinical utility of these drugs. An oral version of amphotericin B exists to treat or prevent oral fungal infections, but systemic distribution of the drug is not achieved. A novel lipid-based formulation for oral delivery is currently under development by iCo Therapeutics, Canada (iCo Therapeutics—oral delivery system: amphotericin B) and nebulized liposomal amphotericin B has been shown to prevent invasive aspergillosis in patients with haematological malignancy (Rijnders et al. 2008).

Flucytosine

Flucytosine (5-fluorocytosine) is a fluorinated pyrimidine derivative, originally developed as an anti-cancer drug (Figure 46.1). It is active against most *Candida* species, *C. neoformans*, and fungal species causing chromoblastomycosis (Vermes et al. 2000a; Pfaller et al. 2015), and is indicated for treating systemic infections caused by these fungi (Table 46.1). *Candida krusei* is inherently resistant to flucytosine (Pfaller et al. 2015), and 6% *C. albicans* strains, 7% *C. tropicalis*, and 12% *C. lusitaniae* strains appear resistant when epidemiological cut-off values are considered (Pfaller et al. 2015).

5-Flucytosine enters the fungal cell via cytosine permease and is converted to 5-fluorouracil by cytosine deaminase. Incorporation of 5-fluorouracil into RNA inhibits protein synthesis, and further conversion of 5-fluorouracil to fluorodeoxyuridine monophosphate inhibits thymidylate synthase, which interferes with DNA synthesis (Vermes et al. 2000a). Resistance to flucytosine occurs via mutations in any of the enzymes involved in uptake or conversion of flucytosine, with the most common mechanism in *C. albicans* being a point mutation in *FUR1*, the gene encoding the uracil phosphoribosyltransferase enzyme (Hope et al. 2004).

Both the FDA and European Medicines Agency (EMA) recommend the use of flucytosine in combination with amphotericin B for the treatment of systemic candidiasis and cryptococcosis (Table 46.1) due to resistant strains (approximately 10% of strains) and emergence of resistance during therapy (Polak and Scholer 1975). This combination is also superior to amphotericin B alone (Bennett et al. 1979). 5-Flucytosine can be administered orally or intravenously and is rapidly absorbed (Table 46.1).

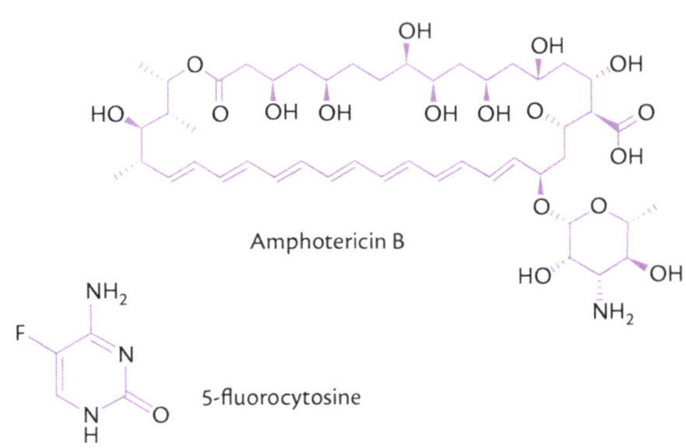

Figure 46.1 Chemical structures of amphotericin B and 5-fluorocytosine.

Table 46.1 Antifungal drugs for treating fungal infections

Name	Manufacturer	Indications	Dosing	Pharmacokinetics/ pharmacodynamics
Amphotericin B				
Fungizone (conventional)	Ben Venue Laboratories, USA, for Bristol-Myers Squibb	Invasive fungal infections (aspergillosis, cryptococcosis, blastomycosis, systemic candidiasis, coccidioidomycosis, histoplasmosis, zygomycosis, sporotrichosis)	Intravenous. Up to 1.5 mg/kg in slow infusion over 2–6 hours	Concentration-dependent killing, maximal activity at concentrations exceeding the MIC from two- to ten-fold. Predictive parameter of efficacy: peak plasma (C_{max})/MIC ratio. Maximal microbiological effect when serum C_{max}/MIC ratio is greater than 40
AmBisome (liposomal)	Gilead Sciences; Astellas Pharma	Systemic and/or deep mycoses (disseminated candidiasis, aspergillosis, mucormycosis, chronic mycetoma, cryptococcal meningitis); presumed fungal infections in febrile neutropenic patients	Intravenous. Daily dose: 1 mg/kg, increased stepwise to 3 mg/kg, as required; administered over 30 min to 2 hours	
Fungisome (liposomal)	Lifecare Innovations, India	Life-threatening fungal infections	Intravenous. Dose: 0.7 mg/kg administered slowly	
Abelcet (lipid complex)	Sigma-Tau Pharmaceuticals, USA	Treatment of invasive fungal infections in patients who fail conventional amphotericin B therapy	Intravenous. Up to 5 mg/kg given as a single infusion, administered at a rate of 2.5 mg/kg/h	
Amphotec (lipid complex)	Ben Venue Laboratories, USA	Invasive aspergillosis, where patients fail on conventional amphotericin B	Intravenous. 3–4 mg/kg once daily; infusion rate: 1 mg/kg/hour	
Ampho-Moronal Suspension	Dermapharm AG, Germany	Oral fungal infection (thrush) (Germany, Switzerland & Austria only)	Oral. 0.5–1 ml (100 mg/ml) four times per day, rinsed around oral cavity, then swallowed	Unknown
5-Fluorocytosine				
Ancobon	Valeant Pharmaceuticals, Canada	Treatment of serious infections caused by *Candida* and *Cryptococcus* only	Capsules. 50–150 mg/kg/day administered in divided doses every 6 hours. Use in combination with amphotericin B for the treatment of systemic candidiasis and cryptococcosis due to resistance	Rapidly and almost completely absorbed when orally administered; peak serum levels within 1–2 hours. Drug efficacy optimal when drug is administered in frequent smaller doses. Excreted via the kidneys; half-life of 2.5–5 hours. Predictive parameter of efficacy: percentage time when drug concentration exceeds MIC. Maximal efficacy when levels exceed MIC for 20–40% dosing interval
Ancotil	Meda Pharmaceuticals, UK	Cryptococcosis, candidiasis, and chromoblastomycosis	Intravenous. 200 mg/kg/day divided into four doses, administered over 20–40 min. Use in combination with amphotericin B for the treatment of systemic candidiasis and cryptococcosis due to resistance	
Azoles				
Nizoral (ketoconazole)	Janssen Pharmaceuticals	Treatment of blastomycosis, coccidioidomycosis, histoplasmosis, chromomycosis, and paracoccidioidomycosis ONLY for patients where other antifungals have failed or are not tolerated	Tablets. Dose: 200 mg once a day for up to 6 months N.B. discontinued in USA, Europe, Australia, and China	Requires acidity for dissolution and absorption. Peak plasma concentration: 1–2 hours after administration. CYP3A4 is the major enzyme involved in metabolism. Mainly excreted via bile.

Table 46.1 (Continued)

Name	Manufacturer	Indications	Dosing	Pharmacokinetics/ pharmacodynamics
Diflucan (fluconazole)	Pfizer	Vaginal candidiasis; oropharyngeal and oesophageal candidiasis; cryptococcal meningitis; coccidioidomycosis, prophylaxis in patients undergoing bone marrow transplantation	Suspension or capsules. Vaginal candidiasis: 150 mg single dose or 300 mg on day 1, followed by 150 mg once daily. Oropharyngeal candidiasis: 200 mg on day 1, followed by 100 mg once daily. Intravenous/oral. Systemic *Candida* infections: up to 400 mg per day. Cryptococcal meningitis: 400 mg on the first day and 200 mg once daily for 10–12 weeks after cerebrospinal fluid becomes culture negative. Coccidioidomycosis: 200–400 mg, once daily for up to 24 months. Prophylaxis: 200–400 mg, once daily.	Similar for oral or intravenous administration. Peak plasma concentrations: 1–2 hours post-administration. Predictive parameter for efficacy: 24 h area under the curve (AUC)/MIC ratio. Value >25 provides the best outcome. Metabolized by CYP2C9 inhibitor and CYP3A4 (moderate).
Sporanox (itraconazole)	Janssen Pharmaceuticals	Empiric therapy of febrile neutropenic patients with suspected fungal infections, blastomycosis, histoplasmosis, and aspergillosis (patients intolerant of or refractory to amphotericin B therapy).	Intravenous. 200 mg twice per day for 48 hours, then 200 mg once daily. Each dose administered slowly over one hour.	Capsules: administer with food; oral suspension: administer before food. Bioavailability differs for capsules and oral suspension; do not use interchangeably. Peak plasma concentrations: 2.5 hours after administration (oral suspension). Steady-state C_{max} values of 2 mg/L reached after daily oral administration of 200 mg. Itraconazole and its major metabolite, hydroxy-itraconazole, inhibit CYP3A4.
Sporanox (itraconazole)	Janssen Pharmaceuticals	Blastomycosis, histoplasmosis, aspergillosis (intolerant of, or refractory to, amphotericin B); dermatophyte nail infections	Capsules. 200 mg twice per day for 48 hours, then 200 mg once daily until infection resolved	
Sporanox (itraconazole)	Janssen Pharmaceuticals	Empiric therapy of suspected fungal infection in febrile neutropenic patients, and oropharyngeal & oesophageal candidiasis	Oral suspension. 200 mg (20 ml) daily for 1–2 weeks—swish 10 mL around mouth, then swallow	
Vfend (voriconazole)	Pfizer	Invasive aspergillosis, candidaemia & deep *Candida* infections, oesophageal candidiasis, scedosporiosis and fusariosis, prophylaxis for stem cell transplant patients	Intravenous. Loading dose: 6 mg/kg every 12 hours for 24 hours; maintenance dose: 4 mg/kg every 12 hours. Treatment for at least 7 days	Pharmacokinetics: non-linear due to metabolism saturation. Inter-individual variability of pharmacokinetics is high. Loading dose establishes steady state within the first 24 hours. Maximum plasma concentrations (C_{max}) are achieved 1–2 hours after dosing. Metabolism via CYP2C19 (highest affinity), followed by CYP2C9, and much lower for CYP3A4.
Vfend (voriconazole)	Pfizer		Suspension or tablets: loading dose: 6 mg/kg every 12 hours for 24 hours Intravenous: maintenance dose: 200 mg every 12 hours. Treatment for at least 7 days	
Noxafil (posaconazole)	Merck Sharp & Dohme	Invasive aspergillosis; fusariosis; chromoblastomycosis and mycetoma; coccidioidomycosis; oropharyngeal candidiasis; prophylaxis in remission-induction chemotherapy patients and haematopoietic stem cell transplant patients	Intravenous. For fungal infections, 300 mg twice a day on the first day followed by 300 mg once a day; duration of treatment depends on the severity of the disease and the patient's response	A correlation between AUC/MIC and clinical outcome is observed, with a critical ratio of 200 required for aspergillosis success. After administration of 300 mg, slowly eliminated with a mean half-life of 27 hours. Potent inhibitor of CYP3A4 and mainly metabolized via UDP-glucuronidation.

(continued)

Table 46.1 (Continued)

Name	Manufacturer	Indications	Dosing	Pharmacokinetics/ pharmacodynamics
Noxafil (posaconazole)	Merck Sharp & Dohme		Oral suspension. Fungal Infections: 400 mg (10 mL) twice a day, or 200 mg (5 mL) four times a day. Oral candidiasis: 200 mg (5 mL) on the first day followed by 100 mg (2.5 mL) once a day for the following 13 days. Prophylaxis: 200 mg (5 mL) three times a day	Peak plasma concentrations reached within 3–4 hours and 4–10 hours in fasted and fed states. AUC can be increased by dividing the total daily dose of 800 mg into either 400 mg twice daily (× 1.7) or 200 mg four times daily (× 2.6). Potent inhibitor of CYP3A4 and mainly metabolized via UDP-glucuronidation.
Noxafil (posaconazole)	Merck Sharp & Dohme		Tablets: 300 mg twice a day on the first day, followed by 300 mg once a day; duration of treatment depends on the severity of the disease and the patient's response	
Cresemba (isavuconazole)	Astellas Pharma & Basilea Pharmaceuticals	Invasive aspergillosis & mucormycosis	Intravenous. Loading dose, 200 mg every 8 hours for 48 hours; maintenance dose, 200 mg daily	Rapidly converted to the active form immediately upon administration—intravenous and oral formulations can be used interchangeably. AUC/MIC ratio is a good predictor of outcome.
Cresemba (isavuconazole)	Astellas Pharma & Basilea Pharmaceuticals	Invasive aspergillosis & mucormycosis	Capsules: loading dose, 200 mg every 8 hours for 48 hours; maintenance dose, 200 mg once daily	Orally administered drug is rapidly absorbed, reaching maximum plasma concentration (C_{max}) 2–3 hours after single and multiple dosing.
Echinocandins				
Cancidas (caspofungin)	Merck, Sharp & Dohme	Invasive candidiasis & aspergillosis (refractory to other treatments), empiric treatment for presumed fungal infections	Intravenous. Loading dose: 70 mg dose, followed by 50–70 mg per day in a single dose. Drug should be administered over 1 hour	Extensively bound to albumin (>92%). Tissue distribution peaks after 1.5–2 days. Plasma elimination is slow (10–12 mL/min). Either C_{max}/MIC or AUC/MIC predict clinical outcome, with a ratio of 10–20 predicting success.
Mycamine (micafungin)	Astellas Pharma; Fujisawa	Invasive and oesophageal candidiasis, prophylaxis of *Candida* infection in patients undergoing stem cell transplantation or neutropenic patients	Intravenous. Invasive candidiasis: 100 mg per day (at least 14 days); oesophageal candidiasis: 150 mg per day; prophylaxis: 50 mg per day. Drug should be administered over one hour	Micafungin remains unmodified in host. Half-life is approximately 10–17 hours. Elimination is primarily non-renal. Either C_{max}/MIC or AUC/MIC predict clinical outcome.
Eraxis/Ecalta (anidulafungin)	Pfizer	Invasive, oesophageal, and intra-abdominal candidiasis and *Candida* peritonitis	Intravenous. Invasive infections: 200 mg loading dose on day 1 (over 3 hours), 100 mg daily maintenance dose (over 1–2 hours) Oesophageal candidiasis: 100 mg loading dose, followed by 50 mg per day (1.1 mg per minute)	Extensively bound (>99%) to human plasma proteins. Half-life: 24 hours. Excretion via the biliary system.

Source: data from US Food and Drug Administration, www.fda.gov; European Medicines Agency, www.ema.europa.eu/; Drugs.com; RxList - the Internet Drug Index for prescription drugs medications and pill identifier, http://www.rxlist.com/.

Azole antifungal drugs

All azole antifungal agents target the fungal cytochrome P450/lanosterol 14-alpha-demethylase enzyme, encoded by *ERG11* or *CYP51*, which functions in ergosterol biosynthesis. Azoles are metabolized by, and inhibitors of, human liver cytochrome P450 enzymes, which leads to significant effects on the metabolism of other drugs (Bruggemann et al. 2009). This is of particular importance in haematology patients and those undergoing solid organ transplants, where azoles administered for antifungal prophylaxis or for treatment of invasive fungal infection can affect levels of immunosuppressants, as well as other drugs used in the care of these patients (Table 46.2). Ketoconazole, itraconazole, and posaconazole are metabolized by CYP3A4, fluconazole by CYP2C9 and

Table 46.2 Examples of drug–azole interactions in haematology and solid organ transplant patients

Drug	Azoles involved	Effects
Immunosuppressants		
Sirolimus, tacrolimus, cyclosporine, everolimus, mycophenolate mofetil, dexamethasone, methylprednisolone	Fluconazole, itraconazole, voriconazole, isavuconazole	Increased levels of immunosuppressant drug in the blood, leading to increased toxicity—requires therapeutic drug monitoring
Sedation & pain relief		
Fentanil	Fluconazole	Increased pharmacological effects and risk of toxicity
Midazolam	Isavuconazole	Increased midazolam levels
Anti-nausea drugs		
Ondansetron	Voriconazole	QT interval prolongation increased
Alprazolam	Voriconazole	Levels increased and prolonged depressant effects persist after antifungal therapy
Antibiotics		
Levofloxacin	Fluconazole	QT interval prolongation increased
Statins		
Atorvastatin	Fluconazole, isavuconazole	Increased atorvastatin levels

Source: data from Fernandez de Palencia Espinosa et al., 2016; Wilson et al., 2016; Lempers et al., 2015.

CYP3A4, isavuconazole by CYP3A4 and CYP3A5, and voriconazole by CYP2C19, CYP2C9, and CYP3A4, with CYP2C19 having a major role in metabolism (Drugs.com; Fung et al. 2008). CYP2C19 is polymorphic, and different genotypes have a major role in the pharmacokinetics of voriconazole (Weiss et al. 2009).

Ketoconazole, a synthetic imidazole which is widely used topically to treat dermatophyte and fungal skin infections, has also been administered orally to treat systemic fungal infections. However, owing to severe liver damage and adrenal gland problems, its use has been suspended in Europe and elsewhere in the world (Table 46.1).

Fluconazole, a fungistatic triazole (Figure 46.2), was developed by Pfizer and was marketed in 1990. It is available in various formulations (Table 46.1). Fluconazole is indicated for oropharyngeal and oesophageal candidiasis, cryptococcal meningitis, and coccidioidomycosis (Table 46.1), and is effective against most *Candida* species, although 7–20% of *C. glabrata, C. tropicalis, C. parapsilosis*, and *C. guilliermondii* strains are resistant (Andes 2013; Pfaller et al. 2013, 2015; Castanheira et al. 2014), with *C. krusei* considered inherently resistant. Fluconazole has no activity against *Aspergillus* and *Fusarium* species (Vermes et al. 2000b).

Itraconazole is a synthetic triazole antifungal (Figure 46.2), available in oral and intravenous formulations (Table 46.1), which was developed by Janssen Pharmaceuticals, although the intravenous formulation is no longer available in the USA. Metabolism by CYP3A4 produces hydroxy-itraconazole, which also has antifungal activity. Itraconazole has broader spectrum activity than fluconazole, being active against *Candida* and *Aspergillus* species, although it is still ineffective against *Fusarium* species and other clinically important moulds (Andes 2013; Pfaller et al. 2013). Resistance occurs infrequently amongst clinical isolates, although a 2015 study reported 8% *C. glabrata* and 20% *C. guilliermondii* isolates to be

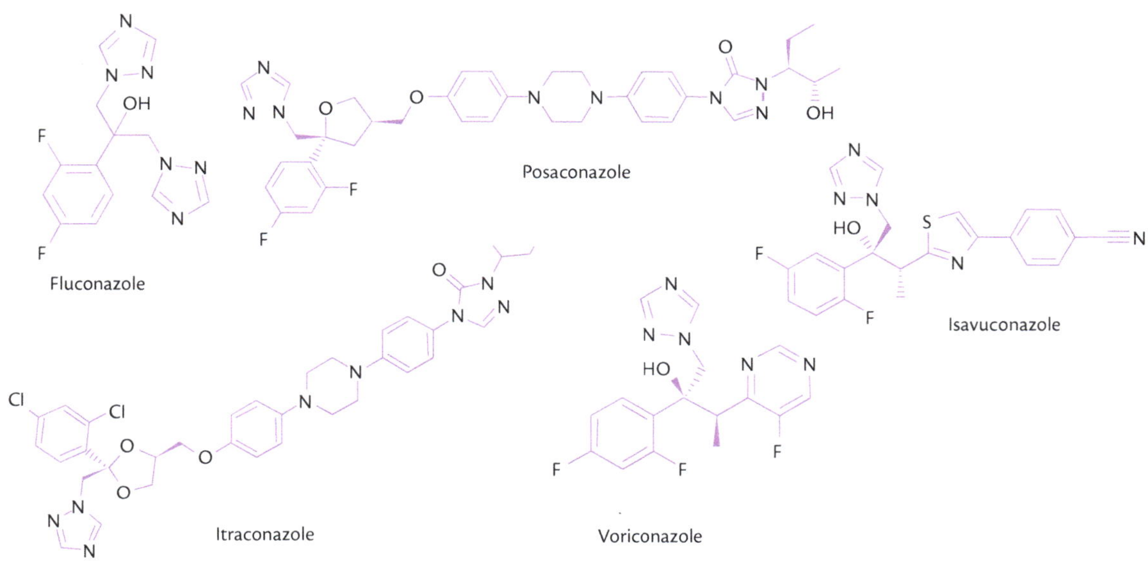

Figure 46.2 Chemical structures of azole antifungal agents.

resistant (Pfaller et al. 2015). Itraconazole is indicated for empiric therapy of suspected fungal infections and for treatment of aspergillosis patients who are intolerant of, or refractory to, amphotericin B therapy (Table 46.1). Itraconazole has been linked to cardiac problems during therapy (Fung et al. 2008).

Voriconazole (Figure 46.2) is a triazole developed by Pfizer and marketed as Vfend in 2002. It has very broad spectrum activity (Andes 2013), with less than 5% resistance seen for most species, with the exception of *C. glabrata* (10%), *C. guilliermondii* (20%), and *C. orthopsilosis* (10%) (Pfaller et al. 2013, 2015; Castanheira et al. 2014). It is available in both oral and intravenous formulations, and is indicated as a first-line therapy for aspergillosis (Table 46.1).

Posaconazole is a triazole (Figure 46.2) marketed as Noxafil by Merck, Sharp & Dohme (UK)/Schering-Plough (USA) in 2005/2006. It is available in multiple formulations and is an extended-spectrum drug (Andes 2013). Incidence of resistance is low, with only *C. guilliermondii* showing significant resistance (20%) (Pfaller et al. 2015). Some resistance in *C. tropicalis* and *C. krusei* has been reported in different regions (Pfaller et al. 2013; Castanheira et al. 2014). Posaconazole is licensed for first-line therapy for invasive aspergillosis, *Fusarium* infections, and chromoblastomycosis (Table 46.1).

Isavuconazole (Figure 46.2), formulated as a pro-drug—isavuconazonium sulphate (Miceli and Kauffman 2015)—was developed by Astellas Pharma/Basilea Pharmaceutica, approved by the FDA and EMA in 2015, and marketed as Cresemba (Table 46.1). Isavuconazole is the newest triazole antifungal agent, shows extended spectrum of activity, and is licensed for treatment of invasive aspergillosis and invasive mucormycosis (Miceli and Kauffman 2015; Pfaller et al. 2015) (Table 46.1). To date, there is little evidence for clinical resistance to isavuconazole (Pfaller et al. 2015), although *C. glabrata* and *C. guilliermondii* show decreased susceptibility to the drug (Pfaller et al. 2015).

Lengthy treatments and the static nature of many azoles allow the development of azole drug resistance (Lopez-Ribot et al. 1998) (see Chapter 47 for more details).

Echinocandin antifungal drugs

Echinocandin antifungals work by inhibiting beta-1,3-D-glucan synthase, leading to reduced beta-glucan levels in the fungal cell wall.

Caspofungin (Figure 46.3) was the first echinocandin antifungal approved by the FDA and EMA in 2001 (Cancidas). It is a semi-synthetic lipopeptide compound synthesized from a fermentation product of *Glarea lozoyensis*, and was licensed for treatment of invasive *Candida* and *Aspergillus* infections (Table 46.1).

Micafungin (Figure 46.3), a semi-synthetic antifungal derived from a *Coleophoma empetri* product, was developed by Astellas Pharma/Fijisawa, and approved by the FDA in 2005 and EMA in 2008 (Mycamine) for prophylaxis for *Candida* infections (Table 46.1).

Anidulafungin (Figure 46.3) is a semi-synthetic antifungal derived from a lipopeptide produced from either *Aspergillus nidulans* or *Aspergillus rugulosus*. It was developed by Pfizer and approved by the FDA as Eraxis in 2006, and as Ecalta by the EMA in 2007, for the treatment of *Candida* infections (Table 46.1).

Echinocandins are fungicidal against yeasts and lyse the growing tip of filamentous fungi. There is little evidence of clinical resistance to echinocandins, although low levels are seen for *C. glabrata* and *C. tropicalis* (Pfaller et al. 2013, 2015; Castanheira et al. 2014). Echinocandin resistance is due to point mutations in *FKS* genes, which encode subunits of the glucan synthase enzyme complex.

Echinocandins are considered safe drugs, with few side effects or drug interactions, but their use is limited by restriction to intravenous formulations only (Table 46.1). However, efforts are being made to develop orally available echinocandin drugs (Apgar et al. 2015).

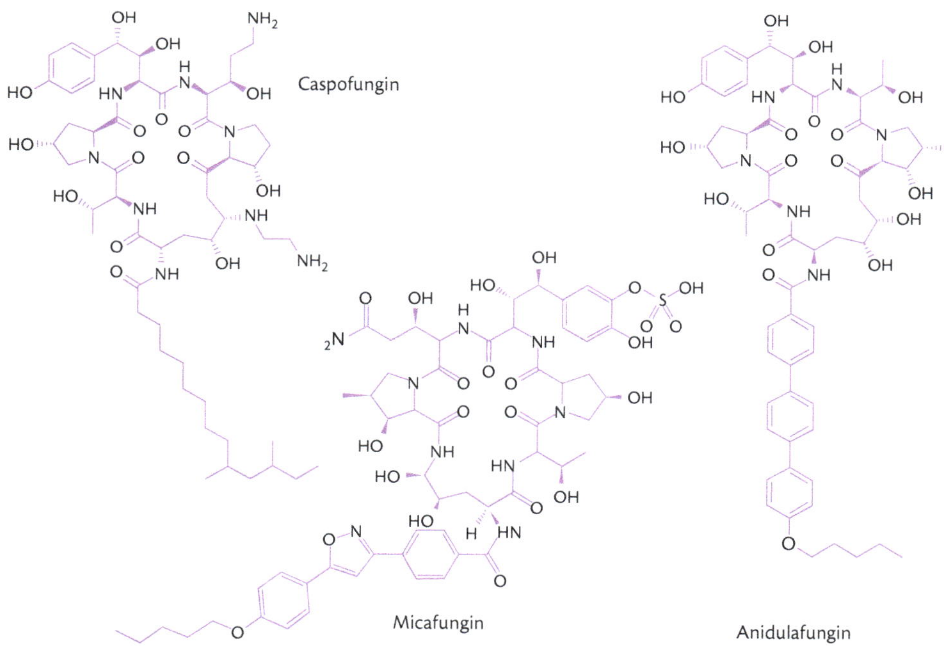

Figure 46.3 Chemical structures of the echinocandins.

Conclusion

A reasonable choice of antifungal agents exists for the treatment of invasive fungal infections, but gaps remain which need to be filled, with *C. glabrata, C. guilliermondii*, and various moulds still difficult to treat with currently available drugs. Further research is required to identify novel antifungals and to develop multiple formulations for clinical use.

References

Drugs.com, http://www.drugs.com/, accessed 1 June 2017.

Rx list—the internet drug index, http://www.rxlist.com, accessed 1 June 2017.

US Food and Drug Administration 2016—last update, http://www.fda.gov/, accessed 1 June 2017.

European Medicines Agency, http://www.ema.europa.eu/, accessed 1 June 2017.

iCo Therapeutics—oral delivery system: amphotericin B, http://www.icotherapeutics.com/_resources/iCo_Corporate_FS_amp_b_v11.pdf, accessed 1 June 2017.

Adler-Moore JP, Gangneux JP and Pappas PG (2016) Comparison between liposomal formulations of amphotericin B. *Med Mycol* 54: 223–31.

Andes D (2013) Optimizing antifungal choice and administration. *Curr Med Res Opin* 29 (Suppl. 4): 13–18.

Apgar JM, Wilkening RR, Greenlee ML, et al. (2015) Novel orally active inhibitors of beta-1,3-glucan synthesis derived from enfumafungin. *Bioorg Med Chem Lett* 25: 5813–18.

Bennett JE, Dismukes WE, Duma RJ, et al. (1979) A comparison of amphotericin B alone and combined with flucytosine in the treatment of cryptococcal meningitis. *N Engl J Med* 301: 126–31.

Bruggemann RJ, Alffenaar JW, Blijlevens NM, et al. (2009) Clinical relevance of the pharmacokinetic interactions of azole antifungal drugs with other coadministered agents. *Clin Infect Dis* 48: 1441–58.

Castanheira M, Messer SA, Jones RN, Farrell DJ and Pfaller MA (2014) Activity of echinocandins and triazoles against a contemporary (2012) worldwide collection of yeast and moulds collected from invasive infections. *Int J Antimicrob Agents* 44: 320–6.

Fernandez de Palencia Espinosa MA, Diaz Carrasco MS, Sanchez Salinas A, de la Rubia Nieto A and Miro AE (2016) Potential drug-drug interactions in hospitalised haematological patients. *J Oncol Pharm Pract* 2016 Aug 10. doi: 10.1177/1078155216664201

Fung SL, Chau CH and Yew WW (2008) Cardiovascular adverse effects during itraconazole therapy. *Eur Respir J* 32: 240.

Gray KC, Palacios DS, Dailey I, et al. (2012) Amphotericin primarily kills yeast by simply binding ergosterol. *Proc Natl Acad Sci U S A* 109: 2234–9.

Hamill RJ (2013) Amphotericin B formulations: a comparative review of efficacy and toxicity. *Drugs* 73: 919–34.

Hope WW, Tabernero L, Denning DW and Anderson MJ (2004) Molecular mechanisms of primary resistance to flucytosine in *Candida albicans*. *Antimicrob Agents Chemother* 48: 4377–86.

Lempers VJ, Martial LC, Schreuder MF, et al. (2015) Drug-interactions of azole antifungals with selected immunosuppressants in transplant patients: strategies for optimal management in clinical practice. *Curr Opin Pharmacol* 24: 38–44.

Lopez-Ribot JL, McAtee RK, Lee LN, et al. (1998) Distinct patterns of gene expression associated with development of fluconazole resistance in serial *Candida albicans* isolates from human immunodeficiency virus-infected patients with oropharyngeal candidiasis. *Antimicrob Agents Chemother* 42: 2932–7.

Mesa-Arango AC, Trevijano-Contador N, Roman E, et al, (2014) The production of reactive oxygen species is a universal action mechanism of amphotericin B against pathogenic yeasts and contributes to the fungicidal effect of this drug. *Antimicrob Agents Chemother* 58: 6627–38.

Miceli MH and Kauffman CA (2015) Isavuconazole: a new broad-spectrum triazole antifungal agent. *Clin Infect Dis* 61: 1558–65.

Pfaller MA, Messer SA, Woosley LN, Jones RN and Castanheira M (2013) Echinocandin and triazole antifungal susceptibility profiles for clinical opportunistic yeast and mold isolates collected from 2010 to 2011: application of new CLSI clinical breakpoints and epidemiological cutoff values for characterization of geographic and temporal trends of antifungal resistance. *J Clin Microbiol* 51: 2571–81.

Pfaller MA, Rhomberg PR, Messer SA, Jones RN and Castanheira M (2015) Isavuconazole, micafungin, and 8 comparator antifungal agents' susceptibility profiles for common and uncommon opportunistic fungi collected in 2013: temporal analysis of antifungal drug resistance using CLSI species-specific clinical breakpoints and proposed epidemiological cutoff values. *Diagn Microbiol Infect Dis* 82: 303–13.

Polak A and Scholer HJ (1975) Mode of action of 5-fluorocytosine and mechanisms of resistance. *Chemotherapy* 21: 113–30.

Rijnders BJ, Cornelissen JJ, Slobbe L, et al. (2008) Aerosolized liposomal amphotericin B for the prevention of invasive pulmonary aspergillosis during prolonged neutropenia: a randomized, placebo-controlled trial. *Clin Infect Dis* 46: 1401–8.

Sokol-Anderson ML, Brajtburg J and Medoff G (1986) Amphotericin B-induced oxidative damage and killing of *Candida albicans*. *J Infect Dis* 154: 76–83.

Vermes A, Guchelaar HJ and Dankert J (2000a) Flucytosine: a review of its pharmacology, clinical indications, pharmacokinetics, toxicity and drug interactions. *J Antimicrob Chemother* 46: 171–9.

Vermes A, van Der Sijs H and Guchelaar HJ (2000b) Flucytosine: correlation between toxicity and pharmacokinetic parameters. *Chemotherapy* 46: 86–94.

Weiss J, Ten Hoevel MM, Burhenne J, et al. (2009) CYP2C19 genotype is a major factor contributing to the highly variable pharmacokinetics of voriconazole. *J Clin Pharmacol* 49: 196–204.

Wilson DT, Dimondi VP, Johnson SW, Jones TM and Drew RH (2016) Role of isavuconazole in the treatment of invasive fungal infections. *Ther Clin Risk Manag* 12: 1197–206.

CHAPTER 47

Antifungal susceptibility testing and resistance

Elizabeth M. Johnson

Introduction to antifungal susceptibility testing and resistance

Clinicians have a choice of systemically active antifungal agents, and following the proliferation in the number of fungal species implicated in invasive disease, they are increasingly looking for guidance from clinical laboratory results to help select the most appropriate agent. There are well-established and predictable patterns of innate *in vitro* resistance to one or more antifungal agents associated with many yeast and mould species (Pfaller and Diekema 2004). However, if identification is delayed, then susceptibility testing of the isolate may yield useful information. In addition, there is the less predictable recognition of emergent resistance in initially susceptible yeast and mould strains during prolonged treatment in the face of persistent infection (Bueid et al. 2010; Jensen et al. 2013). There has also been the recent phenomenon of the emergence of resistance in *Aspergillus fumigatus* strains to the widely used agricultural azole drugs, leading to cross-resistance to one or more of the azole drugs used in clinical practice, thus potentially compromising a first-line treatment option for invasive aspergillosis (Verweij et al. 2009; Vermeulen et al. 2013). All of these trends reinforce the need for timely, accurate, and reproducible susceptibility testing that produces results which correlate with clinical outcome.

Role of standardized *in vitro* susceptibility testing:

- Assessment of a drug's potency against a test organism
- Detection of outlier organisms displaying reduced *in vitro* susceptibility
- Detection of the development of drug resistance during therapy
- Comparison of *in vitro* potency of comparator drugs
- Analysis of the spectrum of activity of antifungal agents
- Assessment of the *in vitro* potency of new agents and those in development

Minimum inhibitory concentration

The minimum inhibitory concentration (MIC) is an *in vitro* assessment of the lowest concentration of an antimicrobial agent that can inhibit the growth of a microorganism, and is a measure of the potency of that agent. Once methods have been standardized, relative potencies of different antifungal agents can be assessed and breakpoints can be established for given drug–organism combinations to help predict the likely clinical outcome.

Minimum fungicidal/lethal concentration

Antifungal agents that are fungicidal at concentrations that can be achieved *in vivo* may be more effective than those which are fungistatic, and thus rely on some host phagocytic cell activity to remove the remaining viable pathogens. Thus, assessment of the concentration at which an agent causes cell death may also be useful. This is usually established by attempting to sub-culture viable organisms from wells or tubes containing inhibitory concentrations of the agent (Pfaller et al. 2004).

Correlation of antifungal susceptibility testing results with clinical outcome

Many factors influence the outcome of antifungal treatment, of which the *in vitro* susceptibility of the causative organism is one. Consideration also has to be given to host factors such as underlying condition and immune status, the site of infection and the infecting organism's propensity to disseminate or form biofilms, the pharmacokinetics and pharmacodynamics of the drug, and the timing of treatment in relation to disease progression. The amenability to surgical or clinical intervention, such as removal of prosthetic material or manipulation of the immune status of the host with cytokine therapy or granulocyte infusions, may also have an influence. It is not therefore a simple algorithm. Susceptibility testing may not guarantee a successful outcome, but the finding of resistance should indicate a higher probability of clinical failure. With certain exceptions, this is the status that susceptibility testing has now achieved with most antifungal agents (Johnson and Cavling-Arendrup 2015).

Clinical resistance and clinical breakpoint setting

Wild-type distribution

Any group of organisms tested by a defined method with any given drug will yield a distribution of MIC results, with the majority concentrated within a small number of concentrations. Graphic representations will usually reveal modal or bimodal distributions, and less susceptible outlier organisms to this wild-type distribution can be readily identified. In the absence of clinical breakpoints, these wild-type distributions and epidemiological cut-off (ECOFF) concentrations are a useful indicator of likely activity (Espinel-Ingroff et al. 2010). Commonly used parameters for defining drug activity against a given species are the range of MIC values encountered and the values at which 50% (MIC_{50}) and 90% (MIC_{90}) of the strains are inhibited.

Clinical breakpoint setting

Although wild-type distributions and associated ECOFF concentrations are helpful if there are insufficient clinical data, the most accurate predictor of likely outcome will be the clinical breakpoint; this is based on an analysis of normal MIC ranges for the infecting species and likely blood or tissue levels of the drug under consideration, backed up by clinical outcome data. The earliest attempt at defining clinical breakpoints was for *Candida* species with fluconazole and itraconazole, predominantly with mucosal oropharyngeal isolates from HIV-infected individuals, although breakpoints derived in this way also held true for bloodstream infections. At this time, breakpoints were suggested that defined MIC ranges as susceptible (S), or likely to respond, resistant (R), or less likely to respond, and susceptible–dose-dependent (SDD), which were likely to respond if the blood antifungal concentration was sufficiently high (Rex et al. 1997). These are the only drugs where the enhanced outcome for the SDD group was proved in those patients with higher blood levels. For most drugs, the terminology of intermediate (I) is used for those MICs above the truly susceptible range and below the MIC defined as resistant.

Recently, breakpoints for most antifungal drugs have been redefined to allow harmonization between the Clinical Laboratory Standards Institute (CLSI) and the European Committee on Antimicrobial Susceptibility Testing (EUCAST). This has been achieved for almost all drug-organism combinations; where differences remain, this is mainly due to differences in the endpoints achieved by the two methods. These are species-specific breakpoints which have been developed for the major systemically active antifungal classes with the most common yeast pathogens and some *Aspergillus* species (Table 47.1). As breakpoints are species-specific, it makes accurate species identification a vital part of breakpoint interpretation.

Table 47.1 CLSI and EUCAST breakpoints for *Candida* species and *Aspergillus fumigatus*. Breakpoints are presented as S: ≤X, R: >Y (values between S and R breakpoints can be evaluated as I) (Johnson and Cavling-Arendrup 2015; CLSI 2012; http://www.eucast.org/fileadmin/src/media/PDFs/EUCAST_files/AFST/Antifungal_breakpoints_v_7.0.pdf)

Agent	CLSI M27-S4 Species-specific breakpoints (mg/L)	EUCAST Species-specific breakpoints (mg/L)
Amphotericin B		≤1, >2.0 *Candida* spp. *Aspergillus fumigatus*
Anidulafungin	≤0.25; >0.5 *C. albicans* *C. krusei* *C. tropicalis* ≤0.125; >0.25 *C. glabrata* ≤2; >4 *C. parapsilosis*	≤0.03; >0.03 *C. albicans* ≤0.06; >0.06 *C. glabrata* *C. krusei* *C. tropicalis* ≤0.002; 4 *C. parapsilosis**
Caspofungin	As for anidulafungin	Not established for caspofungin owing to unacceptable MIC variation
Micafungin	≤0.25; >0.5 *C. albicans* *C. krusei* *C. tropicalis* ≤0.06; >0.125 *C. glabrata* ≤2; >4 *C. parapsilosis*	≤0.016; >0.03 *C. albicans* ≤0.03; >0.03 *C. glabrata* ≤0.002; 2 *C. parapsilosis**
Fluconazole	≤2; >4 *C. albicans* *C. parapsilosis* *C. tropicalis* SDD: ≤32; >32 *C. glabrata***	≤2; >4 *C. albicans* *C. parapsilosis* *C. tropicalis* ≤0.02; 32 *C. glabrata****
Itraconazole		≤1, 2.0 *Aspergillus fumigatus*
Posaconazole	–	≤0.06; >0.06 *C. albicans* *C. parapsilosis* *C. tropicalis* ≤0.125; 0.25 *Aspergillus fumigatus*
Voriconazole	≤0.125; >0.5 *C. albicans* *C. parapsilosis* *C. tropicalis* ≤0.5; >1 *C. krusei*	≤0.125; >0.125 *C. albicans* *C. parapsilosis* *C. tropicalis* ≤1, 2.0 *Aspergillus fumigatus*

* Wild-type population classified as intermediate to anidulafungin and micafungin.

** Wild-type population classified as susceptible dose dependent (SDD) to fluconazole.

*** Wild-type population classified as intermediate to fluconazole.

Methods for antifungal susceptibility testing

Since the earliest attempts at *in vitro* susceptibility testing of yeasts and moulds it has been recognized that interpretation of endpoints is highly influenced by a large number of methodological variables. These include: the test format, solubility, and stability of the antifungal agents under investigation; preparation and size of the inoculum; formulation and pH of the basal medium; and temperature and duration of incubation; as well as the way in which the endpoints are assessed (Johnson 2008). Moreover, yeast and mould are very different growth forms which require different methods of handling and endpoint interpretation. In addition, some antifungal agents cause partial inhibition of growth over a wide concentration range, so rules of interpretation must be formulated. Thus, methods have to be standardized to yield reproducible results even before consideration of whether the results obtained *in vitro* reflect the likely treatment outcome.

The first standardized broth dilution method (National Committee for Clinical Laboratory Standards [NCCLS] M27-P, 1992) was published in the early 1990s. This macrodilution methodology was modified to include a microdilution method conducted in a microtitre plate. Currently accepted reference methods for yeasts (CLSI M27-A3, 2008a) and moulds (CLSI M38-A2, 2008b) have been published by the CLSI. The subcommittee on antifungal susceptibility testing of the EUCAST has also developed broth microdilution methods for fermentative yeast (Edef 7.2) (Arendrup et al. 2012) and for conidia-forming moulds (Edef 9.1) (Rodriquez-Tudela et al. 2008). Since both methods now allow reading after 24 hours' incubation, the main differences are that

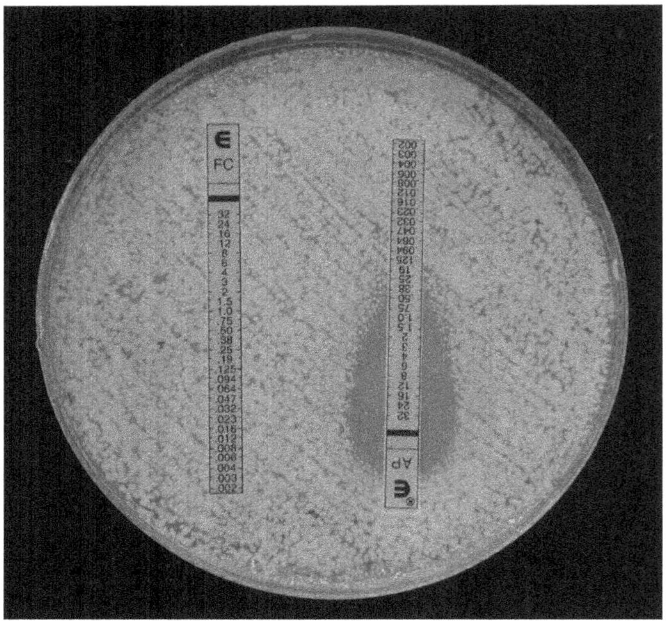

Figure 47.1 Antifungal gradient strips (Etest) on a pre-inoculated agar plate. This isolate is resistant to flucytosine (FC) growing right up to the strip, whereas there is a good zone of inhibition with amphotericin B (AP).

the EUCAST method utilizes more glucose in the basal medium to allow faster growth and is conducted in flat-bottomed microtitre plates to allow an objective spectrophotometric end-point determination for yeast isolates. The CLSI has also developed disc diffusion methods for yeasts (CLSI M44-A2, 2009a) and moulds (CLSI M51-A, 2010). A number of manufacturers produce commercial drug impregnated discs, but care must be taken to employ the correct agar medium to avoid drug antagonism. Zones of inhibition produced under standardized condition can be correlated with MIC for some yeast species (CLSI 2009b).

There are a number of commercial methods of assessing MIC, which include those that employ the microtitre plate format, such as Sensititre (TREK Diagnostics) and Micronaut-AM (Merlin Diagnostika). These incorporate a chromogenic medium in order to facilitate assessment of endpoints. There are also gradient strip methodologies in which a gradient of antifungal drug concentration is incorporated into a strip which is then placed on the surface of an inoculated agar plate. The MIC can be read as the concentration at which the resulting zone of inhibition intersects the strip. Such methods can be used for yeast and mould isolates (Johnson and Cavling-Arendrup 2015) (Figure 47.1).

Proteomic and molecular methods of antifungal susceptibility testing

As the protein composition of fungal cells varies in relation to the inhibition of cell growth in different drug concentrations, proteomic methods can be used to detect the presence of resistance. Minimal profile change concentration endpoints represent the lowest drug concentration at which mass spectrum profile changes can be detected (Marinach et al. 2009). Currently, such approaches remain as labour intensive and time-consuming as microtitre plate reference methods; however, if they can be adapted to breakpoint testing it may provide a useful objective resistance surveillance mechanism.

The presence of multiple azole-resistance mechanisms in *Candida* species complicates molecular detection. Some are due to up-regulation of housekeeping genes, and mechanisms are often acquired in a step-wise manner with one or more present in the same cell. Thus, any method for molecular determination of resistance must be a multiplex system and must also be capable of determining up-regulation of housekeeping genes. In contrast, yeast resistance to echinocandins is often associated with mutations of specific hot spot regions of the *FSK* genes, which are easier to detect by DNA sequencing (Alexander et al. 2013). In *Aspergillus*, resistance to azole drugs may arise owing to long-term treatment of chronic infections, and this scenario gives rise to many and varied resistance mutations (Bueid et al. 2010). The recent emergence of *Aspergillus fumigatus* clades with one of two resistance mechanisms that appear to have arisen in response to agricultural azoles can readily be detected by molecular methods (Vermeulen et al. 2013). However, molecular techniques will be unable to detect previously uncharacterized mechanisms of resistance, so susceptibility cannot be inferred by their absence and should always be confirmed by phenotypic testing.

Resistance to antifungal agents

Two forms of resistance are recognized: clinical resistance, in which there is therapeutic failure irrespective of the MIC of the infecting organism, and *in vitro* resistance, which is the failure of a drug to suppress the growth of an organism under specific test conditions. The latter may or may not correlate with clinical failure. Organisms may display inherent (also known as innate or primary) resistance, which is a phenomenon recognized in particular fungal species, or in a naturally occurring proportion of variants in an otherwise susceptible species, against certain antifungal agents and is often predictable and defines the spectrum of activity of an agent. Examples of innate resistance include *Candida krusei* to fluconazole, *Aspergillus terreus* to amphotericin B, and *in vitro* resistance of *Lomentospora* (previously *Scedosporium*) *prolificans* to all currently available antifungal agents.

Alternatively, organisms may develop secondary (otherwise known as emergent or acquired) resistance following long-term exposure to an agent during treatment of chronic infections, often with low doses in the face of persistent infection. This was first recognized in *Candida albicans* isolates from patients treated with oral ketoconazole for chronic mucocutaneous candidiasis. There were numerous reports during the early stages of the AIDS epidemic in which oropharyngeal candidiasis was treated with low-dose oral fluconazole, and resistance emerged in isolates of *C. albicans, C. dubliniensis, C. glabrata,* and, less frequently, *Cryptococcus neoformans* from cases of meningitis. More recently, resistance has emerged in *Aspergillus fumigatus* isolates from patients treated with oral azole therapy for chronic aspergillosis, and there has been the development of resistance to agricultural azoles, leading to resistance to clinical azoles (Vermeulen et al. 2013). A recent report from the Netherlands has found rates of voriconazole resistance to be as high as 16.2% of *A. fumigatus* isolates from high-risk patients, thus highlighting the need for antifungal susceptibility testing prior to azole therapy (Fuhren et al. 2015).

Mechanisms of resistance to azole antifungal drugs

Azole antifungal agents inhibit the activity of the cytochrome P450 lanosterol 14α-demethylase enzymes, encoded by the *ERG11* gene in yeast, which converts lanosterol to ergosterol, which is the major sterol in fungal cell membranes. Without this sterol there is disruption of the membrane structure and the function of membrane-bound enzymes, leading to inhibition of fungal cell growth; thus, azoles are most often fungistatic, although some also demonstrate fungicidal activity against certain moulds.

Multiple resistance mechanisms to azoles have been reported in the diploid yeast *Candida albicans* (for an excellent overview of antifungal resistance, see Perlin [2015]). In patients on long-term therapy, different resistance mutations are often accumulated in a step-wise manner. In *C. glabrata,* which is a haploid yeast, a single-point mutation can lead to resistance.

Azole resistance mechanisms include:

- membrane changes, leading to reduced uptake of azole drugs
- mutation of the target enzyme
- over-production of the target enzyme
- modification of the ergosterol biosynthesis pathway
- increased efflux due to up-regulation of housekeeping genes encoding efflux pumps:
  - ATP-binding cassette (ABC) transporters, which transport all azoles, leading to cross-resistance
  - multi-facilitator superfamily (MFS) transporters, which transport mainly fluconazole
- biofilm formation, leading to the development of persister cells

There are multiple resistance mutations documented in isolates of *A. fumigatus* from chronic infections treated with azoles (Bueid et al. 2010). These are mainly genetic modifications in *CYP51A*, which codes for lanosterol 14α-demethylase in *Aspergillus*. In contrast, the isolates that have developed resistance to agricultural azoles which are cross-resistant to one or more clinical azoles often display one of two mutations (TR_{34}/L98H or TR_{46}/Y121F/T289A) (Vermeulen et al. 2013). Such isolates have become widespread in the environment, especially in certain countries such as the Netherlands and Belgium, where they are also regularly isolated from immunocompromised patients with invasive disease (Fuhren et al. 2015). They have also been reported from numerous European countries, India, Iran, and China.

Mechanisms of resistance to polyenes

Resistance to the polyene agent amphotericin B remains rare and is often linked to reduced ergosterol levels in the fungal cell membrane, as amphotericin complexes with this membrane sterol to form cross-membrane pores, leading to leakage of cellular constituents and ultimately cell death. Resistance has also been linked to increased intracellular levels of catalase, thus reducing the oxidative killing potential of amphotericin B. Notably, innate resistance to amphotericin B is encountered in some isolates of *Candida lusitaniae, Aspergillus terreus, Scedosporium* spp., *Lomentospora prolificans*, and *Purpureocillium lilacinum*. As amphotericin B is fungicidal, emergent resistance is rare as cells are killed rather than being bathed in a fungistatic agent, allowing mutation to resistance, although this has been observed in some yeast species such as *Candida guilliermondii* (Johnson 2008).

Mechanisms of resistance to flucytosine (5-fluorocytosine)

The spectrum of activity of flucytosine includes most yeast species and some darkly pigmented moulds. To be susceptible, the fungal cell must have a cascade of active enzymes, cytosine permease to take up the drug, and cytosine deaminase and phosphorylase to metabolize it to its toxic form, at which point it disrupts RNA and DNA synthesis. Loss or reduction in activity of any one of the enzymes, but most commonly the latter, leads to primary or emergent resistance (Scholer and Polak 1984). The phenomenon of emergent resistance amongst yeast species during treatment is common, and for this reason flucytosine is rarely used as monotherapy.

Mechanisms of resistance to echinocandins

Echinocandins inhibit the membrane-bound enzyme glucan synthase, which synthesizes beta-glucan, a structural component in fungal cell walls. Without beta-glucan, cells lose their structural integrity. For yeast cells, this results in cell death by lysis, and in moulds lysis of the growing mycelial tips results in fungistatic activity. Although many clinically significant mould species, apart from *Aspergillus* species, are either innately resistant or have reduced susceptibility to the echinocandins, most *Candida* species are susceptible. Members of the *Candida parapsilosis* species complex are innately less susceptible to the echinocandins as they have a proline-alanine mutation at position 660 in the Fks1 protein, but as they often respond clinically, they also have higher echinocandin breakpoints than most other yeast species (Table 47.1). Various resistance mutations have been identified in hot-spot areas in the *FKS1* gene, and less commonly in the *FKS2* and *FKS3* genes, all of which encode the target enzyme, and up-regulation of chitin synthesis—another component of fungal cell wall—has been reported as a rescue mechanism (Rogers et al. 2007; Walker et al. 2008; Pham et al. 2014).

Conclusion

Standardized antifungal susceptibility testing has reached a level of intra- and inter-laboratory reproducibility at which global data can be evaluated to allow breakpoint setting to be correlated with clinical outcome, and can define the antifungal spectrum for most systemically active agents. There are some species with well-recognized innate resistance to one or more agents, but increasingly, common fungal pathogens are encountered in which there is the emergence of resistance to one or more agents. Ongoing surveillance is required to delineate the scale of the problem and specific susceptibility testing is recommended for isolates from invasive or refractory infections.

References

Alexander BD, Johnson MD, Pfeiffer CD et al. (2013) Increasing echinocandin resistance in *Candida glabrata*: clinical failure correlates with presence of *FKS* mutations and elevated minimum inhibitory concentrations. *Clin Infect Dis* 56: 1724–32.

Arendrup MC, Cuenca-Estrella M, Lass-Florl C, Hope W and the EUCAST-AFST (2012) EUCAST technical note on the EUCAST definitive document EDef 7.2: method for the determination of broth dilution minimum inhibitory concentrations of antifungal agents for yeasts EDef 7.2 (EUCAST-AFST). *Clin Microbiol Infect* 18: E246–7.

Bueid A, Howard SJ, Moore CB, et al. (2010) Azole antifungal resistance in *Aspergillus fumigatus*: 2008 and 2009. *J Antimicrob Chemother* 65: 2116–18.

Clinical and Laboratory Standards Institute (CLSI) (2008a) *Reference method for broth dilution antifungal susceptibility testing of yeasts; Approved standard*—3rd edn; CLSI document M27-A3. Wayne, PA: CLSI.

Clinical and Laboratory Standards Institute (CLSI) (2008b) *Reference method for broth dilution antifungal susceptibility testing of filamentous fungi; Approved standard*—2nd edn. NCCLS document M38-A2. Wayne, PA: CLSI.

Clinical and Laboratory Standards Institute (CSLI) (2009a) *Method for antifungal disk diffusion susceptibility testing of yeasts; Approved guideline*—2nd edn. Document M44-A2. Wayne, PA: CLSI.

Clinical and Laboratory Standards Institute (CLSI) (2009b) *Zone diameter interpretive standards and corresponding minimal inhibitory concentration (MIC) interpretive breakpoints.* Informational Supplement M44S3. Wayne, PA: CLSI.

Clinical and Laboratory Standards Institute (CLSI) (2010) *Method for antifungal disk diffusion susceptibility testing of non-dermatophyte filamentous fungi. Approved standard* CLSI document M51-A1. Wayne, PA: CLSI.

Clinical and Laboratory Standards Institute (CLSI) (2012) *Reference method for broth dilution antifungal susceptibility testing of yeast; 4th Informational Supplement. Approved standard* CLSI document M27-S4. Wayne, PA: CLSI.

Espinel-Ingroff A, Diekema DJ, Fothergill A, et al. (2010) Wild-type distributions and epidemiological cutoff values for the triazoles and six *Aspergillus* spp. for the CLSI broth microdilution method (M38-A2 document). *J Clin Microbiol* 48: 3251–7.

Fuhren J, Voskuil WS, Boel CHE, et al. (2015) High prevalence of azole resistance in *Aspergillus funigatus* isolates from high-risk patients. *J Antimicrob Chemother* 70: 2894–8.

Jensen RH, Johansen HK and Arendrup MC (2013) Stepwise development of a homozygous S80P substitution in Fks1p, conferring echinocandin resistance in *Candida tropicalis*. *Antimicrob Agents Chemother* 57: 614–17.

Johnson EM (2008) Issues in antifungal susceptibility testing. *J Antimicrob Chemother* 61 (Suppl. 1): i13–8.

Johnson EM and Cavling-Arendrup M (2015) Susceptibility test methods: yeasts and filamentous fungi, *in*: JH Jorgensen, MA Pfaller, KC Carroll, et al., eds, *Manual of Clinical Microbiology* (11th edn, Washington: ASM Press), 2255–81.

Marinach C, Alanio A, Palous M, et al. (2009) MALDI-TOF MS-based drug susceptibility testing of pathogens: the example of *Candida albicans* and fluconazole. *Proteomics* 9: 4627–31.

NCCLS (1992) Reference method for broth dilution antifungal susceptibility testing of yeasts; proposed standard NCCLS document M27-P. Wayne, PA: National Committee for Clinical and Laboratory Standards.

Perlin DS (2015) Mechanisms of resistance to antifungal agents, *in*: JH Jorgensen, MA Pfaller, KC Carroll, et al., eds, *Manual of Clinical Microbiology* (11th edn, Washington: ASM Press), 2236–54.

Pfaller MA and Diekema DJ (2004) Minireview. Rare and emerging opportunistic fungal pathogens: concern for resistance beyond *Candida albicans* and *Aspergillus fumigatus*. *J Clin Microbiol* 42: 4419–31.

Pfaller MA, Sheehan DJ and Rex JH (2004) Determination of fungicidal activity against yeasts and moulds: lessons learned from bactericidal testing and the need for standardization. *Clin Microbiol Rev* 17: 268–80.

Pham CD, Bolden CB, Kuykendall RJ and Lockhart SR (2014) Development of a luminex-based multiplex assay for detection of mutations conferring resistance to echinocandins in *Candida glabrata*. *J Clin Microbiol* 52: 790–5.

Rex JH, Pfaller MA, Galgiani JN, et al. (1997) Development of interpretive breakpoints for antifungal susceptibility testing—conceptual framework of *in vitro* and *in vivo* correlation data for fluconazole, itraconazole and *Candida* infections. *Clin Infect Dis* 24: 235–47.

Rodriquez-Tudela JL, Donnelly JP, Arendrup MC, et al. (2008) EUCAST Technical Note on the method for the determination of broth dilution minimum inhibitory concentrations of antifungal agents for conidia-forming mould. *Clin Microbiol Infect* 14: 982–4.

Rogers TR, Johnson EM and Munro CA (2007) Echinocandin drug resistance. *The J Invasive Fungal Infect* 1: 99–105.

Scholer HJ and Polak A (1984) Resistance to systemic antifungal agents, *in*: LE Bryan, ed., *Antimicrobial Drug Resistance* (Orlando, FL: Academic Press), 393–460.

Vermeulen E, Lagrou K and Verweij PE (2013) Azole resistance in *Aspergillus fumigatus*: a growing public health concern. *Curr Opin Infect Dis* 26: 493–500.

Verweij PE, Snelders E, Kema GHJ, et al. (2009) Azole resistance in *Aspergillus fumigatus*: a side-effect of environmental fungicide use? *Lancet Infect Dis* 9: 789–95.

Walker LA, Munro CA, de Bruijn I, Lenardon MD, McKinnon A and Gow NA (2008) Stimulation of chitin synthesis rescues *Candida albicans* from echinocandins. *PLoS Pathog* 4: e1000040.

CHAPTER 48

Antifungal therapeutic drug monitoring

H. Ruth Ashbee

Introduction to therapeutic drug monitoring

Therapeutic drug monitoring (TDM) is the process of measuring drug concentrations at specified intervals to ensure that concentration remains within the active and non-toxic range for that drug (Kang and Lee 2009). TDM is required when there is a relationship between the concentration of a drug and its efficacy and/or toxicity, and the drug has: 1) unpredictable absorption, 2) unpredictable metabolism, or 3) drug interactions which alter the drug concentrations (Ali et al. 2013). These conditions are fulfilled by several antifungals, and TDM may improve their efficacy in clinical practice.

Unpredictable absorption is usually due to food effects or gastric pH for orally administered drugs, with some drugs requiring either fasting or intake with food for maximal absorption.

Differences in the metabolism of a drug between individuals may be related to many factors. These can include age, gender, or genetic makeup, and in clinical practice it may be difficult to predict who will metabolize drugs more quickly than others, unless detailed genetic analysis is carried out.

Lastly, drug interactions can lead to large variations in the concentration of a drug within a patient. For antifungal drugs, this is mainly seen with the azoles. Azoles are inhibitors of the cytochrome P450 (CYP 450) system, a superfamily of enzymes involved in steroid synthesis, breakdown of metabolic products, and drug metabolism (Guengerich 2008). Some azoles are substrates of the CYP enzymes and are extensively metabolized by them. Because the CYP enzymes are responsible for metabolizing many drugs, any drug which inhibits or induces these enzymes can have a significant impact on concentrations of concomitant drugs.

Methods for TDM

Both serum and plasma can be used in TDM assays, and in most cases the concentration measured will be the same. However, as plasma retains various proteins, this may be relevant when measuring highly-protein-bound drugs. Additionally, the presence of an anticoagulant in plasma and the increased likelihood of haemolysis in serum may impact on the assay (Uges 1988).

Historically, bioassays were used to measure antifungal concentrations. They are cheap and simple to perform, requiring little equipment, but inherently are lacking in reproducibility and subject to interference and have been largely replaced by other methods.

High-performance liquid chromatography (HPLC) is now widely used for TDM as the equipment is commonly available, commercial kits have been developed, and multiple drugs can be quantified in a single sample. However, HPLC is subject to interference, and the extraction procedure and run times may be lengthy.

Recently, various mass spectrometry methods have been used to determine antifungal drug concentrations. The advantages of mass spectrometry-based methods are that they are very sensitive and specific, can quantify multiple drugs in a single sample, and have less interference than HPLC. However, the equipment is very expensive and not widely available and the process is technically demanding.

External quality assurance schemes (EQAS) are important in determining the reliability of any TDM assay and there are now UK or international schemes which cover various antifungal drugs and provide information on the assay performance.

TDM of specific antifungal drugs

TDM of antifungal drugs is an evolving area. Initially, many drugs were not thought to require TDM, but clinical experience has shown that it may be required. The recommendations presented here may change over time, but this chapter will review what is currently advised (Table 48.1).

Amphotericin B

Amphotericin B is widely used to treat systemic mycoses, mainly as one of the lipid formulations which overcome much of the toxicity associated with use of amphotericin B deoxycholate, the older form of the drug. The drug is administered intravenously, with the total dose being absorbed. Peak concentrations of 2 mg/L are obtained after an infusion of 1 mg/kg amphotericin B deoxycholate (Drew 2010), which exceeds the minimum inhibitory concentration (MIC) of most organisms. As yet, no concentration–toxicity relationship has been described, although nephrotoxicity is related to dosing regimen (Fisher et al. 1989). Because the drug is given intravenously, serum concentrations are predictable, and there is no toxicity–concentration relationship, TDM is not recommended for this antifungal (Ashbee et al. 2014).

Echinocandins

Echinocandins are the newest class of antifungals and have a fungal-specific target, inhibiting the Fks1p subunit of β-1,3-D-glucan

Table 48.1 Current recommendations for therapeutic drug monitoring (TDM) of antifungal agents

Antifungal drug	Recommendation for routine TDM	Target concentration (mg/L)	Comments
Amphotericin B	Not recommended	–	–
Echinocandins	Not recommended	–	–
Flucytosine	Recommended	Trough: >20–40 Peak: 50–100	–
Fluconazole	Not recommended	–	May be helpful in specific circumstances, e.g. patients in ICUs or paediatric patients unresponsive to therapy
Itraconazole	Recommended	Trough: >0.5–1 Peak: <5	–
Voriconazole	Recommended	Trough: >1–2 Peak: <4–6	–
Posaconazole	Recommended	Prophylaxis trough: >0.7 Treatment trough: >1	Requirement for TDM with tablets is evolving, but bioavailability appears to be significantly less variable and concentrations are higher than for the suspension

synthase, an enzyme with no human analogue. They are all large cyclic lipopeptides with little or no oral absorption, and hence are delivered intravenously. Mean trough concentrations range from >1 mg/L for caspofungin to 2 mg/L or greater for anidulafungin and micafungin (Kofla and Ruhnke 2011). All echinocandins have good toxicity profiles and toxicity does not correlate with drug concentration. Thus, at the moment, there is no evidence to suggest that TDM is required during echinocandin therapy.

Flucytosine

Flucytosine (5-fluorocytosine) is a pyrimidine analogue, which inhibits fungal DNA and protein synthesis. It is an old antifungal, but is still important in treating cryptococcal meningitis where it is used in combination with either amphotericin B or fluconazole. It has good oral bioavailability (75–90%) and is predominantly eliminated via the kidneys, necessitating a dose reduction in patients with renal impairment (Vermes et al. 2000). *In vitro* low concentrations of flucytosine have been associated with the development of resistance (Normark & Schönebeck 1972), so there is a theoretical risk of isolates developing resistance in patients with low flucytosine concentrations. Toxicity with flucytosine use includes hepatotoxicity and bone marrow suppression, which occur particularly when serum concentrations exceed 100 mg/L. Variability in flucytosine concentrations in patients has been documented in both adults and children, with significant numbers of samples either too high or too low (Soltani et al. 2006; Pasqualotto et al. 2007).

Because of a strong relationship between concentration and toxicity, and a potential relationship between concentration and the development of resistance, TDM is recommended for most patients receiving flucytosine and has been an accepted part of management for many years (Warnock et al. 1982). Recent recommendations reiterate that most patients receiving flucytosine should have TDM performed within the first 72 hours of therapy and that the trough concentrations should be >20–40 mg/L, with peak concentrations of 50–100 mg/L (Ashbee et al. 2014).

Fluconazole

Fluconazole, the first triazole introduced into clinical practice, is active against most species of *Candida* (except *C. krusei* and with variable activity against *C. glabrata*), *Cryptococcus*, and various endemic moulds, but has no activity against *Aspergillus*.

Fluconazole has excellent, predictable oral bioavailability (>95%) which is not affected by food intake or gastric pH. Fluconazole is mainly excreted in urine via glomerular filtration and there is minimal hepatic metabolism. Because of its renal clearance, doses of fluconazole need to be modified in renal dysfunction (Bellmann 2007). There is limited toxicity associated with fluconazole use, including hepatotoxicity, headache, and nausea, but this is not concentration-dependent.

Although fluconazole is not a substrate for the CYP enzymes, it is an inhibitor of CYP 2C9, and to a lesser extent, 2C19 and 3A4. Because of this, it can increase the concentrations of various drugs, including some antihistamines and immunosuppressants, which are metabolized by these CYP enzymes (Bruggemann et al. 2009).

For routine use, there are no indications to support the use of TDM for fluconazole. It has linear pharmacokinetics, good oral bioavailability, and no suggestion that toxicity is concentration-dependent. However, there may be some circumstances in which TDM is helpful. In critically ill patients, drug pharmacokinetics may be significantly different because of changes in the physiology of the patients, so drugs which can normally be used with a standard dosing may require TDM to optimize exposure (Felton et al. 2014). For example, 40% of paediatric cancer patients had subtherapeutic concentrations of fluconazole in a recent study (van der Elst et al. 2014), so TDM may be helpful in monitoring paediatric patients not responding to treatment.

Itraconazole

Itraconazole was the next azole to come into clinical use, and importantly, has activity against *Aspergillus*. It has been used for both prophylaxis and treatment of mycoses. There are several oral formulations of itraconazole and absorption varies significantly between them. The capsules have relatively poor bioavailability, which is improved when taken with food (Barone et al. 1993) and/or an acidic beverage (Jaruratanasirikul and Kleepkaew 1997). In contrast, itraconazole solution has approximately 30% greater bioavailability than the capsules (Barone et al. 1998), but needs to be taken whilst fasting.

There are many toxicities associated with itraconazole use, although most are relatively minor. They include nausea and vomiting (particularly seen with the suspension and probably due to the cyclodextrin vehicle), rash, headache, hypokalaemia, and liver dysfunction (Lestner and Hope 2013).

Itraconazole is mainly metabolized in the liver by the CYP450 system, predominantly CYP 3A4. Around 30 metabolites are produced, including hydroxy-itraconazole, which is microbiologically active (Heykants et al. 1989). Itraconazole and many of its metabolites are also potent inhibitors of CYP 3A4 (Isoherranen et al. 2004), resulting in multiple clinically significant drug interactions with steroids, statins, benzodiazepines, vinca alkaloids, various immunosuppressants, and antivirals (Bruggemann et al. 2009).

In addition to issues with absorption and drug interactions, there is some evidence that efficacy and toxicity are concentration-dependent. Early prophylactic studies suggested there was a relationship between efficacy and drug exposure, with breakthrough infections more common in patients with serum concentrations of <0.25 mg/L (Boogaerts et al. 1989) or <0.5 mg/L (Glasmacher et al. 1999). Patient responses in aspergillosis (Denning et al. 1989a), cryptococcosis (Denning et al. 1989b), and oral candidiasis (Cartledge et al. 1997) were also improved at higher serum concentrations. Conversely, high serum concentrations have been correlated with increased likelihood of toxicity. Patients with mean concentrations above 17.1 mg/L (measured by bioassay) developed toxicity more frequently (86%) than those with mean concentrations <17.1 mg/L (31%; Lestner et al. 2009).

Factors supporting the routine use of TDM for itraconazole are: variable absorption, many drug interactions, and both efficacy and toxicity–concentration relationships. Therefore, TDM is recommended for all patients receiving itraconazole for prophylaxis or treatment of systemic infections. Serum trough concentrations above 0.5–1 mg/L and below 5 mg/L are generally accepted as maximizing efficacy whilst reducing the likelihood of toxicity (Ashbee et al. 2014).

Voriconazole

Voriconazole, a synthetic derivative of fluconazole, is a broad-spectrum triazole with activity against *Candida, Cryptococcus, Aspergillus, Fusarium*, and *Scedosporium* (Johnson and Kauffman 2003). Initial studies demonstrated an oral bioavailability of 80–85%, but it may only be 60% (Pascual et al. 2012).

Voriconazole is eliminated mainly by hepatic metabolism, predominantly CYP2C19, and to a lesser extent 3A4 and 2C9 (Roffey et al. 2003). CYP2C19 has many allelic variants, whose incidence varies with ethnicity, resulting in poor metabolizer and extensive metabolizer phenotypes (Wijnen et al. 2007). In poor metabolizer phenotypes, serum concentrations of voriconazole can be four- to five-fold higher than those in extensive metabolizers. Genetic polymorphisms in CYP2C19 account for 49% of the variance in clearance of voriconazole (Weiss et al. 2009) and hence play a major role in the variations in pharmacokinetics seen in patients.

Voriconazole is a potent inhibitor of 2C9, 2C19, and 3A4 (Jeong et al. 2009), leading to many of its drug interactions, including those with tacrolimus, cyclosporin, vincristine, midazolam, and rifabutin (Bruggemann et al. 2009). Toxicity associated with voriconazole can be significant and includes visual disturbances, hepatotoxicity, phototoxicity, and squamous cell carcinoma. There are compelling data that toxicity is associated with elevated concentrations of voriconazole, particularly for liver toxicity (Matsumoto et al. 2009), neurotoxicity (Pascual et al. 2012), and skin malignancy, which appears to correlate with duration of voriconazole use, rather than serum concentrations (Epaulard et al. 2013).

An efficacy–concentration relationship has been reported in several studies, with voriconazole trough concentrations above 1–2 mg/L correlating with improved patient outcomes (Smith et al. 2006; Pascual et al. 2008).

Voriconazole has variable metabolism depending on the patient's genotype, variable oral bioavailability, and significant drug interactions. The evidence is also strong for concentration–efficacy and concentration–toxicity relationships, so TDM is strongly recommended for all patients receiving voriconazole. The target therapeutic range is above 1–2 mg/L and below 4–6 mg/L (Ashbee et al. 2014).

Posaconazole

Posaconazole is a synthetic analogue of itraconazole, but has a broader spectrum of activity, including mucoraceous moulds. Posaconazole was initially marketed as an oral suspension, where oral bioavailability is significantly improved with food (168% compared with a fasted state), especially high fat food (290% compared with a fasted state) (Courtney et al. 2004). Absorption is further improved by splitting the dose or administration with a nutritional supplement (Sansone-Parsons et al. 2006; Krishna et al. 2009), whilst agents reducing gastric acidity decrease absorption (Alffenaar et al. 2009). Recently, delayed-release tablets and an intravenous formulation have been released. The tablets have approximately three-fold better oral bioavailability and are less affected by alterations in gastric pH (Guarascio and Slain 2015) or intake of fatty foods (Kersemaekers et al. 2015) than the suspension.

Excretion mainly occurs unchanged in the faeces, with about 14% excreted in the urine after glucuronidation. Posaconazole has limited interaction with the CYP 450 enzymes as it is not a substrate for them and hence has fewer drug interactions than itraconazole or voriconazole, although it does inhibit CYP 3A4 (Bellmann 2007).

Toxicity is limited and includes nausea, vomiting, and liver dysfunction, but there are no data to suggest that this is concentration-dependent.

There is increasing evidence of an efficacy–concentration relationship for posaconazole, with improved response rates at higher serum concentrations in the salvage setting for aspergillosis (Walsh et al. 2007) and in prophylaxis (Dolton et al. 2012). However, accumulation of posaconazole in epithelial cell membranes *in vitro* at concentrations higher than serum suggests that there may be cellular reservoirs of posaconazole and that serum concentrations may not accurately reflect tissue concentrations (Campoli et al. 2013). Limited data from human tissues also suggest that posaconazole accumulates in the heart, lung, liver, and kidneys (Blennow et al. 2014).

Current recommendations are to perform TDM for posaconazole in most patients, aiming for a prophylactic trough concentration of >0.7 mg/L and a treatment trough concentration of >1 mg/L (Ashbee et al. 2014). The use of delayed-release tablets improves oral bioavailability and enhances drug exposure (Cumpston et al. 2015), and in future this may negate the need for posaconazole TDM, particularly if serum concentrations are confirmed to be poor predictors of tissue concentrations.

Conclusions and future perspectives

Our understanding of antifungal pharmacokinetics and pharmacodynamics is improving rapidly and the factors which govern patient treatment outcomes are being unravelled. Pharmacodynamic studies are defining the parameters which produce optimal responses for various drugs. For different drug classes, the ratios of drug exposure:MIC, time of drug concentration above MIC, or ratio of maximum concentration:MIC have all been shown to predict treatment efficacy and may inform TDM in some patients. However, for many patients the aetiological agent is never recovered and no MIC can be determined to guide therapy. For those patients, determining serum concentrations of antifungals may remain the only surrogate marker of drug exposure available and hence TDM is likely to remain an important component of antifungal therapy.

References

Alffenaar JW, van AS, van der Werf TS, Kosterink JG and Uges DR (2009) Omeprazole significantly reduces posaconazole serum trough level. *Clin Infect Dis* 48: 839.

Ali AS, Abdel-Rahman MS, Rahman ABA and Osman OH (2013) Basic principles of therapeutic drug monitoring. *J Appl Biopharm Pharmacokinet* 1: 87–95.

Ashbee HR, Barnes RA, Johnson EM, Richardson MD, Gorton R and Hope WW (2014) Therapeutic drug monitoring (TDM) of antifungal agents: guidelines from the British Society for Medical Mycology. *J Antimicrob Chemother* 69: 1162–76.

Barone JS, Koh JG, Bierman RH, et al. (1993) Food interaction and steady-state pharmacokinetics of itraconazole capsules in healthy male volunteers. *Antimicrob Agents Chemother* 37: 778–84.

Barone JS, Moskovitz BL, Guarnieri J, et al. (1998) Enhanced bioavailability of itraconazole in hydroxypropyl-β-cyclodextrin solution versus capsules in healthy volunteers. *Antimicrob Agents Chemother* 42: 1862–5.

Bellmann R (2007) Clinical pharmacokinetics of systemically administered antimycotics. *Curr Clin Pharmacol* 2: 37–58.

Blennow O, Eliasson E, Pettersson T, et al. (2014) Posaconazole concentrations in human tissues after allogeneic stem cell transplantation. *Antimicrob Agents Chemother* 58: 4941–3.

Boogaerts MA, Verhoef GE, Zachee P, Demuynck H, Verbist L and De Beule K (1989) Antifungal prophylaxis with itraconazole in prolonger neutropenia: correlation with plasma levels. *Mycoses* 32 (Suppl. 1): 103–8.

Bruggemann RJM, Alffenaar JWC, Blijlevens NMA, et al. (2009) Clinical relevance of the pharmacokinetic interactions of azole antifungal drugs with other coadministered agents. *Clin Infect Dis* 48: 1441–58.

Campoli P, Perlin DS, Kristof AS, White TC, Filler SG and Sheppard DC (2013) Pharmacokinetics of posaconazole within epithelial cells and fungi: insights into potential mechanisms of action during treatment and prophylaxis. *J Infect Dis* 208: 1717–28.

Cartledge JD, Midgley J and Gazzard BG (1997) Itraconazole solution: higher serum drug concentrations and better clinical response rates than the capsule formulation in acquired immunodeficiency syndrome patients with candidosis. *J Clin Pathol* 50: 477–80.

Courtney R, Wexler D, Radwanski E, Lim J and Laughlin M (2004) Effect of food on the relative bioavailability of two oral formulations of posaconazole in healthy adults. *Br J Clin Pharmacol* 57: 218–22.

Cumpston A, Caddell R, Shillingburg A, et al. (2015) Superior serum concentrations with posaconazole delayed-release tablets compared to suspension formulation in hematological malignancies. *Antimicrob Agents Chemother* 59: 4424–8.

Denning DW, Tucker RM, Hanson LH and Stevens DA (1989a) Treatment of invasive aspergillosis with itraconazole. *Am J Med* 86: 791–800.

Denning DW, Tucker RM, Hanson LH, Hamilton JR and Stevens DA (1989b) Itraconazole therapy for cryptococcal meningitis and cryptococcosis. *Arch Intern Med* 149: 2301–8.

Dolton MJ, Ray JE, Chen SC-A, Ng K, Pont L and McLachlan AJ (2012) Multicenter study of posaconazole therapeutic drug monitoring: exposure-response relationship and factors affecting concentration. *Antimicrob Agents Chemother* 56: 5503–10.

Drew RH (2010) Polyenes for prevention and treatment of invasive fungal infections, *in*: MA Ghannoum and JR Perfect, eds, *Antifungal Therapy* (London: Informa Healthcare), 163–83.

Epaulard O, Villier C, Ravaud P, et al. (2013) A multistep voriconazole-related phototoxic pathway may lead to skin carcinoma: results from a French nationwide study. *Clin Infect Dis* 57: e182–8.

Felton TW, Hope WW and Roberts JA (2014) How severe is antimicrobial pharmacokinetic variability in critically ill patients and what can be done about it? *Diagn Microbiol Infect Dis* 79: 441–7.

Fisher MA, Talbot GH, Maislin G, McKeon BP, Tynan KP and Strom BL (1989) Risk factors for Amphotericin B-associated nephrotoxicity. *Am J Med* 87: 547–52.

Glasmacher A, Hahn C, Leutner C, et al. (1999) Breakthrough invasive fungal infections in neutropenic patients after prophylaxis with itraconazole. *Mycoses* 42: 443–51.

Guarascio AJ and Slain D (2015) Review of the new delayed-release oral tablet and intravenous dosage forms of posaconazole. *Pharmacotherapy* 35: 208–19.

Guengerich FP (2008) Cytochrome P450 and chemical toxicology. *Chem Res Toxicol* 21: 70–83.

Heykants J, Van Peer A, Van de Velde V, et al. (1989) The clinical pharmacokinetics of itraconazole: an overview. *Mycoses* 32 (Suppl. 1): 67–87.

Isoherranen N, Kunze KL, Allen KE, Nelson WL and Thummel KE (2004) Role of itraconazole metabolites in CYP3A4 inhibition. *Drug Metab Dispos* 32: 1121–31.

Jaruratanasirikul S and Kleepkaew A (1997) Influence of an acidic beverage (Coca-Cola) on the absorption of itraconazole. *Eur J Clin Pharmacol* 52: 235–7.

Jeong S, Nguyen PD and Desta Z (2009) Comprehensive in vitro analysis of voriconazole inhibition of eight cytochrome P450 (CYP) enzymes: major effect on CYPs 2B6, 2C9, 2C19, and 3A. *Antimicrob Agents Chemother* 53: 541–51.

Johnson LB and Kauffman CA (2003) Voriconazole: a new triazole antifungal agent. *Clin Infect Dis* 36: 630–7.

Kang J and Lee M (2009) Overview of therapeutic drug monitoring. *Korean J Intern Med* 24: 1–10.

Kersemaekers WM, Dogterom P, Xu J, Marcantonio EE, de Greef R, Waskin H and van Iersel MLPS (2015) Effect of a high-fat meal on the pharmacokinetics of 300-milligram posaconazole in a solid oral tablet formulation. *Antimicrob Agents Chemother* 59: 3385–9.

Kofla G and Ruhnke M (2011) Pharmacology and metabolism of anidulafungin, caspofungin and micafungin in the treatment of invasive candidosis—review of the literature. *Eur J Med Res* 16: 159–66.

Krishna G, Moton A, Ma L, Medlock MM and McLeod J (2009) Pharmacokinetics and absorption of posaconazole oral suspension under various gastric conditions in healthy volunteers. *Antimicrob Agents Chemother* 53: 958–66.

Lestner J and Hope WW (2013) Itraconazole: an update on pharmacology and clinical use for treatment of invasive and allergic fungal infections. *Expert Opin Drug Metab Toxicol* 9: 911–26.

Lestner JM, Roberts SA, Moore CB, et al. (2009) Toxicodynamics of itraconazole: implications for therapeutic drug monitoring. *Clin Infect Dis* 49: 928–30.

Matsumoto K, Ikawa K, Abematsu K, et al. (2009) Correlation between voriconazole trough plasma concentration and hepatotoxicity in patients with different CYP2C19 genotypes. *Int J Antimicrob Agents* 34: 91–4.

Normark S and J Schönebeck (1972) *In vitro* studies of 5-fluorocytosine resistance in *Candida albicans* and *Torulopsis glabrata*. *Antimicrob Agents Chemother* 2: 14–21.

Pascual A, Calandra T, Bolay S, Buclin T, Bille J and Marchetti O (2008) Voriconazole therapeutic drug monitoring in patients with invasive mycoses improves efficacy and safety outcomes. *Clin Infect Dis* 46: 201–11.

Pascual A, Csajka C, Buclin T, et al. (2012) Challenging recommended oral and intravenous voriconazole doses for improved efficacy and safety: population pharmacokinetics-based analysis of adult patients with invasive fungal infections. *Clin Infect Dis* 55: 381–90.

Pasqualotto AC, Howard SJ, Moore CB and Denning DW (2007) Flucytosine therapeutic monitoring: 15 years' experience from the UK. *J Antimicrob Chemother* 59: 791–3.

Roffey SJ, Cole S, Comby P, et al. (2003) The disposition of voriconazole in mouse, rat, rabbit, guinea pig, dog and human. *Drug Metab Dispos* 31: 731–41.

Sansone-Parsons A, Krishna G, Calzetta A, et al. (2006) Effect of a nutritional supplement on posaconazole pharmacokinetics following oral administration to healthy volunteers. *Antimicrob Agents Chemother* 50: 1881–3.

Soltani M, Tobin CM, Bowker KE, Sunderland J, MacGowan AP and Lovering AM (2006) Evidence of excessive concentrations of 5-flucytosine in children aged below 12 years: a 12-year review of serum concentrations from a UK clinical assay reference laboratory. *Int J Antimicrob Agents* 28: 574–7.

Smith J, Safdar N, Knasinski V, et al. (2006) Voriconazole therapeutic drug monitoring. *Antimicrob Agents Chemother* 50: 1570–2.

Uges DR (1988) Plasma or serum in therapeutic drug monitoring and clinical toxicology. *Pharm Weekbl Sci* 10: 185–8.

van der Elst KCM, Pereboom M, van den Heuvel ER, Kosterink JGW, Schölvinck EH and Alffenaar J-WC (2014) Insufficient fluconazole exposure in pediatric cancer patients and the need for therapeutic drug monitoring in critically ill children. *Clin Infect Dis* 59: 1527–33.

Vermes A, Guchelaar H.-J and Dankert J (2000) Flucytosine: a review of its pharmacology, clinical indications, pharmacokinetics, toxicity and drug interactions. *J Antimicrob Chemother* 46: 171–9.

Walsh TJ, Raad I, Patterson TF, et al. (2007) Treatment of invasive aspergillosis with posaconazole in patients who are refractory to or intolerant of conventional therapy: an externally controlled trial. *Clin Infect Dis* 44: 2–12.

Warnock DW, Richardson MD and Turner A (1982) High performance liquid chromatographic (HPLC) and other non-biological methods for quantification of antifungal drugs. *J Antimicrob Chemother* 10: 467–78.

Weiss J, ten Hoevel MM, Burhenne J, et al. (2009) CYP2C19 genotype is a major factor contributing to the highly variable pharmacokinetics of voriconazole. *J Clin Pharmacol* 49: 196–204.

Wijnen PA, Op den Buijsch RA, Drent M, et al. (2007) Review article: the prevalence and clinical relevance of cytochrome P450 polymorphisms. *Aliment Pharmacol Ther* 26 (Suppl. 2): 211–19.

CHAPTER 49

Antifungal treatment guidelines

Laura Cottom and Brian L. Jones

Introduction to antifungal treatment guidelines

In the modern complex medical environment, guidelines serve to aid clinicians in decision-making processes. Guidelines have existed in medicine since antiquity. However, more recently, they were defined as 'systematically developed statements' (Eccles et al. 2012), the common goal being to provide comprehensive guidance to facilitate best practice.

It is axiomatic that guidelines should be evidence-based. The development of an unbiased, independent, high-quality guideline should involve a multidisciplinary process that reviews and re-evaluates evidence. Unfortunately, good-quality evidence from randomized controlled trials (RCTs) is frequently lacking, with significant variation in the quality of both design and reporting. To address these issues the Consolidated Standards of Reporting Trials statement (CONSORT 2010; http://consort-statement.org) was developed, allowing readers to develop a better understanding of trial design, conduct, analysis, interpretation, and validity of results (Schulz et al. 2010). Guidelines should ideally follow a consistent set of principles to allow reliable inter-user independent assessment of the recommendations. The Grades of Recommendations, Assessment, Development and Evaluation (GRADE) system (US GRADE 2017; http://www.gradeworkinggroup.org/) provides a robust assessment of the strength of recommendation (SoR) based on the quality of evidence (QoE) available (Guyatt et al. 2008) (Table 49.1). The SoR is a synthesis and interplay of several factors—including patients' values and preferences; balance between benefits, harms and burdens; resources; and cost implications—in addition to quality or certainty of evidence.

Important attributes of any guideline include validity, reliability, reproducibility, and clinical applicability (Institute of Medicine Committee to Advise the Public Health Service on Clinical Practice Guidelines, 1990) and these can vary widely between different guidelines. The AGREE (Appraisal of Guidelines for Research & Evaluation) instrument is a generic tool for the evaluation of reliability and validity of guidelines. It assesses guidelines in six domains: scope and purpose, stakeholder involvement, rigour of development, clarity and presentation, application, and editorial independence (AGREE 2010; http://www.agreetrust.org). Recommendations for antifungal treatment in haemato-oncology patients have been reviewed using the AGREE instrument (Agrawal et al. 2012).

It is important to remember that guidelines do not represent a standard of care. Clinical decisions must consider all available evidence and guidelines provide a useful way of consolidating this information. However, they must be interpreted in light of individual patient findings. This is best summarized by the Scottish Intercollegiate Guideline Network (SIGN 2015; http://www.sign.ac.uk): 'A guideline is not to be construed or to serve as a standard of care. Standards of care are determined on the basis of all clinical data available for an individual case and are subject to change as scientific knowledge and technology advance and patterns of care evolve. Adherence to guideline recommendations will not ensure a successful outcome in every case, nor should they be construed as including all proper methods of care or excluding other acceptable methods of care aimed at the same results. The ultimate judgement must be made by the appropriate healthcare professional(s) responsible for clinical decisions regarding a particular clinical procedure or treatment plan. This judgement should only be arrived at following discussion of the options with the patient, covering

Table 49.1 Overview of Grading of Recommendations, Assessment, Development and Evaluation (GRADE) methodology

Category, grade	Determinants	Definition, implications
Strength of Recommendation (SoR)		
Strong recommendation (SR)	Quality (certainty) of evidence Balance between benefits, harms, and burdens Patients' values & preferences Resources and cost	Population: Most people in this situation would want the recommended course of action. Healthcare workers: Most people should receive the recommended course of action. Policy makers: The recommendation can be adapted as a policy in most situations.
Weak recommendation (WR)		Population: The majority of people in this situation would want the recommended course of action, but many would not. Healthcare workers: Be prepared to help people to make a decision that is consistent with their own values/decision aids and shared decision making. Policy makers: There is need for substantial debate and involvement of stakeholders.

Table 49.1 (Continued)

Category, grade	Determinants	Definition, implications
Quality of Evidence (QoE)		
High quality (HQ)	Randomized trials ◆ High initial confidence in an estimate of effect Observational studies	⊕⊕⊕⊕ Randomized trials enter the GRADE system as high-quality evidence; this design is assumed to beat lower risk of bias than observational studies*.
Moderate quality (MQ)	◆ Low initial confidence in an estimate of effect Justifications for considering raising confidence	⊕⊕⊕
Low quality (LQ)	◆ Large effect ◆ Dose response ◆ All plausible confounding & bias would	⊕⊕ Observational studies enter the GRADE system as low-quality evidence; these designs are assumed to be at higher risk of bias*.
Very low quality (VLQ)	• reduce a demonstrated effect, or • suggest a spurious effect if no effect was observed Justifications for considering lowering confidence: ◆ risk of bias ◆ inconsistency ◆ indirectness ◆ imprecision ◆ publication bias *The QoE may be raised or lowered in relation to the categories outlined above.	⊕

Source: data from GRADE working group, www.gradeworkinggroup.org/

the diagnostic and treatment choices available. It is advised, however, that significant departures from the national guideline, or any local guidelines derived from it, should be fully documented in the patient's case notes at the time the relevant decision is made.'

Fungal guidelines

Guidelines may be local, network, regional, national, or international in their scope and may focus on individual organisms applicable to all patient groups or be directed at specific target groups, such as haemato-oncology patients. Over the last decade a number of fungal guidelines have been published, including those from the Infectious Diseases Society of America (IDSA), European Society of Clinical Microbiology and Infectious Diseases (ESCMID), the British Committee for Standards in Haematology (BCSH), and the European Conference on Infections in Leukaemia (ECIL). Major national and international guidelines for the management of invasive fungal infection are listed in Table 49.2.

This chapter will evaluate the major European (ESCMID) and American (IDSA) guidelines for the treatment of *Candida* and

Table 49.2 Guidelines for the management of invasive fungal infection

Disease	Guideline	Date published	Evidence rating	Target group
Candidiasis	IDSA (Pappas et al.) Clinical Practice Guideline for the Management of Candidiasis: 2016 Update	2016	Grading of Recommendations Assessment, Development and Evaluation (GRADE) methodology	All patient groups
Candidiasis Aspergillosis	DGHO (Mousset et al.) Infectious Diseases Working Party (AGIHO) of the German Society of Haematology and Oncology (DGHO): Treatment of invasive fungal infections in cancer patients	2014	IDSA & US Public Health Service Grading System Adapted from GRADE methodology	Haematological & oncology patients
Candidiasis Aspergillosis	ECIL 4 (Groll et al.) Paediatric Group Considerations for Fungal Diseases and Antifungal Treatment in Children	2014	CDC Grading System	Paediatric haematological patients
Aspergillosis	Expert panel recommendations (Al-Abdely et al.) Clinical practice guidelines for the treatment of invasive *Aspergillus* infections in adults in the Middle-East region	2014	Three-tier grading system adapted from the IDSA & US Public Health Service Grading System	All adult patient groups in the Middle East

(continued)

Table 49.2 (Continued)

Disease	Guideline	Date published	Evidence rating	Target group
Candidiasis Aspergillosis	ECIL-5 (Maertens et al.) Update of the ECIL guidelines for antifungal therapy in leukaemia and haematopoietic stem cell transplantation (HSCT)	2013	CDC Grading System	Adult haematological patients
Candidiasis Aspergillosis	NCCN guidelines (Baden et al.) National Comprehensive Cancer Network (NCCN) Prevention and Treatment of Cancer-Related Infections	2012	NCCN Categories of Evidence and Consensus	Haematological & oncology patients
Candidiasis	ESCMID (Ullmann et al.; Cornely et al.) ESCMID guideline for the diagnosis and management of *Candida* diseases 2012	2012	Four-tier grading system based on the Canadian Task Force of the Periodic Health Examination and the 2008 IDSA & US Public Health Service Grading System	All patient groups
Aspergillosis	IDSA (Walsh et al.) Treatment of Aspergillosis: Clinical Practice Guidelines	2008	IDSA & US Public Health Service Grading System	All patient groups
Candidiasis Aspergillosis	National consensus working group Australia (Thursky et al.) Recommendations for the treatment of established fungal infections	2008	IDSA & US Public Health Service Grading System	Adult haematological & oncology patients
Candidiasis Aspergillosis	BCSH (Prentice et al.) Guidelines on the management of invasive fungal infection during therapy for haematological malignancy	2010 Archived	US Agency for Health Care Policy and Research (AHCPR)	Haematological patients

Aspergillus infection, highlighting important discrepancies, differences in evidence interpretation, and gaps in our knowledge base.

Differences in guideline preparation method and the grading systems for recommendations are evident. The 2016 IDSA and 2012 ESCMID *Candida* guidelines outline in detail the mechanism by which the review committee met, evaluated evidence, and reached conclusions. This is lacking for the IDSA 2008 aspergillosis guideline. The method for grading the SoR and QoE also differs between the three guidelines (for an overview of IDSA & ESCMID grading systems, see Appendices 1–3).

The GRADE methodology was adopted by IDSA in 2008. ESCMID utilized an adaptation of the GRADE methodology (Table 49.3). The SoR is assigned according to a four-category grading system, differentiating between 'strongly supported' to 'recommended against'. The assignment of a recommendation against a given intervention or treatment (Category D) was absent in the 2008 IDSA methodology (Table 49.4) (Walsh et al. 2008).

For paediatric patients, the 2012 ESCMID guideline (see Chapter 35) specifically grades each drug–syndrome combination based on the evidence for efficacy, safety, and pharmacokinetic data.

Recognition of the pharmacodynamic/pharmacokinetic differences and the limited data on optimal dosing in paediatric patients is discussed by both the IDSA and ESCMID guidelines (see Chapter 35). Incorporation of guidance with diagnostic algorithms and risk stratification is recommended by both guidelines.

Table 49.3 Overview of the ESCMID grading methodology based on the Canadian Task Force of the Periodic Health Examination and the 2008 IDSA-US Public Health Service Grading System

Category, grade	Definition
Strength of Recommendation (SoR)	
A	ESCMID strongly supports a recommendation for use
B	ESCMID moderately supports a recommendation for use
C	ESMID marginally supports a recommendation for use
D	ESCMID supports a recommendation against use
Quality of Evidence (QoE)	
I	Evidence from ≥1 properly designed randomized controlled trial
II	Evidence from ≥1 well-designed clinical trial, without randomization; from cohort or case-controlled analytic studies (preferably from >1 centre); from multiple time-series; or from dramatic results from uncontrolled experiments
III	Evidence from opinions of respected authorities, based on clinical experience, descriptive case studies

Table 49.4 Overview of the 2008 IDSA-US Public Health Service grading system used for categorizing recommendations in clinical guidelines (Walsh et al. 2008)

Category, grade	Definition
Strength of Recommendation (SoR)	
A	Good evidence to support a recommendation for use
B	Moderate evidence to support a recommendation for use
C	Poor evidence to support a recommendation
Quality of Evidence (QoE)	
I	Evidence from ≥1 properly randomized, controlled trial
II	Evidence from ≥1 well-designed clinical trial, without randomization; from cohort or case-controlled analytical studies (preferably from >1 centre); from multiple time-series; or from dramatic results from uncontrolled experiments
III	Evidence from opinions of respected authorities, based on clinical experience, descriptive studies, or reports of expert committees

The ECIL guidelines (Groll et al. 2014) also advocate this approach in their recommendations for prophylaxis and empirical antifungal therapy.

The IDSA and ESCMID recommendations for the management of candidiasis and aspergillosis in adults are summarized in Appendices 4–11.

Evaluation of candidiasis guideline recommendations

Candidaemia

To date, there are no adequately powered RCTs for the treatment of candidaemia in neutropenic patients. Current data have largely been derived from single-arm studies or small subsets of RCTs that have enrolled mostly non-neutropenic patients.

Both the 2016 IDSA and 2012 ESCMID guidelines (Table 49.5) recommend 14 days of treatment post-clearance from the bloodstream, as assessed by daily blood culture. Furthermore, both recommend fundoscopic assessment to ensure no ocular involvement. ESCMID guidance, but not the IDSA guidance, recommends transoesophageal echocardiography to assess cardiac involvement. Both guidelines recommend the removal of central venous catheters if they can be safely removed.

Finally, both guidelines focus on the use of echinocandins as first-line treatment options. Previous guidelines recommended amphotericin B in its various formulations.

Table 49.5 Summary of candidaemia guideline recommendations

Condition or Treatment Group Adult	IDSA				ESCMID			
	Primary recommendations	**SoR QoE**	**Alternative recommendations**	**SoR QoE**	**Primary recommendations**	**SoR QoE**	**Alternative recommendations**	**SoR QoE**
Non-neutropenic	Echinocandin: Caspofungin (loading 70 mg, then 50 mg daily) Micafungin 100 mg daily Anidulafungin (loading 200 mg, then 100 mg daily)	SR-HQ	Fluconazole 800 mg (12 mg/kg) loading dose, then 400 mg (6 mg/kg) daily In selected patients who are nor critically ill and are unlikely to have a fluconazole-resistant *Candida* species	SR-HQ	Anidulafungin 200/100 mg Caspofungin 70/50 mg Micafungin 100 mg	A-I A-I A-I	L-AmB 3 mg/kg Voriconazole 6/3 mg/kg/day Fluconazole 400–800 mg ABLC 5 mg/kg	B-I B-I C-I C-II
Not recommended					AmB-D AmB-D + fluconazole AmB + 5-fluorocytosine	D-I D-I D-II	Efungumab + ABLC ABCD Itraconazole Posaconazole	D-II D-II D-II D-III
Neutropenic adult	Echinocandin: Caspofungin (loading 70 mg, then 50 mg daily) Micafungin 100 mg daily Anidulafungin (loading 200 mg, then 100 mg daily)	SR-HQ	L-AmB 3–5 mg daily Less attractive option owing to potential for toxicity Fluconazole 800 mg (12 mg/kg) loading dose, then 400 mg (6 mg/kg) daily	SR-MQ WR-LQ	Caspofungin Micafungin Anidulafungin L-AmB	A-II A-II B-II B-II	L-AmB Voriconazole Fluconazole ABLC ABCD	B-II C-II C-II C-II C-III

(continued)

Table 49.5 (Continued)

Condition or Treatment Group Adult	IDSA				ESCMID			
	Primary recommendations	**SoR QoE**	**Alternative recommendations**	**SoR QoE**	**Primary recommendations**	**SoR QoE**	**Alternative recommendations**	**SoR QoE**
			In patients who are nor critically ill and have had no azole exposure Voriconazole 400 mg (6 mg/kg) twice daily for two doses, then 200–300 mg (4 mg/kg) twice daily Can be used when additional mould cover is desired	 WR-LQ				
Not recommended					Itraconazole AmB-D	D-III D-II	Posaconazole	D-III

Table 49.6 Summary of suspected candidiasis guideline recommendations

Condition or Treatment Group Adult	IDSA				ESCMID			
	Primary recommendations	**SoR QoE**	**Alternative recommendations**	**SoR QoE**	**Primary recommendations**	**SoR QoE**	**Alternative recommendations**	**SoR QoE**
Non-neutropenic Adult ICU patient	Echinocandin: Caspofungin (loading 70 mg, then 50 mg daily) Micafungin 100 mg daily Anidulafungin (loading 200 mg, then 100 mg daily)	SR-MQ	Fluconazole 800 mg (12 mg/kg) loading dose, then 400 mg (6 mg/kg) daily In patients with no recent azole exposure and not colonized with azole-resistant *Candida* spp. L-AmB 3–5 mg daily If intolerant of other agents	SR-MQ SR-LQ	Fluconazole	C-II	Echinocandin	C-II
ICU patients with positive (1→3)-β-D-glucan test					Any antifungal	C-II		
Not recommended								
Adult ICU patients with fever despite broad-spectrum antibiotics and APACHE II >16 to resolve fever					Fluconazole 800 mg/daily	D-I		
ICU patients with *Candida* isolated from respiratory secretions					Any antifungal	D-II		

Table 49.6 (Continued)

Condition or Treatment Group Adult	IDSA				ESCMID			
	Primary recommendations	SoR QoE	Alternative recommendations	SoR QoE	Primary recommendations	SoR QoE	Alternative recommendations	SoR QoE
Neutropenic adult					Caspofungin 70 mg loading dose then 50 mg daily	A-I	Itraconazole 200 mg	B-I
					L-AmB 3 mg/kg/day	A-I	Micafungin 100 mg	B-II
					ABLC 5 mg/kg/day	B-I	ABCD 4 mg/kg/day	C-I
					Voriconazole 6 mg/kg b.d. day 1, then 3 mg/kg b.d. thereafter	B-I	Fluconazole 400 mg/day	C-I
Not recommended					AmB-D	D-II		

Suspected candidiasis

Criteria for starting empirical antifungal therapy in non-neutropenic patients remain poorly defined (Table 49.6). Early initiation of therapy may reduce morbidity, mortality, and length of stay in critically ill patients, but the widespread use of these agents must be balanced against the risk of toxicity, costs, and the emergence of resistance.

An echinocandin is recommended in haemodynamically unstable patients, in patients previously exposed to an azole, and in those colonized with azole-resistant *Candida* spp. Liposomal amphotericin (L-AmB) and amphotericin B-deoxycholate (AmB-D) are accepted alternative agents but are considered to have a greater toxicity profile. Empirical therapy with fluconazole may be considered in non-critically-ill patients known to be colonized with an azole-susceptible *Candida* species or in those with no prior exposure to azoles. Both the IDSA and ESCMID guidance discuss the role of prophylaxis in the ICU setting for the prevention of invasive candidiasis. Both guidelines highlight the weak evidence for this approach but emphasize its role with particular focus on high-risk patients. Both recommend fluconazole or an echinocandin for prophylaxis.

Candida urinary tract infection

Current guidance consensus (Table 49.7) recommends that identification of yeasts in urine must be evaluated in the context of the

Table 49.7 Summary of *Candida* urinary tract infection guideline recommendations

Condition or Treatment Group Adult	IDSA				ESCMID			
	Primary recommendations	SoR QoE	Alternative recommendations	SoR QoE	Primary recommendations	SoR QoE	Alternative recommendations	SoR QoE
Asymptomatic	Therapy not usually indicated, unless patients are at high risk or undergoing urological procedures	SR-LQ	Removal in indwelling bladder catheters	SR-LQ	No treatment	A-II		
Asymptomatic cystitis undergoing urology procedure	Fluconazole 400 mg (6 mg/kg) daily 7 days before and after procedure	SR-LQ	AmB-D 0.3–0.6 mg/kg 7 days before and after procedure	SR-LQ	Removal of urinary catheter	B-I	AmB-D bladder irrigation	C-II
					Fluconazole 200 mg for 14 days	C-I		
Symptomatic cystitis	Fluconazole 200 mg (3 mg/kg) daily for 2 weeks	SR-LQ	AmB-D 0.3–0.6 mg/kg for 1–7 days; or flucytosine 25 mg/kg q.i.d. for 7–10 days	SR-LQ	Fluconazole	A-III	AmB-D +/− flucytosine	B-III
	Removal of indwelling bladder catheters	SR-LQ	AmB-D bladder irrigation	WR-LQ				
Pyelonephritis	Fluconazole 200–400 mg (3–6 mg/kg) daily for 2 weeks	SR-LQ	AmB-D 0.5–0.7 mg/kg daily with or without 5-FC 25 mg/kg q.i.d;	SR-LQ	Fluconazole +/− flucytosine	A-III	Caspofungin 70/50 mg for 9–28 days	C-III
			5-FC alone for 2 weeks	WR-LQ	L-AmB +/− flucytosine	A-III		

(*continued*)

Table 49.7 (Continued)

Condition or Treatment Group Adult	IDSA				ESCMID			
	Primary recommendations	SoR QoE	Alternative recommendations	SoR QoE	Primary recommendations	SoR QoE	Alternative recommendations	SoR QoE
Urinary fungus balls	Surgical removal strongly recommended Treatment as per pyelonephritis (above)	SR-LQ SR-LQ	Irrigation via nephrostomy tube if available AmB-D 25–50 mg in 200–500 ml water	SR-LQ	Surgical intervention	A-III		

clinical setting. If no risk factors are present in an asymptomatic patient, observation is advised. Modifying risk factors, such as removal of an indwelling catheter, may be sufficient to eliminate candiduria without antifungal therapy. Certain patient groups, such as low birth weight neonates and severely immunocompromised patients with fever, require a more proactive approach with disseminated candidiasis being considered.

Observational studies of untreated asymptomatic candiduria with long-term follow-up have reported no adverse outcomes. Multiple studies have demonstrated that candiduria does not usually lead to candidaemia. These studies have shown, however, that candiduria is a marker for greater mortality One well-designed trial demonstrated fluconazole to be superior to placebo in clearing candiduria, but at the two-week follow-up, candiduria rates

Table 49.8 Summary of *Candida* osteoarticular infection guideline recommendations

Condition or Treatment Group Adult	IDSA				ESCMID			
	Primary recommendation	SoR QoE	Alternative recommendation	SoR QoE	Primary recommendation	SoR QoE	Alternative recommendation	SoR QoE
Osteomyelitis / spondylodiscitis	Surgical debridement in selected cases Fluconazole 400 mg (6 mg/kg) daily for 6–12 months Echinocandin for 2 weeks, then fluconazole for 6–12 months	SR-LQ SR-LQ SR-LQ	L-AmB 3–5 mg/kg daily for several weeks, then fluconazole for 6–12 months	WR-LQ	Surgical debridement Fluconazole 400 mg for 6–12 months Liposomal amphotericin B 3 mg/kg or amphotericin B lipid complex 5 mg/kg for 2–6 weeks followed by fluconazole 400 mg for 5–11 months	C-III A-II A-II	Voriconazole 12/6 mg/kg for 6–12 weeks Caspofungin 100 mg for 3 weeks, followed by fluconazole 400 mg for ≥4 weeks Posaconazole 800 mg for ≥6 weeks	B-II B-II C-III
Septic arthritis	Surgical debridement Fluconazole 400 mg (6 mg/kg) daily for at least 6 weeks or echinocandin for 2 weeks followed by fluconazole for 4 weeks	SR-MQ SR-L1Q	L-AmB 3–5 mg/kg daily for 2 weeks then fluconazole for 4 weeks	WR-LQ	Liposomal AmB 3 mg/kg/ABLC 5 mg/kg for 2 weeks, followed by fluconazole 400 mg for ≥4 weeks Fluconazole 400 mg for ≥6 weeks	A-II A-II	Voriconazole 12/6 mg/kg for ≥6 weeks Caspofungin 70/50 mg for 6 weeks	B-III C-II
Prosthetic joint infection	Surgical removal of prosthetic device + Treat as above	SR-MQ			Prosthesis removal + treat as above	A-III		
Prosthetic joint infection with prosthesis retention	Fluconazole 400 mg, lifelong if isolate is susceptible	SR-LQ			Fluconazole 400 mg, lifelong	A-III		

were similar between both groups, thus conferring only a transient benefit.

Removal of the urinary catheter was the most promising single intervention for candiduria. In the rare cases of fungal balls, surgical intervention is the only recommended treatment option, as discussed in both the IDSA and ESCMID guidance. Echinocandins do not achieve high urine concentrations and are, thus, not recommended in either guideline.

Candida osteoarticular infection

As no RCTs have been conducted, evidence for the best therapeutic approach is limited (Table 49.8). Approaches to bone and joint infections are based on case reports and open-label series. First-line therapy recommendations are largely similar between the two guidelines, with second-line ones varying more widely.

Central nervous system candidiasis

Most cases are due to *C. albicans*, with very few reports of *C. glabrata* and other species causing infection.

No RCTs have been performed to evaluate the most appropriate treatment. Single cases and small case series reported treatment with AmB-D, with or without flucytosine (5-fluorocytosine). Expert panels favour L-AmB because of the decreased risk of nephrotoxicity (Table 49.9). L-AmB has also been shown to attain higher levels in the brain than amphotericin B lipid complex and AmB-D in a *Candida* meningoencephalitis animal model. Furthermore, there is some clinical experience with use of this formulation for neonatal *Candida* meningitis. The recommended combination of AmB and flucytosine is appealing because of the *in vitro* synergism noted and excellent CSF concentrations achieved by flucytosine. However, the duration of therapy with AmB, alone or in combination with flucytosine, has not been defined.

Candida infection of the cardiovascular system

Medical therapy of endocarditis has occasionally been curative, but the optimum therapy for both native and prosthetic valve endocarditis in adults is considered to be a combination of valve replacement and a prolonged course of antifungal therapy (Table 49.10). Most of the cases reported in the literature have been treated with AmB-D, with or without flucytosine. Azoles, usually fluconazole, have been used for completion of therapy. Because of reduced toxicity and the ability to administer higher dosages, L-AmB is currently favoured over AmB-D. A prospective, open-label clinical trial and several case reports show a role for the echinocandins in the treatment of endocarditis.

Table 49.9 Summary of CNS candidiasis guideline recommendations

Condition or Treatment Group Adult	IDSA				ESCMID			
	Primary recommendation	SoR QoE	Alternative recommendation	SoR QoE	Primary recommendation	SoR QoE	Alternative recommendation	SoR QoE
All patients	L-AmB 5 mg/kg with or without 5-FC 25 mg/kg q.i.d.,	SR-LQ	For patients in whom a ventricular device cannot be removed: AmB-D administered through device into ventricle at dosage ranging from 0.01 mg to 0.5 mg in 2 ml 5% dextrose in water	WR-LQ	L-AmB 3 mg/kg for 10 weeks + flucytosine 150 mg/kg for 10 weeks, followed by fluconazole 3 mg/kg for 5 weeks	B-III	Voriconazole 12/6 mg/kg	C-III
	Followed by step-down to fluconazole 400–800 mg (6–12 mg/kg) daily	SR-LQ			L-AmB 3 mg/kg for 4 weeks + fluconazole 6 mg/kg for 4 weeks	B-III	Fluconazole 800 mg	C-III
	Therapy should continue until all signs, symptoms, and CSF & radiological abnormalities have resolved	SR-LQ						
	Infected CNS devices, including drains, shunts, stimulators, prosthetic devices, and biopolymer wafers, should be removed	SR-LQ						
Not recommended					AmB-D 0.5–1.0 mg/kg for >2 weeks +/− flucytosine 30–120 mg/kg for >2 weeks	D-II	Caspofungin 70/50 mg for 4 weeks, followed by fluconazole 400 mg for 2 weeks	D-III

Table 49.10 Summary of *Candida* infection of the cardiovascular system treatment recommendations

Condition or Treatment Group	IDSA				ESCMID			
	Primary recommendation	**SoR QoE**	**Alternative recommendation**	**SoR QoE**	**Primary recommendation**	**SoR QoE**	**Alternative recommendation**	**SoR QoE**
Endocarditis native valve	Valve replacement Followed by at least 6 weeks therapy as detailed below. Initial therapy L-AmB 3–5 mg/kg with or without 5-FC 25 mg/kg q.i.d; *or* High-dose echinocandin caspofingin 150 mg daily, micafungin 150 mg daily, Anidulafungin 200 mg daily. Step-down to fluconazole 400–800 mg (6–12 mg/kg) daily for susceptible isolates in patients who are clinically stable and have cleared *Candida* from bloodstream	SR-LQ SR-LQ SR-LQ	For patients who cannot undergo valve replacement long term Fluconazole 400–800 mg (6–12 mg/kg) daily for susceptible isolates Voriconazole 200–300 mg (3–4 mg/kg) twice daily or posaconazole 300 mg daily as step-down agents for those isolates not sensitive to fluconazole	SR-LQ WR-VLQ	Surgery within 1 week Combined with L-AmB +/– flucytosine for 6–8 weeks, followed by fluconazole *or* caspofungin +/– flucytosine	A-II B-II C-II		
Endocarditis Prosthetic valve	As above but with subsequent lifelong suppressive therapy Fluconazole 400–800 mg (6–12 mg/kg) daily lifelong	SR-LQ SR-LQ			As above			
Endocarditis Prosthetic valve (retained)	As above but with subsequent lifelong suppressive therapy	SR-LQ			L-AmB 5 mg/kg Caspofungin 70/50 mg B	B-III B-III	Suppression with lifelong fluconazole 400–800 mg/daily	C-III
Infected Pacemaker, ICD, or VAD	Device removal followed by treatment as per native valve endocarditis for 6 weeks	SR-LQ	For devices that cannot be removed, the treatment regime is the same as retained native/prosthetic valve	SR-LQ	Device removal combined with systemic treatment as above	A-II		

Candida chorioretinitis and endophthalmitis

There are no prospective studies for the treatment of *Candida* endophthalmitis. The majority of published cases report the use of intravenous and/or intra-vitreal AmB-D, with or without oral flucytosine, as initial therapy (Table 49.11).

Oral or intravenous fluconazole has also been used successfully as initial, salvage, and transition therapy. Although the data are very limited, L-AmB, the echinocandins, and voriconazole are reasonable options for second-line treatment. However, caution is advised with echinocandin therapy given their poor ocular penetration. Voriconazole at a dose of 3–4 mg/kg twice daily appears to be an established safe approach, achieving excellent intra-vitreal levels.

Early surgical intervention with a partial vitrectomy is an essential adjunct to antifungal therapy in more advanced cases and can be a sight-saving procedure. The value of intraocular

Table 49.11 Summary of *Candida* chorioretinitis and endophthalmitis treatment recommendations

Condition or Treatment Group	IDSA				ESCMID			
	Primary recommendation	**SoR QoE**	**Alternative recommendation**	**SoR QoE**	**Primary recommendation**	**SoR QoE**	**Alternative recommendation**	**SoR QoE**
Susceptibility of isolate unknown	AmB-D 0.7–1 mg/kg with or without 5-FC 25 mg/kg q.i.d.	SR-LQ			L-AmB 5 mg/kg Liposomal amphotericin B plus flucytosine Amphotericin B lipid complex plus flucytosine	B-III B-III B-III	AmB-D 0.6–1.0 mg/kg Amphotericin B lipid complex 5 mg/kg Amphotericin B deoxycholate plus flucytosine	C-II C-III C-III
Not recommended					Caspofungin 50–100 mg	D-II		
Susceptible isolate	Fluconazole 800 mg (12 mg/kg) loading dose followed by 400–800 mg (6–12 mg/kg) daily	SR-LQ	Voriconazole 400 mg loading dose (6 mg/kg) × 2 then 300 mg (4 mg/kg) twice daily	SR-LQ	Fluconazole 400–800 mg	A-II	Voriconazole 12/6 mg/kg IV, followed by 400 mg PO	A-II
Vitreal involvement Endophthalmitis requires local and systemic treatment plus surgery	AmB-D 5–10 μg intravitreal injection	SR-LQ	Voriconazole 100 μg intravitreal injection	SR-LQ	AmB-D 5–10 μg intravitreal injection Vitrectomy plus intravitreal amphotericin B 5–10 μg, fluconazole 400 mg for 12 weeks	B-II B-II	Voriconazole 100 μg intravitreal injection	B-III

instillation of antifungals at the time of vitrectomy has not been well studied. The optimal duration of antifungal therapy has also not been determined, but most expert panels advise at least six weeks of systemic treatment and continuation of treatment until all clinical evidence of intraocular infection has resolved.

Evaluation of aspergillosis guideline recommendations

Most expert panels recommend treating invasive *Aspergillus* infection until resolution or stabilization of all clinical and radiographic features (Table 49.12). The duration of therapy for most diseases,

Table 49.12 Summary of IDSA aspergillosis guidance

Condition or Treatment Group	IDSA			
	Primary recommendation	**SoR QoE**	**Alternative recommendation**	**SoR QoE**
Invasive pulmonary aspergillosis	Voriconazole (6 mg/kg IV every 12 h for 1 day, followed by 4 mg/kg IV every 12 h; oral dosage is 200 mg every 12 h)	A-I	L-AmB (3–5 mg/kg/day IV) ABLC (5 mg/kg/day IV), caspofungin (70 mg day 1 IV and 50 mg/day IV thereafter) Micafungin (IV 100–150 mg/day; dose not established), Posaconazole (200 mg q.i.d.initially, then 400 mg b.i.d. PO after stabilization of disease), Itraconazole (dosage depends upon formulation)	A-I A-II B-II B-II B-II
Tracheobronchial aspergillosis	Similar to invasive pulmonary aspergillosis		Similar to invasive pulmonary aspergillosis	

(continued)

Table 49.12 (Continued)

Condition or Treatment Group	IDSA			
	Primary recommendation	**SoR QoE**	**Alternative recommendation**	**SoR QoE**
Invasive sinus aspergillosis	Similar to invasive pulmonary aspergillosis		Similar to invasive pulmonary aspergillosis	
Chronic necrotizing pulmonary aspergillosis	Similar to invasive pulmonary aspergillosis		Similar to invasive pulmonary aspergillosis	
Aspergillosis of the CNS	Similar to invasive pulmonary aspergillosis		Similar to invasive pulmonary aspergillosis	
Aspergillus infections of the heart (endocarditis, pericarditis, and myocarditis)	Voriconazole		Similar to invasive pulmonary aspergillosis	
Aspergillus osteomyelitis and septic arthritis	Voriconazole		Similar to invasive pulmonary aspergillosis	
Aspergillus infections of the eye (endophthalmitis and keratitis)	Intraocular AmB indicated with partial vitrectomy		Similar to invasive pulmonary aspergillosis; limited data with echinocandins	
Cutaneous aspergillosis	Voriconazole		Similar to invasive pulmonary aspergillosis	
Aspergillus peritonitis	Voriconazole		Similar to invasive pulmonary aspergillosis	
Prophylaxis against invasive aspergillosis	Posaconazole (200 mg t.i.d.)		Itraconazole Micafungin	

however, has not been optimally defined. Factors such as site of infection (e.g. osteomyelitis), level of immunosuppression, and extent of disease should always be evaluated when considering management. Reversal of immunosuppression, where possible, is generally regarded to improve the chances of a favourable outcome for invasive aspergillosis.

In *Aspergillus* infections of the heart, osteomyelitis, septic arthritis, cutaneous aspergillosis, and *Aspergillus* peritonitis, most patients in individual case reports have been treated primarily with AmB-D. Voriconazole use in randomized trials typically relates only to the treatment of pulmonary invasive aspergillosis. Expert opinion recommends voriconazole as primary therapy for extrapulmonary and disseminated infection on the basis of successful treatment in case reports. Currently, guidelines do not recommend combination therapy for the treatment of invasive *Aspergillus* infections.

References

Agrawal S, Jones B, Barnes R, et al. (2012) A practical critique of antifungal treatment guidelines for haemato-oncologists. *Crit Rev Microbiol* 38: 203–16.

Al-Abdely HM, Alothman AF, Salman JA, et al. (2014) Clinical practice guidelines for the treatment of invasive *Aspergillus* infections in adults in the Middle East region: expert panel recommendations. *J Infect Public Health* 7: 20–31.

Baden LR, Bensinger W, Angarone M, et al (2012) Prevention and treatment of cancer-related infections. *J Natl Compr Canc Netw* 10: 1412–45.

Cornely OA, Bassetti M, Calandra T, et al. (2012) ESCMID* guideline for the diagnosis and management of *Candida* diseases 2012: non-neutropenic adult patients. *Clin Microbiol Infect* 18 (Suppl. 7): 19–37.

Eccles MP, Grimshaw JM, Shekelle P, Schünemann HJ and Woolf S (2012) Developing clinical practice guidelines: target audiences, identifying topics for guidelines, guideline group composition and functioning and conflicts of interest. *Implement Sci* 7: 60.

Groll AH, Castagnola E, Cesaro S, et al. (2014) Fourth European Conference on Infections in Leukaemia (ECIL-4): guidelines for diagnosis, prevention, and treatment of invasive fungal diseases in paediatric patients with cancer or allogeneic haemopoietic stem-cell transplantation. *Lancet Oncol* 15: e327–40.

Guyatt GH, Oxman AD, Vist GE, et al. (2008) GRADE: an emerging consensus on rating quality of evidence and strength of recommendations. *BMJ* 336: 924–6.

Institute of Medicine (US) Committee to Advise the Public Health Service on Clinical Practice Guidelines (1990) *Clinical Practice Guidelines: Directions for a New Program*. Washington (DC): National Academies Press (US).

Maertens J, Girmenia C, Duarte R and Ribaud P (2013) ECIL 5: primary antifungal prophylaxis, https://www.ebmt.org/Contents/Resources/Library/ECIL/Pages/ECIL.aspx, accessed 30 September 2017.

Maertens J, Marchetti O, Herbrecht R, et al. (2011) European guidelines for antifungal management in leukemia and hematopoietic stem cell transplant recipients: summary of the ECIL 3—2009 update. *Bone Marrow Transplant* 46: 709–18.

Mousset S, Buchheidt D, Heinz W, et al. (2014) Treatment of invasive fungal infections in cancer patients—updated recommendations of the Infectious Diseases Working Party (AGIHO) of the German Society of Hematology and Oncology (DGHO). *Annals Hematol* 93: 13–32.

Pappas PG, Kauffman CA, Andes D, et al. (2009) Clinical practice guidelines for the management of candidiasis: 2009 update by the Infectious Diseases Society of America. *Clin Infect Dis* 48: 503–35.

Pappas PG, Kauffman CA, Andes DR, et al. (2016) Clinical practice guideline for the management of candidiasis: 2016 update by the Infectious Diseases Society of America. *Clin Infect Dis* 62: e1–50.

Prentice AG, Glasmacher A, Hobson RP, et al. (2010) Guidelines on the management of invasive fungal infection during therapy for haematological malignancy, *British Committee for Standards in Haematology*.

Schulz KF, Altman DG, Moher D, for the CONSORT Group (2010) CONSORT 2010 Statement: updated guidelines for reporting parallel group randomised trials. *Ann Intern Med* 152: 726–32.

Scottish Intercollegiate Guidelines Network (SIGN), http://www.sign.ac.uk, accessed 20 June 2017.

Thursky KA, Playford EG, Seymour JF, et al. (2008) Recommendations for the treatment of established fungal infections. *Intern Med J* 38: 496–520.

Ullmann AJ, Akova M, Herbrecht R, et al. (2012) ESCMID* guideline for the diagnosis and management of *Candida* diseases 2012: adults with haematological malignancies and after haematopoietic stem cell transplantation (HCT). *Clin Microbiol Infect* 18 (Suppl. 7): 53–67.

US GRADE Network. Approach and implications to rating the quality of evidence and strength of recommendations using the GRADE methodology, http://www.gradeworkinggroup.org, accessed 1 June 2017.

Walsh TJ, Anaissie EJ, Denning DW, et al. (2008) Treatment of aspergillosis: clinical practice guidelines of the Infectious Diseases Society of America. *Clin Infect Dis* 46: 327–60.

Index

Tables, figures, and boxes are indicated by an italic *t*, *f*, and *b* following the page number.